MEDICAL ABBREVIATIONS:

28,000 Conveniences at the Expense of Communication and Safety

13th Edition

Neil M Davis, MS, PharmD, FASHP

Professor Emeritus, Temple University
    School of Pharmacy, Philadelphia, PA,
Editor Emeritus, Hospital Pharmacy
President, Safe Medication Practices
    Consulting, Inc.

published by

Neil M Davis Associates
2049 Stout Drive, B-3
Warminster, PA 18974-3861

Phone (215) 442-7430 or (888) 333-1862
    (9 AM-4 PM EST, Mon-Fri)
FAX (215) 442-7432 or (888) 333-4915
E-mail med@neilmdavis.com
Secure Website www.medabbrev.com

First edition, 1983, titled, "1700 Medical Abbreviations:
  Conveniences at the Expense of Communications and Safety"

Second edition, 1985, titled, "Medical Abbreviations: 2300
  Conveniences ..."
Third edition, 1987, titled, "Medical Abbreviations: 4200 ..."
Fourth edition, 1988, titled, "Medical Abbreviations: 5500 ..."
Fifth edition, 1990, titled, "Medical Abbreviations: 7000 ..."
Sixth edition, 1993, titled, "Medical Abbreviations 8600 ..."
Seventh edition, 1995, titled, "Medical Abbreviations 10,000 ..."
Eighth edition, 1997, titled, "Medical Abbreviations: 12,000 ..."
Ninth edition, 1999, titled, "Medical Abbreviations: 14,000 ..."
Tenth edition, 2001, titled, "Medical Abbreviations: 15,000 ..."
Eleventh edition, 2003, titled, "Medical Abbreviations: 24,000 ..."
Twelfth edition, 2005, titled, "Medical Abbreviations: 26,000 ..."

Library of Congress Catalog Card Number 2006906921

ISBN 0-931431-13-1

Warning: The user must exercise care in that the meaning shown in this book may not be the one intended by the writer of the medical abbreviation. When there is doubt, the writer must be contacted for clarification.

Permissions: To photocopy, print, or otherwise use portions of either this work or its electronic counterpart, in accordance with federal copyright law, contact Dr Neil M Davis, 2049 Stout Drive, B-3, Warminster, Pa 18974 or med@neilmdavis.com

Printed in Canada.

Contents

Dedication

This book is dedicated to Julie, my wife, for her support, patience, assistance, and love.

Acknowledgments

The assistance of Evelyn Canizares, Vicki Bell, Ann Sandt Kishbaugh, Matthew Davis, Robin Miller, and Ben Miller is gratefully acknowledged.

I would like to express my deep appreciation for the many contributions received from readers for their suggested additions and corrections. Please continue to send these to—

Dr. Neil M Davis
2049 Stout Drive, B-3
Warminster, PA 18974

FAX (215) 442-7432 or (888) 333-4915
E-mail   med@neilmdavis.com
Secure Website www.neilmdavis.com

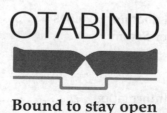

OTABIND

Bound to stay open

The pages in this book open easily and lie flat, a result of the Otabind bookbinding process. Otabind combines advanced adhesive technology and a free-floating cover to achieve books that last longer and are bound to stay open.

Preface
Website-Version Access Information

Along with the purchase of each book, the book owner, at no extra cost, is entitled to a single-user license for access to the Internet version of this 13th edition. This license is valid for 24 months from the date of the initial log-in. Internet Explorer 4.0, Netscape 4.0, or AOL 5.0 can meet the minimum browser requirement.

Features of the Web-Version

- Updated monthly (suggestions from users are welcomed and will be incorporated).
- Can instantaneously search for the meanings of abbreviations and acronyms.
- Has a reverse-search feature, for example, looking for all the abbreviations that contain the word "laparoscopic."
- Can search for cross-referenced generic and brand names of drugs.
- Can search through the listings of symbols, lists, and normal adult laboratory values.
- Quick access to a "Do Not Use" list of dangerous abbreviations, an explanation as to why they are dangerous, and suggested alternatives to be used. For those facilities that obtain multi-user licenses, they may substitute their own "Do Not Use" list, which they can control and update.
- Can read the full-text of the introductory chapters of the book.

Initial One-time Log-in

- Access the Website at *www.medabbrev.com*
- Click the **Register** button (on the top-left of the screen)
- You must agree to the Single-User License Agreement which is presented.
- You will be asked for the 8-letter access code that appears on the front inside cover of the book. This will be the only time you are asked for this code.
- At this point just follow the directions.
- Note your sign-in name and your self-assigned password. This name/password will only permit one access at a time, so keep this information confidential to ensure your ready access to the site.

Multi-user site licenses are available. A copy of the Multi-User Site License agreement and its price list is available by clicking the "Submit Suggestions" button on *www.medabbrev.com* where you can type a request to receive it or by calling 1 888 333 1862 or 1 215 442 7430.

Searching for the Meaning of an Abbreviation on the Web-version

- Use upper OR lower case letters as the search engine is NOT case sensitive.
- Use normal upper OR lower case letters as the search engine is NOT sensitive to whether the letters are **bold-face** or *italicized.*
- Superscripts and subscripts are to be entered as regular text.
- For other details, just follow the simple instructions shown on the Website. The Web-version of the book is essentially the same as the print version except for the fact that it is searchable and is updated monthly with about 80 new entries.

Additions, Corrections, and Suggestions are Welcomed

Please send them via any means shown below:

Neil M Davis
2049 Stout Drive, B-3
Warminster PA 18974-3861

FAX 1 888 333 4915 or 1 215 442 7432
Email med@neilmdavis.com
Web site www.medabbrev.com

Thank you for your help in the past.

Have You Used the Web-Version of This Book?

- It is instantaneously searchable for the meanings of abbreviations
- It is reverse searchable (search for all the abbreviations containing a particular word)
- Each month, about 80 new entries are added

See the preface (page vii) for access instructions. A two-year, single-user access is included in the purchase price of the book.

PDA Versions are Available

See pricing and ordering information in the pricing section on page 357.

Multi-User Site Licenses are Available

Medical facilities can substitute their own "Do Not Use" list of dangerous abbreviations for the one present. The ability also exists to list abbreviations that are unique to your region and/or organization which would normally not appear in any national list. These lists would be controlled by the facility. Demonstrations and pricing information are available by calling 1 888 333 1862 or 1 215 442 7430 or via an e-mail request to ev@neilmdavis.com

Chapter 1
Introduction

L isted are current acronyms, symbols, and other abbreviations and 28,000 of their possible meanings. This list has been compiled to assist individuals in reading and transcribing medical records, medically-related communications, and prescriptions. The list, although current and comprehensive, represents a portion of abbreviations in use and their many possible meanings as new ones are being coined every day.

WARNING

Abbreviations are a convenience, a time saver, a space saver, and a way of avoiding the possibility of misspelling words. However, a price can be paid for their use. Abbreviations are sometimes not understood. They can be misread, or are interpreted incorrectly. Their use lengthens the time needed to train individuals in the health fields, wastes the time of healthcare workers in tracking down their meaning, at times delays the patient's care, and occasionally results in patient harm.

The publication of this list of abbreviations is not an endorsement of their legitimacy. It is not a guarantee that the intended meaning has been correctly captured, nor is it an indication that the abbreviation is commonly used. The person who uses an abbreviation must take responsibility for making sure that it is properly interpreted. When an uncommon or ambiguous abbreviation is used and it may not be understood correctly, it should be defined by the writer. Where uncertainty exists, the one who wrote the abbreviation must be contacted for clarification.

There are many variations in how an abbreviation can be expressed. Anterior-posterior has been written as AP, A.P., ap, and A/P. Since there are few standards and those who use abbreviations do not necessarily follow these standards, this book only shows anterior-posterior as AP. This is done to make it easier to find the meaning of an abbreviation as all the meanings of AP are listed together. This elimination of unnecessary duplication also keeps the book at a convenient size, thus enabling it to be sold at a reasonable price.

When an abbreviation is made up of a series of abbreviations, it may not be listed as such. In such instances, the meaning may be determined by looking up each set of abbreviations, as in the example of DTP$_a$-HIB-PNU-MEN, which means, diphtheria, tetanus toxoids, acellular pertussis; *Haemophilus influenzae* type b conjugate; pneumococcal (*Streptococcus pneumoniae*) conjugate; meningococcal (*Neisseria meningitidis*) conjugate (serogroups unspecified) vaccine.

Lower case letters are used when firm custom dictates as in Ag, Na, mCi, etc. The first letter of brand names are capitalized, whereas nonproprietary names appear in lower case.

The abbreviation AP is listed as meaning doxorubicin and cisplatin. The reason for this apparent disparity is that the official generic names (United States Adopted Names) are shown rather than the brand names Adriamycin and Platinol. In the case of LSD, the official name, lysergide, is given, rather than the chemical name, lysergic acid diethylamide. The Latin derivations for older medical and pharmaceutical abbreviations (*t.i.d., ter in die,* three times daily) may be found in *Remington*.[1]

Some abbreviations which have been encountered or that have been suggested for addition to the book have not been added. Some were obscene or completely insensitive.

Abbreviations for medical facility names create problems as they are usually not recognized by the readers in other geographic areas. A clue to the fact that one is dealing with such an abbreviation is when it ends with MC, for Medical Center; HS, for Health System; MH, for Memorial Hospital; CH, for Community Hospital; UH, for University Hospital; and H, for Hospital.

When an abbreviation which ends with "s" can not be found it might be a plural form of a listed abbreviation.

When an abbreviation cannot be found in this book or when the listed meaning(s) do not make sense, there is a possibility that the abbreviation has been misread. As an example, a reader could not find the meaning of HHTS. On closer examination it really was +HTS, not HHTS. Also EWT could not be identified because it was really ENT.

Some common French and Spanish abbreviations are listed in the book. Because of language structure differences, these abbreviations are often reversed, as in the case of HIV, which in Spanish and French is abbreviated as VIH.

Chapter 4 presents a list of 275 of the most commonly used abbreviations. The purpose of this list is to serve as a primer for whose entering a health-related field.

Chapter 8 contains a cross-referenced list of 3,400 generic and brand drug names. The list contains names of commonly prescribed and new drugs. Brand names have their first letter capitalized whereas generic names are in lower case. This list will enable readers to obtain the generic name for brand name products or brand names for generic names. It will also serve as a spelling check.

Coded drug names and abbreviations for drug names are found in the chapter on abbreviations (Chapter 5).

Chapter 9 is a table of normal laboratory values. Both the conventional and international values are listed. Each laboratory publishes a list of its normal values. These local lists should be reviewed to see if there are significant differences.

The Council of Biology Editors (CBE), in their 1983 edition of the *CBE Style Manual* listed about 600 abbreviations gathered from 15 internationally recognized authorities and organizations.[2] The majority of these symbols and abbreviations tend to be more scientifically oriented than those which would appear in medical records. In the few situations where the CBE abbreviations differ from what is presented in this book, the CBE abbreviation has been placed in parentheses after the meaning. As is the practice in the United States, mL has been used rather than ml and the spelling of liter, meter, etc. is used rather than litre and metre, even though ml, litre, and metre are listed in the *CBE Style Manual*. A new edition of the *CBE Style Manual* was published in 1995.[3] Again, in this edition, emphasis is placed on scientific abbreviations.

Only a few of the acronyms and abbreviations for the major cardiologic trials, such as, TIMI-Thrombosis In Myocardial Infarction (trial), have been included in this book. For a list of 4,200 of these acronyms and abbreviations, consult reference number 4.

An examination of the abbreviations, acronyms, symbols, and their 28,000 meanings is a testimonial to the problems and dangers associated with most undefined abbreviations.

References

1. Hendrickson R, ed. Remington's The Science and Practice of Pharmacy, 21st ed. Phila., PA: Lippincott Williams and Wilkins, 2006.
2. CBE Style Manual, 5th ed. Bethesda, MD: Council of Biology Editors; 1983.
3. Scientific Style and Format: The CBE Manual for Authors, Editors, and Publishers, 6th Ed. Council of Biological Editors-Cambridge University Press. Cambridge UK, New York, Victoria Australia: 1995.
4. Cheng TO, Julian D. Acronyms of cardiologic trials-2002. Int J Cardiol 2003;91:261–351.

Chapter 2

Dangerous, Contradictory, and/or Ambiguous Abbreviations

Healthcare organizations are directed by the Joint Commission on Accreditation of Healthcare Organizations to formulate a "Do Not Use" list of dangerous abbreviations which should NOT be used. An example of such a list, which has been adopted from the Institute of Safe Medication Practice Inc. (ISMP) list, is shown as Table 1.

Many inherent problems associated with abbreviations contribute to or cause errors. Reports of such errors have been published routinely.[1-5]

Abbreviations and symbols can easily be misread or interpreted in an unintended manner. For example:

(1) "HCT250 mg" was intended to mean hydrocortisone 250 mg but was interpreted as hydrochlorothiazide 50 mg (HCTZ50 mg).

(2) Flucytosine was improperly abbreviated as 5 FU, causing it to be read as fluorouracil. Flucytosine is abbreviated 5 FC and fluorouracil is 5 FU.

(3) Floxuridine was improperly abbreviated as 5 FU, causing it to be read as fluorouracil. Floxuridine is abbreviated FUDR and fluorouracil is 5 FU.

(4) MTX was thought to be mechlorethamine. MTX is methotrexate and mechlorethamine is abbreviated HN2.

(5) **The abbreviation "U" for unit is the most dangerous one in the book, having caused numerous ten-fold insulin and heparin overdoses. The word unit should never be abbreviated.** The handwritten U for unit has been mistaken for a zero, causing tenfold errors. The handwritten U has also been read as the number four, six, and as "cc."

(6) OD, meant to signify once daily, has caused Lugol's solution to be given in the right eye.

(7) OJ meant to signify orange juice, looked like OS and caused saturated solution of potassium iodide to be given in the left eye.

(8) IVP, meant to signify intravenous push (Lasix 20 mg IVP), caused a patient to be given an intravenous pyelogram which is the usual meaning of this abbreviation.

(9) Na Warfarin (sodium warfarin) was read as "No Warfarin."

(10) The abbreviation "s" for "without" has been thought to mean "with" (c).

(11) The order for PT, intended to signify a laboratory test order for prothrombin time, resulted in the ordering of a physical therapy consultation.

(12) The abbreviation "TAB," meant to signify Triple Antibiotic (a coined name for a hospital sterile topical antibiotic mixture), caused patients to have their wounds irrigated with a diet soda. At another facility, with the same set of circumstances, they did not have TAB®, so they used Diet Shasta.®

(13) A slash mark (/) has been mistaken for a one, causing a patient to receive a 100 unit overdose of NPH insulin when the slash was used to separate an order for two insulin doses:
6 units regular insulin/20 units NPH insulin

(14) Vidarabine, an antiviral agent, was ordered as ara-A; however, ara-C, which is cytarabine, an antineoplastic agent, was given.

Table 1. Dangerous abbreviations and dosage designations

Problem term	Reason	Suggested term
O.D. for once daily	Interpreted as right eye	Write "once daily"
q.o.d. for every other day	Interpreted as meaning "every once a day" or read as q.i.d.	Write "every other day"
q.d. for once daily	Read or interpreted as q.i.d.	Write "once daily"
q.n. for every night	Read as every hour	Write "every night," "HS" or nightly
q hs for once daily at bedtime, each day	Read as every hour	Use "HS" or "at bedtime"
TIW for three times a week	Interpeted as T/W (Tuesday & Wednesday); as twice a week; as TID (three times daily)	Write "three times a week"
U for Unit	Read as 0, 4, 6, or cc	Write "unit"
O.J. for orange juice	Read as OD or OS	Write "orange juice"
μg (microgram)	When handwritten, misread as mg	Write "mcg"
sq or sub q for subcutaneous	The q is read as every	Use "subcut"
IU for international unit	Misread as IV (intravenous) also the I is is read as a one (6 IU is read as 61 units)	Use "units" or spell out "international units," using a lowercase i.
AU for each ear	Read as OU (each eye)	Spell out "each ear"
ss for sliding scale or half in the Apothecary system	Read as the number 55	Spell out "sliding scale" or "1/2"
Chemical symbols	Not understood or misunderstood	Write full name
cc for expressing liquid measurements	Read as u (unit)	Write "mL" when expressing liquid measurements (drugs, urine, blood, etc.)

4

Table 1. Dangerous abbreviations and dosage designations (continued)

Problem term	Reason	Suggested term
Lettered abbreviations for drug names such as MS and MSO4 for morphine sulfate or DPH, ASA, APAP, AZT, CPZ, and others and for protocols	Not understood or misunderstood	Use generic or brand name(s). For protocols, follow the facility's procedures.
Apothecary symbols or terms	Not understood or misunderstood	Use metric system
per os for by mouth	OS read as left eye	Use "by mouth," "orally," or "PO"
D/C for discharge	Interpreted as discontinue (orders for discharge medications result in premature discontinuance of current medication)	Write "discharge"
T/d for one per day	Read as t.i.d.	Use "once daily"
/ (a slash mark) for with, and, or per	Read as a one	Use, "and," "with," or "per"
Roman numerals	Not understood or misinterpreted (iv read as intravenous rather than 4; iii, X, L, and C, are not understood)	Use Arabic numerals (4, 3, 10, 50, 100, etc.)
> and <	Not understood or the meaning is reversed	Use "greater than" or "less than"
Drug name and dosage not separated by space	Inderal40 mg misread as Inderal 140 mg	Always leave a space between a drug name, dose, and unit of measure
Trailing zeros; 1.0 mg	Decimal point not seen causing tenfold overdose	Omit zero; 1 mg
Naked decimal point; .5 mL	Decimal point not seen causing tenfold overdose	Add zero; 0.5 mL

5

(15) On several occasions, pediatric strength diphtheria-tetanus toxoids (DT) have been confused with adult strength tetanus-diphtheria toxoids (Td).

(16) DTP is commonly understood to refer to diphtheria-tetanus-pertussis vaccine, but in some hospitals it is also used as shorthand for a sedative cocktail of Demerol, Thorazine, and Phenergan. Several cases have occurred where a child was vaccinated rather than given the sedative mixture.

(17) What does the abbreviation MR mean? Some will guess measles-rubella vaccine (M-R-Vax II, Merck), while others will assume mumps-rubella vaccine (Biavax II, Merck).

(18) The abbreviation TIW (three times a week) was thought to mean Tuesday and Wednesday when the I was read as a slash mark. Due to confirmation bias (you see what you know), this uncommon abbreviation is seen as the more commonly used TID (three times a day).

(19) PCA, meant to be procainamide, was interpreted as patient-controlled analgesia.

(20) PGE$_1$ (alprostadil, Caverject) was read as P6 E1 (Alcon's ophthalmic 6% pilocarpine and 1% epinephrine solution).

(21) A nurse transcribed an oral order for the antibiotic aztreonam as AZT, which was subsequently thought to be the antiviral drug zidovudine.

(22) An order for TAC 0.1%, intended to mean triamcinolone cream, was interpreted as tetracaine, Adrenalin, and cocaine solution.

(23) An order for SPA (salt poor albumin) was overlooked because it was not recognized as a drug order.

(24) Therapy was delayed and considerable professional time was wasted when an order for "Bactrim SS q 12 h on S/S" had to be clarified (Bactrim Single Strength every 12 hours on Saturday and Sunday).

(25) A physician wrote an order stating "may take own supply of EPO". The physician meant evening primrose oil, not Epogen (epoetin alfa).

(26) 4-MP was recommended to treat ethylene glycol poisoning. The medical resident mistakenly interpreted this as 6-MP (6-mercaptopurine). 4-MP is fomepizole (4 methylpyrazole) and 6-MP is mercaptopurine (6-mercaptopurine).

(27) An order for lomustine stated it was to be given at "hs". This was misinterpreted as to mean every night. After continuous administration, toxicity resulted in the patient's death. The drug is normally given once every 6 weeks. State complete orders such as "HS × 1 dose today," "HS nightly," or "HS nightly PRN for sleep."

(28) The directions for an order for Cortisporin Otic Solution indicated "Three drops in ® ear TID." The patient was given the drops in the rear rather than the right ear.

(29) There have been mix-ups between IL-2 and IL-11 when IL-2 is expressed as IL-II (Roman numeral 2). The II has been read as "IL eleven," and vice versa. IL-2 (interleukin 2) is aldesleukin (Proleukin) and IL-11 is oprelvekin (Neumega).

(30) A drug was ordered "Q 10 h." It was read as QID (four times daily). Drugs should not be ordered at unusual hourly intervals such as every 10, 18, or 36 hours, as this has resulted in a host of errors. Standard times are every 2, 3, 4, 6, 8, or 12 hours; once, twice, three, or four times daily; every other day, or Monday, Wednesday, and Friday and once weekly.

(31) 6 IU was read 61 units instead of the intended 6 international units.

(32) A dose of phenytoin was modified and expressed as mg/Kg/d. The d was read as "dose" rather than the intended "day" resulting in 3 extra doses being given.

(33) An order appeared as "If no BM in PM, give MOM in AM p.r.n."

(34) Sometimes ambiguous abbreviations cause financial losses to health providers. For example, an insurance provider may pay less for an office visit for mental retardation than it does for mitral regurgitation. This can happen if the coder is faced with the abbreviation MR.

Table 2. Examples of abbreviations that have contradictory or ambiguous meanings

ABP = ambulatory blood pressure
arterial blood pressure

AC = anticoagulant
anticonvulsant

ACU = acute receiving unit
ambulatory care unit

AMI = amifostine
amitriptyline

APC = advanced pancreatic cancer
advanced prostate cancer

ATR = atropine
atracurium

AZT = zidovudine
azathioprine

BM = bone metastases
brain metastases

BNO = bladder neck obstruction
bowels not open

BO = bowel open
bowel obstruction

BT = bladder tumor
brain tumor
breast tumor

CARBO = Carbocaine
carboplatin (Paraplatin)

CAS = carotid artery stenosis
cerebral arteriosclerosis
coronary artery stenosis

CIA = chemotherapy-induced
amenorrhea
chemotherapy-induced anemia

CLD = chronic liver disease
chronic lung disease

CPM = cyclophosphamide
chlorpheniramine maleate

CPZ = chlorpromazine
Compazine

CRU = cardiac rehabilitation unit
catheterization recovery unit
clinical research unit

DW = dextrose in water
distilled water
deionized water

DXM = dexamethasone
dextromethorphan

ESLD = end-stage liver disease
end-stage lung disease

FA = folic acid
folinic acid (Leucovorin calcium)

FEC = fluorouracil, epirubicin, and
cyclophosphamide
fluorouracil, etoposide, and
cisplatin

FGAs = first generation antihistamines
first generation antipsychotics

FLU = fluconazole (Diflucan)
fludarabine (Fludara)
flunisolide (Aero Bid)
fluoxetine (Prozac)
fluticasone propionate (Flonase)
influenza

GD = Graves disease
Gaucher disease

GEM = gemfibrozil
gemcitabine

HD = Hansen disease
Hirschsprung disease
Hodgkin disease
Huntington disease

HRF = hypertensive renal failure
hypoxic respiratory failure

ICA = internal carotid artery
intracranial abscess
intracranial aneurysm

IAI = intra-abdominal infection
intra-abdominal injury
intra-amniotic infection

7

Table 2. Examples of abbreviations that have contradictory or ambiguous meanings (*continued*)

I & D	= incision and drainage irrigation and debridement		mitral stenosis musculoskeletal medical student minimal support muscle strength
IRDM	= insulin-required diabetes mellitus Insulin resistant diabetes mellitus		
IT	= intrathecal intratracheal intratumoral	MTD	= maximum tolerated dose minimum toxic dose
KET	= ketamine ketoconazole	MTZ	= mirtazapine mitoxantrone
LAPC	= locally-advanced pancreatic cancer locally-advanced prostatic cancer	MV	= mechanical ventilation manual ventilation
		NBM	= no bowel movement normal bowel movement nothing by mouth
LFD	= lactose-free diet low fat diet low fiber diet	NE	= no effect no enlargement not evaluated
LL	= left leg left lung lower lid lower limb lower lip	NITRO	= nitroglycerin sodium nitroprusside
LNE	= lymph node enlargement lymph node excision	OLB	= open-liver biopsy open-lung biopsy
LNU	= learned nonuse (splint) lower and upper (heard as L & U)	PBL	= primary breast lymphoma primary brain lymphoma
Ltx	= liver transplant Lung transplant	PBZ	= phenylbutazone pyribenzamine phenoxybenzamine
MBC	= male breast cancer metastatic breast cancer	PCU	= palliative care unit primary care unit progressive care unit protective care unit
MP	= melphalan; prednisone mitoxantrone; prednisone		
MPM	= malignant peritoneal mesothe- lioma malignant pleural mesothelioma	PD	= Paget disease panic disorder Parkinson disease personality disorder
MS	= mental status milk shake mitral sound morning stiffness morphine sulfate multiple sclerosis	PORT	= postoperative radiotherapy postoperative respiratory therapy
		PVO	= peripheral vascular occlusion portal vein occlusion pulmonary venous occlusion

Table 2. Examples of abbreviations that have contradictory or ambiguous meanings (*continued*)

RS	= Reiter syndrome Rett syndrome Reye syndrome Raynaud disease (syndrome) rumination syndrome	T/E	= testosterone to epitestosterone (ratio) testosterone to estrogen (ratio) trunk-to-extremity skinfold thickness (index)
S & S	= swish and spit swish and swallow	TICU	= thoracic intensive care unit transplant intensive care unit trauma intensive care unit
SA	= suicide alert suicide attempt	TMZ	= temazepam temozolomide
SAD	= schizoaffective disorder social anxiety disorder seasonal affective disorder	TS	= Tay-Sachs (disease) Tourette syndrome Turner syndrome
SDBP	= seated, standing, or supine diastolic blood pressure	VAD	= vincristine, doxorubicin, (Adriamycin) and dexamethasone vincristine, doxorubicin (Adriamycin) and dactinomycin
SGAs	= second generation antihistamines second generation antipsychotics		
SJS	– Schwartz-Jampel syndrome Stevens-Johnson syndrome Swyer-James syndrome	VAP	= vincristine, Adriamycin, and prednisone vincristine, Adriamycin, and procarbazine vincristine, actinomycin D, and Platinol AQ vincristine, asparaginase, and prednisone
SSE	= saline solution enema soapsuds enema		
STF	= special tube feeding standard tube feeding		
TAC	= tetracaine, Adrenalin, and cocaine solution triamcinolone cream		

The author would appreciate receiving other examples of abbreviations that have been misinterpreted causing error or delays so that this section can be expanded.

A prescription could be written with directions as follows: "OD OD OD," to mean one drop in the right eye once daily!

Abbreviations should not be used for drug names as they are particularly dangerous. As previously illustrated, there is the possibility that the writer may, through mental error, confuse two abbreviations and use the wrong one. Similarly, the reader may attribute the wrong meaning to an abbreviation. To further confound the problem, some drug name abbreviations have multiple meanings (see ATR, CPM, CPZ, FLU, GEM, NITRO, and PBZ in Table 2). The abbreviation AC has been used for three different cancer chemotherapy combinations to mean Adriamycin and either cyclophosphamide, carmustine, or cisplatin.

Beside causing medication errors and incorrect interpretation of medical records, abbreviations can create problems because treatment is delayed while a health professional seeks clarification for the meaning of the abbreviation used. Abbreviations should not be used to designate drugs or combinations of drugs.

Certain meanings of abbreviations in the book are followed by a warning, "this is a dangerous abbreviation." This warning could be placed after many abbreviations, but was reserved for situations where errors have been published because these abbreviations were used or where the meaning is critical and not likely to be known. If no alternative abbreviation is suggested, then the term should be spelled out rather than abbreviated. Such warning statements should also appear after every abbreviation for a drug or drug combination.

References

1. Davis NM, Cohen MR. Medication errors: causes and prevention. Huntingdon Valley, PA: Neil M Davis Associates; 1983.
2. Cohen MR. Medication error reports. Hosp Pharm (appears monthly from 1975 to the present).
3. Cohen MR. Medication errors. Nursing 2005 (appears monthly, starting in Nursing 77, to the present).
4. Davis NM. Med Errors. Am J Nursing (appears monthly from 1994 to 1995).
5. Cohen MR. Medication Errors. American Pharmacists Assoc. Wash. DC, 2006.

Chapter 3

A Healthcare Controlled Vocabulary

Presently there are no standards for abbreviations used in prescribers' orders, consultations, written prescriptions, standing orders, computer order sets, nurse's medication administration records, pharmacy profiles, hospital formularies, etc. Because in the healthcare field everyone does their own thing, there are many variations. These variations in the way abbreviations are expressed are not always understood and at times are misinterpreted. They cause delays in initiating therapy, cause accidents, waste time for everyone in clarifying these documents, lengthen the time it takes to train those working in the healthcare field, lengthen hospital stays, and waste money.

A controlled vocabulary similar to what is used in the aviation industry is needed. Everyone in the aviation industry "follows the book," and uses a controlled vocabulary. All pilots and air traffic controllers say, "alfa", "bravo", "charlie." See Table 1, the phonetic alphabet. They do not go off on their own and say "adam", "beef", "candy!" They say "one three," not thirteen, because thirteen sounds like thirty. Radio transmission in the aviation industry is not easy to decipher, yet because precision is critical everything possible is done to eliminate error. To prevent errors all radio transmissions are given only in English, every transmission is given in the same order and must be immediately repeated by the receiver to make sure it was heard correctly. Written and oral communication in the medical professions are just as critical and are also not easy to decipher, so establishing a controlled vocabulary is also necessary in this industry.

Listed below are six organizations that have ongoing projects related to standardizing medical terminology:

Computer-Based Patient Record Institute, Inc.
1000 East Woodfield Rd. Suite 102
Schuamburg, IL 60173-5921
http://www.CPRI.org

The United States Pharmacopeial Convention, Inc.
12601 Twinbrook Parkway
Rockville, MD, 20852

National Library of Medicine
Unified Medical Language Systems
8600 Rockville Pike
Bethesda, MD, 20894

Council of Biological Editors, through their Scientific Style and Format: The CBE Manual for Authors, Editors, and Publishers, 6th Ed. Council of Biological Editors; Cambridge University Press, Cambridge UK, New York, Victoria Australia: 1995

American Medical Association, through their American Medical Assoc. Manual of Style, 9th Edition. AMA, Chicago, 1998

American Association of Medical Transcriptionists through their AAMT Book of Style for Medical Transcriptions, 2nd Edition. American Assoc. for Medical Transcriptions, Modesta CA, 2002

Listed below (Table 2) is the start of a Healthcare Controlled Vocabulary. The basis for this controlled vocabulary is established standard terminology and the result of 39 years of studying medical errors by this author.

It is anticipated that a Healthcare Controlled Vocabulary, with professional organizations' input and backing, will grow and someday evolve into an "official standard." Your suggestions and comments are vital to this growth and eventual recognition. It is always safest to avoid the use of abbreviations unless they are well known in your work environment.

Table 1. Phonetic Alphabet

The International Civil Aviation Organization phonetic alphabet is used by the aviation industry when communications conditions are such that the information cannot be readily received without their use. Health professionals also should use it when it is necessary to orally spell critical information.

Character	Telephony	Phonic
A	Alfa	(AL-FAH)
B	Bravo	(BRAH-VOH)
C	Charlie	(CHAR-LEE) or (SHAR-LEE)
D	Delta	(DELL-TA)
E	Echo	(ECK-OH)
F	Foxtrot	(FOKS-TROT)
G	Golf	(GOLF)
H	Hotel	(HOH-TEL)
I	India	(IN-DEE-AH)
J	Juliett	(JEW-LEE-ETT)
K	Kilo	(KEY-LOH)
L	Lima	(LEE-MAH)
M	Mike	(MIKE)
N	November	(NO-VEM-BER)
O	Oscar	(OSS-CAH)
P	Papa	(PAH-PAH)
Q	Quebec	(KEH-BECK)
R	Romeo	(ROW-ME-OH)
S	Sierra	(SEE-AIR-RAH)
T	Tango	(TANG-GO)
U	Uniform	(YOU-NEE-FORM) or (OO-NEE-FORM)
V	Victor	(VIK-TAH)
W	Whiskey	(WIS-KEY)
X	X-ray	(ECKS-RAY)
Y	Yankee	(YANG-KEY)
Z	Zulu	(ZOO-LOO)
1	One	(WUN)
2	Two	(TOO)
3	Three	(TREE)
4	Four	(FOW-ER)
5	Five	(FIFE)
6	Six	(SIX)
7	Seven	(SEV-EN)
8	Eight	(AIT)
9	Nine	(NIN-ER)
0	Zero	(ZEE-RO)

Table 2. Examples of a Controlled Vocabulary

Standard	What **not** to use or do	Comments
100 mg (100 space mg)	100mg (100 no space mg)	The USP* standard way of expressing a strength is to leave a space between the number and its units. Leaving this space makes it easier to read the number as can be seen below.
		1mg 1 mg 10mg 10 mg 100mg 100 mg
1 mg	1.0 mg	This is a USP standard. When a trailing zero is used, the decimal point is sometimes not seen thus causing a tenfold overdose. These overdoses have caused injury and death.
0.1 mL	.1 mL	When the decimal point is not seen, this is read as 1 mL, causing a ten fold overdose.
once daily (Do not abbreviate.)	The abbreviation OD	The classic meaning for OD is right eye. Liquids intended to be given once daily are mistakenly given in the right eye.
	The abbreviation QD	When the Q in QD is dotted too aggressively it looks like Q.I.D. and the medication is given four times daily. When a lower case q is used, the tail of the q has come up between the q and the d to make it look like qid. In the United Kingdom, Q.D. means four times daily
unit (Do not abbreviate. Write "unit" using a lower-case u)	The abbreviation U	The handwritten U is mistaken for a zero when poorly written causing a 10 fold overdose (i.e. 6 U regular insulin is read as 60). The poorly written U has also been read as a 4, 6, and cc. Write "unit," leaving a space between the number and the word unit.
mg (lower case mg with no period)	mg., Mg., Mg, MG, mgm, mgs	The USP standard expression is the mg
mL (lower case m with a capital L, no period)	mL, ml, mL., mls, mLs, cc	The USP standard expression is the mL for the measurement of liquids

14

Table 2. (cont.)

Standard	What **not** to use or do	Comments
Use generic names or brand names	Do not abbreviate drug names or combinations of drugs, such as CPZ, PBZ, NTG, MS, MSO4, 5FC, MTX, 6MP, MOPP, ASA, HCTZ, etc. Do not use shortened names or chemical names in patient-related documents	Abbreviated drug names and acronyms are not always known to the reader; at times they have more than one possible meaning, or are thought to be another drug. When the chemical name "6 mercaptopurine" has been used, six doses of mercaptopurine have been mistakenly administered. The generic name, mercaptopurine, should be used. MgSO4 has been read as morphine sulfate. When an unofficial shortened version of the name norfloxacin, norflox was used, Norflex was mistakenly given. An order for Aredia was read as Adriamycin, as some professionals abbreviated the name Adriamycin as "Adria" which looks like Aredia.
The metric system	The apothecary system (grains, drams, minims, ounces, etc.)	The Apothecary system is so rarely used it is not recognized or understood. The symbol for minim ($\mathfrak{m}$) is read as mL; the symbol for one dram ($\mathfrak{z}$ T) is read as 3 tablespoons, and gr (grain) is read as gram.
Use properly placed commas for numbers above 9999, as in 10,000, or 5,000,000.	5000000	Some healthcare workers have difficulty in reading large numbers such as 5000000. The use of commas helps the reader to read these numbers correctly.
600 mg When possible, do not use decimal expressions. 25 mcg	0.6 g 0.025 mg	A USP standard. The elimination of decimals lessens the chance for error. Mistakes are made when reading numbers less than 1 with decimals.
Use specific concentrations and the time in which intravenous potassium chloride should be administered.	Do not use the term "bolus" in conjunction with the administration of potassium chloride injection.	Some physicians will erroneously indicate that potassium chloride injection should be "bolused" or be given "IV push," vaguely meaning that it should not be dripped in slowly. Many deaths have been reported when prescribers have been taken literally and the potassium chloride was given by bolus or IV push for fluid-restricted patients. Orders should be specific such as, "20 mEq of potassium chloride in 50 mL of 5% dextrose to run over 30 minutes."

(continued)

Table 2. (cont.)

Standard	What **not** to use or do	Comments
use "and"	Do not use a slash (/) mark or the symbol "&"	A slash mark looks like a one. An order written "6 units regular insulin/20 units NPH insulin," was read as 120 units of NPH insulin. The symbol "&" has been read as a 4.
Orally transmitted medical orders should be read back as heard for verification.	Do not assume that one has spoken or heard correctly.	During oral communications, speakers misspeak and/or transcribers mishear. To minimize these errors, the transmitter must speak clearly and slowly, the transcriber must repeat what was transcribed, and the transmitter must listen attentively when this is being done. Errors are less likely to occur when the prescription is complete. When spelling out words, use the phonetic alphabet shown in Table 1. Oral orders should be avoided whenever possible.
When prescriptions are written or orally transmitted they must be complete. • dosage form must be specified • strength must be specified • directions must be specified • included in the directions must be the purpose or indication.	Incomplete orders	Prescribers on occasion think of one drug and mistakenly order another. Nurses and pharmacists on occasion misread prescriptions because of error, poor handwriting or poor oral communications, or look-alike or sound-alike drugs.[1] When the prescription is complete and the purpose or indication is included, these errors are less likely to occur. Listing the purpose or indication on the prescription label will assist in increasing patient adherence.
Written communications must be legible.	Illegible handwriting	Those who cannot or will not write legibly must print (if this would be legible), type, use a computer, or have an employee write for them and then immediately verify and sign the document.
Prescribe specific doses.	Do not prescribe 2 ampuls or 2 vials	There is often more than one size or concentration of drug available. Failing to be specific will lead to unintended doses being administered.
As required by the Joint Commission on Accreditation of Healthcare Organizations, establish a list of dangerous abbreviations which should not be used	Use dangerous abbreviations.	See Chapter 2 of this book "Dangerous, Contradictory, and/or Ambiguous Abbreviations."

Table 2. (cont.)

Standard	What **not** to use or do	Comments
Use h or hr for hour	°	An order written as q 4° has been read as q 40 or the symbol ° has not been understood.
Specify amount of drug to be given in a single dose.[2]	Specify total amount of drug to be administered over a period of time.	Orders such as . . . . 1,600 mg over 4 days have caused death when mistakenly given as a single dose. Order should state . . . . 400 mg once daily for four days (2-1-C6 to 2-4-06)

*USP = United States Pharmacopeia
1. Davis NM. Look-alike and sound alike drug names. Hosp Pharm 2006, Supplement Wall-chart (Call 1-800-223-0554)
2. Kohler D. Standardizing the expression & nomenclature of cancer treatment regimens. Am J Health-System Pharm. 1998;55;137–44

17

Additions, Corrections, and Suggestions are Welcomed

Please send them via any means shown below:

Neil M Davis
2049 Stout Drive, B-3
Warminster PA 18974-3861

FAX 1 888 333 4915 or 1 215 442 7432
Email med@neilmdavis.com
Web site www.medabbrev.com

Thank you for your help in the past.

Have You Used the Web-Version of This Book?

- It is instantaneously searchable for the meanings of abbreviations
- It is reverse searchable (search for all the abbreviations containing a particular word)
- Each month, about 80 new entries are added

See the preface (page vii) for access instructions. A two-year, single-user access is included in the purchase price of the book.

PDA Versions are Available

See pricing and ordering information in the pricing section on page 357.

Multi-User Site Licenses are Available

Medical facilities can substitute their own "Do Not Use" list of dangerous abbreviations for the one present. The ability also exists to list abbreviations that are unique to your region and/or organization which would normally not appear in any national list. These lists would be controlled by the facility. Demonstrations and pricing information are available by calling 1 888 333 1862 or 1 215 442 7430 or via an e-mail request to ev@neilmdavis.com

Chapter 4
Medical Abbreviation Primer

When first entering a medically related field, one must learn the language in order to function. Part of learning this language is to learn the meaning of the abbreviations, acronyms, and symbols in use. This chapter is intended to introduce newcomers to this commonly used medically related shorthand.

The determination of which abbreviations (refers also to acronyms and symbols) are most commonly used is based on the selection by the author with the consultation of experts in various health-related fields. The categorizing of the abbreviations is arbitrary, but is intended to represent the most common use, as the abbreviations could have been placed in many different categories.

This list could have been expanded to include many hundreds-more commonly used abbreviations, but then the list would have been too long to serve as a primer. The absence of an abbreviation from this listing does not mean it is not in common use. Each area of practice and specialty could have added their own commonly used abbreviations.

A few of the abbreviations below have more than one meaning listed. This was done when several meanings are in common use. Many abbreviations have more than one meaning and they must be viewed in their clinical context to arrive at their intended meaning. See Chapter 5 of this book for additional meanings for the abbreviations listed below.

In practice, there are inconsistencies as to how abbreviations are written. They may appear in all capital letters, lower case, or in capital letters and lower case. They may or may not have periods after each letter.

The readers are urged to read Chapter 2, Dangerous, Contradictory, and/or Ambiguous Abbreviations.

Two Hundred and Seventy-Five Commonly Used Medical Abbreviations Arranged by Category—a Primer

Physical Examination, History Portion of the Medical Record, and Discharge Summary

C/O	complains of	DTR	deep tendon reflex
CC	chief complaint(s)	EOMI	extraocular muscles intact
CTA	clear to auscultation	HJR	hepatojugular reflux
Dx	diagnosis	JVD	jugular venous distention
F/U	follow-up	IBW	ideal body weight
FH	family history	LBW	lean body weight
H/O	history of	BSA	body surface area
HPI	history of present illness	LMP	last menstrual period
Hx	history	NAD	no apparent distress
PE	physical examination		no apparent disease
	pelvic examination	NC/AT	normocephalic, atraumatic
	pulmonary embolism	NKA	no known allergies
PH/SH	personal and social history	NKDA	no known drug allergies
PI	present illness	OD	right eye
PMH	past medical history	OS	left eye
ROS	review of systems	OU	both eyes
SH	social history	PERRLA	pupils equal, round, reactive to
Tx	treatment		light and accommodation
CV	cardiovascular	IOP	intraocular pressure
GI	gastrointestinal	ROM	range of motion
GU	genitourinary	VS	vital signs
EENT	ears, eyes, nose, and throat	P	pulse
HEENT	head, ears, eyes, nose, and throat	T	temperature
Ob/Gyn	obstetrics and gynecology	RR	respiratory rate; recovery room
Peds	pediatrics	HR	heart rate
UCD	usual childhood diseases	RRR	regular rate and rhythm (heart)
A & P	auscultation and percussion	WDWNWM	well developed, well nourished,
ADL	activities of daily living		white male (also there are
CN III	third cranial nerve (there are CN I to XII)		abbreviations for females and other races [WF = white female;
RCM	right costal margin (there is also a LCM)		AAF = African-American female]
RUQ	right upper quadrant (also there is RLQ, LUQ, and LLQ)	YO	year old
		DOB	date of birth
TM	tympanic membrane	+	positive; present; plus
AAO X 3	awake and oriented to time, place, and person	−	negative; absent; minus
		c̄	with
BM	bowel movement	ō	negative; without
BP	blood pressure	W/O	without
CVAT	costovertebral angle tenderness		

Diseases and Symptoms

AD	Alzheimer disease
AIDS	acquired immunodeficiency syndrome
HIV	human immuno-deficiency virus
AMI	acute myocardial infarction
MI	myocardial infarction
CHF	congestive heart failure
ACS	acute coronary syndrome
HT	hypertension (also HTN) height
DM	diabetes mellitus
AODM	adult onset diabetes mellitus
IDDM	insulin dependent diabetes mellitus
NIDDM	noninsulin-dependent diabetes mellitus
PD	Parkinson disease
AOM	acute otitis media
Ca	cancer
COAD	chronic obstructive airway disease
COPD	chronic obstructive pulmonary disease
DOE	dyspnea on exertion
SOB	shortness of breath
URI	upper respiratory infection
TB	tuberculosis
CVA	cerebrovascular accident; costovertebral angle
DVT	deep vein thrombosis
NV	nausea and vomiting
NVD	nausea, vomiting, and diarrhea neck vein distention
PONV	postoperative nausea and vomiting
PUD	peptic ulcer disease
GERD	gastroesophageal reflux disease
RA	rheumatoid arthritis
OA	osteoarthritis
SLE	systemic lupus erythematosus
TIA	transient ischemic attack
HA	headache
BPH	benign prostatic hypertrophy (hyperplasia)
UTI	urinary tract infection
STD	sexually transmitted disease
MVA	motor vehicle accident

Clinical Laboratory

ANA	antinuclear antibody
Alb	albumin
ALT	alanine aminotransferase
LFT	liver function test
aPTT	activated partial thromboplastin time
AST	aspartate aminotransferase
BG	blood glucose; blood gases
BS	blood sugar
	bowel sounds
	breath sounds
BUN	blood urea nitrogen
CK-MB	creatine kinase, MB fraction
CO_2	carbon dioxide
CPK	creatinine phosphokinase
CrCl	creatinine clearance
SCr	serum creatinine
C & S	culture and sensitivity
ESR	erythrocyte sedimentation rate
Gluc	glucose
FBS	fasting blood sugar
HbA_{1c}	glycosylated hemoglobin
CHOL	cholesterol
HDL	high-density lipoprotein
LDL	low-density lipoprotein
LDH	lactic dehydrogenase
Trig	triglycerides
INR	international normalized ratio
DB	direct bilirubin
TB	total bilirubin
TP	total protein
Ca	Calcium (also Ca^{++})
Cl	Chloride (also Cl^-)
K	Potassium (also K^+)
Mg	Magnesium (also Mg^{++})
Na	Sodium (also Na^+)
OGTT	oral glucose tolerance test
PSA	prostate-specific antigen
UA	urinalysis
VDRL	Venereal Disease Research Laboratory (test for syphilis)
CBC	complete blood count
Diff	differential (blood count)
Eos	eosinophil
Fe	iron
Hct	hematocrit
Hgb	hemoglobin
Plt	platelets
MCV	mean corpuscular volume
RBC	red blood cell (count)
Segs	segmented neutrophils
WBC	white blood cell (count)
ABG	arterial blood gases
WNL	within normal limits

Other Diagnostic Tests, Procedures, and Treatments

ECG	electrocardiogram	CT	computer tomography
EEG	electroencephalogram	IVP	intravenous pyelogram
FEV$_1$	forced expiratory volume in one second	MRI	magnetic resonance imaging
		PET	positron emission tomography
IPPB	intermittent positive-pressure breathing	US	ultrasound
		CABG	coronary artery bypass graft
PFT	pulmonary function tests	PCTA	percutaneous transluminal coronary angioplasty
PEEP	positive end-expiratory pressure		
MUGA	multigated (radionuclide) angiogram	PT	physical therapy
		D & C	dilatation and curettage

Physicians' Orders and Prescriptions

ASAP	as soon as possible	i	one
OOB	out of bed	ii	two
BRP	bathroom privileges	q	*every (as in q 6 hours)*
CPR	cardiopulmonary resuscitation	h	hour(s)
DNR	do not resuscitate	b.i.d.	*twice daily*
DAW	dispense as written	t.i.d.	*three times daily*
DC or D/C	discharge	q.i.d.	*four times daily*
	discontinue	QAM	every morning
I/O	intake and output	QPM	every evening
LD	loading dose	AC	*before meals*
NAS	no salt added	PC	*after meals*
NPO	nothing by mouth	HS	*bedtime*
PO	by mouth; postoperative	NR	no refills (prescriptions)
IM	intramuscular	PRN	*as required; whenever necessary*
IV	intravenous	MRx1	may repeat one time
SC	subcutaneous	Rx	*prescription*
SQ	subcutaneous (SC preferred)		*pharmacy*
PICC	percutaneous indwelling central catheter	OTC	over-the-counter (no prescription required)
IVPB	intravenous piggyback	Stat	*immediately*
NGT	nasogastric tube	TKO	to keep (vein) open
cap	capsule	TO	telephone order
tab	tablet	VO	verbal order
inj	injection		

Drug Names (It is dangerous to abbreviate drug names)

APAP	acetaminophen	KCl	potassium chloride
ASA	aspirin	MgSO$_4$	magnesium sulfate
5D/W	dextrose 5% injection (in water)	MOM	milk of magnesia
Dig	digoxin	NaCl	sodium chloride
ETOH	alcohol (ethyl alcohol)	NS	normal saline (0.9% sodium chloride; same as NSS)
FeSO$_4$	ferrous sulfate		
H$_2$O	water	NSS	normal saline solution (0.9% sodium chloride)
H$_2$O$_2$	hydrogen peroxide		
HCl	hydrochloride (when following a drug name, as in thiamine HCl [thiamine hydrochloride])	O$_2$	oxygen
		PCN	penicillin
		tPA	tissue plasminogen activator
		IVF	intravenous fluids
	hydrochloric acid (when it appears separately [not as part of a drug name])	TPN	total parenteral nutrition
		lytes	electrolytes (sodium, potassium, chloride, etc.)

Drug Classes

ABX	antibiotic(s)	PPI	proton pump inhibitor
COX-2 I	cyclooxygenase-2 inhibitor	SSRI	selective serotonin reuptake
MOAI	monoamine oxidase inhibitor		inhibitor
NSAID	nonsteroidal anti-inflammatory drug	TCA	tricyclic antidepressant
OC	oral contraceptive		

Units of Measure

cm	centimeter (2.54 cm = 1 inch)	mEq	milliequivalent
g	gram (28.35 g = 1 ounce)	mg	milligram (1,000 mg = 1 gram [g])
Kg	kilogram (1 Kg = 2.2 pounds)	mL	milliliter (1,000 mL = 1 liter [L])
L	liter (l L = 1,000 mL = 1 quart plus about 2 ounces)	mmHg	millimeters of mercury
		°C	degrees Centigrade
lb	pound (1 lb = 0.454 Kg)	°F	degrees Fahrenheit
mcg	microgram (1,000 mcg = 1 milligram [mg])		

Hospital Locations

CCU	cardiac care unit	OB	obstetrics
DR	delivery room	OR	operating room
ED	emergency department	PACU	postanesthesia care unit
ER	emergency room (same as ED)	PICU	pediatric intensive care unit
ICU	intensive care unit		pulmonary intensive care unit
L & D	labor and delivery	RD	radiology department
LDR	labor, delivery, and recovery	SICU	surgical intensive care
MICU	medical intensive care unit		unit
NICU	neonatal intensive care unit		

Miscellaneous

ARNP	Advanced Registered Nurse Practitioner	MD	Doctor of Medicine
		OD	Doctor of Osteopathy
LPN	Licensed Practical Nurse	PA	Physician Assistant
MA	Medical Assistant	RPh	Registered Pharmacist
MAR	medication administration record	RN	Registered Nurse

Additions, Corrections, and Suggestions are Welcomed

Please send them via any means shown below:

Neil M Davis
2049 Stout Drive, B-3
Warminster PA 18974-3861

FAX 1 888 333 4915 or 1 215 442 7432
Email med@neilmdavis.com
Web site www.medabbrev.com

Thank you for your help in the past.

Have You Used the Web-Version of This Book?

- It is instantaneously searchable for the meanings of abbreviations
- It is reverse searchable (search for all the abbreviations containing a particular word)
- Each month, about 80 new entries are added

See the preface (page vii) for access instructions. A two-year, single-user access is included in the purchase price of the book.

PDA Versions are Available

See pricing and ordering information in the pricing section on page 357.

Multi-User Site Licenses are Available

Medical facilities can substitute their own "Do Not Use" list of dangerous abbreviations for the one present. The ability also exists to list abbreviations that are unique to your region and/or organization which would normally not appear in any national list. These lists would be controlled by the facility. Demonstrations and pricing information are available by calling 1 888 333 1862 or 1 215 442 7430 or via an e-mail request to ev@neilmdavis.com

Chapter 5

Lettered Abbreviations and Acronyms

When an abbreviation contains numbers, symbols, punctuation, spaces, etc., they are *not* considered during alphabetizing. When looking for 6MP, it will be found after the MP listings and H_2O will be found after HO. Abbreviations that only contain numbers (no letters) are found in chapter 6, Symbols and Numbers. Entries beginning with a *Greek letter* are alphabetized where the name of the letter would be found alphabetically.

The letter-by-letter (dictionary) system of alphabetizing is used ("*ad lib*" is listed under ADL).

Brand names (proprietary names) have their first letter capitalized, whereas nonproprietary (generic) names are in lower-case letters.

Drug names should not be abbreviated as the meaning may not be known to the reader or interpreted as intended.

The listing of symbols, numbers, and Greek letters can be found in Chapter 6.

See WARNING in chapter 1.

A

A	accommodation
	Acinetobacter
	adenosine
	age
	alive
	ambulatory
	angioplasty
	anterior
	anxiety
	apical
	arterial
	artery
	Asian
	assessment
	auscultation
A+	blood type A positive (A positive is preferred)
A−	blood type A negative (A negative is preferred)
A′	ankle

@	at
(a)	axillary temperature
ā	before
A_1	aortic first heart sound
A_2	aortic second sound
A250	5% albumin 250 mL
A1000	5% albumin 1000 mL
A II	angiotensin II
AA	accelerated approval (FDA)
	acetic acid
	achievement age
	active assistive
	acute asthma
	affected area
	affirmative action
	African American
	Alcoholics Anonymous
	alcohol abuse
	alopecia areata
	alveolar-arterial gradient
	amino acid
	anaplastic astrocytoma
	androgenetic alopecia
	anesthesiologist assistant

anti-aerobic
antiarrhythmic agent
aortic aneurysm
aplastic anemia
arachidonic acid
arm ankle (pulse ratio)
ascending aorta
ascorbic acid (vitamin C)
audiologic assessment
Australia antigen
authorized absence
automobile accident
cytarabine (ara-C) and doxorubicin (Adriamycin)

aa of each

A&A aid and attendance
albuterol and ipratropium bromide (Atrovent) (this combination is available as Combivent Aerosol and DuoNab inhalation solution)
arthroscopy and arthrotomy
awake and aware

A-a alveolar arterial (gradient)

a/A arterial-alveolar (gradient)

AIIA Angiotensin II antagonist

AAA abdominal aortic aneurysmectomy (aneurysm)
acute anxiety attack
Area Agencies on Aging
aromatic amino acids
arterio-arterial anastomosis

A&AA active and active assistive

AAAASF American Association for Accreditation of Ambulatory Surgery Facilities

AAAE amino acid activating enzyme

AAAHC Accreditation Association of Ambulatory Health Care

AABB American Association of Blood Banks

AABR automated auditory brainstem response

AAC Adrenalin, atropine, and cocaine
advanced adrenocortical cancer
antimicrobial agent-associated colitis
augmentative and alternative communication

AACD aging-associated cognitive decline

AACG acute-angle closure glaucoma

AACLR arthroscopic anterior cruciate ligament reconstruction

AAD acid-ash diet
antibiotic-associated diarrhea

A_1AD alpha$_1$-antitrypsin deficiency

AADA Abbreviated Antibiotic Drug Application

[A-a]Do$_2$ alveolar-arterial oxygen tension gradient

AAE active assistance exercise
acute allergic encephalitis

AAECS amino acid enriched cardioplegic solution

A/AEX active assistive exercise

AAF African-American female
altered auditory feedback

AAFB alcohol acid-fast bacilli

AAFO active ankle-foot orthoses

AAG alpha-1-acid glycoprotein

AAH acute alcoholic hepatitis
atypical adenomatous hyperplasia

AAI acute alcohol intoxication
arm-ankle index
atlantoaxial instability
atrial demand-inhibited (pacemaker)

AAK atlantoaxial kyphosis

AAL anterior axillary line

AALNC Legal Nurse Consultant (American Association of Legal Nurse Consultants)

AAM African-American male
amino acid mixture

AAMI age-associated memory impairment

AAMS acute aseptic meningitis syndrome

AAN AIDS-associated neutropenia
analgesic abuse nephropathy
analgesic-associated nephropathy
attending's admission notes

AANA American Association of Nurse Anesthetists

AAO alert, awake, & oriented

AAO × 3 awake and oriented to time, place, and person

AAOC antacid of choice

AAP acute anterior poliomyelitis
American Academy of Pediatrics (guidelines)
assessment adjustment pass

AAPC antibiotic-associated pseudomembranous colitis

AAPMC antibiotic-associated pseudomembranous colitis

a/ApO$_2$ arterial-alveolar oxygen tension ratio

AAPSA age-adjusted prostate-specific antigen

AAR antigen-antiglobulin reaction
automated anesthesia record

AARF atlantoaxial rotatory fixation (subluxation; dislocation)

AAROM active-assistive range of motion

AAS acute abdominal series
allergic Aspergillus sinusitis
androgenic-anabolic steroid
Ann Arbor stage (Hodgkin disease staging system)
aortic arch syndrome

Associate's Degree, Applied Science
atlantoaxis subluxation
atomic absorption spectroscopy
atypical absence seizure

AASCRN amino acid screen

AASH adrenal androgen-stimulating
hormone

AAST American Association for the
Surgery of Trauma (trauma
grading)

AAST- American Association for the
OIS Surgery of Trauma—Organ
Injury Scale

AASV antibody-associated systemic
vasculitis

AAT activity as tolerated
alpha-antitrypsin
androgen ablation therapy
at all times
atrial demand-triggered (pacemaker)
atypical antibody titer
automatic atrial tachycardia

A_1AT alpha$_1$-antitrypsin

A_1AT-P_i alpha$_1$-antitrypsin (phenotyping)

AAU acute anterior uveitis

AAV adeno-associated vector
adeno-associated virus

AAVV accumulated alveolar ventilatory
volume

AAWD antiandrogen withdrawal

AB abortion
Ace® bandage
antibiotic
antibody
Aphasia Battery
apical beat
armboard
attentional blink
products meeting bioequivalence
requirements for generic
pharmaceuticals

Aβ beta-amyloid peptide

A/B acid-base ratio
apnea/bradycardia

A > B air greater than bone (conduction)

A & B apnea and bradycardia
assault and battery

AB+ AB positive blood type
(AB positive preferred)

AB− AB negative blood type
(AB negative preferred)

ABA applied behavioral analysis

ABBI Advanced Breast Biopsy
Instrumentation

ABC abacavir (Ziagen)
abbreviated blood count
Aberrant Behavior Checklist
absolute band counts

absolute basophil count
activity-based costing
advanced breast cancer
airway, breathing, and circulation
all but code (resuscitation order)
aneurysmal bone cyst
antigen-binding capacity
apnea, bradycardia, and cyanosis
applesauce, bananas, and
cereal (diet)
argon-beam coagulator
aspiration, biopsy and cytology
artificial beta cells
automated blood count
(no differential)
avidin-biotin complex

ABCD amphotericin B cholesteryl
sulfate complex (Amphotec;
amphotericin B colloid dispersion)
asymmetry, border irregularity,
color variation, and diameter more
than 6 mm (melanoma warning
signs in a mole)
automated blood count (differential
done manually)

ABCDE botulism toxoid pentavalent

ABCS automated blood count, STKR
(differential done by machine)

ABD after bronchodilator
automated border detection
detection
type of plain gauze dressing

Abd abdomen
abdominal
abductor

ABDCT atrial bolus dynamic computer
tomography

ABD GR abdominal girth

ABD PB abductor pollicis brevis

ABD PL abductor pollicis longus

ABE acute bacteria endocarditis
adult basic education
average bioequivalence
botulism equine trivalent antitoxin

ABECB acute bacterial exacerbations of
chronic bronchitis

ABEP auditory brain stem-evoked
potentials
aortic blood flow

A-beta42 beta-amyloid 42

ABF aortobifemoral (bypass)

ABG air/bone gap
aortoiliac bypass graft
arterial blood gases
axiobuccogingival

ABH Ativan, Benadryl, and Haldol

ABI ankle brachial index (ankle-to-arm
systolic blood pressure ratio)

	atherothrombotic brain infarction
	auditory brainstem implant
ABID	antibody identification
A Big	atrial bigeminy
ABK	aphakic bullous keratopathy
ABL	abetalipoproteinemia
	allograft bound lymphocytes
	axiobuccolingual
ABLB	alternate binaural loudness balance
ABLC	amphotericin B lipid complex (Abelcet)
ABLV	Australian bat lyssavirus
A/B Mods	apnea/bradycardia moderate stimulation
ABMS	acute bacterial maxillary sinusitis
	autologous bone marrow support
A/B MS	apnea/bradycardia mild stimulation
ABMT	autologous bone marrow transplantation
ABN	abnormality(ies)
	Advance Beneficiary Notice
abnl bld	abnormal bleeding
ABNM	American Board of Nuclear Medicine
abnor.	abnormal
ABO	absent bed occupant
	blood group system (A, AB, B, and O)
ABP	ambulatory blood pressure
	androgen-binding protein
	arterial blood pressure
ABPA	allergic bronchopulmonary aspergillosis
ABPB	axillary brachial plexus block
ABPI	Association of the British Pharmaceutical Industry
ABPM	axillary brachial plexus block
ABPM	allergic bronchopulmonary mycosis
	ambulatory blood pressure monitoring
ABQAURP	American Board of Quality Assurance and Utilization Review Physicians
ABR	absolute bed rest
	auditory brain-stem response
ABRS	acute bacterial rhinosinusitis
ABS	absent
	absorbed
	absorption
	Accuchek® blood sugar
	acute brain syndrome
	admitting blood sugar
	Alterman-Bishop stent
	antibody screen
	at bedside
ABSS	Anderson Behavioral State Scale
A/B SS	apnea/bradycardia self-stimulation

ABT	aminopyrine breath test
	antibiotic therapy
	autologous blood therapy
ABVD	doxorubicin (Adriamycin)®, bleomycin, vinblastine, and dacarbazine (DTIC)
ABW	actual body weight
ABx	antibiotics
AC	abdominal circumference
	acceleration capacity (heart)
	acetate
	acromioclavicular
	activated charcoal
	acute
	African Caribbean
	air conditioned
	air conduction
	anchored catheter
	antecubital
	anticoagulant
	anticonvulsant
	arm circumference
	assist control
	autologous cell
	before meals (a.c. preferred)
	doxorubicin (Adriamycin) and cyclophosphamide
a.c.	before meals
A-C	Astler-Coller (stages of colorectal cancer
A/C	anterior chamber of the eye
	assist/control
A & C	alert and cooperative
A1C	glycosylated hemoglobin A1C
5-AC	azacitidine (Vidaza)
9AC	rubitecan (9-aminocamptothecin; Orathecin)
ACA	acrodermatitis chronica atrophicans
	acyclovir
	adenocarcinoma
	against clinical advice
	aminocaproic acid (Amicar)
	anterior cerebral artery
	anterior communicating artery
	anticanalicular antibodies
AC/A	accommodation convergence–accommodation (ratio)
ACABS	acute community-acquired bacterial sinusitis
ACAD	anterior circulation arterial dissection
ACAS	acute community-acquired sinusitis
	asymptomatic carotid artery study
ACAT	acyl coenzyme A: cholesterol acyltransferase
ACB	alveolar-capillary block
	antibody-coated bacteria
	aortocoronary bypass
	before breakfast

AcB	assist with bath
AC & BC	air and bone conduction
ACBE	air contrast barium enema
ACBG	aortocoronary bypass graft
ACBT	active cycle of breathing techniques
ACC	acalculous cholecystitis
	accident
	accommodation
	adenoid cystic carcinomas
	administrative control center
	advanced colorectal cancer
	ambulatory care center
	American College of Cardiology (guidelines)
	amylase creatinine clearance
	anterior cingulate cortex
	automated cell count
ACCE	Academic Clinical Coordinator Educator
ACC-NCDR	American College of Cardiology-National Cardiovascular Data Registry
AcCoA	acetyl-coenzyme A
ACCP	American College of Chest Physicians
ACCR	amylase creatinine clearance ratio
ACCU	acute coronary care unit
ACCU✔	Accucheck® (blood glucose monitoring)
ACD	absolute cardiac dullness
	absorbent cover dressing
	acid-citrate-dextrose
	advanced cervical dilation
	allergic contact dermatitis
	anemia of chronic disease
	anterior cervical diskectomy
	anterior chamber depth
	anterior chamber diameter
	anterior chest diameter
	average cost per day
	before dinner
	dactinomycin (actinomycin D; Cosmegen)
ACDC	antibody complement-dependent cytolysis
AC-DC	bisexual (homo- and heterosexual)
ACDDS	Alcoholism/Chemical Dependency Detoxification Service
ACDF	anterior cervical diskectomy and fusion
ACDFs	adult children from dysfunctional families
ACDK	acquired cystic disease of the kidney
ACDs	anticonvulsant drugs
ACE	adrenocortical extract
	adverse clinical event
	aerosol-cloud enhancer
	angiotensin-converting enzyme

	antegrade colonic enema
	antegrade continence enema
	doxorubicin (Adriamycin), cyclophosphamide, and etoposide
ACEI	angiotensin-converting enzyme inhibitor
ACF	aberrant crypt focus
	accessory clinical findings
	acute care facility
	anterior cervical fusion
ACG	accelerography
	adjusted clinical groups
	angiocardiography
ACGME	Accreditation Council for Graduate Medical Education
ACH	adrenal cortical hormone
	aftercoming head
	arm girth, chest depth, and hip width
ACh	acetylcholine
ACHA	air-conduction hearing aid
AChE	acetylcholinesterase
AChEIs	acetylcholinesterase inhibitors
ACHES	abdominal pain, chest pain, headache, eye problems, and severe leg pains (early danger signs of oral contraceptive adverse effects)
AC & HS	before meals and at bedtime
ACI	acceleration index
	adrenal cortical insufficiency
	aftercare instructions
	anabolic-catabolic index
	anemia of chronic illness
	autologous chondrocyte implantation
ACIOL	anterior chamber intraocular lens
ACIP	Advisory Committee on Immunization Practices (of the Centers for Disease Control and Prevention)
ACIS	automated cellular imaging system
ACJ	acromioclavicular joint
A/CK	Accuchek®
ACL	accessory collateral ligament (hand)
	American cutaneous leishmaniasis
	anterior cruciate ligament (knee)
aCL	anticardiolipin (antibody)
ACLA	aclarubicin
ACLF	adult congregate living facility
ACLR	anterior cruciate ligament repair
ACLS	advanced cardiac (cardiopulmonary) life support
	Allen Cognitive Level Screen
ACM	alternative/complementary medicine
	Arnold-Chiari malformation
ACME	arginine catabolic mobile element
	aphakic cystoid macular edema
	Automated Classification of Medical Entities

ACMT	advanced combined modality therapy
ACMV	assist-controlled mechanical ventilation
ACN	acute conditioned neurosis
ACNP	Acute Care Nurse Practitioner
ACNU	nimustine HCl (Nidran; Acnu)
ACO	anterior capsular opacification
ACOA	Adult Children of Alcoholics
ACOG	American College of Obstetricians and Gynecologists
A COMM A	anterior communicating artery
ACOS-OG	American College of Surgeons Oncology Group
ACP	accessory conduction pathway
	acid phosphatase
	adamantinomatous craniopharyngioma
	adenocarcinoma of the prostate
	ambulatory care program
	anesthesia-care provider
	anterior cervical plate
	antrochoanal polyp
ACPA	anticytoplasmic antibodies
AC-PC line	anterior commissure-posterior commissure line
AC-PH	acid phosphatase
ACPO	acute colonic pseudo-obstruction
ACPP	adrenocorticopolypeptide
ACPPD	average cost per patient day
ACPP PF	acid phosphatase prostatic fluid
ACPS	anterior cervical plate stabilization
ACQ	acquired
	Areas of Change Questionnaire
ACR	adenomatosis of the colon and rectum
	albumin to creatinine ratio
	American College of Rheumatology
	anterior chamber reformation
	anticonstipation regimen
ACR20	American College of Rheumatology rating scale (20% or more improvement)
ACRC	advanced colorectal cancer
ACRES	amplification created restriction enzyme site
ACRN	AIDS-Certified Registered Nurse
ACS	anterior compartment syndrome
	acute confusional state
	acute coronary syndromes
	American Cancer Society
	anodal-closing sound
	automated corneal shaper
	before supper
ACSF	anterior cervical spine fixation
	artificial cerebrospinal fluid
ACSL	automatic computerized solvent litholysis

ACSVBG	aortocoronary saphenous vein bypass graft
ACSW	Academy of Certified Social Workers
ACT	activated clotting time
	aggressive comfort treatment
	allergen challenge test
	anticoagulant therapy
	artemisinin-based combination therapy
	assertive community treatment (program)
	doxorubicin (adriamycin), cyclophosphamide, and paclitaxel (Taxol)
ACT-D	dactinomycin (Cosmegen)
Act Ex	active exercise
ACTG	AIDS Clinical Trial Group
ACTH	corticotropin (adrenocorticotropic hormone)
ACT-Post	activated clotting time post-filter
ACT-Pre	activated clotting time pre-filter
ACTSEB	anterior chamber tube shunt encircling band
ACU	ambulatory care unit
ACUP	adenocarcinoma of unknown primary (origin)
ACUV	air-contrast ultrasound venography
ACV	acyclovir (Zovirax)
	amifostine, cisplatin, and vinblastine
	assist control ventilation
	atrial/carotid/ventricular
A-C-V	A wave, C wave, and V wave
ACVBP	doxorubicin (Adriamycin), cyclophosphamide, vindesine, bleomycin, and prednisone
ACVD	acute cardiovascular disease
ACVP	doxorubicin (Adriamycin), cyclophosphamide, vincristine, and prednisone
ACW	anterior chest wall
	apply to chest wall
acyl-CoA	acyl coenzyme A
AD	accident dispensary
	admitting diagnosis
	advance directive (living will)
	air dyne
	alternating days (this is a dangerous abbreviation)
	Alzheimer disease
	androgen deprivation
	antidepressant
	assistive device
	atopic dermatitis
	autistic disorder
	axillary dissection
	axis deviation
	right ear

A&D	admission and discharge	ADFT	atrial defibrillation threshold
	alcohol and drug	ADFU	agar diffusion for fungus
	ascending and descending	ADG	atrial diastolic gallop
	vitamins A and D		axiodistogingival
ADA	adenosine deaminase	ADH	antidiuretic hormone
	American Dental Association		atypical ductal hyperplasia
	American Diabetes Association	ADHD	attention-deficit hyperactivity
	Americans with Disabilities Act		disorder
	anterior descending artery	ADHF	acute decompensated heart failure
	awareness during anesthesia	ADI	acute diaphragmatic injury
ADAM	adjustment disorder with anxious		AIDS (acquired immunodeficiency
	mood		symdrome) defining illness
ADAS	Alzheimer Disease Assessment Scale		allowable (acceptable) daily intake
ADAS-	Alzheimer Disease Assessment		axiodistoincisal
COG	Scale-Cognitive Subscale	A-DIC	doxorubicin (Adriamycin) and
ADAT	advance diet as tolerated		dacarbazine
ADAU	adolescent drug abuse unit	Adj Dis	adjustment disorder
ADB	amorous disinhibited behavior	Adj D/O	adjustment disorder
ADC	Aid to Dependent Children	ADL	activities of daily living
	AIDS (acquired immune deficiency	ADLG	average duration of life gained
	syndrome) dementia complex	*ad lib*	as desired
	anxiety disorder clinic		at liberty
	apparent diffusion coefficient	ADM	abductor digiti minimi (muscle)
	(radiology)		acceptance of disability modified
	average daily census		administered (dose)
	average daily consumption		admission
ADCA	autosomal dominant cerebellar ataxia		adrenomedullin
ADCC	antibody-dependent cellular		doxorubicin (Adriamycin)
	cytotoxicity	ADMA	asymmetrical dimethyl arginine
A.D.C.	mnemonic for formatting	ADME	absorption, distribution, metabolism,
VAAN	physician orders:		and excretion
DIML	**A**dmit, **D**iagnosis, **C**ondition, **V**itals,	ADO	axiodisto-occlusal
	Activity, **A**llergies, **N**ursing	Ad-OAP	doxorubicin (Adriamycin),
	procedures, **D**iet, **I**ns and outs,		vincristine, (Oncovin) cytarabine,
	Medication, **L**abs		(Ara C) and prednisone
ADD	adduction	ADOL	adolescent
	annual disability density	ADON	Assistant Director of Nursing
	arrest in dilation/descent	ADP	arterial demand pacing
	attention-deficit disorder		adenosine diphosphate
	average daily dose	ADPKD	autosomal dominant polycystic
ADDH	attention-deficit disorder with		kidney disease
	hyperactivity	ADPV	anomaly of drainage of pulmonary
ADDL	additional		vein
ADDM	adjustment disorder with depressed	ADQ	abductor digiti quinti
	mood		adequate
ADDP	adductor pollicis	ADR	acute dystonic reaction
ADDs	AIDS (acquired immune deficiency		adverse drug reaction
	syndrome)-defining diseases		alternative dispute resolution
ADDU	alcohol and drug dependence		doxorubicin (Adriamycin)
	unit	ADRB2	beta-2 adrenergic receptor
ADE	acute disseminated encephalitis	ADRD	Alzheimer disease and related
	adverse drug event		disorders
ADEM	acute disseminating	ADRIA	doxorubicin (Adriamycin)
	encephalomyelitis	ADRV	adult diarrhea rotavirus
ADE-	adenocarcinoma	ADS	admission day surgery
NOCA			anatomical dead space
ADEPT	antibody-directed enzyme		anonymous donor's sperm
	prodrug therapy		antibody deficiency syndrome

ADs	advance directives (living wills)	AEDP	assisted end-diastolic pressure
AdSD	adductor spasmodic dysphonia		automated external defibrillator
ADSU	ambulatory diagnostic surgery unit		pacemaker
ADT	admission, discharge, and transfer	AEE	asthma-exacerbation episodes
	alternate-day therapy	AEEU	admission entrance and evaluation
	androgen deprivation treatment		unit
	(therapy)	AEG	air encephalogram
	anticipate discharge tomorrow		Alcohol Education Group
	any damn thing (a placebo)	AEIOU	mnemonic for the diagnosis of
	Auditory Discrimination Test	TIPS	coma: Alcohol, Encephalopathy,
ADTP	Adolescent Day Treatment Program		Insulin, Opiates, Uremia, Trauma,
	Alcohol-Dependence Treatment		Infection, Psychiatric, and
	Program		Syncope
ADTR	Academy of Dance Therapists,	AELBM	after each loose bowel movement
	Registered	AEM	active electrode monitor
ADU	automated dispensing unit		ambulatory electrogram monitor
ADV	adenovirus vaccine, not otherwise		antiepileptic medication
	specified	AEP	auditory evoked potential
adv	adventitious sounds (wheezes and	AEq	age equivalent
	rhonchi)	AER	acoustic evoked response
ADV$_4$	adenovirus vaccine, type 4, live, oral		albumin excretion rate
ADV$_7$	adenovirus vaccine, type 7, live, oral		auditory evoked response
A5D5W	alcohol 5%, dextrose 5% in water	AERD	aspirin-exacerbated respiratory
	for injection		disease
ADX	audiological diagnostic	Aer. M.	aerosol mask
AE	above elbow (amputation)	AERS	adverse event reporting system
	accident and emergency	AERs	adverse event reports
	(department)	Aer. T.	aerosol tent
	acute exacerbation	AES	adult emergency service
	adaptive equipment		anti-embolic stockings
	adverse event	AEs	adverse events
	air entry	AET	alternating esotropia
	androgen excess		atrial ectopic tachycardia
	anoxic encephalopathy	AF	acid-fast
	antiembolitic		afebrile
	arm ergometer		amniotic fluid
	aryepiglottic (fold)		anterior fontanel
A&E	accident and emergency		antifibrinogen
	(department)		aortofemoral
AEA	above-elbow amputation		ascitic fluid
	anti-endomysium		atrial fibrillation
	antibody	AFB	acid-fast bacilli
AEB	as evidenced by		aorto-femoral bypass
	atrial ectopic beat		aspirated foreign body
AEC	absolute (blood) eosinophil	AFB$_1$	aflatoxin B$_1$
	count	AFBG	aortofemoral bypass graft
	at earliest convenience	AFBY	aortofemoral bypass (graft)
AECB	acute exacerbations of chronic	AFC	adult foster care
	bronchitis		air filled cushions
AECG	ambulatory electrocardiogram		alveolar fluid clearance
AECOPD	acute exacerbation of chronic	AFDC	Aid to Families with Dependent
	obstructive pulmonary disease		Children
AED	antiepileptic drug	AFE	amniotic fluid embolization
	automated (automatic) external	AFEB	afebrile
	defibrillator	AFEU	ante partum fetal evaluation unit
AEDD	anterior extradural defects	AF/FL	atrial fibrillation/atrial flutter
AEDF	absent end-diastolic flow (umbilical-	aFGF	acidic fibroblast growth factor
	artery Doppler ultrasonography)	AFH	adult family home

	angiomatoid fibrous histiocytoma
	anterior facial height
AFI	acute febrile illness
	amniotic fluid index
A fib	atrial fibrillation
AFIP	Armed Forces Institute of Pathology
AFKO	ankle-foot-knee orthosis
AFL	air/fluid level
	atrial flutter
AFLP	acute fatty liver of pregnancy
	amplified fragment length polymorphism
A Flu	atrial flutter
AFM	active fetal movement
	acute *Plasmodium falciparum* malaria
	aerosol face mask
	atomic force microscopy
	doxorubicin (Adriamycin), fluorouracil, and methotrexate
AFM×2	double-aerosol face mask
AFO	ankle-fixation orthotic
	ankle-foot orthosis
AFOF	anterior fontanelõopen and flat
AFP	acute flaccid paralysis
	alpha-fetoprotein
	anterior faucial pillar
	ascending frontal parietal
AFQT	Armed Forces Qualification Test
AFRD	acute febrile respiratory disease
AFRIMS	Armed Forces Research Institute of Medical Sciences
AFRRI	Armed Forces Radiological Research Institute
AFRS	allergic fungal rhinosinusitis
AFS	allergic fungal sinusitis
	atomic fluorescence spectrometry
Aft/Dis	aftercare/discharge
AFV	amniotic fluid volume
AFVSS	afebrile, vital signs stable
AFX	air-fluid exchange
AG	abdominal girth
	adrenogenital
	aminoglycoside
	Amsler grid
	anaplastic glioma
	anion gap
	antigen
	antigravity
	atrial gallop
Ag	silver
A/G	albumin to globulin ratio
AGA	accelerated growth area
	acute gonococcal arthritis
	androgenetic alopecia
	antigliadin antibody
	appropriate for gestational age
	average gestational age

AGAS	accelerated graft atherosclerosis
AG/BL	aminoglycoside/beta-lactam
AGC	absolute granulocyte count
	advanced gastric cancer
	atypical glandular cells
AGCUS	atypical glandular cells of undetermined significance
AGD	agar gel diffusion
AGE	acute gastroenteritis
	advanced glycation end product(s)
	angle of greatest extension
	anterior gastroenterostomy
	arterial gas embolism
AGECAT	automatic geriatric examination for computer-assisted taxonomy
AGF	angle of greatest flexion
AGG	agammaglobulinemia
aggl.	agglutination
AGI	alpha-glucosidase inhibitor
AGIB	acute gastrointestinal bleeding
AGL	acute granulocytic leukemia
A GLAC-TO-LK	alpha galactoside leukocytes
AGN	acute glomerulonephritis
AGNB	aerobic gram-negative bacilli
$AgNO_3$	silver nitrate
AgNORs	argyrophilic nucleolar organizer regions (staining)
α_1-AGP	alpha$_1$-acid glycoprotein
AGPT	agar-gel precipitation test
AGS	adrenogenital syndrome
	Alagille syndrome
	American Geriatric Society (guidelines)
AG SYND	adrenogenital syndrome
AGT	alanine-glyoxylate aminotransferase
	angiotensinogen
AGTT	abnormal glucose tolerance test
AGU	aspartylglycosaminuria
AGUS	atypical glandular cells of uncertain significance
AGV	Ahmed glaucoma valve
AGVHD	acute graft-versus-host disease
AGVI	Ahmed glaucoma valve implantation
AH	abdominal hysterectomy
	amenorrhea and hirsutism
	amenorrhea-hyperprolactinemia
	antihyaluronidase
	auditory hallucinations
A&H	accident and health (insurance)
AHA	acetohydroxamic acid (Lithostat®)
	acquired hemolytic anemia
	American Health Association (guidelines)
	autoimmune hemolytic anemia
AHAs	alpha hydroxy acids
AHase	antihyaluronidase
AHB_c	hepatitis B core antibody

AHC	acute hemorrhagic conjunctivitis	AHSG	fetuin-A (alpha2-Heremans Schmid
	acute hemorrhagic cystitis		glycoprotein
	Adolescent Health Center	AHSP	alpha hemoglobin stabilizing protein
	alternating hemiplegia of childhood	AHST	autologous hematopoietic stem cell
	avoidable hospitalization conditions		transplantation
AHCA	Agency for Healthcare	AHT	alternating hypertropia
	Administration		autoantibodies to human
	American Healthcare Association		thyroglobulin
AHCPR	Agency for Health Care	AHTG	antihuman thymocyte globulin
	Policy and Research	AI	accidentally incurred
AHCs	academic health centers		accommodative insufficiency
AHD	alien-hand syndrome		allelic imbalance
	antecedent hematological disorder		American Indian
	arteriosclerotic heart disease		allergy index
	autoimmune hemolytic disease		aortic insufficiency
AHE	acute hemorrhagic encephalomyelitis		apical impulse
	amygdalo-hippocampectomy		artificial insemination
AHEC	Area Health Education Center		artificial intelligence
AHF	antihemophilic factor	A & I	Allergy and Immunology
	Argentine hemorrhagic fever		(department)
	(Junin virus) vaccine		auscultation and inspection
AHF-M	antihemophilic factor (human),	AIA	Accommodation Independence
	method M, (monoclonal purified)		Assessment
AHFS	American Hospital Formulary		allergen-induced asthma
	Service		allyl isopropyl acetamide
AHG	antihemophilic globulin		anti-insulin antibody
AHGS	acute herpetic gingival stomatitis		aspirin-induced asthma
AHHD	arteriosclerotic hypertensive heart	AI-Ab	anti-insulin antibody
	disease	AIBF	anterior interbody fusion
AHI	apnea-hypopnea index	AICA	anterior inferior cerebellar artery
AHJ	artificial hip joint		anterior inferior communicating
AHL	apparent half-life		artery
AHM	ambulatory Holter monitoring	AICBG	anterior interbody cervical bone
AHMO	anterior horizontal mandibular		graft
	osteotomy	AICD	activation-induced cell death
AHN	adenomatous hyperplastic nodule		automatic implantable cardioverter/
	Assistant Head Nurse		defibrillator
AHO	Albright hereditary osteodystrophy	AICM	anti-inflammatory controller
AHP	acute hemorrhagic pancreatitis		medication
	acute hepatic panel (see page 298)	AICS	acute ischemic coronary syndromes
	American Herbal Pharmacopeia	AID	absolute iron deficiency
	and Therapeutic Compendium		acute infectious disease
AHPB	adjusted historic payment base		aortoiliac disease
AhpF	alkyl hydroperoxide reductase,		artificial insemination donor
	F isomer		automatic implantable defibrillator
AHR	adjusted hazard ratios	AIDH	artificial insemination donor husband
	airway hyperresponsiveness	AIDKS	acquired immune deficiency
AHRE	atrial high-rate event		syndrome with Kaposi sarcoma
AHRF	acute hypoxemic respiratory failure	AIDP	acute inflammatory demyelinating
AHS	adaptive hand skills		polyradiculoneuropathy
	allopurinol hypersensitivity syndrome	AIDS	acquired immunodeficiency
	Alpers-Huttenlocher syndrome		syndrome
	anticonvulsant hypersensitivity	AIE	acute inclusion body encephalitis
	syndrome	AIED	autoimmune inner-ear Disease
AHSA	Assistant Health Services	AIEOP	Italian Association of Pediatric
	Administrator		Hematology and Oncology (cancer
AHSCT	autologous hemopoietic stem-cell		study group)
	transplantation	AIF	aortic-iliac-femoral

AIGHL anterior band of the inferior glenohumeral ligament
AIH artificial insemination with husband's sperm
autoimmune hepatitis
AIHA autoimmune hemolytic anemia
AIHD acquired immune hemolytic disease
AIIS anterior inferior iliac spine
AILD angioimmunoblastic lymphadenopathy with dysproteinemia
AILT angioimmunoblastic T-cell lymphoma
AIM anti-inflammatory medication
AIMS Abnormal Involuntary Movement Scale
Arthritis Impact Measurement Scales
AIN acute interstitial nephritis
anal intraepithelial neoplasia
anterior interosseous nerve
AINS anti-inflammatory non-steroidal
AIO all-in-one (lipid emulsion, protein, carbohydrate, and electrolytes combined total parenteral nutrition)
AIOD aortoiliac occlusive disease
AION anterior ischemic optic neuropathy
AIP acute infectious polyneuritis
acute intermittent porphyria
acute interstitial pneumonia
asymptomatic inflammatory prostatitis
autoimmune pancreatitis
AIPC androgen-independent prostate cancer
AIR accelerated idioventricular rhythm
acetylcholine-induced relaxation
acute insulin response
AIRE autoimmune regulator (gene)
AIRR acute infusion-related reaction
AIS Abbreviated Injury Score
acute ischemic stroke
adolescent idiopathic scoliosis
anti-insulin serum
AISA acquired idiopathic sideroblastic anemia
AIS/ISS Abbreviated Injury Scale/ Injury Severity Score
AIT adoptive immunotherapy
Advanced Individual Training (Army)
auditory integration therapy
AITD autoimmune thyroiditis
AITN acute interstitial tubular nephritis
AITP autoimmune thrombocytopenia purpura

AIU absolute iodine uptake
adolescent inpatient unit
AIVC absence of the inferior vena cava
AIVR accelerated idioventricular rhythm
AJ ankle jerk
AJCC American Joint Committee on Cancer
AJO apple juice only
AJR abnormal jugular reflex
AK above-knee (amputation)
actinic keratosis
artificial kidney
AKA above-knee amputation
alcoholic ketoacidosis
all known allergies
also known as
a.k.a. also known as
AKP anterior knee pain
AKS alcoholic Korsakoff syndrome
arthroscopic knee surgery
AKU artificial kidney unit
AL acute leukemia
argon laser
artemether-lumefantrine (antimalarial drug combination [Riamet; Coartem])
arterial line
assisted living
attachment level (dental)
axial length
left ear
Al aluminum
ALA adrenalin (epinephrine), lidocaine, and amethocaine (tetracaine)
alpha-linolenic acid (α-linolenic acid)
alpha-lipoic acid
amebic liver abscess
aminolevulinic acid (Levulan)
antileukotriene agent
antilymphocyte antibody
as long as
ALAC antibiotic-loaded acrylic cement
ALAD abnormal left axis deviation
ALA-GLN alanyl-glutamine
ALARA as low as reasonably achievable
ALAT alanine aminotransferase (also ALT; SGPT)
ALAX apical long axis
ALB albumin
albuterol
anterior lenticular bevel
ALBUMS aldehyde linker-based ultrasensitive mismatch scanning
ALC acute lethal catatonia
alcohol
alcoholic liver cirrhosis
allogeneic lymphocyte cytotoxicity

35

	alternate level of care	ALP	alkaline phosphatase
	Alternate Lifestyle Checklist		argon laser photocoagulation
	axiolinguocervical		Alupent
ALCA	anomalous left coronary artery	ALPS	autoimmune lymphoproliferative
ALCL	anaplastic large-cell lymphoma		syndrome
ALC R	alcohol rub	ALPSA	anterior labroligamentous periosteal
ALD	adrenoleukodystrophy		sleeve avulsion
	alcoholic liver disease	ALPZ	alprazolam (Xanax)
	aldolase	ALR	adductor leg raise
ALDH	aldehyde dehydrogenase	ALRI	acute lower-respiratory-tract
ALDO	aldosterone		infection
ALDOST	aldosterone		anterolateral rotary instability
ALF	acute liver failure	ALS	acid-labile subunit
	arterial line filter		acute lateral sclerosis
	assisted living facility		advanced life support
ALFT	abnormal liver function tests		amyotrophic lateral sclerosis
ALG	antilymphoblast globulin		antilymphocyte serum
	antilymphocyte globulin	ALSG	Australian Leukemia Study Group
ALGB	adjustable laparoscopic gastric	ALT	alanine aminotransferase(SGPT)
	banding		antibiotic lock technique
ALH	atypical lobular hyperplasia		(catheter infection prevention)
ALI	Abbott Laboratories, Inc.		argon laser trabeculoplasty
	acute lung injury		autolymphocyte therapy
	argon laser iridotomy	2 *alt*	every other day (this is a dangerous
ALIF	anterior lumbar interbody fusion		abbreviation)
A-line	arterial catheter	ALTB	acute laryngotracheobronchitis
ALJ	administrative law judge	ALTE	acute (aberrant, apparent) life
ALK	alkaline		threatening event
	automated lamellar keratoplasy	ALTF	anterolateral thigh flap
ALK Ø	alkaline phosphatase	*alt hor*	every other hour (this is a dangerous
ALK ISO	alkaline phosphatase isoenzymes		abbreviation)
ALK-P	alkaline phosphatase	ALTP	argon laser trabeculoplasty
ALK PHOS	alkaline phosphatase isoenzyme	ALUP	Alupent
ISO		ALv	attachment level (dental)
ALL	acute lymphoblastic leukemia	ALVAD	abdominal left ventricular assist
	acute lymphocytic leukemia		device
	allergy	ALWMI	anterolateral wall myocardial
ALLD	arthroscopic lumbar laser diskectomy		infarct
ALLO	allogeneic	ALZ	Alzheimer disease
Allo-BMT	allogeneic bone marrow	AM	adult male
	transplantation		aerosol mask
Allo-HCT	allogenic hematopoietic cell		amalgam
	transplant		anovulatory menstruation
ALM	acral lentiginous melanoma		anterior midpapillary
	alveolar lining material		morning (a.m.)
	autoclave-killed *Leishmania*		myopic astigmatism
	major	AMA	advanced maternal age
ALMI	anterolateral myocardial infarction		against medical advice
ALN	anterior lower neck		American Medical Association
	anterior lymph node		antimitochondrial antibody
	axillary lymph nodes	AMAC	adults molested as children
ALND	axillary lymph node dissection	AMAD	activity median aerodynamic
ALNM	axillary lymph node metastasis		diameter
ALO	apraxia of eyelid opening	AMBI	acute multiple brain infarcts
	axilinguo-occlusal	AM Care	brushing teeth, washing
ALOC	altered level of consciousness		face and hands
Al(OH)₃	aluminum hydroxide	AMAD	morning admission
ALOS	average length of stay	AM/ADM	morning admission

AMAG	adrenal medullary autograft
AMAL	amalgam
AMAN	acute motor axonal neuropathy
AMAP	American Medical Accreditation Program
	as much as possible
Amask	aerosol mask
AMAT	anti-malignant antibody test
	Arm Motor Ability Test
A-MAT	amorphous material
AMB	ambulate
	ambulatory
	amphotericin B (Fungizone)
	as manifested by
AMBER	advanced multiple beam equalization radiography
AMC	arm muscle circumference
	arthrogryposis multiplex congenita
AM/CR	amylase to creatinine ratio
AMD	age-related macular degeneration
	arthroscopic microdiskectomy
	axiomesiodistal
	dactinomycin (actinomycin D; Cosmegen)
	methyldopa (alpha methyldopa)
AMDR	acceptable macronutrient distribution range
AME	agreed medical examination
	anthrax meningoencephalitis
	apparent mineralocorticoid excess (syndrome)
	Aviation Medical Examiner
AMegL	acute megokaryoblastic leukemia
AMES-LAN	American sign language
AMF	aerobic metabolism facilitator
	amifostine (Ethyol)
	autocrine motility factor
AMG	acoustic myography
	aminoglycoside
	axiomesiogingival
	Federal Republic of Germany's equivalent to United States Food, Drug, and Cosmetic Act
AMGA	American Medical Group Association
AMI	acute myocardial infarction
	amifostine (Ethyol)
	amitriptyline
	axiomesioincisal
AMKL	acute megakaryocytic leukemia
AML	acute myelogenous leukemia
	angiomyolipoma
	anterior mitral leaflet
AMLOS	arithmetic mean length of stay
AMLR	auditory midlatency response
	Marketing Authorization Application (French)

AMM	agnogenic myeloid metaplasia
AMML	acute myelomonocytic leukemia
AMMOL	acute myelomonoblastic leukemia
AMN	adrenomyeloneuropathy
amnio	amniocentesis
AMN SC	amniotic fluid scan
AMOL	acute monoblastic leukemia
AMOVA	analysis of molecular variance
AMP	adenosine monophosphate
	ampere
	ampicillin
	ampul
	amputation
	antipressure mattress
AMPLE	allergies, medications, past medical history, last meal, events leading to admission (used for history and physical examination)
AMPPE	acute multifocal placoid pigment epitheliopathy
A-M pr	Austin-Moore prosthesis
AMPS	Assessment of Motor and Process Skills
AMPT	metyrosine (alphamethylpara tyrosine)
AMR	acoustic muscle reflex
	alternating motion rates
	amrubicin
AMRI	anterior medial rotary instability
AMS	accelerator mass spectrometry
	acute maxillary sinusitis
	acute mountain sickness
	aggravated in military service
	altered mental status
	amylase
	aseptic meningitis syndrome
	atypical mole syndrome
	auditory memory span
m-AMSA	amsacrine (acridinyl anisidide)
AMSAN	acute motor sensory axonal neuropathy
AMSIT	portion of the mental status examination: A—appearance, M—mood, S—sensorium, I—intelligence, T—thought process
AMT	abbreviated mental test
	Adolph's Meat Tenderizer
	allogeneic (bone) marrow transplant
	alpha-methyltryptamine
	aminopterin
	amniotic membrane transplantation
	amount
AMTS	Abbreviated Mental Test Score
AMU	accessory-muscle use
AMV	alveolar minute ventilation

	assisted mechanical ventilation	ANT	anterior
AMY	amylase		anthrax vaccine, not otherwise specified
AMY/CR	amylase/creatinine ratio		
AN	acoustic neuromas		enpheptin (2-amino-5-nitrothiazol)
	Alaska Native	ANT_a	anthrax vaccine, absorbed
	amyl nitrate	*ante*	before
	anorexia nervosa	ANTI	anti–blood group A antiglobulin test
	anticipatory nausea	A:AGT	
	Associate Nurse	Anti bx	antibiotic
	avascular necrosis	anti-D	anti-D immune globulin
ANA	American Nurses Association	anti-GAD	antibodies to glutamic acid decarboxylase
	antinuclear antibody		
ANAD	anorexia nervosa and associated disorders	anti-HBc	antibody to hepatitis B core antigen (HBcAg)
ANADA	Abbreviated New Animal Drug Application	anti-HBe	antibody to hepatitis B e antigen (HBeAg)
ANAG	acute narrow angle glaucoma	anti-HBs	antibody to hepatitis B surface antigen (HBsAg)
ANA SWAB	anaerobic swab		
		ant sag D	anterior sagittal diameter
ANC	absolute neutrophil count	ANTU	alpha naphthylthiourea
ANCA	antineutrophil cytoplasmic antibody	ANUG	acute necrotizing ulcerative gingivitis
anch	anchored		
ANCN	absolute neutrophil count nadir	ANV	acute nausea and vomiting
ANCOVA	analysis of covariance	ANX	anxiety
AND	anterior nasal discharge		anxious
	Associate's Degree in Nursing	ANZDATA	Australia and New Zealand Dialysis and Transplant Registry
	axillary node dissection		
ANDA	Abbreviated New Drug Application		
anes	anesthesia	AO	abdominal obesity
ANF	antinuclear factor		acridine orange (stain)
	atrial natriuretic factor		Agent Orange
ANG	angiogram		anaplastic oligodendrogliomas
ANG II	angiotensin II		anterior oblique
ANGIO	angiogram		aorta
ANH	acute normovolemic hemodilution		aortic opening
	artificial nutrition and hydration		aortography
	assisted nutrition and hydration		axio-occlusal
ANISO	anisocytosis		plate, screw (orthopedics)
ANK	ankle		right ear
	appointment not kept	A-O	atlanto-occipital (joint)
ANLL	acute nonlymphoblastic leukemia	A/O	alert and oriented
ANM	Assistant Nurse Manager	A & O	alert and oriented
ANN	artificial neural network(s)	A&O × 3	awake and oriented to person, place, and time
	axillary node-negative		
ANNA	artificial neural network analysis	A&O × 4	awake and oriented to person, place, time, and object
ANOVA	analysis of variance		
ANP	Adult Nurse Practitioner	AOA	anaplastic oligoastrocytoma
	atrial natriuretic peptide (anaritide acetate)	AOAA	aminooxoacetic acid
		AOAP	as often as possible
	axillary node–positive	AOAs	adult offspring of alcoholics
ANPR	advanced notice of proposed rule making	AOB	alcohol on breath
		AOBC	aortic occlusion balloon catheter
ANS	answer	AOBS	acute organic brain syndrome
	autonomic nervous system	AOC	abridged ocular chart
ANSER	Aggregate Neurobehavioral Student Health and Education Review		advanced ovarian cancer
			amoxicillin, omeprazole, and clarithromycin
ANSI	American National Standards Institute		anode opening contraction

	antacid of choice
	area of concern
AOCD	anemia of chronic disease
AOCL	anodal opening clonus
AOCN	Advanced Oncology Certified Nurse
AOD	adult-onset diabetes
	alcohol and (and/or) other drugs
	alleged onset date
	anaplastic oligodendroglioma
	arterial occlusive disease
	Assistant-Officer-of-the-Day
AODA	alcohol and other drug abuse
AODM	adult-onset diabetes mellitus
AOE	acute otitis externa
A of 1	assistance of one
A of 2	assistance of two
AOI	area of induration
ao-il	aorta-iliac
AOIVM	angiographically occult intracranial vascular malformation
AOL	augmentation of labor
AOLC	acridine-orange leukocyte cytospin
AOLD	automated open lumbar diskectomy
AOM	acute otitis media
	alternatives of management
AONAD	alert, oriented, and no acute distress
AOO	anodal opening odor
	continuous arterial asynchronous pacing
AOP	anemia of prematurity
	anodal opening picture
	aortic pressure
	apnea of prematurity
AOR	adjusted odds ratio
	Alvarado Orthopedic Research
	at own risk
	auditory oculogyric reflex
AORT REGURG	aortic regurgitation
AORT STEN	aortic stenosis
AOS	ambulatory outpatient surgery
	anode opening sound
	antibiotic order sheet
	aortic ostial stenoses
	arrived on scene
AOSC	acute obstructive suppurative cholangiotomy
AOSD	adult-onset Still disease
AOTB	alcohol on the breath
AOTe	anodal opening tetanus
AP	abdominal pain
	abdominoperineal
	acute pancreatitis
	aerosol pentamidine
	alkaline phosphatase
	angina pectoris
	antepartum

	anterior-posterior (x-ray)
	apical periodontitis
	apical pulse
	appendectomy
	appendicitis
	arterial pressure
	arthritis panel (see page 298)
	atrial pacing
	attending physician
	doxorubicin (Adriamycin); cisplatin (Platinol)
A&P	active and present
	anterior and posterior
	assessment and plans
	auscultation and percussion
A/P	accounts payable
	ascites/plasma ratio
$A_2 > P_2$	second aortic sound greater than second pulmonic sound
APA	aldosterone-producing adenoma
	American Psychiatric Association
	anticipatory postural adjustment
	antiphospholipid antibody
APAA	anterior parietal artery aneurysm
APAC	acute primary angle closure
APACHE	Acute Physiology and Chronic Health Evaluation
APAD	anterior-posterior abdominal diameter
APAG	antipseudomonal aminoglycosidic
APAP	acetaminophen (N acetylpara-aminophenol; Tylenol; paracetamol)
APB	abductor pollicis brevis
	atrial premature beat
APBI	accelerated partial breast irradiation
APBSCT	autologous peripheral blood stem cell transplantation
APC	absolute phagocyte count
	activated protein C
	acute pharyngoconjunctiivitis (fever)
	adenoidal-pharyngeal-conjunctival
	adenomatous polyposis of the colon and rectum
	advanced pancreatic cancer
	advanced prostate cancer
	Ambulatory Payment Classification
	antigen-presenting cell
	argon plasma coagulator
	aspirin, phenacetin, and caffeine (no longer marketed in the US)
	asymptomatic prostate cancer
	atrial premature contraction
	autologous packed cells
APCD	adult polycystic disease
APCE	affinity probe capillary electrophoresis
APCIs	atrial peptide clearance inhibitors

APCKD	adult polycystic kidney disease
AP-CT	abdominal and pelvic computer tomography
APD	acid peptic disease
	action potential duration
	afferent pupillary defect
	anterior-posterior diameter
	atrial premature depolarization
	automated peritoneal dialysis
	pamidronate disodium (aminohydroxypropylidene diphosphate)
APDC	Anxiety and Panic Disorder Clinic
AP-DRGs	all-patient diagnosis-related groups
APDT	acellular pertussis vaccine with diphtheria and tetanus toxoids
APE	absolute prediction error
	acute psychotic episode
	acute pulmonary edema
	anterior pituitary extract
	doxorubicin (Adriamycin), cisplatin (Platinol-AQ), and etoposide
APECED	autoimmune polyendocrinopathy-candidiasis ectodermal dystrophy
APER	abdominoperineal excision of the rectum
APG	ambulatory patient group
	Apgar (score)
Apgar	appearance (color), pulse (heart rate), grimace (reflex irritability), activity (muscle tone), and respiration (score reflecting condition of newborn)
APH	adult psychiatric hospital
	alcohol-positive history
	antepartum hemorrhage
APhA	American Pharmacists Association
APHIS	Animal and Plant Health Inspection Service
API	active pharmaceutical ingredients
	Asian-Pacific Islander
APIS	Acute Pain Intensity Scale
APIVR	artificial pacemaker-induced ventricular rhythm
APKD	adult polycystic kidney disease
	adult-onset polycystic kidney disease
APL	abductor pollicis longus
	accelerated painless labor
	acute promyelocytic leukemia
	anterior pituitary-like (hormone)
	chorionic gonadotropin
AP & L	anteroposterior and lateral
APLA	antiphospholipid antibody
APLD	automated percutaneous lumbar diskectomy
APLS	antiphospholipid syndrome
APME	acute postinfectious measles encephalitis

APMPPE	acute posterior multifocal placoid pigment epitheliopathy
APMS	acute pain management service
APN	acquired pendular nystagmus
	acute panautonomic neuropathy
	acute pyelonephritis
	Advanced Practice Nurse
APO	adverse patient occurrence
	apolipoprotein A-1
	doxorubicin (Adriamycin), prednisone, and vincristine (Oncovin)
APO(a)	apolipoprotein (A)
APOE	apolipoprotein E
APOE-4	apolipoprotein-E (gene)
APOLT	auxiliary partial orthotopic liver transplantation
APOPPS	adjustable postoperative protective prosthetic socket
APP	alternating pressure pad
	amyloid precursor protein
	appetite
APPG	aqueous procaine penicillin G (dangerous terminology; since it is for intramuscular use only; write as penicillin G procaine)
appr.	approximate
appt.	appointment
APPY	appendectomy
APR	abdominoperineal resection
	acute radiation proctitis
	average payment rate
AP & R	apical and radial (pulses)
APR-DRGs	all-patient refined diagnosis-related groups
APRT	abdominopelvic radiotherapy
APRV	airway pressure release ventilation
APS	acute pain service
	Acute Physiology Scoring (system)
	adult protective services
	Adult Psychiatric Service
	antiphospholipid syndrome
APSAC	anistreplase (anisoylated plasminogen streptokinase activator complex)
APSD	Alzheimer presenile dementia
APSP	assisted peak systolic pressure
APSS	Associated Professional Sleep Societies
aPTT	activated partial thromboplastin time
APU	ambulatory procedure unit
	antepartum unit
APUD	amine precursor uptake and decarboxylation
APV	amprenavir (Agenerase)
APVC	partial anomalous pulmonary venous connection
APVR	aortic pulmonary valve replacement

APW	aortopulmonary window	ARDMS	American Registry of Diagnostic Medical Sonographers
AQ	amodiaquine		
aq	water	ARDS	adult respiratory distress syndrome
AQ	accomplishment quotient	ARE	active-resistive exercises
aq dest	distilled water	ARF	acute renal failure
AQLQ-J	Asthma Quality of Life Questionnaire—Juniper		acute respiratory failure
			acute rheumatic fever
AQLQ-M	Asthma Quality of Life Questionnaire—Marks		amylase-rich food (flour)
		ARFF	at risk for falling
AQOL	acne quality of life	ARG	alkaline reflux gastritis
A quad	atrial quadrageminy		arginine
AR	Achilles reflex	ARGNB	antibiotic-resistant gram-negative bacilli
	acoustic reflex		
	active resistance	ARH	autosomal recessive hypercholesterolemia
	airway resistance		
	alcohol related	ARHL	age-related hearing loss
	allergic rhinitis	ARHNC	advanced resected head and neck cancer
	androgen receptor		
	ankle reflex	ARI	acute renal insufficiency
	aortic regurgitation		acute respiratory infection
	apoptotic rate		aldose reductase inhibitor
	Argyll Robertson (pupil)		arousal index
	assisted respiration	ARIF	arthroscopic reduction and internal fixation
	at risk		
	aural rehabilitation	ARIMA	autoregressive integrated moving average (model)
	autorefractor		
Ar	argon	ARJP	autosomal recessive juvenile parkinsonism
A&R	adenoidectomy with radium		
	advised and released	ARL	acquired immunodeficiency syndrome (AIDS)-related lymphoma
A-R	apical-radial (pulses)		
A/R	accounts receivable		average remaining lifetime
ARA	Action Research Arm (test)	ARLD	alcohol-related liver disease
	adenosine regulating agent	ARM	anxiety reaction, mild
ara-A	vidarabine (Vira-A)		artificial rupture of membranes
ara-AC	fazarabine	ARMD	age-related macular degeneration
ara-C	cytarabine (Cytosar-U)	ARMS	alveolar rhabdomyosarcoma
ARAD	abnormal right axis deviation		amplification refractory mutation system
ARAS	ascending reticular activating system		
	atherosclerotic renal-artery stenosis	ARN	acute retinal necrosis
ARB	angiotensin II receptor blocker	ARND	alcohol-related neurodevelopmental disorder
	antibiotic-resistant bacteria		
	any reliable brand	ARNP	Advanced Registered Nurse Practitioner
ARBOR	arthropod-borne virus		
ARBOW	artificial rupture of bag of water	AROM	active range of motion
ARC	abnormal retinal correspondence		artifical rupture of membranes
	adult residential care	ARP	absolute refractory period
	AIDS-related complex		acute radiation proctitis
	Alcohol Rehabilitation Center		alcohol rehabilitation program
	anomalous retinal correspondence	ARPE	amylase-rich pleural effusion
	American Red Cross	ARPF	anterior release posterior fusion
	autologous red cells	ARPKS	autosomal recessive polycystic kidney disease
ARCBS	American Red Cross Blood Services		
		ARPN	Advanced Practice Registered Nurse
ARD	acute respiratory disease	ARPT	acid reflux provocation test
	adult respiratory distress	ARR	absolute risk reduction
	antibiotic removal device		anterior rectal resection
	antibiotic retrieval device		arrive
	aphakic retinal detachment	aRR	adjusted rate ratio

ARROM	active resistive range of motion	ASA II	A patient with mild to moderate systemic disease
ARRT	American Registry of Radiologic Technologists	ASA III	A patient with severe systemic disease limiting activity but not incapacitating
ARS	antirabies serum		
ART	Accredited Record Technician (for newer title, see RHIT)	ASA IV	A patient with incapacitating systemic disease
	Achilles (tendon) reflex test		
	acoustic reflex threshold(s)	ASA V	Moribund patient not expected to live.
	antiretroviral therapy		
	arterial		(These are American Society of Anesthesiologists' patient classifications. Emergency operations are designated by "E" after the classification.)
	assessment, review, and treatment		
	assisted reproductive technology		
	automated reagin test (for syphilis)		
ARTIC	articulation		
Art T	art therapy	5-ASA	mesalamine (5-aminosalicylic acid; Asacol; Rowasa) (this is a dangerous abbreviation as it is mistaken for five aspirin tablets)
ARU	acute receiving unit		
	alcohol rehabilitation unit		
ARV	AIDS-related virus		
	antiretroviral	ASAA	acquired severe aplastic anemia
ARVC	arrhythmogenic right ventricular cardiomyopathy	ASACL	American Society of Anesthesiologists Classification (see ASA I)
ARVD	arrhythmogenic right ventricular dysplasia		
		ASAD	arthroscopic subacromial decompression
	atherosclerotic renovascular disease		
ARVMB	anomalous right ventricular muscle bundles	AS/AI	aortic stenosis/aortic insufficiency
		A's & B's	apnea and bradycardia
ARVs	antiretroviral drugs	ASAM	Patient Placement Criteria published by the American Society of Addiction Medicine, Second Edition
ARW	Accredited Rehabilitation Worker	PPC-2	
ARWY	airway		
AS	activated sleep		
	alpha-synuclein	ASAP	Alcohol and Substance Abuse Program
	American Samoa		
	anabolic steroid		as soon as possible
	anal sphincter	ASAT	aspartate aminotransferase (also AST; SGOT)
	androgen suppression		
	Angelman syndromes	ASB	anesthesia standby
	ankylosing spondylitis		asymptomatic bacteriuria
	anterior synechia	ASBO	adhesive small-bowel obstruction
	anxiety sensitivity	ASBS	American Society of Bariatric Surgery
	aortic stenosis		
	artesunate (an antimalarial agent)	ASBs	artificially sweetened beverages
	Asperger syndrome	ASC	altered state of consciousness
	atherosclerosis		ambulatory surgery (surgical) center
	atropine sulfate		anterior subcapsular cataract
	AutoSuture®		antimony sulfur colloid
	doctor called through answering service		apocrine skin carcinoma
			ascorbic acid (vitamin C)
	left ear	ASCA	antisaccharomyces cerevisiae
ASA	American Society of Anesthesiologists	ASCAD	atherosclerotic coronary artery disease
	American Statistical Association		
	argininosuccinate	ASCCC	advanced squamous cell cervical carcinoma
	aspirin (acetylsalicylic acid)		
	as soon as	ASCCHN	advanced squamous cell carcinoma of the head and neck
	atrial septal aneurysm		
ASA I	**American Society of anesthesiologists' classification**	ASCI	acute spinal cord injury
		ASCO	American Society of Clinical Oncology
	Healthy patient with localized pathological process	ASCR	autologous stem cell rescue

ASCS	autologous stem cell support
ASCT	allogeneic stem cell transplantation
	autologous stem cell transplantation
ASCUS	atypical squamous cell of undetermined significance
ASCVD	arteriosclerotic cardiovascular disease
ASCVR	arteriosclerotic cardiovascular renal disease
ASD	air-space disease
	aldosterone secretion defect
	androstenedione
	annual summary dose (ionizing radiation)
	atrial septal defect
	autism spectrum disorder(s)
ASD I	atrial septal defect, primum
ASD II	atrial septal defect, secundum
ASDA	American Sleep Disorders Association (criteria)
ASDH	acute subdural hematoma
ASDPs	antisocial personality disorders
ASE	abstinence symptom evaluation
	acute stress erosion
ASEX	Arizona Sexual Experiences (sexual dysfunction scale)
ASF	anterior spinal fusion
	asymmetric screen film (radiology)
ASFR	age-specific fertility rate
ASG	atrial septal graft
ASH	American Society of Hematology (guidelines)
	asymmetric septal hypertrophy
AsH	hypermetropic astigmatism
ASHD	arteriosclerotic heart disease
ASI	active specific immunotherapy
	Anxiety Status Inventory
	Arterial Stiffness Index
aSi	amorphous silicon
ASIA	**American Spinal Injury Association (Score)**
	A-Complete—No preservation of any motor and/or sensory function below the zone of injury
	B-Incomplete—Preserved sensation
	C-Incomplete—Preserved motor (nonfunctional)
	D-Incomplete—Preserved motor (functional)
	E-Complete Recovery
ASIH	absent, sick in hospital
ASIMC	absent, sick in medical center
ASIS	anterior superior iliac spine
ASK	antistreptokinase
ASKase	antistreptokinase
ASL	American Sign Language
	antistreptolysin (titer)

ASLO	antistreptolysin-O
ASLV	avian sarcoma and leukosis virus (Rous virus)
AsM	myopic astigmatism
ASMA	antismooth-muscle antibody
ASMI	anteroseptal myocardial infarction
ASN	Associate's of Science in Nursing
ASO	accessory sinus ostia
	administrative services only (contract)
	AIDS (acquired immunodeficiency syndrome) service organization(s)
	aldicarb sulfoxide
	allele-specific oligodeoxy-nucleotide (probes)
	Amplatzer Septal Occluder
	antisense oligonucleotides
	antistreptolysin-O titer
	arterial switch operation
	arteriosclerosis obliterans
	automatic stop order
As_2O_3	arsenic trioxide (Trisenox)
ASOT	antistreptolysin-O titer
ASOTP	Affiliate Sex Offender Treatment Provider
ASP	acute suppurative parotitis
	acute symmetric polyarthritis
	antisocial personality
	application service provider
	asparaginase
	aspartic acid
ASPDV	anterior superior pancreaticoduodenal vein
ASPVD	arteriosclerotic peripheral vascular disease
ASR	aldosterone secretion rate
	automatic speech recognition
ASRA	Alcohol Severity Rating Scale
ASS	anterior superior supine
	aspirin (some European countries)
	assessment
ASST	autologous serum skin test
asst	assistant
AST	allergy skin test
	Aphasia Screening Test
	aspartate aminotransferase (SGOT)
	astemizole (Hismanal)
	astigmatism
AstdVe	assisted ventilation
ASTH	asthenopia
ASTI	acute soft tissue injury
AS TOL	as tolerated
ASTIG	astigmatism
ASTM	American Society for Testing and Materials
ASTRO	American Society for Therapeutic Radiation and Oncology
	astrocytoma

ASTZ	antistreptozyme test		anterior temporal lobectomy
ASU	acute stroke unit		anterior tricuspid leaflet
	ambulatory surgical unit		antitension line
ASV	antisnake venom		atypical lymphocytes
ASVD	arteriosclerotic vessel disease	ATLL	adult T-cell leukemia lymphoma
ASYM	asymmetric(al)	ATLP	anterior thoracolumbar locking (implant) plate
ASX	asymptomatic		
AT	abdominothoracic	ATLS	acute tumor lysis syndrome
	activity therapy (therapist)		advanced trauma life support
	Addiction Therapist	ATM	acute transverse myelitis
	anaerobic threshold		ataxia telangiectasia mutated (gene)
	antithrombin		atmosphere
	applanation tonometry	At ma	atrial milliamp
	ataxia-telangiectasia	ATN	acute tubular necrosis
	atraumatic	ATNC	atraumatic normocephalic
	atrial tachycardia	aTNM	autopsy staging of cancer
AT1	angiotensin II type 1	ATNR	asymmetrical tonic neck reflex
AT 10	dihydrotachysterol (Hytakerol; DHT®)	ATO	arsenic trioxide (Trisenox)
		ATOD-C	Alcohol, Tobacco and Drugs, Certified
ATA	atmosphere absolute		
	authority to administer	ATP	according-to-protocol
ATB	antibiotic		addiction treatment program
	aquatic therapy bar		adenosine triphosphate
	atypical tuberculosis		anterior tonsillar pillar
ATBF	African tick-bite fever		autoimmune thrombocytopenia purpura
ATC	acute toxic class		
	aerosol treatment chamber	ATP III	Adult Treatment Panel III
	alcoholism therapy classes	ATPase	adenosine triphosphatase
	all-terrain cycle	ATPS	ambient temperature & pressure, saturated with water vapor
	antituberculous chemoprophylaxis		
	around-the-clock	ATR	Achilles tendon reflex
	Arthritis Treatment Center		atracurium (Tracrium)
	Athletic Trainer, Certified		atrial
ATCC	American Type Culture Collection		atropine
ATCCS	acute traumatic central cord syndrome	ATRA	all-*trans* retinoic acid (tretinoin-Vesanoid)
ATD	antithyroid drug(s)	atr fib	atrial fibrillation
	anticipated time of discharge	ATRO	atropine
	aqueous tear deficiency	ATRX	acute transfusion reaction
	asphyxiating thoracic dystrophy	ATU	alcohol treatment unit
	autoimmune thyroid disease	ATUE	abbreviated therapeutic use exemption
ATE	adipose tissue extraction		
AT-EI	assistive technology and environmental interventions	ATV	all-terrain vehicle
		ATS	American Thoracic Society (guidelines)
ATEM	analytical transmission electron microscopy		antimony trisulfide
ATEs	arterial thromboembolic events		antitetanic serum (tetanus antitoxin)
ATF	Alcohol, Tobacco, and Firearms (Bureau)		anxiety tension state
At Fib	atrial fibrillation	ATSO	admit to (the) service of
ATFL	anterior talofibular ligament	ATSO4	atropine sulfate
AT III FUN	antithrombin III functional	ATSP	asked to see patient
ATG	antithymocyte globulin	ATT	alternating triple therapy
ATHR	angina threshold heart rate		antitetanus toxoid
ATI	Abdominal Trauma Index		arginine tolerance test
	acute traumatic ischemia	ATTN	attention
ATL	Achilles tendon lengthening	ATTR	amyloid transtyretin
	adult T-cell leukemia	at. wt	atomic weight
		ATX	atelectasis

ATZ	anal transitional zone
AU	allergenic (allergy) units
	arbitrary units
	both ears (this is a dangerous abbreviation, as it may be seen as OU [both eyes])
Au	gold
A/U	at umbilicus
198Au	radioactive gold
AUA score	American Urological Association—pertains to benign prostatic hypertrophy symptoms
AUB	abnormal uterine bleeding
AuBMT	autologous bone marrow transplant
AUC	area under the curve
AUC$_t$	area under the curve to last time point
AUD	amplifiable units of DNA (deoxyribonucleic acid)
	arthritis of unknown diagnosis
	auditory
AUD COMP	auditory comprehension
AUDIT	Alcohol Use Disorders Identification Test
AUG	acute ulcerative gingivitis
AUGIB	acute upper gastrointestinal bleeding
AUIC	area under the inhibitory curve
AUL	acute undifferentiated leukemia
AUR	acute urinary retention
AUS	acute urethral syndrome
	artificial urinary sphincter
	auscultation
AutD	autistic disorder
AUTO	autologous
AUTO SP	automatic speech
AV	anteverted
	anticipatory vomiting
	arteriovenous
	atrioventricular
	auditory visual
	auriculoventricular
A:V	arterial-venous (ratio in fundi)
AVA	anthrax vaccine, adsorbed
	aortic valve atresia
	arteriovenous anastomosis
AVB	atrioventricular block
	Aventis Behring
AVC	acrylic veneer crown
	aortic valve classification
	atrioventricular conduction
AVD	aortic valve disease
	apparent volume of distribution
	arteriosclerotic vascular disease
	atrioventricular delay
	cerebrovascular accident (French, Spanish)

AVDP	asparaginase, vincristine, daunorubicin, and prednisone
	avoirdupois
AVDO$_2$	arteriovenous oxygen difference
AVE	aortic valve echocardiogram
	atrioventricular extrasystole
AVED	ataxia with isolated vitamin E deficiency
AVF	arteriovenous fistula
	augmented unipolar foot (left leg)
avg	average
AVGS	autologous vein graft stent
AVGs	ambulatory visit groups
AVH	acute viral hepatitis
AVHB	atrioventricular heart block
AVJA	atrioventricular junction ablation
AVJR	atrioventricular junctional rhythm
AVL	American visceral leishmaniasis
	augmented unipolar left (left arm)
AVLT	auditory verbal learning test
AVM	arteriovenous malformation
AVN	arteriovenous nicking
	atrioventricular node
	avascular necrosis
AVNB	atrioventricular nodal block
AVNR	atrioventricular nodal re-entry
AVNRT	atrioventricular node recovery time
	atrioventricular nodal re-entry tachycardia
A-VO$_2$	arteriovenous oxygen difference
AVOC	avocation
AVP	arginine vasopressin
	Aventis Pasteur
AVPU	alert, (responds to) verbal (stimuli), (responds to) painful (stimuli), unresponsive (mnemonic used by EMTs to judge patients' level of consciousness)
AVR	aortic valve replacement
	augmented unipolar right (right arm)
AVRP	atrioventricular refractory period
AVRT	atrioventricular reciprocating tachycardia
AVS	aortic valve sclerosis
	atriovenous shunt
AVSD	atrioventricular septal defect
AVSS	afebrile, vital signs stable
AVT	atrioventricular tachycardia
	atypical ventricular tachycardia
AvWS	acquired von Willebrand syndrome
AW	abdominal wall
	abnormal wave
	airway
A/W	able to work
A&W	alive and well
AWA	alcohol withdrawal assessment
	as well as

A waves	atrial contraction wave
AWB	autologous whole blood
AWD	alcohol withdrawal delirium
	alive with disease
AWDW	assault with a deadly weapon
AWE	acetowhite epithelium
AWI	anterior wall infarct
AWMI	anterior wall myocardial infarction
AWO	airway obstruction
AWOL	absent without leave
AWP	airway pressure
	average wholesale price
AWRU	active wrist rotation unit
AWS	alcohol withdrawal seizures
	(syndrome)
AWSA	Alcohol Withdrawal Severity
	Assessment (scale)
AWU	alcohol withdrawal unit
ax	axillary
AXB	axillary block
AXC	aortic cross clamp
ax-fem.fem.	axilla-femoral-femoral (graft)
AXND	axillary node dissection
AXR	abdomen x-ray
AxSYM®	immunodiagnostic testing equipment
AXT	alternating exotropia
AY	acrocyanotic (infant color)
AZA	azathioprine (Imuran)
5 AZA-CdR	5-Aza-2'-deoxycitidine (decitabine; Dacogen)
5-AZC	azacitidine (Vidaza)
AzdU	azidouridine
AZE	azelastine hydrochloride (Astelin)
AZM	acquisition zoom magnification
	azithromycin (Zithromaz; Z-Pak)
AZOOR	acute zonal occult outer retinopathy
AZQ	diaziquone
AZT	zidovudine (azidothymidine; Retrovir)
A-Z test	Aschheim-Zondek test (diagnostic test for pregnancy)

B

B	bacillus
	bands
	bilateral
	black
	bloody
	bolus
	both
	botulism (Vaccine B is botulism toxoid)
	brother
	buccal
	See "Plan B"
Ⓑ	both
B+	blood type B positive (B positive is preferred)
B−	blood type B negative (B negative is preferred)
B₁	thiamine HCl
B I	Billroth I (gastric surgery)
B II	Billroth II (gastric surgery)
B₂	riboflavin
B₃	nicotinic acid
b/4	before
B₅	pantothenic acid
B₆	pyridoxine HCl
B₇	biotin
B₈	adenosine phosphate
B₉	benign
B₁₂	cyanocobalamin
B19	parvovirus B19
BA	backache
	Baker Act (Florida mental health act enabling involuntary commitment)
	Baptist
	benzyl alcohol
	bile acid
	biliary atresia
	bioavailability
	blood agar
	blood alcohol
	bone age
	Bourns assist
	branchial artery
	broken appointment
	bronchial asthma
	buccoaxial
	butyric acid
Ba	barium
B > A	bone greater than air
B < A	bone less than air
B & A	brisk and active
BAA	beta-adrenergic agonist
BAAM	Beck airway airflow monitor

Bab	Babinski
BAC	Bacterial Artficial Chromosome
	benzalkonium chloride
	blood-alcohol concentration
	bronchioloalveolar carcinoma
	buccoaxiocervical
BACCA	basal cell cancer
BACE	beta-site APP (amyloid precursor protein)-cleaving enzyme
BACI	bovine anti-cryptosporidium immunoglobulin
BACM	blocking agent corticosteroid myopathy
BACON	bleomycin, doxorubicin, lomustine, vincristine, and mechlorethamine
BACOP	bleomycin, doxorubicin (Adriamycin), cyclophosphamide, vincristine, and prednisone
BACPAC	Bulk Activities Post Approval Change
BACs	bacterial artificial chromosomes
BACT	bacteria
	base-activated clotting time
BAD	Benadryl, Ativan, and Decadron
	bipolar affective disorder
	blunt aortic disruption
BADL	basic activities of daily living
BADLS	Bristol Activities of Daily Living Scale
BaE	barium enema
BAE	bronchial artery embolization
BAEDP	balloon aortic end diastolic pressure
BAEP	brain stem auditory evoked potential
BAERs	brain stem auditory evoked responses
BaEV	baboon endogenous virus
BAG	buccoaxiogingival
BAHA	bone-anchored hearing aid
BAI	blunt abdominal injury
	breath-actuated inhalers
	Brief Assessment Interview
BAIQ	below average intelligence quotient
BAK cage	an interbody fusion system used to stabilize the spine
BAL	balance
	blood-alcohol level
	British antilewisite (dimercaprol)
	bronchoalveolar lavage
BALB	binaural alternate loudness balance
BALF	bronchoalveolar lavage fluid
B-ALL	B cell acute lymphoblastic leukemia
BALP	baseline bone alkaline phosphatase
BALT	bronchus-associated lymphoid tissue
BAM	bony acetabular morphology
	Brain Acoustic Monitor
BaM	barium meal

BAMS	bioaerosol mass spectrometry
BAN	British Approved Name
BAND	band neutrophil (stab)
BANS	back, arm, neck and scalp
BAO	basal acid output
BAoV	bicuspid aortic valve
BAP	blood agar plate
BAPS	balance activation proprioceptive system
	biomechanical ankle platform system
BAPT	Baptist
baPWV	brachial-ankle pulse wave velocity
BAR	biofragmentable anastomotic ring
Barb	barbiturate
BARN	bilateral acute retinal necrosis
BAR Troche	Benadryl, Ativan, and Reglan troche
BAS	balloon atrial septostomy
	Barnes Akathisia Scale
	behavioral activation system
	bile acid sequestrants
	boric acid solution
	bronchial asthma (in) status
BaS	barium swallow
BASA	baby aspirin (81 mg chewable tablets of aspirin)
BASIS	Basic Achievement Skills Individual Screener
BASK	basket cells
BASMI	Bath Ankylosing Spondylitis Metrology Index
baso.	basophil
BASO STIP	basophilic stippling
BAT	Behavioral Avoidance Test
	best available therapy
	blunt abdominal trauma
	borreliacidal-antibody test
	brightness acuity tester
BATF	Bureau of Alcohol, Tobacco and Firearms
BATO	boronic acid adduct of technetium oxime
batt	battery
BAVP	balloon aortic valvuloplasty
BAU	bioequivalent allergy units
BAV	bicuspid aortic valve
BAW	bronchoalveolar washing
BB	baby boy
	backboard
	back to back
	bad breath
	bed bath
	bed board
	beta-blocker
	blanket bath
	blood bank
	blow bottle

	blue bloaters
	body belts
	both bones
	breakthrough bleeding
	breast biopsy
	bronchial brushing
	brush biopsy
	buffer base
B&B	bismuth and bourbon
	bowel and bladder
B/B	backward bending
BBA	born before arrival
BBAS	blade and balloon atrial septostomy
BBB	baseball bat beating
	blood-brain barrier
	bundle branch block
BBBB	bilateral bundle branch block
BBC	bilateral breast cancer
	Brown-Buerger cystoscope
BBD	baby born dead
	before bronchodilator
	benign breast disease
BBE	biofield breast examination
BBFA	both bones forearm
BBFF	both bone foreman fracture
BBFP	blood and body fluid precautions
BBI	Bowman Birk inhibitor
BBIC	Bowman Birk inhibitor concentrate
BBL	bottle blood loss
BBM	banked breast milk
BBOW	bulging bag of water
BBP	blood-borne pathogen
	butyl benzyl phthalate
BBR	bibasilar rales
BBS	Berg Balance Scale
	bilateral breath sounds
BBSE	bilateral breath sounds equal
BBSI	Brigance Basic Skills Inventory
BBT	basal body temperature
	Buteyko breathing technique
BB to MM	belly button to medial malleolus
B Bx	breast biopsy
BC	back care
	basket catheter
	battered child
	bed and chair
	beta carotene
	bicycle
	birth control
	bladder cancer
	blood culture
	Blue Cross
	bone conduction
	Bourn control
	breast cancer
	buccocervical
	buffalo cap (cap for intravenous line)

B/C	because
	blood urea nitrogen/creatinine ratio
B&C	bed and chair
	biopsy and curettage
	board and care
	breathed and cried
BCA	balloon catheter angioplasty
	basal cell atypia
	bichloracetic acid
	bicinchoninic acid
	brachiocephalic artery
BCAA	branched-chain amino acids
BC < AC	bone conduction less than air conduction
BC > AC	bone conduction greater than air conduction
B. cat	*Branhamella catarrhalis*
B-CAVe	bleomycin, lomustine (CCNU), doxorubicin (Adriamycin), and vinblastine (Velban)
BCB	Brilliant cresyl blue (stain)
BCBR	bilateral carotid body resection
BC/BS	Blue Cross/Blue Shield
BCC	basal cell carcinoma
	birth control clinic
BCCa	basal cell carcinoma
BCD	basal cell dysplasia
	bleomycin, cyclophosphamide, and dactinomycin
	borderline of cardial dullness
BCDCSW	Board Certified Diplomate in Clinical Social Work
BCDH	bilateral congenital dislocated hip
BCE	basal cell epithelioma
	beneficial clinical event
BCEDP	breast cancer early detection program
B cell	B lymphocyte
BCETS	Board Certified Expert in Traumatic Stress
BCF	basic conditioning factor
	Baylor core formula
BCG	bacille Calmette-Guérin vaccine
	bicolor guaiac
BCH	benign cephalic histiocytosis
	benign coital headache
BCHA	bone-conduction hearing aid
BChE	butyrylcholinesterase
BCI	blunt carotid injury
BCIE	bullous congenital ichthyosiform erythroderma
BCIR	Barnett continent intestinal reservoir
BCL	basic cycle length
	bio-chemoluminescence
B/C/L	BUN,(blood urea nitrogen), creatinine, lytes (electrolytes)
B-CLL	B-cell chronic lymphocytic leukemia
BCLP	bilateral cleft lip and palate

BCLS	basic cardiac life support		twice daily (in the United Kingdom, Australia, and elsewhere)
BCM	below costal margin		
	birth control medication	bd	twice daily (in the United Kingdom, Australia, and elsewhere)
	birth control method		
	body cell mass	B-D	Becton Dickinson and Company
BCMA	bar-code medication administration	BDAE	Boston Diagnostic Aphasia Examination
BCME	bis (chloromethyl) ether		
BCNP	Board Certified Nuclear Pharmacist	BDAS	balloon dilation atrial septostomy
BCNU	bacteria-controlled nursing unit	BDBS	Bonnet-Dechaume-Blanc syndrome
	carmustine (BiCNU; Gliadel)	BDC	burn-dressing change
BCOC	bowel care of choice	BDCM	bromodichloromethane
	bowel cathartic of choice	BDD	body dysmorphic disorder
BCP	biochemical profile		bronchodilator drugs
	birth control pills	BDE	bile duct exploration
	blood cell profile	BDF	bilateral distal femoral
	carmustine, cyclophosphamide, and prednisone		black divorced female
		BDI	Beck Depression Inventory
BCPAP	Broun continuous positive airway pressure		bile duct incision
			bile duct injury
BCPNN	Bayesian Confidence Propagation Neural Network	BDI SF	Beck Depression Inventory-Short Form
BCQ	breast central quadrantectomy	BDL	below detectable limits
BCR	bicaudate ratio		bile duct ligation
	breakpoint cluster region (gene)	B-DLCL	diffuse large B-cell lymphoma
	bulbocavernosus reflex	BDM	black divorced male
BCRE	black cohosh root extract	BDNF	brain-derived neurotrophic factor
BCRS	Brief Cognitive Rate Scale	BDOD	brain-dead organ donor
BCRT	breast-conservation followed by radiation therapy	B-DOPA	bleomycin, dacarbazine, vincristine (Oncovin), prednisone, and doxorubicin (Adriamycin)
BCS	battered child syndrome		
	breast-conserving surgery	BDP	beclomethasone dipropionate (Beconase AQ; QVAR)
	Budd-Chiari syndrome		
BCSF	bone cell stimulating factor		best demonstrated practice
BCSS	bone cell stimulating substance	BDR	background diabetic retinopathy
BCT	Bag Carrying Test		black dot ringworm
	breast-conserving therapy		bronchodilator response
	broad complex tachycardias		bulk dose regimen
BCTP	bi-component triton tri-n-butyl phosphate	BDS	bile duct stone(s)
		BDV	Borna disease virus
BCU	burn care unit	BE	bacterial endocarditis
BCUG	bilateral cystourethrogram		barium enema
BCVA	best corrected visual acuity		Barrett esophagus
BCVI	blunt cerebrovascular injury		base excess
BD	band neutrophil		below elbow
	base deficit		bioequivalence
	base down		bread equivalent
	behavior disorder		breast examination
	Behçet disease	B ↑ E	both upper extremities
	bile duct	B ↓ E	both lower extremities
	bipolar disorder(s)	B & E	brisk and equal
	birth date	BEA	below-elbow amputation
	birth defect	BEAC	carmustine (BiCNU), etoposide, cytarabine (ara-C), and cyclophosphamide
	blood donor		
	brain dead		
	bronchial drainage	BEACOPP	bleomycin, etoposide, doxorubicin (Adriamycin), cyclophosphamide, vincristine (Oncovin), procarbazine, and prednisone
	bronchodilator		
	buccodistal		
	1,4-butanediol		

BEAM	brain electrical activity mapping carmustine BCNU), etoposide, cytarabine (ara-C), and methotrexate
BEAR	Bourn electronic adult respirator
BEP	benign essential blepharospasm
BEC	bacterial endocarditis
BECs	bronchial epithelial cells
BECT	barium enema computed tomography
BED	binge-eating disorder
	biochemical evidence of disease
	biological effective dose
	biological equivalent dose
BEE	basal energy expenditure
BEF	bronchoesophageal fistula
BEGA	best estimate of gestational age
BEH	behavior
	benign essential hypertension
Beh Sp	behavior specialist
BEI	bioelectric impedance
	butanol-extractable iodine
BEL	blood ethanol level
BEP	bleomycin, etoposide, and cisplatin (Platinol)
	brain stem evoked potentials
BE-PEG	balanced electrolyte with polyethylene glycol
BEST	bio-electrical stimulation therapy
BET	bacterial endotoxins test
BEV	billion electron volts
	bleeding esophageal varices
BF	biofeedback
	black female
	bone fragment
	boyfriend
	breakfast fed
	breast-fed
B/F	bound-to-free ratio
B & F	back and forth
%BF	percentage of body fat
BFA	baby for adoption
	basilic forearm
	bifemoral arteriogram
BFC	benign febrile convulsion
BFD	blackfoot disease
BFEC	benign focal epilepsy of childhood
bFGF	basic fibroblast growth factor
BFI	Brief Fatigue Inventory
BFL	breast firm and lactating
B-FLY	butterfly
BFM	Berlin-Frankfurt-Munster(cancer study group)
	black married female
	body fat mass
	bright field microscope
BFNC	benign familial neonatal convulsions
BFP	biologic false positive
	blue fluorescent protein

BFR	Backward Functional Reach (test)
	blood filtration rate
	blood flow rate
B. frag	Bacillus fragilis
BFT	bentonite flocculation test
	biofeedback training
BFU$_e$	erythroid burst-forming unit
BG	baby girl
	basal ganglia
	blood glucose
	bone graft
B-G	Bender-Gestalt (test)
BGA	Bundesgesundheitsamt (German drug regulatory agency)
B-GA-LACTO	beta galactosidase
BGC	basal-ganglion calcification
BGCT	benign glandular cell tumor
BGDC	Bartholin gland duct cyst
BGDR	background diabetic retinopathy
BGL	blood glucose level
BGM	blood glucose monitoring
bGS	biopsy Gleason score
BGT	Bender-Gestalt test
	blood glucose testing
BGTT	borderline glucose tolerance test
BH	bowel habits
	breath holding
BHA	butylated hydroxyanisole
BHC	benzene hexachloride
	Braxton Hicks contractions
bHCG	beta human chorionic gonadotropin
BHD	carmustine, hydroxyurea, and dacarbazine
BHDS	Birt-Hogg-Dube syndrome
B-HEXOS-A-LK	beta hexosaminidase A leukocytes
BHGI	The Breast Health Global Initiative
BHI	biosynthetic human insulin
	brain-heart infusion
BHMCO	behavioral health managed care organization
BHN	bridging hepatic necrosis
BHR	bronchial hyperresponsiveness (hyperactivity)
BHP	boarding home placement
	British Herbal Pharmacopeia
BHS	Beck Hopelessness Scale
	beta-hemolytic streptococci
	breath-holding spell
BHT	borderline hypertensive
	breath hydrogen test
	butylated hydroxytoluene
BI	Barthel Index
	base in
	bleeding index (dental)
	Boehringer Ingelheim Pharmaceuticals, Inc.

	bowel impaction	BIS	behavioral inhibition system
	brain injury		Bispectral Index
Bi	bismuth	Bi-SLT	bilateral, sequential single lung
BIA	bioelectrical impedance analysis		transplantation
	biospecific interaction analysis	bisp	bispinous diameter
BIB	brought in by	BIT	behavioral inattention test
BIBA	brought in by ambulance	BITA	bilateral internal thoracic artery
BIC	brain injury center	BiV	biventricular pacing
BICAP	bipolar electrocoagulation therapy	BIVAD	bilateral ventricular (biventricular)
bicarb	bicarbonate		assist device
BiCNU®	carmustine	BIW	twice a week (this is a dangerous
BICROS	bilateral contralateral routing of		abbreviation)
	signals	BIZ-PLT	bizarre platelets
BICU	burn intensive care unit	BJ	Bence Jones (protein)
BID	brought in dead		biceps jerk
BID	twice daily (b.i.d. preferred)		body jacket
b.i.d.	twice daily		bone and joint
BIDA	amonafide	BJE	bone and joint examination
BiDil®	hydralazine and isosorbide		bones, joints, and extremities
	dinitrate	BJI	bone and joint infection
BIDS	bedtime insulin, daytime	BJLO	Benton Judgment Line Orientation
	sulfonylurea		(test)
BIF	bifocal	BJM	bones, joints, and muscles
BIG	botulism immune globulin	BJOA	basal joint osteoarthritis
	Breast International Group	BJP	Bence Jones protein
BIGEM	bigeminal	BK	below knee (amputation)
BIG-IV	botulism immune globulin		bradykinin
	intravenous (human)		bullous keratopathy
BIH	benign intracranial hypertension	BKA	below-knee amputation
	bilateral inguinal hernia	BKC	blepharokeratoconjunctivitis
BIL	bilateral	bkft	breakfast
	brother-in-law	Bkg	background
BILAT SLC	bilateral short leg case	BKTT	below-knee to toe (cast)
BILAT SXO	bilateral salpingo-	BKWC	below-knee walking cast
	oophorectomy	BKWP	below-knee walking plaster
Bili	bilirubin		(cast)
BILI-C	conjugated bilirubin	BL	baseline (fetal heart rate)
BIL MRY	bilateral myringotomy		bioluminescence
BIMA	bilateral internal mammary arteries		bland
BIN	twice a night (this is a dangerous		blast cells
	abbreviation)		blood level
BIND	Biological Investigational New		blood loss
	Drug		blue
BIO	binocular indirect ophthalmoscopy		bronchial lavage
BIOF	biofeedback		Burkitt lymphoma
BIP	bipolar affective disorder	B/L	brother-in-law
	bleomycin, ifosfamide, and cisplatin	BLA	Biological License Application
	(Platinol)	BLB	Boothby-Lovelace-Bulbulian
	brain injury program		(oxygen mask)
BIPA	Benefits Improvement and Protection		bronchoscopic lung biopsy
	Act	BLBK	blood bank
BiPAP	bilevel (biphasic) positive airway	BLBS	bilateral breath sounds
	pressure	BL = BS	bilateral equal breath sounds
BiPD	biparietal diameter	bl cult	blood culture
BIPP	bismuth iodoform paraffin paste	B-L-D	breakfast, lunch, and dinner
BIR	back internal rotation	bldg	bleeding
BIRB	Biomedical Institutional Review	bld tm	bleeding time
	Board	BLE	both lower extremities

BLEED	ongoing *b*leeding, *l*ow blood pressure, *e*levated prothrombin time, *e*rratic mental status, and unstable comorbid *d*isease (risk factors for continued gastrointestinal bleeding)	BME	basal medium Eagle (diploid cell culture)
			biomedical engineering
			brief maximal effort
		BMET	basic metabolic panel (see page 298)
BLEO	bleomycin sulfate	BMF	between meal feedings
BLESS	bath, laxative, enema, shampoo, and shower		black married female
		BMFDS	Burke-Marsden-Fahn dystonia rating scale
BLG	bovine beta-lactoglobulin	BMG	benign monoclonal gammapathy
BLI	blast lung injury	BMH	bone marrow harvest
BLIC	beta-lactamase inhibitor combination	BMI	body mass index
		BMJ	bones, muscles, joints
BLIP	beta-lactamase inhibiting protein	BMK	birthmark
BLL	bilateral lower lobe	BMM	black married male
	blood lead level		bone marrow metastases
	brows, lids, and lashes		bone marrow micrometastases
BLLS	bilateral leg strength	BMMC	bone marrow mononuclear T cells
BLM	bleomycin sulfate	BMMM	bone marrow micrometastases
BLN	bronchial lymph nodes	B-MODE	brightness modulation
BLOBS	bladder obstruction	BMP	basic metabolic profile (panel) (see page 298)
BLOC	brief loss of consciousness		
BLPB	beta-lactamase-producing bacteria		behavior management plan
BLPO	beta-lactamase-producing organism		bone morphogenetic protein
BLQ	both lower quadrants	BMPC	bone marrow plasmacytosis
BLR	blood flow rate	BMPs	bone-morphogenic proteins
BLS	basic life support	BMR	basal metabolic rate
	Bureau of Labor Statistics		best motor response
BLT	bilateral lung transplantation	BMRM	bilateral modified radical mastectomy
	blood-clot lysis time	BMS	bare-metal stents
	brow left transverse		Bristol-Myers Squibb Company
B.L. unit	Bessey-Lowry units		burning mouth syndrome
BLV	bovine leukemia virus	BMSC	bone marrow-derived stem cells
BM	bacterial meningitis	BMT	bilateral myringotomy and tubes
	black male		bismuth subsalicylate, metronidazole, and tetracycline
	bone marrow		
	bone metastases		bone marrow transplant
	bowel movement	BMTH	bismuth, metronidazole, tetracycline, and a histamine H_2-receptor antagonist
	brain metastases		
	breast milk		
	bullous myringitis	BMTN	bone marrow transplant neutropenia
BMA	biomedical application	BMTT	bilateral myringotomy with tympanic tubes
	bismuth subsalicylate, metronidazole, and amoxicillin		
		BMTU	bone marrow transplant unit
	bone marrow aspirate	BMU	basic multicellular unit
	British Medical Association	BMY	Bristol-Myers Squibb
BMAT	basic motor ability test(s)	BN	battalions
BMB	bone marrow biopsy		bladder neck
BMBF	German Ministry of Education and Research		bulimia nervosa
		BNBAS	Brazelton Neonatal Behavioral Assessment
BMC	bone marrow cells	BNC	binasal cannula
	bone marrow culture		bladder neck contracture
	bone mineral content	BNCT	boron neutron capture therapy
BMD	Becker muscular dystrophy	BNE	but not exceeding
	benchmark dose	BNF	British National Formulary
	bone marrow depression	BNI	blind nasal intubation
	bone mineral density	BNL	below normal limits
BMDC	bone marrow-derived (stem) cells		

	breast needle localization
Bn M	bone marrow
B-NHL	B-cell non-Hodgkin lymphoma
BNO	bladder neck obstruction
	bowels not open
BNP	brain natriuretic peptide
	B-type natriuretic peptide (nesiritide [Natrecor])
BNPA	binasal pharyngeal airway
BNR	bladder neck retraction
BNS	benign nephrosclerosis
BNT	back to normal
	Boston Naming Test
BO	base out
	because of
	behavior objective
	body odor
	bowel obstruction
	bowel open
	bucco-occlusal
B & O	belladonna & opium (suppositories)
BOA	behavioral observation audiometry
	born on arrival
	born out of ascpsis
BOB	ball-on-back
BOC	beats of clonus
BOD	bilateral orbital decompression
	burden of disease
Bod Units	Bodansky units
BOE	bilateral otitis externa
BOH	Board of Health
	bundle of His
BOLD	bleomycin, vincristine (Oncovin), lomustine, and dacarbazine
	blood oxygenation level-dependent
BOM	benign ovarian mass
	bilateral otitis media
BOMA	bilateral otitis media, acute
BOME	bilateral otitis media with effusion
BOMP	bleomycin, vincristine (Oncovin), mitomycin, and cisplatin (Platinol)
BOO	bladder outlet obstruction
BOOP	bronchitis obliterans-organized pneumonia
BOP	bleeding on probing
BOR	bortezomib (Velcade)
	bowels open regularly
	bronchia-oto-renal (syndrome)
BORN	State Board of Registration in Nursing
BORospA	borreliosis (Lyme disease, *Borrelia* sp.) vaccine, outer surface protein A
BOS	base of support
	bronchiolitis obliterans syndrome
BOSS	Becker orthopedic spinal system
BOT	base of tongue
	borderline ovarian tumors

BOU	burning on urination
BOUGIE	bougienage
BOVR	Bureau of Vocational Rehabilitation
BOW	bag of water
BOW-I	bag of water–intact
BOW-R	bag of water–ruptured
BP	bathroom privileges
	bed pan
	bench press
	benzoyl peroxide
	bipolar
	birthplace
	blood pressure
	bodily pain
	body powder
	British Pharmacopeia
	bullous pemphigoid
	bypass
bp	base pair(s) (genetics)
BP-200	Bourn Infant Pressure Ventilator
BPA	birch pollen allergy
BPAD	bipolar affective disorder
BPAR	biopsy-proven actue rejection
BPb	whole blood lead concentration
BPCF	bronchopleural cutaneous fistula
BPI	bipolar disorder, Type I
BPII	bipolar type II disorder
BPD	benzoporphyrin derivative
	biparietal diameter
	borderline personality disorder
	bronchopulmonary dysplasia
BPd	diastolic blood pressure
BPD/DS	biliopancreatic diversion with a duodenal switch (surgery for obesity)
BPE	benign enlargement of the prostate
BPF	Brazilian purpuric fever
	bronchopleural fistula
BPH	benign prostatic hypertrophy
BPG	bypass graft
	penicillin G benzathine (Bicillin L-A; Permapen) for IM use only
BPI	bactericidal/permeability increasing (protein)
	Brief Pain Inventory
BPIG	bacterial polysaccharide immune globulin
BPL	benzylpenicilloylpolylysine
	bone probing length (dental)
BPLA	blood pressure, left arm
BPLND	bilateral pelvic lymph node dissection
BPM	beats per minute
	breaths per minute
BPN	bacitracin, polymyxin B, and neomycin sulfate
BPO	benign prostatic obstruction
	benzoyl peroxide

	bilateral partial oophorectomy		Baylor rapid autologous transfuser
BPOC	barcode point-of-care		blunt thoracic abdominal trauma
BPOP	bizarre parosteal	BRATT	bananas, rice (rice cereal),
	osteochondromatous proliferation		applesauce, tea, and toast
	(Nora's Lesion)	BRB	blood-retinal barrier
BPP	biophysical profile		bright red blood
BPPP	bilateral pedal pulses present	BRBR	bright red blood per rectum
BP,P,R,T,	blood pressure, pulse, respiration,	BRBPR	bright red blood per rectum
	and temperature	BRC	bladder reconstruction
BPPV	benign paroxysmal positional vertigo	BrCa	breast cancer
BPR	beeper	BRCM	below right costal margin
	blood per rectum	BrdU	bromodeoxyuridine
	blood pressure recorder	BRex	breathing exercise
BPRS	Brief Psychiatric Rating Scale	Br Fdg	breast-feeding
BPS	bilateral partial salpingectomy	BRFS	biochemical relapse-free survival
	blood pump speed	BRFSS	Behavioral Risk Factor Surveillance
BPs	systolic blood pressure		System
BPSD	behavioral and psychological	BRJ	brachial radialis jerk
	symptoms of dementia	BRM	biological response modifiers
	bronchopulmonary segmental	BRN	brown
	drainage	BRO	brother
BPSO	bilateral prophylactic salpingo-	BROM	back range of motion
	oophorectomy	BRONK	bronchoscopy
BPT	BioPort Corporation	BRP	bathroom privileges
BPV	benign paroxysmal vertigo	BRR	Bannayan-Riley-Ruvalcaba
	benign positional vertigo		(syndrome)
	bovine papilloma virus	BR RAO	branch retinal artery occlusion
Bq	becquerel	BR RVO	branch retinal vein occlusion
BQL	below quantifiable levels	BRS	baroreceptor reflex sensitivity
BQR	brequinar sodium	BrS	breath sounds
BR	bathroom	BRSV	bovine respiratory syncytial virus
	bedrest	BRU	basic remodeling unit (osteon)
	Benzing retrograde		brucellosis (*Brucella melitensis*)
	birthing room		vaccine
	blink rate	BRVO	branch retinal vein occlusion
	blink reflex	BS	barium swallow
	bowel rest		bedside
	brachioradialis		before sleep
	breast		Behçet syndrome
	breast reconstruction		Bennett seal
	breech		blind spot
	bridge		blood sugar
	bright red		Blue Shield
	brown		bone scan
Br	bromide		bowel sounds
	bromine		breath sounds
BRA	bananas, rice (rice cereal), and	B & S	Bartholin and Skene (glands)
	applesauce		bending and stooping
	brain		Brown and Sharp (suture sizes)
BrAC	breath alcohol content	BS×4	bowel sounds in all four quadrants
BRCA1	breast cancer gene 1	BSA	body surface area
BRCA2	breast cancer gene 2		bowel sounds active
BRADY	bradycardia		Brief Scale of Anxiety
BRANCH	branch chain amino acids	BSAB	Balthazar Scales of Adaptive
BRAO	branch retinal artery occlusion		Behavior
BRAS	bilateral renal artery stenosis	BSAb	broad-spectrum antibiotics
BRAT	bananas, rice (rice cereal),	BSAP	bone-specific alkaline phosphatase
	applesauce, and toast	BSB	bedside bag

	body surface burned	BSS	Baltimore Sepsis Scale
BSC	basosquamous (cell) carcinoma		bedside scale
	bedside care		bismuth subsalicylate
	bedside commode		black silk sutures
	best supportive care	BSS®	balanced salt solution
	biological safety cabinet	BSSG	sitogluside
	Biomedical Science Corps	BSSO	bilateral sagittal split osteotomy
	burn scar contracture	BSSRO	bilateral sagittal split-ramus osteotomy
BSCC	bedside commode chair		
	Bjork-Shiley convexo-concave (valves)	BSSS	benign sporadic sleep spikes
BSCVA	best spectacle-corrected visual acuity	BSST	breast self-stimulation test
BSD	baby soft diet	BST	bedside testing
	bedside drainage		bovine somatotropin
BSE	bovine spongiform encephalopathy		brief stimulus therapy
	breast self-examination	BSU	Bartholin, Skene, urethra (glands)
BSEC	bedside easy chair		behavioral science unit
BSepF	black separated female	BSu	blood sugar
BSepM	black separated male	BSUTD	baby shots up to date
BSER	brain stem evoked responses		Base Service Unit
BSF	black single female	BSW	Bachelor of Social Work
	busulfan (Myleran)		bedscale weight
BSG	Bagolini striated glasses	BT	bedtime
	brain stem gliomas		behavioral therapy
BSGA	beta streptococcus group A		bituberous
BSGI	breast-specific gamma imaging		bladder tumor
BSI	bloodstream infection		Blalock-Taussig (shunt)
	body substance isolation		bleeding time
	brain stem injury		blood transfusion
	Brief Symptom Inventory		blood type
BSL	baseline		blunt trauma
	Biological Safety Level		brain tumor
	blood sugar level		breast tumor
BSL-1	Biosafety Level 1		bowel tones
BS L base	breath sounds diminished, left base	Bt	*Bacillus thuringiensis*
		B-T	Blalock-Taussig (shunt)
BSM	black single male	B/T	between
	blood safety module	Bt#	bottle number
BSN	Bachelor of Science in Nursing	BTA	below the ankle
	bowel sounds normal		bladder tumor antigen
BSNA	bowel sounds normal and active		bladder tumor associated analytes
BSNMT	Bachelor of Science in Nuclear Medicine Technology		botulinum toxic type A (Botox)
BSNT	breast soft and nontender	BTA-A	botulinum toxin type A (Botox)
BSNUTD	baby shots not up to date	BTB	back to bed
BSO	bilateral salpingo-oophorectomy		beat-to-beat (variability)
	l-buthionine sulfoximine		breakthrough bleeding
bSOD	bovine superoxide dismutase	BTBV	beat-to-beat variability
BSOM	bilateral serous otitis media	BTC	bilateral tubal cautery
BSP	body substance precautions		biliary tract cancer
	bone sialoprotein		bladder tumor check
	Bromsulphalein®		by the clock
BSPA	bowel sounds present and active	BTE	Baltimore Therapeutic Equipment
BSPM	body surface potential mapping		behind-the-ear (hearing aid)
BSR	body stereotactic radiosurgery		bisected, totally embedded
	bowels sounds regular	BTF	blenderized tube feeding
BSRI	Bem Sex Role Inventory	BTFS	breast tumor frozen section
BSRT (R)	Bachelor of Science in Radiologic Technology (Registered)	BTG	beta thromboglobulin
		B-Thal	beta thalassemia

BTHOOM	beats the hell out of me (better stated as "differed diagnosis")	BVF	bulboventricular foramen
BTI	biliary tract infection	BVH	biventricular hypertrophy
	bitubal interruption	BVL	bilateral vas ligation
BTKA	bilateral total knee arthroplasty	BVM	bag valve mask
BTL	bilateral tubal ligation	BVMG	Bender Visual-Motor Gestalt (test)
BTM	bilateral tympanic membranes	BVO	branch vein occlusion
	bismuth subcitrate, tetracycline, and metronidazole	BVR	Bureau of Vocational Rehabilitation
		BVRO	bilateral vertical ramus osteotomy
BTMEAL	between meals	BVRT	Benton Visual Retention Test
BTO	bilateral tubal occlusion	BVT	bilateral ventilation tubes
BTP	bismuth tribromophenate	BVZ	bevacizumab (Avastin)
	breakthrough pain	BW	bandwidth (radiology)
BTPABA	bentiromide		birth weight
BTPS	body temperature pressure saturated		bite-wing (radiograph)
BTR	bladder tumor recheck		body water
BTS	Blalock-Taussig shunt		body weight
BTSH	bovine thyrotropin	B & W	Black and White (milk of magnesia & aromatic cascara fluidextract)
BTU	behavior therapy unit		
BTW	back to work	BWA	bed-wetter admission
	between	BWC	bladder-wash cytology
BTW M	between meals	BWCS	bagged white cell study
BTX	Botulinum toxin type A (Botox)	BWF	Blackwater fever
BtxA	botulinum toxin type A (Botox)	BWFI	bacteriostatic water for injection
BU	base up (prism)	BWidF	black widowed female
	below umbilicus	BWidM	black widowed male
	Bodansky units	BWS	battered woman syndrome
	burn unit		Beckwith-Wiedemann syndrome
	busulfan (Myleran)	BWs	bite-wing (x-rays)
BUA	broadband ultrasound attenuation	BWSE	black widow spider envenomation
BUCAT	busulfan, carboplatin, and thiotepa	BWSTT	body weight-supported treadmill training
BuCy	busulfan and cyclophosphamide		
BUD	budesonide (Rhinocort)	BWT	bowel wall thickness
BUdR	bromodeoxyuridine	BWX	bite-wing x-ray
BUE	both upper extremities	Bx	behavior
BUFA	baby up for adoption		biopsy
BULB	bilateral upper lid blepharoplasty	B × B	back-to-back
BUN	blood urea nitrogen	BX BS	Blue Cross and Blue Shield
	bunion	BXM	B-cell crossmatch
BUO	bleeding of undetermined origin	BXO	balanitis xerotica obliterans
BUR	back-up rate (ventilator)	ΦBZ	phenylbutazone
Burd	Burdick suction	BZD	benzodiazepine
BUS	Bartholin, urethral, and Skene glands	BZDZ	benzodiazepine
	bladder ultrasound		
	bulbourethral sling		
BUSV	Bartholin urethral Skeins vagina		
BUT	biopsy urease test		
	break up time		
BV	bacterial vaginitis		
	bevacizumab (Avastin)		
	biological value		
	blood volume		
BVAD	biventricular assist device		
BVAS	Birmingham Vasculitis Activity Score		
BVD	bovine viral diarrhea		
BVDU	bromovinlydeoxyuridine (brivudin)		
BVE	blood volume expander		

C

C   ascorbic acid (Vitamin C)
carbohydrate
Catholic
Caucasian
Celsius
centigrade
Chlamydia
clubbing
conjunctiva
constricted
cyanosis
cytidine
hundred

$\bar{c}$ with
C′   cervical spine
C+   with contrast
C−   without contrast
C 1   cyclopentolate 1% ophthalmic
     solution (Cyclogyl)
C_1–C_7 cervical vertebra 1 through 7
C_1–C_8 cervical nerves 1 through 8
C_1–C_9 precursor molecules of the
     complement system
C_1–C_{12} cranial nerves 1 to 12
C3   complement C3
C4   complement C4
CI CV   Drug Enforcement Agency scheduled
     substances class one through five
C_{II} second cranial nerve
CA   cancelled appointment
Candida albicans
carcinoma
cardiac arrest
carotid artery
celiac artery
cellulose acetate (filter)
Certified Acupuncturist
chronologic age
Cocaine Anonymous
community-acquired
compressed air
continuous aerosol
coronary angioplasty
coronary artery
Ca   calcium
C/A   conscious, alert
Ca++   calcification
calcium
CA 125   cancer antigen 125
C&A   Clinitest® and Acetest®
CAA   cerebral amyloid angiopathy
coloanal anastomosis
crystalline amino acids

CAAP-1   Certified Associate Addiction
     Professional Level 1
CAB   catheter-associated bacteriuria
cellulose acetate butyrate
combined androgen blockade
complete atrioventricular block
coronary artery bypass
CAB-BAGE   coronary artery bypass graft
CABG   coronary artery bypass graft
CaBI   calcium bone index
CaBP   calcium-binding protein
CABS   coronary artery bypass surgery
CAC   cardioacceleratory center
Certified Alcohol Counselor
Community Action Center
computer-assisted coding
computerized autocoding
coronary artery calcification
CACI   computer-assisted continuous
     infusion
$CaCl_2$ calcium chloride
$CaCO_3$ calcium carbonate
CACP   cisplatin
CACS   cancer-related anorexia/cachexia
CAD   cadaver (kidney donor)
calcium alginate dressing
computer-aided diagnosis
computer-aided dispatch
coronary atherosclerotic disease
coronary artery disease
CaD   calcium and vitamin D (fortified
     milk)
CADAC   Certified Alcohol and Drug Abuse
     Counselor
CADASIL   cerebral autosomal dominant
     arteriopathy with subcortical
     infarcts and leukoencephalopathy
CADD®   Computerized Ambulatory Drug
     Delivery (pump)
CADL   communication activities of daily
     living (speech/ cognitive test)
CADP   computer-assisted design of
     prosthesis
CADRF   coronary artery disease risk factors
CADXPL   cadaver transplant
CAE   cellulose acetate electrophoresis
coronary artery endarterectomy
cyclophosphamide, doxorubicin
     (Adriamycin), and etoposide
CAEC   cardiac arrhythmia evaluation center
Cook airway exchange catheter
CaEDTA   calcium disodium edetate
CAF   chronic atrial fibrillation
controlled atrial flutter/fibrillation
cyclophosphamide, doxorubicin
     (Adriamycin), and fluorouracil
CAFF   controlled atrial fibrillation/flutter

CAFT	Clinitron® air fluidized therapy
CAG	chronic atrophic gastritis
	closed angle glaucoma
	continuous ambulatory gamma globin (infusion)
	coronary arteriography
CaG	calcium gluconate
CAGE	a questionnaire for alcoholism evaluation C Have you ever felt the need to cut down on your drinking? A Have you ever felt annoyed by criticism of your drinking? G Have you ever felt guilty abut your drinking? E Have you ever taken a drink (eye opener) first thing in the morning?
CAH	chronic active hepatitis
	chronic aggressive hepatitis
	congenital adrenal hyperplasia
CAHB	chronic active hepatitis B
CAI	carbonic anhydrase inhibitors
	carboxyamide aminoimidazoles
	carotid artery injury
	computer-assisted instructions
'caid	Medicaid
CAIV	cold-adapted influenza virus vaccine
CAL	callus
	calories (cal)
	chronic airflow limitation
	clinical attachment level (dental)
C_{alb}	albumin clearance
cal ct	calorie count
CALD	chronic active liver disease
CALGB	Cancer and Leukemia Group B
CALI	chromophore-assisted laser inactivation
CALLA	common acute lymphoblastic leukemia antigen
CAM	campylobacter vaccine
	Caucasian adult male
	cell adhesion molecules
	child abuse management
	complementary and alternative medicine
	confusion assessment method
	controlled ankle motion
	cystic adenomatoid malformation
CAMA	Chronic and Acute Medical Assistance
	corrected-arm-muscle area
CAMCOG	Cambridge Cognitive Examination
CAMD	computer-aided molecular design
CAMF	cyclophosphamide, Adriamycin, methotrexate, and fluorouracil
CAMP	cyclophosphamide, doxorubicin (Adriamycin), methotrexate, and procarbazine

cAMP	cyclic adenosine monophosphate
CA-MRSA	community-associated methicillin-resistant *Staphylococcus aureus*
CAMs	cell adhesion molecules
CAN	cardiovascular autonomic neuropathy
	Certified Nurse Assistant
	chronic allograft nephropathy
	contrast-associated nephropathy
	cord around neck
CA/N	child abuse and neglect
CAN-A	Certified Nursing Assistant-Advanced
CANC	cancelled
c-ANCA	antineutrophil cytoplasmic antibody
CANDA	computer-assisted new drug application
CAN-KLB	*Candida albicans, Klebsiella pneumoniae* vaccine
CANP	Certified Adult Nurse Practitioner
CAO	chronic airway (airflow) obstruction
CaO_2	arterial oxygen concentration
CAOS	computer-assisted orthopedic surgery
CaOx	calcium oxalate
CAP	cancer of the prostate
	capsule
	cellulose acetate phthalate
	Certified Addiction Professional
	cervical acid phosphatase
	chaotic atrial tachycardia
	chemistry admission profile
	chloramphenicol
	community-acquired pneumonia
	compound action potentials
	cyclophosphamide, doxorubicin (Adriamycin), and cisplatin
CaP	cancer of the prostate
Ca/P	calcium to phosphorus ratio
CA4P	combretastatin A4 prodrug
CAPA	Certified Ambulatory Perianesthesia Nurse
	Corrective and Preventive Action (related to FDA)
CAPB	central auditory processing battery
CAPD	central auditory processing disorder
	continuous ambulatory peritoneal dialysis
CAPLA	computer-assisted product license application
CaPPS	calcium pentosan polysulfate
CAPS	aspects of cognition, affective state, physical condition, and social factors (patient assessment; parameters)
	caffeine, alcohol, pepper, and spicy food (dietary restrictions)
CAPWA	computerized arterial pulse waveform analysis
CAR	cancer-associated retinopathy

	cardiac ambulation routine	CATS	catecholamines
	carotid artery repair	CATT	card agglutination test with stained trypanosomes
	carotid artery rupture		
	coronary artery revascularization	CAU	Caucasian
	Coxsackie adenovirus receptor	CAUTI	catheter-associated urinary tract infection
CA-RA	common adductor-rectus abdominis		
CARB	carbohydrate	CAV	cardiac allograft vasculopathy
CARBO	Carbocaine		computer-aided ventilation
	carboplatin (Paraplatin)		congenital absence of vagina
CARD	Cardiac Automatic Resuscitative Device		cyclophosphamide, doxorubicin (Adriamycin), and vincristine
CARES	Cancer Rehabilitation Evaluation System	CAV-1	canine adenovirus type 1
		CAVB	complete atrioventricular block
CARF	Commission on Accreditation of Rehabilitation Facilities	CAVC	common artrioventricular canal
		CAVE	Content Analysis of Verbatim Explanation
CARM	Centre for Adverse Reactions Monitoring (New Zealand)		cyclophosphamide, doxorubicin, (Adriamycin) vincristine, and etoposide
C-arm	fluoroscopy image intensifier		
CARN	Certified Addiction Registered Nurse		
CARN-AP	Certified Addictions Registered Nurse - Advanced Practice	CAVH	continuous arteriovenous hemofiltration
CARS	Childhood Autism Rating Scale	CAVHD	continuous arteriovenous hemodialysis
CART	classification and regression tree		
CARTI	community-acquired respiratory tract infection(s)	CAVM	cerebral arteriovenous malformation
		CAV-P-VP	cyclophosphamide, doxorubicin (Adriamycin), vincristine, cisplatin, and etoposide
CAS	carotid angioplasty and stenting		
	carotid artery stenosis (stenting)		
	cerebral arteriosclerosis	CAVR	continuous arteriovenous rewarming
	Chemical Abstracts Service	CAVS	calcific valve stenosis
	Clinical Asthma Score	CAVU	continuous arteriovenous ultrafiltration
	combined androgen suppression		
	computer-assisted surgery	CAW	carbonaceous-activated water (Willard Water)
	coronary artery stenosis		
CASA	cancer-associated serum antigen	CAX	central axis
	Center on Addiction and Substance Abuse	Ca x P	calcium times phosphorus product
		CB	cesarean birth
	computer-assisted semen analysis		chronic bronchitis
CaSC	carcinoma of the sigmoid colon		code blue
CASH	chemotherapy-associated steatohepatitis		conjugated bilirubin (direct)
			(umbilical) cord blood
CASHD	coronary arteriosclerotic heart disease	c/b	complicated by
		C & B	chair and bed
CASL	continuous arterial spin labeled		crown and bridge
CASP	Child Analytic Study Program	CB1	cannabinoid receptor, type 1
CASS	computer-aided sleep system	CBA	chronic bronchitis and asthma
CAST®	color allergy screening test		cost-benefit analysis
CASWCM	Certified Advanced Social Work Case Manager		County Board of Assistance
		CBAPF	Certified Board of Addiction Professionals
CAT	Cardiac Arrest Team		
	carnitine acetyl transferase	CBASP	Cognitive Behavioral Analysis System of Psychotherapy
	cataract		
	Children's Apperception Test	CBAVD	congenital bilateral absence of the vas deferens
	coital alignment technique		
	computed axial tomography	CBC	carbenicillin
	methcatinone		complete blood count
CATH	catheter		contralateral breast cancer
	catheterization	CBCDA	carboplatin
	Catholic	CBCL	Child Behavior Checklist

C

59

CBCT	community based clinical trials	cerebral concussion
CBD	closed bladder drainage	cervical cancer
	common bile duct	chart check (as in 24 hour CC)
	corticobasal degeneration	chief complaint
CBDE	common bile duct exploration	choriocarcinoma
CBDS	common bile duct stone(s)	chronic complainer
CBE	charting by exception	circulatory collapse
	child birth education	clean catch (urine)
	clinical breast examination	comfort care
CBER	Center for Biologics Evaluation and Research (FDA)	complications and comorbidity
		coracoclavicular
CBF	cerebral blood flow	cord compression
CBFS	cerebral blood flow studies	corpus callosum
CBFV	cerebral blood flow velocity	creatinine clearance
CBG	capillary blood glucose	critical condition
CBGM	capillary blood glucose monitor	cubic centimeter (cc), (mL); Note, mL is preferred as a poorly written cc looks like the dangerous abbreviation for unit, "u"
CBH	collimated beam handpiece (for laser)	
CBI	Caregiver Burden Index	
	continuous bladder irrigation	with correction (with glasses)
CBLI	cumulative blood lead index	
CBM	cryopreserved bone marrow	C_c concentration of drug in the central compartment
CBN	chronic benign neutropenia	
	collected by nurse	C/C cholecystectomy and operative cholangiogram
CBP	chronic benign pain	
	copper-binding protein	complete upper and lower dentures
CBPP	contagious bovine pleuropneumonia	CCII Clinical Clerk–2nd year
CBPS	congenital bilateral perisylvian syndrome	C & C cold and clammy
		CCA calcium-channel antagonist
	coronary bypass surgery	Certified Coding Associate
CBR	carotid bodies resected	cholangiocarcinoma
	chronic bedrest	circumflex coronary artery
	clinical benefit rate	common carotid artery
	clinical benefit responders	concentrated care area
	complete bedrest	countercurrent chromatography
CBRAM	controlled partial rebreathing-anesthesia method	critical care area
		CCAM congenital cystic adenomatoid malformation (of the lung)
CBRN	chemical, biological, radiological, or nuclear (agents)	
		CCAP capsule cartilage articular preservation
CB RRR s M/R/G	cardiac beat, regular rhythm and rate without murmurs, rubs, or gallops	
		CCAT common carotid artery thrombosis
		C-CATODSW Certified Clinical Alcohol, Tobacco and Other Drugs Social Worker
CBrS	clear breath sounds	
CBS	Caregiver Burden Screen	
	Charles Bonnet syndrome	CCAVC complete common atrioventricular canal
	chronic brain syndrome	
	coarse breath sounds	CCB calcium channel blocker(s)
	corticobasal syndrome	Community Care Board
	Cruveilhier-Baumgarten syndrome	corn, callus, and bunion
CBT	cognitive behavioral therapy	CCBT Certified Cognitive Behavioral Therapist
CBU	cumulative breath units	
CBV	central blood volume	CCC Cancer Care Center
	cyclophosphamide, carmustine (BiCNu), and etoposide (VePesid)	central corneal clouding (Grade 0+ to 4+)
		Certificate of Clinical Competency
CBZ	carbamazepine (Tegretol)	
CBZE	carbamazepine epoxide	child care clinic
CC	cardiac catheterization	cholangiocellular carcinoma
	Catholic	circulating cancer cells

	closed chest compressions
	Comprehensive Cancer Center
	continuous curvilinear
	capsulorrhexis
C/cc	colonies per cubic centimeter
CC & C	colony count and culture
CCC-A	Certificate of Clinical Competence
	in Audiology
CCCE	Clinical Center Coordinator Educator
CCCN	Certified Continence Care Nurse
CCC-SP	Certificate of Clinical Competence
	in Speech-Language Pathology
CCD	charged-coupled device
	childhood celiac disease
	chin-chest distance
	clinical cardiovascular disease
CCDC	Certified Chemical Dependency
	Counselor
CCDC-1	Certified Chemical Dependency
	Counselor, Level One
CCDS	color-coded duplex sonography
CCE	clubbing, cyanosis, and edema
	countercurrent electrophoresis
CC-EMG	corpus cavernosum
	electromyography
CCF	cephalin cholesterol flocculation
	Cleveland Clinic Foundation
	compound comminuted fracture
	congestive cardiac failure
	crystal-induced chemotactic factor
CCFA	cycloserine cefoxitin fructose agar
CCFE	cyclophosphamide, cisplatin,
	fluorouracil, and estramustine
CCFs	chronic-care facilities
CCG	Children's Cancer Group
CCH	chronic community care home
	Cook County Hospital
	cluster headache
CCHB	congenital complete heart block
CCHD	complex congenital heart disease
	cyanotic congenital heart disease
CCHF	Congo-Crimean
	hemorrhagic fever
CCHS	congenital central hypoventilation
	syndrome
CCI	chronic coronary insufficiency
	Correct Coding Initiative
	corrected count increment
CCJAP	Certified Criminal Justice Addiction
	Professional
CCJAS	Certified Criminal Justice Addiction
	Specialist
CCK	cholecystokinin
CCK-OP	cholecystokinin octapeptide
CCK-PZ	cholecystokinin pancreozymin
CCL	cardiac catheterization laboratory
	critical condition list
CCl_4	carbon tetrachloride

CCLE	chronic cutaneous lupus
	erythematosus
CCM	calcium citrate malate
	cerebral cavernous malformation
	Certified Case Manager
	children's case management
	country coordinating mechanism
	cyclophosphamide, lomustine
	(CCNU; CeeNU), and
	methotrexate
CCMHC	Certified Clinical Mental Health
	Counselor
CCMSU	clean catch midstream urine
CCMU	critical care medicine unit
CCN	continuing care nursery
	cyr61, ctfg, nov (family of proteins)
CCNS	cell cycle-nonspecific
	Certified Clinical Nurse Specialist
CCNU	lomustine (CeeNu)
CCO	continuous cardiac output
	Corporate Compliance Officer
CCOHTA	Canadian Coordinating Office for
	Health Technology Assessment
C-collar	cervical collar
CCP	crystalloid cardioplegia
CCPD	continuous cycling (cyclical)
	peritoneal dialysis
CCPs	Corporate Compliance Programs
CCR	California Cancer Registry
	cardiac catheterization recovery
	complete cytogenetic remission
	Continuity of Care Record
	continuous complete remission
	counterclockwise rotation
C_{cr}	creatinine clearance
cCR	complete clinical remission
CCRC	Certified Clinical Research
	Coordinator
	continuing care residential
	community
CC-RCC	clear-cell renal-cell carcinoma
CCRN	Certified Critical Care Registered
	Nurse
CCRT	combined chemoradiotherapy
CCRU	critical care recovery unit
CCS	cell cycle-specific
	certified coding specialist
	color contrast sensitivity
CC & S	cornea, conjunctiva, and sclera
CCSA	Canadian Cardiovascular Society
	Angina (score)
CCSK	clear cell sarcoma of the kidney
CCSP	Certified Chiropractic Sports
	Physician
	Clara cell secretory protein
CCS-P	Certified Coding Specialist,
	Physician-Based
CCSS	Childhood Cancer Survivor Study

C

CCSV	cell-cultured smallpox vaccine		concentration of drug
CCT	calcitriol	C/D	cigarettes per day
	carotid compression tomography		cup-to-disc ratio
	central corneal thickness	CD4	antigenic marker on helper/inducer
	Certified Cardiographic Technician		T cells (also called OKT 4, T4,
	closed cerebral trauma		and Leu3)
	closed cranial trauma	CD8	antigenic marker on suppressor/
	collision cell technology		cytotoxic T cells (also called
	congenitally corrected transposition		OKT 8, T8, and Leu 8)
	(of the great vessels)	C&D	curettage and desiccation
	Critical Care Technician		cystectomy and diversion
	crude coal tar		cytoscopy and dilatation
CCTGA	congenitally corrected transposition	CDA	Certified Dental Assistant
	of the great arteries		chenodeoxycholic acid (chenodiol)
CCT in PET	crude coal tar in		congenital dyserythropoietic anemia
	petroleum	2-CDA	cladribine (Leustatin;
CCTV	closed circuit television		chlorodeoxyadenosine)
CCU	coronary care unit	CDAD	*Clostridium difficile*-associated
	critical care unit		diarrhea
CCUA	clean catch urinalysis	CDAI	Crohn Disease Activity Index
CCUP	colpocystourethropexy	CDAK	Cordis Dow Artificial Kidney
CCV	Critical Care Ventilator (Ohio)	CDAP	continuous distended airway pressure
	critical closing volume	CDB	cough and deep breath
CCW	childcare worker	CDC	calculated day of confinement
	counterclockwise		cancer detection center
CCWR	counterclockwise rotation		carboplatin, doxorubicin, and
CCX	complications		cyclophosphamide
CCY	cholecystectomy		Centers for Disease Control and
CD	cadaver donor		Prevention
	candela		Certified Drug Counselor
	Castleman disease		chenodeoxycholic acid (chenodiol)
	celiac disease		*Clostridium difficile* colitis
	cervical dystonia	CDCA	chenodeoxycholic acid (chenodiol)
	cesarean delivery	CDCP	Centers for Disease Control and
	character disorder		Prevention (CDC is official
	chemical dependency		abbreviation)
	childhood disease	CDCR	conjunctivodacryocystorhinostomy
	chlorproguanil-dapsone (Lapdap)	CDD	Certificate of Disability for
	chronic dialysis		Discharge
	circular dichroism		*Clostridium difficile* disease
	closed drainage		cytidine deaminase
	Clostridium difficile	CDDN	Certified Developmental Disabilities
	clusters of differentiation		Nurse
	common duct	CDDP	cisplatin (Platinol)
	communication disorders	CDE	canine distemper encephalitis
	complementarity-determining		Certified Diabetes Educator
	complicated delivery		common data element
	conjugate diameter		common duct exploration
	contact dermatitis	CDER	Center for Drug Evaluation and
	continuous drainage		Research (FDA)
	conventional denture	CDFI	color Doppler flow imaging
	convulsive disorder	CDG	carbohydrate-deficient glycoprotein
	cortical dysplasia		congenital disorders of
	Crohn disease		glycosylation
	cumulative doses	CDGE	constant denaturant gel
	cyclodextran		electrophoresis
	cytarabine and daunorubicin	CDGP	constitutional delay of growth and
Cd	cadmium		puberty

CDGS	carbohydrate-deficient glycoprotein syndrome	CDSPIES	congestive heart failure, drugs, spasm, pneumothorax, infection, embolism, and secretions (differential diagnosis mnemonic)
CDH	chronic daily headache		
	congenital diaphragmatic hernia		
	congenital dislocation of hip	CDSR	Cochrane Database of Systematic Reviews
	congenital dysplasia of the hip		
CDHP	5-chloro-2 4-dihydroxypyridine	CDSS	Cervical Dystonia Severity Scale
CDI	Children's Depression Inventory	CDSSs	clinical decision support systems
	clean, dry, and intact	CDT	carbohydrate-deficient transferrin
	color Doppler imaging		catheter-directed thrombolysis
	conformation-dependent immunoassay		Chemical Dependency Technician
			clinical development team
	Cotrel Duobosset Instrumentation		Clock-Drawing Test
CDIC	*Clostridium difficile*-induced colitis		complete decongestive therapy (for lymphedema)
C Dif	*Clostridium difficile*		
C Diff	*Clostridium difficile*		connecting discourse tracking (measure of speech perception)
CDJ	choledochojejunostomy		
CDK	climatic droplet keratopathy		cystic dysplasia of the testis
	cyclin-dependent kinase		current dental terminology
CDKI	cyclin-dependent kinase inhibitor		cytolethal distending toxin
CDK2	cyclin-depenent kinases 2	CDTA	cyclohexane-1,2-diaminetetraacetic acid
CDLC	continuous double-loop closure		
CDLE	chronic discoid lupus erythematosus	CDTM	collaborative drug therapy management
CdLS	Cornelia de Lange syndrome		
CDM	charge description master	CDU	chemical dependency unit
	clinical development monitor		color-coded duplex ultrasonography
CDMS	Certified Disability Management Specialist	CDV	canine distemper virus
			cardiovascular
	clinically definite multiple sclerosis		cyclophosphamide, doxorubicin, and vincristine
CDO	cartilage disorder		
CDONA/ LTC	Certified Director of Nursing Administration in Long-Term Care	CDX	chlordiazepoxide (Librim)
		cDXA	central dual-energy X-ray absorptiometry
CDP	cancer detection program		
	chemical dependence profile	cdyn	dynamic compliance
	Chemical Dependency Professional	CE	California encephalitis
	Child Development Program		capillary electrophoresis
	clinical development plan		capsule endoscopy
	complete decongestive physiotherapy		carboplatin and etoposide
	crystalline degradation product		cardiac enlargement
	cytidine diphosphate		cardiac enzymes
CDQ	corrected development quotient		cardioesophageal
CDR	clinical data repository		Carpentier-Edwards (heart-valve prosthesis)
	Clinical Dementia Rating		
	cognitive dietary restraint		cataract extraction
	continuing disability review		central episiotomy
CDRH	Center for Devices and Radiological Health		chemoembolization
			chest expansion
CDR(H)	cup-to-disc ratio horizontal		cholesterol ester
CDRs	complementary determining regions		community education
CDRS	Children's Depression Rating Scale		conjugated estrogens
CDR(V)	cup-to-disc ratio vertical		consultative examination
CDS	Chemical Dependency Specialist		continuing education
	Chronic Disease Score		contrast echocardiology
	closed-door seclusion		cystic echinococcosis
	color Doppler sonography	C&E	consultation and examination
	continuous dopamine stimulation		cough and exercise
CDSC	Communicable Disease Surveillance Centre (United Kingdom)		curettage and electrodesiccation
		CEA	carcinoembryonic antigen

C

	carotid endarterectomy	CEPE	cataract extraction by
	cost-effectiveness analysis		phacoemulsification
CEB	calcium entry blocker	CEPH	cephalic
	carboplatin, etoposide, and bleomycin		cephalosporin
CEBV	chronic Epstein-Barr virus	CEPH FLOC	cephalin flocculation
CEC	capillary electrochromatography		
	Council for Exceptional Children	CEPP (B)	cyclophosphamide, etopside,
CECA	Childhood Experience of Care and		procarbazine, prednisone, and
	Abuse (interview)		bleomycin
CECD	congenital endothelial corneal	CER	conditioned emotional response
	dystrophy	CE&R	central episiotomy and repair
CEc̄/IOL	cataract extraction with intraocular	CERA	cortical evoked response audiometry
	lens	CERAD	Consortium to Establish a Registry
CECT	contrast-enhanced computed		for Alzheimer Disease
	tomography	CERD	chronic end-stage renal disease
CED	Camurati-Engelmann disease	CERT	Comprehensive Error Rate Testing
	clinically effective dose	CERULO	ceruloplasmin
	cystoscopy-endoscopy dilation	CERV	cervical
CEDS	Certified Eating Disorders Specialist	CES	Cauda equina syndrome
CEE	Central European encephalitis		central excitatory state
	conjugated equine estrogen		cognitive environmental stimulation
	(Premarin; conjugated estrogen)		estrogen, conjugated (conjugated
CEF	chick embryo fibroblast		estrogen substance)
	cyclophosphamide, epirubicin, and	CESB	chronic electrical stimulation of the
	fluorouracil		brain
CEFM	continuous external fetal monitoring	CES-D	Center for Epidemiologic Studies –
CEFOT	cefotaxime (Claforan)		Depression
CEFOX	cefoxitin (Mefoxtin)	CESI	cervical epidural steroid injection
CEFTAZ	ceftazidime	CET	common extensor tendon
CEFUR	cefuroxime	CETC	circulating epithelial tumor cells
CEI	continuous extravascular infusion	CETN	Certified Enterostomal Therapy
	converting enzyme inhibitor		Nurse
CEJ	cementoenamel junction (dental)	CETP	cholesterol ester transfer protein
	cervical-enamel junction (dental)	CEU	Utah residents with ancestry from
CEL	cardiac exercise laboratory		northern and western European
CELIP	Claims Expansion Line-item		ancestry (populations included in
	Processing		HapMap - see HapMap)
CELP	chronic erosive lichen planus	CEV	cyclophosphamide, etoposide, and
CEM	Clinical Event Manager		vincristine
CEMD	consultative examination by	CE w/IOL	cataract extraction with
	physician		intraocular lens
ceMRI	contrast-enhanced magnetic	CF	calcium leucovorin (citrovorum
	resonance imaging		factor)
CEN	Certified Emergency Nurse		cancer-free
	European Committee for		cardiac failure
	Standardization		Caucasian female
CENOG	computerized electroneuro-		Christmas factor
	ophthalmogram		cisplatin and fluorouracil
CEO	chief executive officer		complement fixation
CEOT	calcifying epithelial odontogenic		contractile force
	tumor		count fingers
CEP	cardiac enzyme panel		cystic fibrosis
	chronic eosinophilic pneumonia	C&F	cell and flare
	cognitive evoked potential		chills and fever
	congenital erythropoietic porphyria	CFA	common femoral artery
	countercurrent electrophoresis		complete Freund adjuvant
	cyclophosphamide, etoposide, and		cryptogenic fibrosing alveolitis
	cisplatin (Platinol AQ)		cystic fibrosis anthropathy

C

CFAC	complement-fixing antibody consumption	CFU-S	colony-forming unit–spleen
C-factor	cleverness factor	CFV	common femoral vein
CFCF	carbon fiber composite frame cage	CFVR	coronary flow velocity reserve
CFCs	chlorofluorocarbons	CFX	circumflex artery
CFD	color-flow Doppler	CG	cardiogreen (dye)
	computational fluid dynamics		caregiver
CFEOM	congenital fibrosis of the extraocular		cholecystogram
	muscles		contact guarding
CFF	critical fusion (flicker) frequency		contralateral groin
CFFT	critical flicker fusion threshold	CGA	clonal group A
CFH	chemical fume hood		comprehensive geriatric assessment
CFI	chemotherapy-free intervals		contact guard assist
	confrontation fields intact		corrected gestation age
CFIDS	chronic fatigue immune dysfunction syndrome	CGB	chronic gastrointestinal (tract) bleeding
CFL	cadaveric fascia lata	CGCG	central giant-cell granuloma
	calcaneofibular ligament	CGCR	Clinical Global Consensus Rating
	cisplatin, fluorouracil, and leucovorin calcium	CGD	chronic glycogen deficit
			chronic granulomatous disease
			cobalt gray equivalent
CFLX	ciprofloxacin (Cipro)	CGF	continuous gavage feeding (infant feeding)
	circumflex		
CFM	cerebral function monitor	CGI	Clinical Global Impressions (scale)
	close fitting mask	CGIC	Clinical Global Impression of Change
	craniofacial microsomia		
	cyclophosphamide, fluorouracil, and mitoxantrone	CGI-S	Clinical Global Impressions, Severity of Illness
CFNS	chills, fever, and night sweats	CGL	chronic granulocytic leukemia
CFP	cystic fibrosis protein		with correction/with glasses
CFPT	cyclophosphamide, fluorouracil, prednisone, and tamoxifen	CGM	continuous glucose monitoring
			cortical gray matter
CFR	case-fatality rates	CGMP	Current Good Manufacturing Practices
	Code of Federal Regulations		
	coronary flow reserve	cGMP	cyclic guanine monophosphate
CFRB	critical findings read back	CGN	Certified Gastroenterology Nurse
CFRN	Certified Flight Registered Nurse		chronic glomerulonephritis
CFRP	carbon-fiber reinforced polymer	cGN	crescentic glomerulonephritis
CFS	cancer family syndrome	C-GRD	coffee-ground
	Child and Family Service	CGRN	Certified Gastroenterology Registered Nurse
	childhood febrile seizures		
	chronic fatigue syndrome	CGRP	calcitonin gene-related peptide
	congenital fibrosarcoma	CGS	cardiogenic shock
	craniofacial surgery		catgut suture
CFSAN	Center for Food Safety and Applied Nutrition (FDA)		centimeter-gram-second system
		CGTT	cortisol glucose tolerance test
CFT	capillary filling time	cGVHD	chronic graft-versus-host disease
	chronic follicular tonsillitis	cGy	centigray
	complement fixation test	CH	Caribbean Hispanic
CFTR	cystic fibrosis transmembrane (conductance) regulator		chest
			chief
	cystic fibrosis transmembrane receptor		child (children)
			chronic
CFU	colony-forming units		cluster headache
CFU-E	colony-forming unit–erythroid		concentric hypertrophy
CFU-G	colony-forming unit–granulocyte		congenital hypothyroidism
CFU-G/M	colony-forming unit– granulocyte/macrophage		convalescent hospital
			crown-heal
CFU-M	colony-forming unit–macrophage	C_h	hepatic clearance

ch[1]	Christ Church chromosone		concentric hypertrophic cardiomyopathy
CH_{50}	total hemolytic complement		
C&H	cocaine and heroin	CH_3-	semustine
CHA	compound hypermetropic astigmatism	CCNU	
		CHCT	caffeine-halothane contracture test
	congenital hypoplastic anemia	cHct	central hematocrit
CHAD	cyclophosphamide, altretamine, (hexamethylmelamine), doxorubicin (Adriamycin), and cisplatin (DDP)	CHD	center hemodialysis
			changed diaper
			childhood diseases
			chronic hemodialysis
CHADS	an index that quantifies baseline risk of stroke for individuals with atrial fibrillation (congestive heart failure, hypertension, age greater than 75, diabetic, and history of stroke)		common hepatic duct
			congenital heart disease
			coordinate home care
		CHE	chronic hepatic encephalopathy
			comprehensive health examination
		CHEDDAR	Chief Compliant; History: social and physical as well as contributing factors; Examination; Details of problems and complaints; Drugs and dosage—list current meds; Assessment, diagnostic process, total impression; Return visit information or referral (format of documentation)
CHAI	Commission for Healthcare Audit and Inspection (United Kingdom)		
	continuous hepatic artery infusion		
CHAID	Chi Square Automatic Interaction Detection		
CHAM-OCA	cyclophosphamide, hydroxyurea, dactinomycin, methotrexate, vincristine, leucovorin, and doxorubicin		
CHAM-PUS	Civilian Health and Medical Program of the Uniformed Services	CHEF	clamped homogeneous electric field
		ChEI	cholinesterase inhibitor
		CHEM 7	see page 298
CHAMPVA	Civilian Health and Medical Program-Veterans Administration	CHEMO	chemotherapy
		ChemoRx	chemotherapy
		CHEOPS	Children's Hospital of Eastern Ontario Pain Scale
CHAP	child health associate practitioner		
	cyclophosphamide, altretamine, (hexamethylmelamine), doxorubicin (Adriamycin), and cisplatin (Platinol)	CHESS	chemical shift suppression
		CHF	congestive heart failure
			Crimean hemorrhagic fever
CHAQ	childhood health assessment questionnaire	CHFV	combined high-frequency of ventilation
CHARGE	coloboma (of eyes), hearing deficit, choanal atresia, retardation of growth, genital defects (males only), and endocardial cushion defect	CHG	change
			chlorhexidine gluconate
		CHI	chikungunya virus vaccine
			closed head injury
			Consolidated Health Informatics
CHART	complaint, history, assessment, Rx (treatment), transport		contrast harmonic imaging
			creatinine-height index
	continuous hyperfractionated accelerated radiotherapy	CHID	Combined Health Information Database
	Craig Handicap Assessment and Reporting Technique	CHIK	Chikungunya (virus)
CHB	chronic hepatitis B	CHILD	congenital hemidysplasia with ichthyosiform nevus and limb defects (syndrome)
	complete heart block		
	congenital heart block	CHIN	community health information network
	Han Chinese from Beijing (populations included in HapMap - see HapMap)	CHIP	Children's Health Insurance Program
			comprehensive health insurance plan
			iproplatin
CHBHA	congenital Heinz body hemolytic anemia	CHIR	Chiron Corporation
		Chix	chickenpox
CHC	community health center	CHL	conductive hearing loss

CHLC	Cooperative Human Linkage Center		Certified Hypnotherapist
ChloMP	chlorambucil, mitoxantrone, and prednisolone		chemotherapy
			closed head trauma
ChlVPP	chlorambucil, vinblastine, procarbazine, and prednisone	ChT	chemotherapy
		CHTN	chronic hypertension
CHM	complete hydatidiform mole	CHU	closed head unit
CHMP	Committee for Medicinal Products for Human Use (EMEA)	CHUC	Certified Health Unit Coordinator
		CHVP	cyclophosphamide, doxorubicin (hydroxydaunorubicin), teniposide (VM26), and prednisone
CHN	central hemorrhagic necrosis		
	Certified Hemodialysis Nurse		
	Chinese herb nephropathy	CHW	community health workers
	Community Health Nurse	CHWG	chewing gum
	community nursing home	CHX	chlorhexidine (Peridex; Periogard)
CHO	carbohydrate	CI	cardiac index
	Chemical Hygiene Officer		cerebral infarction
	Chinese hamster ovary		cesium implant
C_{H_2O}	free-water clearance		Clinical Instructor
CHO_a	cholera vaccine, attenuated live (oral)		cochlear implant
			cognitively impaired
CHO_{cn}- LPS	cholera vaccine, lipopolysaccharide-toxin conjugate		colon inertia
			commercial insurance
$C_2 H_5 OH$	alcohol (ethyl alcohol)		complete iridectomy
CHO_{i-w}	cholera vaccine, inactivated whole cell		confidence interval
			continuous infusion
CHO_{i-w-BS}	cholera vaccine, inactivated whole cell, B subunit		contraindications
			convergence insufficiency
chol	cholesterol		core imprint (cytology)
c̄ hold	withhold		coronary insufficiency
CHO_o	cholera, oral vaccine	Ci	curie(s)
CHOP	cyclophosphamide, doxorubicin (hydroxy-daunorubicin), vincristine (Oncovin), prednisone	CI30	cumulative incidence at 30 years
		CIA	calcaneal insufficiency avulsion
			chemotherapy-induced amenorrhea
CHOP- Bleo	cyclophosphamide, doxorubicin (hydroxydaunorubicin), vincristine (Oncovin), prednisone, and bleomycin		chemotherapy-induced anemia
			chronic idiopathic anhidrosis
			collagen-induced arthritis
		CIAA	competitive insulin autoantibodies
		CIAED	collagen-induced autoimmune ear disease
CHO_{tox}	cholera toxin/toxoid vaccine		
CHPB	Canadian Health Protection Branch (the equivalent of the U.S. Food and Drug Administration)	CIB	Carnation Instant Breakfast®
			crying-induced bronchospasm
			cytomegalic inclusion bodies
CHPN	Certified Hospice and Palliative Nurse	CIBD	chronic inflammatory bowel disease
		CIBI	Clinician Interview-Based Impression (of change)
CHPX	chickenpox		
CHR	Cercaria-Hullen reaction	CIBIC	Clinician Interview-Based Impression of Change
	chronic		
	complete hematological response	CIBIC- plus	Clinician Interview- Based Impression of Change with Caregiver Input
ChronoHAI	circadian-based hepatic artery infusion		
		CIBP	chronic intractable benign pain
CHRN	Certified Hyperbaric Registered Nurse	C-IBS	constipated predominant irritable bowel syndrome
CHRPE	congenital hypertrophy of the retinal pigment epithelium		
		CIC	cardioinhibitory center
CHRS	congenital hereditary retinoschisis		Certified in Infection Control
CHS	Chediak-Higashi syndrome		circulating immune complexes
	contact hypersensitivity		clean intermittent catheterization
CHT	Certified Hand Therapist		completely in-the-canal (hearing aid)
	Certified Hyperbaric Technician		coronary intensive care

CICE	combined intracapsular cataract extraction	CINAHL	Cumulative Index to Nursing and Allied Health
CICU	cardiac intensive care unit	CIND	cognitive impairment, no dementia
CICVC	centrally inserted central venous catheter	CINE	chemotherapy-induced nausea and emesis
CID	Center for Infectious Diseases (CDC)		cineangiogram
	Central Institute for the Deaf	CINV	chemotherapy-induced nausea and vomiting
	cervical immobilization device	CIO	corticosteroid-induced osteoporosis
	chemotherapy-induced diarrhea	CIOMS	The Council for International Organization of Medical Sciences
	combined immunodeficiency		
	cytomegalic inclusion disease	CIP	Cardiac Injury Panel
CIDP	chronic inflammatory demyelinating polyradiculoneuropathy (polyneuropathy)		critical illness polyneuropathy
		CIPD	chronic intermittent peritoneal dialysis
CIDS	cellular immunodeficiency syndrome	CIPN	chemotherapy-induced peripheral neuropathy
	continuous insulin delivery system		
CIE	capillary immunoelectrophoresis	CipRGC	ciprofloxacin-resistant *Neisseria gonorrhoeae*
	chemotherapy-induced emesis	CIR	continent intestinal reservoir
	congenital ichthyosiform erythroderma	CIRB	central institutional review board
	counterimmunoelectrophoresis	Circ	circulation
	crossed immunoelectrophoresis		circumcision
CIEA	continuous infusion epidural analgesia		circumference
			circumflex
CIEF	capillary isoelectric focusing	circ. & sen.	circulation and sensation
CIEP	counterimmunoelectrophoresis	CIRF	cocaine-induced respiratory failure
	crossed immunoelectrophoresis	CIRM	California Institute of Regenerative Medicine
CIFN	chemotherapy-induced fever and neutropenia		
		CIRS-G	Cumulative Illness Rating Scale-Geriatric
CI 5-FU	continuous infusion of fluorouracil	CIRT	carbon ion radiotherapy
CIG	cigarettes	CIS	Cancer Information Service (National Cancer Institute)
CIH	Certified in Industrial Health		
	continuous infusion haloperidol		carcinoma in situ
CIHD	chronic ischemic heart disease		clinically isolated syndrome
CIHI	Canadian Institute for Health Information		Commonwealth of Independent States
CIHR	Canadian Institutes of Health Research		continuous interleaved sampling
		CI&S	conjunctival irritation and swelling
CII	continuous insulin infusion	CISC	clean intermittent self-catheterization
CIIA	common internal iliac artery		
CIL	carbamazepine-induced lupus	CISCA	cisplatin, cyclophosphamide, and doxorubicin (Adriamycin)
CIM	change in menses		
	chemotherapy-induced mucositis	CISCOM	The Centralized Information Service for Complementary Medicine
	constraint-inducedmovement		
	convective interaction media	CISD	critical incident stress debriefing (used by EMTs)
	corticosteroid-induced myopathy		
	critical illness myopathy	Cis-DDP	cisplatin (Platinol)
CIMCU	cardiac intermediate care unit	CISH	chromogen in situ hybridization
CIMT	carotid (artery) intimamedia thickness	CISM	critical incident stress management (debriefing used by EMTs)
	constraint-induced movement therapy	CIS-R	Clinical Interview Schedule, Revised
		CI-Stim	cochlear implant stimulation
CIN	cervical intraepithelial neoplasia	CIT	chemotherapy-induced toxicities
	chemotherapy-induced neutropenia		constraint-induced therapy (protocol)
	chronic interstitial nephritis		conventional immunosuppressive therapy
C_{IN}	insulin clearance		conventional insulin therapy

C

CIT IDS	citation identifiers (National Library of Medicine)	CLASS I	congestive heart failure with no limitation with ordinary activity (New York Heart Association Classification)
CITP	capillary isotachophoresis		
CIU	chronic idiopathic urticaria		
	crisis intervention unit	CLASS II	congestive heart failure with slight limitation of physical activity
CIV	common iliac vein		
	continuous intravenous (infusion)	CLASS III	congestive heart failure with marked limitation of physical activity
CIVI	continuous intravenous infusion		
CIXU	constant infusion excretory urogram	CLASS IV	congestive heart failure with inability to engage in any physical activity without symptoms
CIWA-Ar	Clinical Institute Withdrawal Assessment for Alcohol–revised		
CJD	Creutzfeldt-Jakob disease	Clav	clavicle
cJET	congenital junctional ectopic tachycardia	CLB	chlorambucil (Leukeran) coccidian-like body
CJR	centric jaw relation	CLB_{atx}	*Clostridium botulinum* antitoxin
CJS	chronic joint symptoms	CLBBB	complete left bundle branch block
CK	check	CLBD	cortical Lewy body disease
	conductive keratoplasty	CLBP	chronic low back pain
	creatine kinase	CLB_{tox}	*Clostridium botulinum* toxoid vaccine
CK-BB	creatine kinase BB band (primarily in brain)		
		CLC	cork leather and celastic (orthotic)
CKC	cold-knife conization	CL/CP	cleft lip and cleft palate
CKD	chronic kidney disease	CLD	central lung distance
CK-ISO	creatine kinase isoenzyme		chronic liver disease
CK-MB	creatine kinase MB fraction (primarily in cardiac muscle)		chronic lung disease
			Clostridium difficile vaccine
CK MM	creatine kinase MM fraction (primarily in skeletal muscle)	Cl_d	dialysis clearance
		CLE	centrilobular emphysema
CKW	clockwise		congenital lobar emphysema
Cl	chloride		constant-load exercise
CL	central line		continuous lumbar epidural (anesthetic)
	chemoluminescence		
	clear liquid	CLED	cysteine lactose electrolyte-deficient (agar)
	cleft lip		
	cloudy	CLEIA	chemiluminescent enzyme immunoassay
	confidence limits		
	contact lens	CLEP	college level examination program
	critical list	CLF	cholesterol-lecithin flocculation
	cutaneous leishmaniasis	CLG	clorgyline
	cycle length	CLH	chronic lobular hepatitis
	lung compliance	C_h	hepatic clearance
C_L	compliance of the lungs	CLI	central lymphatic irradiation
C-L	consultation-liaison		clomipramine (Anafranil)
CLA	community living arrangements		critical leg (limb) ischemia
	congenital lactic acidosis	CLIA	chemiluminescent immunoassay
	congenital laryngeal atresia		Clinical Laboratory Improvement Act
	conjugated linoleic acid		
C lam	cervical laminectomy	Cl_{int}	intrinsic clearance
CLAMSS	cleavage- and ligation-associated mutation-specific sequencing	CLL	chronic lymphocytic leukemia
		CLLE	columnar-lined lower esophagus
CLAP	contact laser ablation of prostate	cl liq	clear liquid
CLARE	contact lens-associated acute red eye	CLM	colorectal liver metastases
		CLN	centrolobular necrosis
CLAS	Cancer Linear Analogue Scale	CLNC	Certified Legal Nurse Consultant
	congenital localized absence of skin	Cl_{nr}	nonrenal clearance
		CLO	*Campylobacter*-like organism
CLASS	computer laser-assisted surgical system		close
			cod liver oil

CLOX — clock-drawing task (cognitive impairment test)
CL & P — cleft lip and palate
CL PSY — closed psychiatry
CLPU — contact lens-induced peripheral ulceration
Cl_r — renal clearance
CLRB — clinical laboratory (results) read back
Cl Red — closed reduction
CLRO — community leave for reorientation
CLS — capillary leak syndrome
    community living skills
CLSE — calf-lung surfactant extract (Infasurf)
CLSM — confocal laser scanning microscopy
CLT — chronic lymphocytic thyroiditis
    complex lymphedema therapy
    cool lace tent
Cl_T — total body clearance
CLV — cutaneous leukocytoclastic vasculitis
CL VOID — clean voided specimen
CLW_c — *Clostridium welchii* type C (Pigbel) toxoid vaccine
clysis — hypodermoclysis
CLZ — clozapine (Clozaril)
cm — centimeter (2.54 cm = 1 inch)
CM — capreomycin (Capastat)
    CarboMedics (heart valve prosthesis)
    cardiac monitor
    cardiomegaly
    cardiomyopathy
    case management
    case manager
    Caucasian male
    centimeter (cm)
    cerebral malaria
    chondromalacia
    cochlear microphonics
    common migraine
    continuous microwave
    continuous murmur
    contrast media
    costal margin
    cow's milk
    culture media
    cutaneous melanoma
    cystic mesothelioma
    tomorrow morning (this is a dangerous abbreviation)
cM — centimorgan (one one-hundredth of a morgan; the unit of distance on a linkage map)
cm1 — circumflex marginal 1
cm2 — circumflex marginal 2
cm^2 — square centimeters
cm^3 — cubic centimeter
CMA — Certified Medical Assistant
    Certified MovementAnalyst
    compound myopic astigmatism
    cost-minimization analysis
    cow's milk allergy
CMAF — centrifuged microaggregate filter
CMAI — Cohen-Mansfield Agitation inventory
CMAP — compound muscle action potential
CMAPs — compound muscle action potentials
C_{max} — maximum concentration of drug
CMB — carbolic methylene blue
CMBBT — cervical mucous basal body temperature
CMC — carboxymethylcellulose
    carpal metacarpal (joint)
    chloramphenicol
    chronic mucocutaneous candidiasis
    clinically meaningful change
    closed mitral commissurotomy
CMCD — carboxymethylcellulose dressing
CMCN — Certified Managed Care Nurse
CMD — congenital muscular dystrophy
    corrected mass defect
    cytomegalic disease
CMDRH — Center for Medical Devices and Radiological Health (of the Food and Drug Administration)
CME — cervicomediastinal exploration (examination)
    continuing medical education
    cystoid macular edema
CMER — current medical evidence of record
CMF — cyclophosphamide, methotrexate and fluorouracil
CMFP — cyclophosphamide, methotrexate, fluorouracil, and prednisone
CMFT — cyclophosphamide, methotrexate, fluorouracil, and tamoxifen
CMFVP — cyclophosphamide, methotrexate, fluorouracil, vincristine, and prednisone
CMG — cystometrogram
CMGM — chronic megakaryocytic granulocytic myelosis
CMGN — chronic membranous glomerulonephritis
CMGs — case-mix groups
CMH — Cochran Mantel Haenszel
    current medical history
CMHC — Certified Mental Health Counselor
    Community Mental Health Center
    Community Migrant Health Center
CMHN — Community Mental Health Nurse
CMI — case mix index
    cell-mediated immunity
    clomipramine (Anafranil)
    Cornell Medical Index
CMID — cytomegalic inclusion disease
C_{min} — minimum concentration of drug
CMIR — cell-mediated immune response

CMJ	carpometacarpal joint		circulation motion sensation
	cervicomedullary junction		chocolate milkshake
CMK	congenital multicystic kidney		constant moderate suction
CML	cell-mediated lympholysis		continuous motion syndrome
	chronic myelogenous leukemia	CMSC	Certified Medical Staff Coordinator
	chronic myeloid leukemia	CMSUA	clean midstream urinalysis
CML5	lower second premolar	CMT	carpometatarsal (joint)
CML-BP	blastic phase chronic		Certified Massage Therapist
	myeloid leukemia		Certified Medication Technician
CMM	Comprehensive Major Medical		Certified Medical Transcriptionist
	(insurance)		Certified Music Therapist
	continuous metabolic monitor		cervical motion tenderness
	cutaneous malignant melanoma		Charot-Marie-Tooth (phenotype)
CMME	chloromethyl methyl ether		(disease)
CMML	chronic myelomacrocytic leukemia		Chiropractic manipulative
CMMS	Columbia Mental Maturity Scale		treatment
CMN	Certificate of Medical Necessity		choline magnesium trisalicylate
	congenital melanocytic nevi		(Trilisate)
	congenital mesoblastic nephroma		combined modality therapy
CMO	cardiac minute output		continuing medication and treatment
	cetyl myristoleate		cutis marmorata telangiectasia
	Chief Medical Officer	CMTX	chemotherapy treatment
	comfort measures only (resuscitation	CMUA	continuous motor unit activity
	order)	CMV	cisplatin, methotrexate, and
	consult made out		vinblastine
CMO 1	corticosterone methyl oxidase type 1		controlled mechanical ventilation
CMOP	cardiomyopathy		conventional mechanical ventilation
C-MOPP	cyclophosphamide, mechloreth-		cool mist vaporizer
	amine, vincristine (Oncovin),		cytomegalovirus
	procarbazine, and prednisone		cytomegalovirus vaccine
CMP	cardiomyopathy	CMVIG	cytomegalovirus immune globulin
	chondromalacia patellae	CMVS	culture midvoid specimen
	comprehensive (complete) metabolic	CN	charge nurse
	profile (see page 298)		congenital nystagmus
	cushion mouthpiece		cranial nerve
CMPA	cow's milk protein allergy		tomorrow night (this is a dangerous
CMPF	cow's milk, protein-free		abbreviation)
CMPS	chronic myofascial pain syndrome	Cn	cyanide
CMPT	cervical mucous penetration test	C/N	contrast-to-noise ratio
CMR	cardiovascular magnetic resonance	CN II–XII	cranial nerves 2 through 12
	cerebral metabolic rate	CNA	Certified in Nursing Administration
	chief medical resident		Certified Nurse Aide
	child (1-4 years) mortality rates		chart not available
	chloroform-methanol residue	C_{Na}	sodium clearance
	crude mortality rate	CNAA	Certified in Nursing Administration,
CMRI	cardiac magnetic resonance imaging		Advanced
CMRIT	combined modality	CNAG	chronic narrow angle glaucoma
	radioimmunotherapy	CNAP	continuous negative airway pressure
CMRNG	chromosomally mediated resistant	CNB	core-needle biopsy
	Neisseria gonorrhoeae	CNC	clinical nurse coordinator
CMRO	chronic multifocal recurrent		Community Nursing Center
	osteomyelitis		Consonant-Vowel Nucleus-
$CMRO_2$	cerebral metabolic rate for oxygen		Consonant (Maryland CNC
CMS	Centers for Medicare and Medicaid		word list)
	Services (replaces Health	CNCbl	cyanocobalamin (vitamin B_{12})
	Care Financing Administration	CND	canned
	[HCFA])		cannot determine
	children's medical services		chronic nausea and dyspepsia

C

CNDC	chronic nonspecific diarrhea of childhood	CNTF	ciliary neurotrophic factor
CNE	Chief Nurse Executive	CNV	choroidal neovascularization
	chronic nervous exhaustion	CNVM	choroidal neovascular membrane
	continuing nursing education	CO	carbon monoxide
	could not establish		cardiac output
	culture-negative endocarditis		castor oil
CNEP	continuous negative extrathoracic pressure		centric occlusion
			Certified Orthoptist
C-NES	conversion nonepileptic seizures		cervical orthosis
CNF	cyclophosphamide, mitoxantrone (Novatantrone), and fluorouracil		corneal opacity
			corn oil
CNH	central neurogenic hypernea		court order
	contract nursing home	Co	cobalt
CNHC	chronodermatitis nodularis helicis chronicus	C/O	check out
			complained of
	community nursing home care		complaints
CNI	calcineurin inhibitors		under care of
CNL	chemonucleolysis	^{60}Co	radioactive isotope of cobalt
	chronic neutrophilic leukemia	CO_2	carbon dioxide
	Connaught Laboratories	CO_3	carbonate
CNLCP	Certified Nurse Life Care Planner	COA	children of alcoholic
CNLD	chronic neonatal lung disease		coenzyme A
CNLSD	condensation nucleation light scattering detection		condition on admission
		CoA	coarctation of the aorta
CNM	certified nurse midwife	COAD	chronic obstructive airway disease
CNMP	chronic nonmalignant pain		chronic obstructive arterial disease
CNMT	Certified Nuclear Medicine Technologist	COAG	chronic open angle glaucoma
		COAGSC	coagulation screen
CNN	Certified in Nephrology Nursing	COAP	cyclophosphamide, vincristine (Oncovin), cytarabine (ara-C), and prednisone
	congenital nevocytic nevus		
CNNP	Certified Neonatal Nurse Practitioner		
CNO	Chief Nursing Officer	COAR	coarctation
	community nursing organization	COARCT	coarctation
CNOP	cyclophosphamide, mitoxantrone (Novantrone), vincristine (Oncovin), and prednisone	COB	cisplatin, vincristine (Oncovin), and bleomycin
			coordination of benefits
CNOR	Certified Nurse, Operating Room	COBE	chronic obstructive bullous emphysema
CNP	capillary nonprofusion		
CNPB	continuous negative pressure breathing	COBRA	Consolidated Omnibus Budget Reconciliation Act of 1985
CNPS	cardiac nuclear probe scan		
CNR	contrast-to-noise ratio (radiology)	COBS	chronic organic brain syndrome
CNRN	Certified Neurosurgical Registered Nurse	COBT	chronic obstruction of biliary tract
		COC	calcifying odontogenic cyst
CNS	central nervous system		chain of custody
	Certified Nutrition Specialist		combination oral contraceptive
	Clinical Nurse Specialist		continuity of care
	coagulase-negative staphylococci	COCCIO	coccidioidomycosis
	Crigler-Najjar syndrome	COCM	congestive cardiomyopathy
CNSD	Certified Nutrition Support Dietitian	COCN	Certified Ostomy Care Nurse
		CoCr	cobalt-chromium alloy
CNSHA	congenital nonspherocytic hemolytic anemia	COD	carotid occlusive disease
			cataract, right eye
CNSN	Certified Nutrition Support Nurse		cause of death
CNT	could not tell		chronic oxygen dependency
	could not test		codeine
CNTA	combined neurosurgical and transfacial approach		coefficient of oxygen delivery
			condition on discharge

CODAS	chronotherapeutic oral drug absorption system	COMP	Committee on Orphan Medicinal Products (EMEA)
CODE 99	patient in cardiac or respiratory arrest		compensation
CODES	Crash Outcome Data Evaluation System (National Highway Traffic Safety Administration-sponsored)		complications
			composite
			compound
			compress
COD-MD	cerebro-oculardysplasia muscular dystrophy		cyclophosphamide, vincristine (Oncovin), methotrexate, and prednisone
CODO	codocytes		
COE	court-ordered examination	COMS	clinical outcomes management system
COEPS	cortically originating extrapyramidal symptoms		
		COMT	catechol-O-methyl-transferase
COER-24	24-hour controlled-onset, extended-release (dosage form)	COMTA	Commission on Message Therapy Accreditation
COFS	cerebro-oculo-facioskeletal	CON	catheter over a needle
COG	center of gravity		certificate of need
	Central Oncology Group		conservatorship
	Children's Oncology Group	CON A	concanavalin A
	cognitive function tests	conc.	concentrated
COGN	cognition	CONG	congenital
COGTT	cortisone-primed oral glucose tolerance test		gallon
COH	carbohydrate	CONJ	conjunctiva
	controlled ovarian hyperstimulation	CONPA-DRI I	cyclophosphamide, vincristine, doxorubicin, and melphalan
COHb	carboxyhemoglobin		
COHN	Certified Occupational Health Nurse	CONPA-DRI II	conpadri I plus high-dose methotrexate
COHN/CM	Certified Occupational Health Nurse/Case Manager	CONPA-DRI III	conpadri I plus intensified doxorubicin
COHN-S	Certified Occupational Health Nurse - Specialist	CoNS	coagulase-negative staphylococci
		CONT	continuous
COHN-S/CM	Certified Occupational Health Nurse - Specialist Case Manager		contusions
		CON-TRAL	contralateral
COI	conflict of interest	CONTU	contusion
Coke	Coca-Cola®	CONV	conversation
	cocaine	Conv. ex.	convergence excess
COL	colonoscopy	ConvRX	conventional therapy
COLD	chronic obstructive lung disease	CO-Ox	Co-oximetry
	Computer Output to Laser Disk	COP	center of pressure
COLD A	cold agglutin titer		change of plaster
Collyr	eye wash		cicatricial ocular pemphigoid
col/ml	colonies per milliliter		Colibacilosis porcina vaccine
colp	colporrhaphy		colloid osmotic pressure
COLTRU	colletotrichum truncatum		complaint of pain
COM	calcium oxalate monohydrate		cryptogenic organizing pneumonia
	center of mass		cycophosphamide, vincristine (Oncovin), and prednisone
	chronic otitis media		
COMBO	combination ultrasound with electrical stimulation	CoP	Communities of Practice
			Conditions of Participation
COME	chronic otitis media with effusion	COP 1	copolymer 1
COMF	comfortable	COPA	cuffed oropharyngeal airway
COMLA	cyclophosphamide, vincristine (Oncovin), methotrexate, calcium leucovorin, and cytarabine (ara-C)	COPAdM	cyclophosphamide, vincristine (Oncovin), prednisone, doxorubicin (Adriamycin) and methotrexate
COMM E	Committee E, a German Federal Health Agency committee for the evaluation of herbal remedies		

COP-BLAM	cyclophosphamide, vincristine (Oncovin), prednisone, bleomycin, doxorubicin (Adriamycin), and procarbazine (Matulane)
COPD	chronic obstructive pulmonary disease
COPE	chronic obstructive pulmonary emphysema
COPP	cyclophosphamide, vincristine, procarbazine, and prednisone
COPS	community outpatient service
COPT	circumoval precipitin test
CoQ10	coenzyme Q_{10}
COR	coefficient of reproducibility
	conditioned orientation response
	coronary
CoR	custodian of records
CORA	conditioned orientation reflex audiometry
CORBA	Common-Object Request Broker Architecture
CORE	cardiac or respiratory emergency
CORF	Comprehensive Outpatient Rehabilitation Facility
CORLN	Certified Otorhinolaryngology and Head/Neck Nurse
COR P	cor pulmonale
CORT	Certified Operating Room Technician
COS	cataract, left eye
	change of shift
	Chief of Staff
	clinically observed seizure
	controlled ovarian stimulation
	Crisis Outpatient Services
C_{osm}	osmolal clearance
COSTART	Coding symbols for a thesaurus of adverse reaction terms
COT	content of thought
	court-ordered treatment
COTA	Certified Occupational Therapy Assistant
COTE	comprehensive occupational therapy evaluation
COTT CH	cottage cheese
COTX	cast-off, to x-ray
COU	cardiac observation unit
	cataracts, both eyes
COV	coefficient of variation
COW	circle of Willis
COWA	controlled oral word association
COWAT	Controlled Oral Word Association Test
COWS	cold to the opposite and warm to the same
COX	Coxsackie virus
	cyclo-oxygenase
	cytochrome C oxidase
COX-2	cyclo-oxygenase-2
CP	centric position
	cerebral palsy
	Certified Paramedic
	chemical peel
	chemistry profiles
	chest pain
	chloroquine-primaquine
	chondromalacia patella
	chronic pain
	chronic pancreatitis
	cleft palate
	clinical pathway
	closing pressure
	cold pack
	convenience package
	cor pulmonale
	creatine phosphokinase
	cyclophosphamide and cisplatin (Platinol)
	cystopanendoscopy
	process capability
C_p	concentration of drug plasma
	phosphate clearance
Cp	*Chlamydia pneumoniae*
C/P	carbohydrate-to-protein ratio
C&P	compensation and pension
	complete and pain-free (range of motion)
	complete and pushing
	cystoscopy and pyelography
CPA	cardiopulmonary arrest
	carotid photoangiography
	cerebellar pontile angle
	chest pain alert
	child protection agency
	color power angiography
	conditioned play audiometry
	costophrenic angle
	cyclophosphamide (Cytoxan)
	cyproterone acetate (Androcur)
CPAF	chlorpropamide-alcohol flush
C_{PAH}	para-amino hippurate clearance
CPAN	Certified Postanesthesia Nurse
CPAP	continuous positive airway pressure
CPB	cardiopulmonary bypass
	cisplatin, cyclophosphamide, and carmustine (BiCNU)
	competitive protein binding
CPBA	competitive protein-binding assay
CPBP	cardiopulmonary bypass
CPC	cancer prevention clinic
	cerebral palsy clinic
	Certified Procedural Coder
	chronic passive congestion
	clinicopathologic conference
	coil planet centrifuge
	continue plan of care

CPC-H	Certified Procedural Coder, Hospital-Based
CP-CML	chronic phase chronic myeloid leukemia
CPCR	cardiopulmonary-cerebral resuscitation
CPCS	clinical pharmacokinetics consulting service
CPD	cephalopelvic disproportion
	chorioretinopathy and pituitary dysfunction
	chronic peritoneal dialysis
	citrate-phosphate-dextrose
CPDA-1	citrate-phosphate-dextrose-adenine-one
CPDA-2	citrate-phosphate-dextrose-adenine-two
CPDD	calcium pyrophosphate deposition disease
CPDG2	carboxypeptidase-G2
CPDN	Certified Peritoneal Dialysis Nurse
CPDR	Center for Prostate Disease Research (Department of Defense)
CPE	cardiogenic pulmonary edema
	chronic pulmonary emphysema
	Clinical Pastoral Education
	clubbing, pitting, or edema
	complete physical examination
	continuing professional education
	cytopathic effect
CPEB	cytoplasmic polyadenylation element binding (protein)
CPE-C	cyclopentenylcytosine
CPEFM	Clear-Plan Easy Fertility Monitor
CPEO	chronic progressive external ophthalmoplegia
CPER	chest pain emergency room
CPET	cardiopulmonary exercise testing
CPETU	chest pain evaluation and treatment unit
CPF	cerebral perfusion pressure
	chlorpyrifos (an insecticide)
CPFT	Certified Pulmonary Function Technologist
CPFX	ciprofloxacin (Cipro)
CPG	clinical practice guidelines
CPG2	carboxypeptidase G2
CPGN	chronic progressive glomerulonephritis
CPH	chronic persistent hepatitis
CPHQ	Certified Professional in Healthcare Quality
CPhT	Certified Pharmacy Technician
CPI	chronic public inebriate
	constitutionally psychopathia inferior
CPID	chronic pelvic inflammatory disease
CPIP	chronic pulmonary insufficiency of prematurity

CPK	creatine phosphokinase (BB, MB, MM are isoenzymes)
CPK-1	creatine phosphokinase MM fraction
CPK-2	creatine phosphokinase MB fraction
CPK-BB	creatine phosphokinase BB fraction
CPKD	childhood polycystic kidney disease
CPK-MB	creatine phosphokinase of muscle band
CPL	criminal procedure law
CPM	cancer pain management
	central pontine myelinolysis
	chlorpheniramine maleate
	chronic progressive myelopathy
	Clinical Practice Model
	continue present management
	continuous passive motion
	counts per minute
	cycles per minute
	cyclophosphamide (Cytoxan)
CPmax	peak serum concentration
CPMDI	computerized pharmacokinetic model-driven drug infusion
CPmin	trough serum concentration
CPMM	constant passive motion machine
CPMP	Committee for Proprietary Medicinal Products (of the European Union)
CPN	Certified Pediatric Nurse
	chronic pyelonephritis
	common peroneal nerve
CPNA	Certified Pediatric Nurse Associate
CPNI	common peroneal nerve injury
CPO	chief privacy officer
	continue present orders
CPOE	computerized physician (prescriber) order entry
CPOM	continuous pulse oximeter monitoring
CPON	Certified Pediatric Oncology Nurse
CPOX	chicken pox
CPP	central precocious puberty
	cerebral perfusion pressure
	chronic pelvic pain
	coronary perfusion pressure
	cryo-poor plasma
CPPB	continuous positive pressure breathing
CPPD	calcium pyrophosphate dihydrate
	cisplatin
CP & PD	chest percussion and postural drainage
CPPS	chronic pelvice pain syndrome
CPPV	continuous positive pressure ventilation
CPQ	Conner Parent Questionnaire
CPR	cardiopulmonary resuscitation
	computer-based patient records
	computerized patient record
	customary, prevailing and reasonable (charge payment method)

	tablet (French)
CPR-1	all measures except cardiopulmonary resuscitation
CPR-2	no extraordinary measures (to resuscitate)
CPR-3	comfort measures only
CPRAM	controlled partial rebreathing anesthesia method
CP/ROMI	chest pain, rule out myocardial infarction
CPRS	Categorical Pain Relief Scale
CPRS-OCS	Comprehensive Psychiatric Rating Scale, Obsessive-Compulsive Subscale
CPS	carbamyl phosphate synthetase
	cardiopulmonary support
	Center for Prevention Services (CDC)
	cervical pedicle screw
	chest pain syndrome
	child protective services
	Chinese paralytic syndrome
	chloroquine-pyrimethamine sulfadoxine
	chronic paranoid schizophrenia
	clinical performance score
	clinical pharmacokinetic service
	CoaguChek® Plus System
	coagulase-positive staphylococci
	complex partial seizures
	counts per second
	cumulative probability of success
CPs	clinical pathways
CPS I	carbamyl phosphate synthetase I
cPSA	complexed prostate-specific antigen
CPSC	Consumer Product Safety Commission
CPSI	Chronic Prostatitis Symptom Index
CPSN	Certified Plastic Surgical Nurse
CPSP	central post-stroke pain
CPT	camptothecin
	carnitine palmitoyl transferase
	chest physiotherapy
	child protection team
	chromo-perturbation
	chronic paranoid type
	cold pressor test
	Continuous Performance Test
	corticosteroid pulse treatment
	current perception threshold
	Current Procedural Terminology (coding system)
CPT-2007	Current Procedural Terminology, 2007 Edition
CPT-11	irinotecan hydrochloride (Camptosar)
CPTA	Certified Physical Therapy Assistant

CPT/C	current perception threshold, computerized
CPTH	chronic post-traumatic headache
CPU	children's psychiatric unit
	clinical pharmacology unit
CPUE	chest pain of unknown etiology
CPUM	Certified Professional in Utilization Management
CPV	canine parvovirus
	cowpox virus
CPX	complete physical examination
CPZ	chlorpromazine
	Compazine® (CPZ is a dangerous abbreviation as it could be either)
CQ	chloroquine
CQDS	cumulative quality disruption score
CQI	continuous quality improvement
CR	caloric restrictions
	capillary refill
	cardiac rehabilitation
	cardiorespiratory
	case reports
	chief resident
	chorioretinal
	clockwise rotation
	closed reduction
	colon resection
	complete remission
	contact record
	controlled release
	cosmetic rhinoplasty
	creamed
	credentialing
	crutches
	cycloplegia retinoscopy
Cr	caloric restrictions
	chromium
	creatinine
C/R	conscious, rational
C & R	convalescence and rehabilitation
	cystoscopy and retrograde
CR₁	first cranial nerve
CRA	central retinal artery
	chronic rheumatoid arthritis
	cis-retinoic acid (isotretinion, Accutane®)
	Clinical Research Associate
	colorectal anastomosis
	Contract Research Assistant
	corticosteroid-resistant asthma
CRABP	cellular retinoic acid binding protein
CRAbs	chelating recombinant antibodies
CRADA	Cooperative Research and Development Agreement (with NIH)
CRAG	cerebral radionuclide angiography
CrAg	cryptococcal antigen

CRAMS	circulation, respiration, abdomen, motor, and speech		CRKL	crackles
CRAN	craniotomy		CRL	crown rump length
CRAO	central retinal artery occlusion		CRM	circumferential resection margins
CRAX	crackers			continual reassessment method
CRB	Clinical Review Board			cream
CRBBB	complete right bundle branch block			cross-reacting mutant
CRBIs	catheter-related bloodstream infections		CRM +	cross-reacting material positive
			CRMD	children with retarded mental development
CRBP	cellular retinol-binding protein		CRN	Certified Radiologic Nurse
CRBSI	catheter-related bloodstream infections			crown
			CRNA	Certified Registered Nurse Anesthetist
CRC	case review committee			
	child-resistant container		CRNFA	Certified Registered Nurse, First Assistant
	clinical research center			
	Clinical Research Coordinator		CRNH	Certified Registered Nurse in Hospice
	colorectal cancer			
CRCLM	colorectal cancer liver metastases		CRNI	Certified Registered Nurse Intravenous
CR & C	closed reduction and cast			
CrCl	creatinine clearance		CRNL	Certified Registered Nurse - Long-Term Care
CRD	childhood rheumatic disease			
	chronic renal disease		CRNO	Certified Registered Nurse in Ophthalmology
	chronic respiratory disease			
	colorectal distension		CRNP	Certified Registered Nurse Practitioner
	cone-rod dystrophy			
	congenital rubella deafness		CRO	cathode ray oscilloscope
	crown-rump distance			contract research organization(s)
CRE	cumulative radiation effect		CROM	cervical range of motion
CREAT	serum creatinine			chronic refractory osteomyelitis
CREC	ciprofloxacin-resistant *Escherichia coli*		CROMY	chronic refractory osteomyelitis
			CROS	contralateral routing of signals
CREF	cycloplegic refraction		CRP	canalith repositioning procedure
CRELM	screening tests for Congo-Crimean, Rift Valley, Ebola, Lassa, and Marburg fevers			chronic relapsing pancreatitis
				coronary rehabilitation program
				C-reactive protein
CREP	crepitation		C&RP	curettage and root planning
CREST	calcinosis, Raynaud disease, esophageal dysmotility, sclerodactyly, and telangiectasia		CRPA	C-reactive protein agglutinins
			CRPC	castration-refractory prostate cancer
			CRPD	chronic restrictive pulmonary disease
CRF	cancer-related fatigue		CRPF	chloroquine-resistant *Plasmodium falciparum*
	cardiac risk factors			
	case report form		CRPP	closed reduction and percutaneous pinning
	chronic renal failure			
CRG-L2	Cancer related gene-Liver 2		CRPS	complex regional pain syndromes
CRH	corticotropic-releasing hormone		CRPS I	complex regional pain syndrome type I
CRFZ	closed reduction of fractured zygoma			
CRH	corticotropin-releasing hormone		CRQ	Chronic Respiratory (Disease) Questionnaire
CRHCa	cancer-related hypercalcemia			
CRI	Cardiac Risk Index		CRR	community rehabilitation residence
	catheter-related infection		CRRN	Certified Rehabilitation Registered Nurse
	chronic renal insufficiency			
CRIB	Clinical Risk Index for Babies		CRRN-A	Certified Rehabilitation Registered Nurse - Advanced
CRIE	crossed radioimmunoelectrophoresis			
CRIF	closed reduction and internal fixation		CRRT	continuous renal replacement therapy
CRIMF	closed reduction/intermaxillary fixation			
			CRS	Carroll Self-Rating Scale
CRIS	controlled-release infusion system			catheter-related sepsis
crit	hematocrit			Center for Scientific Review (NIH)

	Chemical Reference Substances
	child restraint system(s)
	Chinese restaurant syndrome
	chronic rhinosinusitis
	cocaine-related seizure(s)
	colon-rectal surgery
	congenital rubella syndrome
	continuous running suture
	cryoreductive surgery
	cytokine-release syndrome
CRSD	circadian rhythm sleep disorder
CRST	calcification, Raynaud phenomenom, scleroderma, and telangiectasia
CRT	cadaver renal transplant
	capillary refill time
	Cardiac Rescue Technician
	cardiac resynchronization therapy
	cartilage roof triangle
	cathode ray tube
	central reaction time
	Certified Rehabilitation Therapist
	chemoradiotherapy
	choice reaction time
	circuit resistance training
	copper reduction test
	cranial radiation therapy
CRT-D	cardiac resynchronization therapy defibrillator
Cr Tr	crutch training
CRTs	case report tabulations
CRTT	Certified Respiratory Therapy Technician
CRTX	cast removed take x-ray
CRU	cardiac rehabilitation unit
	catheterization recovery unit
	clinical research unit
CRV	central retinal vein
CRVF	congestive right ventricular failure
CRVO	central retinal vein occlusion
CRx	chemotherapy
CIIRx	Century II Bicarbonate Dialysis Machine
CRYO	cryoablation
	cryosurgery
CRYST	crystals
CS	cardiogenic shock
	cardioplegia solution
	cat scratch
	cervical spine
	cesarean section
	chest strap
	cholesterol stone
	chlorobenzylidene malononitrile
	cigarette smoker
	clinically significant
	Clinical Specialist
	clinical stage
	close supervision

	conditionally susceptible
	congenital syphilis
	conjunctiva-sclera
	consciousness
	conscious sedation
	consultation
	consultation service
	coronary sinus
	corticosteroid(s)
	cranial setting
	Cushing syndrome
	cycloserine
	o-chlorobenzylidene malononitrile
C&S	conjunctiva and sclera
	cough and sneeze
	culture and sensitivity
C/S	cesarean section
	consultation
	culture and sensitivity
CSA	central sleep apnea
	childhood sexual abuse
	compressed spectral activity
	Controlled Substances Act
	controlled substance analogue
	corticosteroid-sensitive asthma
	cryosurgical ablation
CsA	cyclosporine (cyclosporin A)
CsA-ME	cyclosporine microemulsion (Neoral)
CSAP	cryosurgical ablation of the prostate
CSB	caffeine sodium benzoate
	Cheyne-Stokes breathing
	Children's Services Board
CSBF	coronary sinus blood flow
CSBO	complete small bowel obstruction
CSC	central serous chorioretinopathy
	cornea, sclera, and conjunctiva
	cryogen spray cooling
	cryopreserved stem cells
CSCI	continuous subcutaneous infusion
CSCR	central serous chorioretinopathy
CSD	cat scratch disease
	celiac sprue disease
	cortical spreading depression
C S&D	cleaned, sutured, and dressed
CSDD	Center for the Study of Drug Development
CSDH	chronic subdural hematoma
	combined systolic and diastolic hypertension
CSE	combined spinal/epidurals
	cross-section echocardiography
CSEA	combined spinal-epidural anesthesia
C sect.	cesarean section
CSF	cerebrospinal fluid
	colony-stimulating factors
CSFELP	cerebrospinal fluid electrophoresis

CSFP	cerebrospinal fluid pressure	CSS	Canadian Stroke Scale (score)
CSGIT	continuous-suture graft-inclusion technique		carotid sinus stimulation

CSFP   cerebrospinal fluid pressure
CSGIT   continuous-suture graft-inclusion technique
C-Sh   chair shower
CSH   carotid sinus hypersensitivity
     chronic subdural hematoma
     combat surgical hospital(s)
CSHQ   Children's Sleep Habits Questionnaire
CSI   chemical shift imaging
     Computerized Severity Index
     continuous subcutaneous infusion
     coronary stent implantation
     corticosteroid injection
     craniospinal irradiation
CsI   cesium iodide
CSICU   cardiac surgery intensive care unit
CSID   congenital sucrase-isomaitase deficiency
CSII   continuous subcutaneous insulin infusion
CSIO   continuous subcutaneous infusion of opiates
CS IV   clinical stage 4
CSL   chemical safety level
CSLO   confocal scanning laser ophthalmoscopy
CSLU   chronic status leg ulcer
CSM   carotid sinus massage
     cerebrospinal meningitis
     cervical spondylotic myelopathy
     circulation, sensation, and movement
     Committee on Safety of Medicines (United Kingdom)
CSME   cotton-spot macular edema
CSMN   chronic sensorimotor neuropathy
CSN   Certified School Nurse
     cystic suppurative necrosis
CSNB   congenital stationary night blindness
CSNRT   corrected sinus node recovery time
CSNS   carotid sinus nerve stimulation
CSO   Chief Security Officer
     Consumer Safety Officer (FDA)
     copied standing orders
CSOM   chronic serous otitis media
     chronic suppurative otitis media
CSP   cellulose sodium phosphate
     cervical spine pain
     chiral stationary phase
C-SPI   Certified Specialist in Poison Information
C-spine   cervical spine
CSR   central supply room
     Cheyne-Stokes respiration
     clinical statistical report
     corrected sedimentation rate
     corrective septorhinoplasty
C-S RT   craniospinal radiotherapy

CSS   Canadian Stroke Scale (score)
     carotid sinus stimulation
     Central Sterile Services
     chemical sensitivity syndrome
     chewing, sucking, and swallowing
     child safety seats
     Churg-Strauss syndrome
C_{ss} concentration of drug at steady-state
CSSD   closed system sterile drainage
CSSSIs   complicated skin and skin-structure infections
CSSU   cardiac short-stay unit
CST   cardiac stress test
     castration
     central sensory conducting time
     cerebroside sulfotransferase
     Certified Surgical Technologist
     cesarean section prior to labor at term
     contraction stress test
     convulsive shock therapy
     cosyntropin stimulation test
     static compliance
C_{STAT} static lung compliance
CSTE   Council of State and Territorial Epidemiologists
CSU   cardiac surgery unit
     cardiac surveillance unit
     cardiovascular surgery unit
     casualty staging unit
     catheter specimen of urine
CSVD   cerebral small-vessel disease
CSVT   cerebral sinovenous thrombosis
CSW   cerebral salt-wasting (syndrome)
     Clinical Social Worker
     commercial sex worker
CSWCM   Certified Social Work Case Manager
CSWs   commercial sex workers
CSWSS   continuous spike-waves during slow sleep
CT   calcitonin
     calf tenderness
     cardiothoracic
     carpal tunnel
     cellulose triacetate (filter)
     cervical traction
     chemotherapy
     chest tube
     Chlamydia trachomatis
     circulation time
     client
     clinical trial
     clotting time
     coagulation time
     coated tablet
     compressed tablet
     computed tomography
     Coomb test

C

	corneal thickness	CTGF	connective tissue growth factor
	corneal transplant	CTH	clot to hold
	corrective therapy	CTHA	computed tomography hepatic
	cytarabine and thioguanine		arteriography
	cytoxic drug	CTI	certification of terminal illness
C_t	concentration of drug in tissue	CTIBL	cancer treatment-induced bone loss
C/T	compared to	CTICU	cardiothoracic intensive care unit
CTA	catamenia (menses)	CTID	chemotherapy-induced diarrhea
	clear to auscultation	CTL	cervical, thoracic, and lumbar
	computed tomographic angiography		chronic tonsillitis
C-TAB	cyanide tablet		control (subjects)
CTAP	clear to auscultation and percussion		cytotoxic T-lymphocytes
	computed tomography during arterial	CTLSO	cervicothoracic-lumbosacral orthosis
	portography	CTM	Chlor-Trimeton
CTB	ceased to breathe		clinical trials materials
	cholera toxin B		computed tomographic myelography
CTC	Cancer Treatment Center	CT/MPR	computed tomography with
	circular tear capsulotomy		multiplanar reconstructions
	circulating tumor cells	CTN	calcitonin
	Clinical Trial Certificate (United		Certified Transcultural Nurse
	Kingdom's equivalent to the	C & T N,	color and temperature
	Investigational New Drug	BLE	normal, both lower extremities
	Application)	cTnC	cardiac troponin C
	Common Toxicity Criteria	cTnI	cardiac troponin I
	computed tomographic colonography	cTNM	clinical-diagnostic staging of cancer
	cyclophosphamide, thiotepa, and	CTnT	cardiac troponin T
	carboplatin	CTO	chronic total (coronary) occlusion
CTCAE	Common Terminology Criteria for	CTP	comprehensive treatment plan
v3.0	Adverse Events, version 3.0	CTPA	clear to percussion and auscultation
	(National Cancer Institute grading	CTPN	central total parenteral nutrition
	system for treatment-related	CTR	carpal tunnel release
	toxicities; grade 1 = mild, grade		carpal tunnel repair
	2 = moderate, grade 3 = severe,		Certified Tumor Registrar
	grade 4 = life-threatening or		cosmetic transdermal reconstruction
	disabling, grade 5 = death related	CTRB	Clinical Trial Review Board
	to adverse event)		critical tests read back
CTCL	cutaneous T-cell lymphoma (mycosis	CTRS	Certified Therapeutic Recreation
	fungoides)		Specialist
CT & DB	cough, turn & deep breath		Conners Teachers Rating Scale
CTD	carboxy-terminal domain	CT-RT	chemo-radiotherapy
	carpal tunnel decompression	CTS	cardiothoracic surgeon
	chest tube drainage		carpal tunnel syndrome
	connective tissue disease		closed-tube sampling
	corneal thickness depth	CTSP	called to see patient
	cumulative trauma disorder	CTT	cotton-thread test
CTDW	continues to do well	CTTH	chronic tension-type headache
CTEP	Cancer Therapy Evaluation Program	CTU	computed tomographic urography
	Center for Therapy Evaluation	CTW	central terminal of Wilson
	Programs (National Cancer	CTX	cerebrotendinous xanthomatosis
	Institute)		cervical traction
CTF	Colorado tick fever		chemotherapy
	continuous tube feeding		cyclophosphamide (Cytoxan)
CTG	cardiotocography	CTXN	contraction
C/TG	cholesterol to triglyceride ratio	CTZ	chemoreceptor trigger zone
CTGA	complete transposition of the great		co-trimoxazole (sulfamethoxazole
	arteries		and trimethoprim)
	corrected transposition of the great	CU	cause undetermined
	arteries		cause unknown

	chronic undifferentiated
	clinical units
	color unit
	convalescent unit
	Cuprophan (filter)
Cu	copper
C_u	urea clear clearance
C/U	checkup
	creatinine/urea ratio
CUA	Certified Urologic Associate
	clean urinalysis
	cost-utility analysis
CUC	chronic ulcerative colitis
	Clinical Unit Clerk
CUCNS	Certified Urologic Clinical Nurse Specialist
CUD	cause undetermined
	controlled unsterile delivery
CUFCM	Century Ultrafiltration Control Machine
CUG	cystourethrogram
Cu-IUD	copper intrauterine device
CUNP	Certified Urologic Nurse Practitioner
CUOG	Canadian Urologic Oncology Group
CUP	carcinoma of unknown primary (site)
CUPS	carcinoma of unknown primary site
CUR	curettage
	cystourethrorectocele
CURN	Certified Urologic Registered Nurse
CUS	carotid ultrasound
	chronic undifferentiated schizophrenia
	compression ultrasonography
	contact urticaria syndrome
CUSA	Cavitron ultrasonic suction aspirator
CUT	chronic undifferentiated type (schizophrenia)
CUTA	congenital urinary tract anomaly
CV	cardiovascular
	cell volume
	cisplatin and etoposide (VePesid)
	coefficient of variation
	color vision
	common ventricle
	consonant vowel
	contrast venography
	curriculum vitae
C/V	cervical/vaginal
CVA	cerebrovascular accident
	costovertebral angle
	cough-variant asthma
CVAAS	cold vapor atomic absorption spectrometry
CVAD	central venous access device
CVAH	congenital virilizing adrenal hyperplasia
CVAT	costovertebral angle tenderness

CVB	chronic villi biopsy
	group B coxsackievirus
CVC	central venous catheter
	chief visual complaint
	consonant-vowel-consonant
CVD	cardiovascular disease
	collagen vascular disease
CVDU	chronic ventilator-dependent unit
CVEB	cisplatin, vinblastine, etoposide, and bleomycin
CVENT	controlled ventilation
CVF	cardiovascular failure
	central visual field
	cervicovaginal fluid
	colovesical fistula
CVG	coronary vein graft
	cutis verticis gyrata
CVHD	chronic valvular heart disease
CVI	carboplatin, etoposide, ifosfamide, and mesna uroprotection
	cerebrovascular insufficiency
	chronic venous insufficiency
	common variable immunodeficiency (disease)
	continuous venous infusion
CVICU	cardiovascular intensive care unit
CVID	common variable immune deficiency
CVINT	cardiovascular intermediate
CVL	central venous line
	cervicovaginal lavage
	clinical vascular laboratory
CVLP	chimeric virus-like particles
CVLT	California Verbal Learning Test
CVM	Center for Veterinary Medicine (NIH)
CVMP	Committee for Medicinal Products for Veterinary Use (EMEA)
CVMT	cervical-vaginal, motion tenderness
CVN	central venous nutrient
	Certified Vascular Nurse
CVNSR	cardiovascular normal sinus rhythm
CVO	central vein occlusion
	conjugate diameter of pelvic inlet
CvO_2	mixed venous oxygen content
CVOD	cerebrovascular obstructive disease
CVOR	cardiovascular operating room
CVP	central venous pressure
	cyclophosphamide, vincristine, and prednisone
CVPP	lomustine, vinblastine, procarbazine, and prednisone
CVR	cerebral vascular resistance
	cerebrovascular resuscitation
	coronary vascular reserve
CVRI	coronary vascular resistance index
CVRS	Cardiovascular-Respiratory Score
CVS	cardiovascular surgery
	cardiovascular system

	challenge virus standard		cylinder axis
	chorionic villi sampling		cystectomy
	clean voided specimen	Cx	consultation
	continuing vegetative state	CXA	circumflex artery
CVSCU	cardiovascular special care unit	CxBx	cervical biopsy
CVSD	congenital ventricular septal defecct	CxMT	cervical motion tenderness
CVST	cardiovascular stress test	CXR	chest x-ray
	cerebral venous sinus thrombosis	CXTX	cervical traction
CVSU	cardiovascular specialty unit	CY	calendar year
CVT	calf vein thrombosis		cyclophosphamide (Cytoxan)
CVTC	central venous tunneled catheter	C&Y	Children with Youth (program)
CVU	clean voided urine	CYA	cover your ass
CVUG	cysto-void urethrogram	CyA	cyclosporine
CVVH	continuous venovenous	CyADIC	cyclophosphamide, doxorubicin
	hemofiltration		(Adriamycin), and dacarbazine
CVVHDF	continuous venovenous	CYC	cyclophosphamide
	hemodiafiltration	Cyclo C	cyclocytidine HCl
CW	careful watch	CYL	cylinder
	case worker	CYP	cytochrome P-450 system
	chest wall	CYP450	cytochrome P450 system
	clockwise	CYRO	cryoprecipitate
	compare with	CYSTA	cystathionine
C/W	consistent with	CYSTO	cystogram
	crutch walking		cystoscopy
CWA	chemical warfare agents	CYT	cyclophosphamide (Cytoxan)
CWAF	Chemical Withdrawal Assessment	CYTA	cytotoxic agent
	Flowsheet	CYVA DIC	cyclophosphamide,
CWAP	continuous wave arthroscopy pump		vincristine, Adriamycin, and
CWCN	Certified Wound Care Nurse		dacarbazine
CWD	canal-wall down	CZE	capillary zone electrophoresis
	cell-wall defective	CZI	crystalline zinc insulin (regular
	change wet dressing		insulin)
	chronic wasting disease	CZP	clonazepam (Klonopin)
CWE	cotton-wool exudates		
CWL	Caldwell-Luc		
CWM	comprehensive weight management		
CWMS	color, warmth, movement, and		
	sensation		
CWOCN	Certified Wound, Ostomy and		
	Continence Nurse		
CWP	centimeters of water pressure		
	childbirth without pain		
	coal worker's pneumoconiosis		
	cold wet packs		
cWPW	concealed Wolff-Parkinson-White		
	syndrome		
CWR	clockwise rotation		
CWS	Certified Wound Care Specialist		
	comfortable walking speed		
	cotton-wool spots		
CWT	compensated work training		
CWV	closed wound vacuum		
CX	cancel		
	cervix		
	chronic		
	circumflex		
	circumflex artery		
	culture		

C

D

D	daughter
	day
	dead
	decay
	dependent
	depression
	dextrose
	dextro
	diarrhea
	diastole
	dictated
	dilated
	diminished
	Dinamap (blood pressure monitor)
	diopter
	distal
	distance
	divorced
	dream
D+	note has been dictated/look for report
D−	note not dictated, save chart for doctor
$D_{0(2/7/07)}$	Day zero (the day treatment begins, February 7th, 2007)
D_1	day one (first day of treatment) first diagonal branch (coronary artery)
D-1 . . . . D-12	dorsal vertebrae 1 to 12 dorsal nerves 1-12
D_2	second diagonal branch (coronary artery) ergocalciferol
2/d	twice a day (this is a dangerous abbreviation)
2-D	two-dimensional
3-D	three-dimensional
D_3	cholecalciferol
D-3+7	cytarabine and daunorubicin
4D	4 prism diopters
4-D	four-dimensional
D5	dextrose 5% injection
5xD	five times a day (this is a dangerous abbreviation)
D-15	Farnsworth panel D-15 color vision test
D50	50% dextrose injection
$D_{5/.45}$	dextrose 5% in 0.45% sodium chloride injection
DA	darbepoetin alfa (Aranesp) dark adaptation (test) Debtors Anonymous degenerative arthritis delivery awareness Dental Assistant

	diagnostic arthroscopy
	diastolic augmentation
	direct admission
	direct agglutination
	disk areas
	diversional activity
	dopamine
	drug addict
	drug aerosol
Da	daltons
D/A	discharge and advise
DAA	dead after arrival dissection aortic aneurysm
DA/A	drug/alcohol addiction
DAB	days after birth diamino benzidine
DABA	Diplomate of the American Board of Anesthesiology
DAC	day activity center decitabine disabled adult child Division of Ambulatory Care
DACL	Depression Adjective Checklists
DACS	density-adjusted cell sorting
DACT	dactinomycin (Cosmegen)
DAD	diffuse alveolar damage diode array detector Disability Assessment of Dementia dispense as directed drug administration device father
DADS	distal acquired demyelinating symmetrical (neuropathy)
DAE	diving air embolism
DAEC	diffuse-adherence *Entamoeba coli*
DAF	decay-accelerating factor delayed auditory feedback
DAFE	Dial-A-Flow Extension®
DAFM	double-aerosol face mask
DAFNE	dose adjustment for normal eating
DAG	diacylglyerol dianhydrogalactitol
DAH	diffuse alveolar hemorrhage disordered action of the heart
DAI	diffuse axonal injury
DAIDS	Division of AIDS (of the National Institute of Allergy and Infectious Diseases, NIH)
DAL	diffuse aggressive lymphomas drug analysis laboratory
DALE	disability-adjusted life expectancy
DALM	dysplasia-associated lesion or mass
DALY	disability-adjusted life year(s)
DAM	diacetylmonoxine
DAMA	discharged against medical advice

DAMP	deficits in attention, motor control, and perception	DAWN	Drug Abuse Warning Network
DAN	diabetic autonomic neuropathy	dB	decibel
DANA	drug-induced antinuclear antibodies	DB	database
DAo	descending aorta		date of birth
DAOM	depressor anguli oris muscle		deep breathe
DAP	dapsone		demonstration bath
	diabetes-associated peptide		dermabrasion
	diastolic augmentation pressure		diaphragmatic breathing
	distending airway pressure		difficulty breathing
	Draw-A-Person		direct bilirubin
			double blind
DAPT	Draw-A-Person Test	DBA	Diamond-Blackfan anemia
DAR	daily affective rhythm	dBA	decibel, weighted according to the A scale
	data, action, response		
DARB	darbepoetin alfa (Aranesp)	DB & C	deep breathing and coughing
DARE	data, action, response, and evaluation	DBD	milolactol (dibromodulicitol)
DARP	drug abuse rehabilitation program	DBDS	Dementia Behavior Disturbance Scale
	drug abuse reporting program		
DARPA	Defense Advanced Research Projects Agency (US Department of Defense)	DBE	deep breathing exercise
		DBED	penicillin G benzathine (for IM use only; Bicillin L-A)
DARQ	diarylquinoline	dBEMCL	decibel effective masking contralateral
D/ART	depression/awareness, recognition and treatment		
		D₅BES	dextrose in balanced electrolyte solution
DAS	day of admission surgery		
	developmental apraxia of speech	DBI	documented by initials
	died at scene	DBI®	phenformin HCl
	distractive auditory stimuli	DBIL	direct bilirubin
	dynamometer anchoring station	DBKT	Diabetes: Basic Knowledge Test
DAs	daily activities	DBL	double beta-lactam
DASE	dobutamine-atropine stress echocardiography	DBM	dibenzoylmethane
		DBMT	displacement bone marrow transplantation
DASH	Dietary Approaches to Stop Hypertension (diet)		
		DBP	D-binding protein
	Disabilities of the Arm, Shoulder and Hand (rating)		diastolic blood pressure
			dibutyl phthalate
DASI	Duke Activity Status Index	DBPCFC	double-blind, placebo-controlled food challenge
DAST	Drug Abuse Screening Test		
DAT	daunorubicin, cytarabine, (ara-C), and thioguanine	DBPT	dacarbazine (DTIC), carmustine (BCNU), cisplatin (Platinol), and tamoxifen
	definitely abnormal tracing (electrocardiogram)		
		DBQ	debrisoquin
	dementia of the Alzheimer type	DBS	deep brain stimulation
	diet as tolerated		desirable body weight
	diphtheria antitoxin		diminished breath sounds
	direct agglutination test		dried blood stain
	direct amplification test	DBT	dialectical behavior therapy
	direct antiglobulin test	DBW	dry body weight
DAU	daughter	DBZ	dibenzamine
	drug abuse urine	DC	daunorubicin and cytarabine
DAUNO	daunorubicin		daycare
DAVA	vindesine sulfate (Eldisine; desacetyl vinblastine amide sulfate)		deceleration capacity (heart)
			decrease
DAVE	The Data Assessment and Verification program		dendritic cells
			dextrocardia
DAVM	dural arteriovenous malformation		diagonal conjugate
DAV SEP	deviated septum		direct Coombs (test)
DAW	dispense as written		direct current

discharge (This is a dangerous abbreviation as it is read as discontinue)

discomfort

Doctor of Chiropractic

D&C dilatation and curettage
direct and consensual

D/C disconnect
discontinue

DCA dichloroacetate
directional coronary atherectomy
disk/condyle adhesion
double-cup arthroplasty
sodium dichloroacetate

DCAG double-coronary artery graft

DCAP-BTLS deformities, contusions, abrasions, and punctures/penetrations, burns, tenderness, lacerations, and swelling (an assessment mnemonic used by EMTs)

DC-ART disease controlling anti-rheumatic therapy

DC&B dilation, currettage, and biopsy

DCBE double-contrast barium enema

DCC day care center(s)
diabetes care clinic
direct current cardioversion

DCCF dural carotid-cavernous fistula

DCCs day care centers

DCCT Diabetes Control and Complications Trial (questionnaire)

DCD developmental coordination disorder
donation after cardiac death

DC'd discontinued

DCE delayed contrast-enhancement
designated compensable event
detection-controlled estimation

DCE-MRI dynamic contrast enhanced magnetic resonance imaging

DCF data collection form
Denomination Commune Francaise (French-approved nonproprietary name)
docetaxel, cisplatin, and fluorouracil
pentostatin (Nipent; 2′ deoxycoformycin)

DCFS Department of Children and Family Services

DCG diagnostic cardiogram

DCH delayed cutaneous hypersensitivity

DCI decompression illness

DCIA deep circumflex iliac artery (flap)

DCIS ductal carcinoma *in situ*

DCL diffuse cutaneous leishmaniasis

DCLHb diaspirin cross-linked hemoglobin

DCM dementia care mapping
dilated cardiomyopathy

DCMP dilated cardiomyopathy

DCMXT dichloromethotrexate

DCN Darvocet N

DCNU chlorozotocin

DCO damage control orthopedics
death certificates only (cases known only from death certificates)
diffusing capacity of carbon monoxide

DCP dynamic compression plate

DCP® calcium phosphate, dibasic

DCPM daunorubicin, cytarabine, prednisolone, and mercaptopurine

DCPN direction-changing positional nystagmus

DCR dacryocystorhinostomy
delayed cutaneous reaction

DCRC disseminated colorectal cancer

DCRF data case report forms

3DCRT three-dimensional conformal radiation therapy

DCS damage-control surgery
decompression sickness
dorsal column stimulator

DCSA double-contrast shoulder arthrography

DCSW Diplomate in Clinical Social Work

DCT daunorubicin, cytarabine, and thioguanine
decisional conflict theory
deep chest therapy
direct (antiglobulin) Coombs test
dynamic contour tonometry

DCTM delay computer tomographic myelography

DCU day care unit

DCUS duplex-color ultrasonography

DCVC dual-channel virus counter

DCW direct care worker

DCYS Department of Children and Youth Services

DD delayed diarrhea
delivery date
dependent drainage
Descemet detachment
detrusor dyssynergia
developmentally delayed
developmental disabilities
developmentally disabled
dialysis dementia
died of the disease
differential diagnosis
disc diameter
discharge diagnosis
Doctor of Divinity
dose-dense
double dose (used by Radiology)
down drain

D

	dry dressing	D_5E_{75}	5% Dextrose and Electrolyte 75
	dual disorder	2-DE	two-dimensional echocardiography
	Duchenne dystrophy		two-dimential gel electrophoresis
	due date	3-DE	three-dimensional echocardiography
	dysthymic disorder	D&E	dilation and evacuation
D/D	diarrhea/dehydration	DEA#	Drug Enforcement Administration
D → D	discharge to duty		number (physician's federal
D & D	debridement and dressing		narcotic number)
	diarrhea and dehydration	DEAE	diethylaminoethyl
	drilling and drainage	DEB	diepoxybutane (test)
DDA	dideoxyadenosine		dystrophic epidermolysis bullosa
DDAH	dimethylarginine	DEC	deciduous (primary teeth)
	dimethylaminohydrolase		decrease
DDAVP®	desmopressin acetate		diethylcarbamazine (Hetrazan)
DDC	dose-dense chemotherapy		Drug Evaluation and Classification
	zalcitabine (dideoxy-cytidine; Hivid)		(a standardized curriculum to train
DDCI	dopadecarboxylase inhibitor		police officers)
DDD	defined daily doses	DECA	nandrolone decanoate (Deca-
	degenerative disk disease		Durabolin)
	dense deposit disease	DECAFS	Department of Children and Family
	fully automatic pacing		Services
DDDR	pacemaker code (D = chamber	DECEL	deceleration
	paced-dual, D = chamber sensed-	decub	decubitus
	dual, D = response to sensing-	DED	diabetic eye disease
	dual, R = programmability-rate		died in emergency department
	modulation)	DEEDS	drugs, exercise, education, diet, and
DDDR-70	dual-chamber rate responsive pacing		self-monitoring
	at 70/minute	DEEG	depth electroencephalogram
DDE	dichlorodiphenylethylene		deteriorating electroencephalogram
DDGB	double-dose gallbladder (test)	DEET	diethyltoluamide
DDH	developmental dysplasia of the hip	DEF	decayed, extracted, or filled
DDHT	double-dissociated hypertropia		defecation
DDI	didanosine (dideoxyinosine; Videx)		deficiency
	dressing dry, intact	2-DEF	two-dimensional echo-derived
DDIs	drug-drug interactions		ejection fraction
DDis	developmental disorder	DEFT	defendant
DDiv	Doctor of Divinity		driven equilibrium Fourier transform
DDMC	diabetes disease management clinic		(technique)
DDNS	digestive disease and nutrition	DEG	diethylene glycol
	service	degen	degenerative
DDP	cisplatin (Platinol)	DEHP	diethylhexyl phthalate
DDRA	dead despite resuscitation attempt	DEJ	dentin-enamel junction
DDRE	Division of Drug Risk Evaluation	DEL	delivered
	(FDA)		delivery
DDRUL	dorsal distal radioulnar ligament		deltoid
DDS	dialysis disequilibrium syndrome	DELM	digital epiluminescence microscopy
	Doctor of Dental Surgery	DEM	drug evaluation matrix
	double-decidual sac (sign)	DEMRI	dynamic enhanced magnetic
	4, 4-diaminodiphenyl-sulfone		resonance imaging
	(dapsone)	Denver II	Denver Developmental Screening
DDST	Denver Development Screening Test		Test - second edition
DDT	chlorophenothane	DEPs	diesel exhaust particles
DDTP	drug dependence treatment program	DEP ST	depressed ST segment
DDx	differential diagnosis	SEG	
DE	dermal epidermal (junction)	DER	disulfiram-ethanol reaction
	digitalis effect	DERM	dermatology
	diminished emotionality	DES	desflurane (Supreme)
D_5E_{48}	5% Dextrose and Electrolyte 48		diethylstilbestrol

	diffuse esophageal spasm
	disequilibrium syndrome
	Dissociative Experience Scale
	drug eluting stent
	dry-eye syndrome
	dysfunctional elimination syndrome (urology)
DESAT	desaturation
DESF	desflurane (Suprane)
DESI	Drug Efficacy Study Implementation
DET	diethyltryptamine
	dipyridamole echocardiography test
DETOX	detoxification
DEV	deviation
	duck embryo vaccine
DEVR	dominant exudative vitreoretinopathy
DEX	dexamethasone
	dexrazoxane (Zinecard)
	dexter (right)
	dexverapamil
DEXA	dual-energy x-ray absorptiometry
DF	day frequency (of voiding)
	decayed and filled
	deferred
	defibrotide
	degree of freedom
	dengue fever
	dexfenfluramine
	diabetic father
	diastolic filling
	dietary fiber
	dorsiflexion
	drug-free
	dye-free
DFA	delayed feedback audiometry
	diet for age
	difficulty falling asleep
	direct fluorescent antibody
	distal forearm
DFCI	Dana-Farber Cancer Institute
DFD	defined formula diets
	degenerative facet disease
DFE	dilated fundus examination
	distal femoral epiphysis
DFG	direct forward gaze
DFI	disease-free interval
DFLE	disability-free life expectancy
DFM	decreased fetal movement
	deep finger massage
	deep friction massage
DFMC	daily fetal movement count
DFMR	daily fetal movement record
DFO	deferoxamine (Desferal)
DFOM	deferoxamine (Desferal)
DFP	diastolic filling period
	isoflurophate (diisopropyl flurophosphate)
DFR	diabetic floor routine

DFRC	deglycerolized frozen red cells
DFS	disease-free survival
	Division of Family Services
	Doppler flow studies
DFSP	dermatofibrosarcoma protuberans
DFT	defibrillation threshold (testing)
DFU	dead fetus in uterus
	diabetic foot ulcer
DFV	D'Aoust Fineman virus
	dengue fever vaccine
	diarrhea, fever, and vomiting
DFW	Dexide face wash
DFWO	dorsiflexory wedge osteotomy
DFYS	Division of Family and Youth Services (government agency)
DG	diagnosis
	dorsal glides
	downward gaze
DGA	DiGeorge anomaly
	disseminated granuloma annulare
DGC	dystrophin-glycoprotein complex
DGE	delayed gastric emptying
DGF	delayed graft function
DGGE	denaturing gradient gel electrophoresis
DGI	disseminated gonococcal infection
DGL	deglycyrrhizinated licorice
DGR	duodenogastric reflux
DGM	ductal glandular mastectomy
DGs	documentation guidelines
DGT	decaffeinated green tea
DH	delayed hypersensitivity
	Dental Hygienist
	dermatitis herpetiformis
	developmental history
	diaphragmatic hernia
D+H	delusions and hallucinations
D-H	Dimon-Hughston (intertrochanteric osteotomy technique)
DHA	dihydroxyacetone
	docosahexaenoic acid
DHAC	dihydro-5-azacytidine
DHAD	mitoxanthrone HCl (Novantrone)
DHANP	Diplomate of the Homeopathic Academy of Naturopathic Physicians
DHAP	dexamethasone, high-dose cytarabine, (ara-A) cisplatin (Platinol)
	docosahexaenoic acid-paclitaxel
DHA-TP	dihydroartemisinin, trimethoprim, and piperaquine
DHBV	duck hepatitis B virus
DHCA	deep hypothermia circulatory arrest
DHCC	dihydroxycholecalciferol
DHD	dissociated horizontal deviation
DHE	dental health education
DHE 45®	dihydroergotamine mesylate

DHEA	dehydroepiandrosterone	DIB	disability insurance benefits
DHEAS	dehydroepiandrosterone sulfate	DIBC	drug-induced blood cytopenias
DHF	dengue hemorrhagic fever	DIBD	drug-induced behavioral disinhibition
	diastolic heart failure	DIB-R	Diagnostic Interview for Borderlines
DHFR	dihydrofolate reductase		(personality disorders)-Revised
DHHS	Department of Health and Human	DIBS	dead-in-bed syndrome
	Services	DIC	dacarbazine (DTIC-Dome)
DHI	Dizziness Handicap Inventory		diagnostic imaging center
	dynamic hyperinflation		differential interference contrast
DHIC	detrusor hyperactivity with impaired		disseminated intravascular
	contractility		coagulation
DHL	diffuse histocytic lymphoma		drug information center
DHP	dihydropyridine	DICC	dynamic infusion cavernosometry
DHP-1	dehydropeptidase-1		and cavernosography
DHPG	ganciclovir	DICE	dexamethasone, ifosfamide, cisplatin,
DHPLC	denaturing high-performance liquid		and etopside, with mesna
	chromatography	DICLOX	dicloxacillin (Dynapen)
DHPR	dihydropteridine reductase	DICP	demyelinated inflammatory chronic
DHPS	dihydopteroate synthase		polyneuropathy
DHR	delayed hypersensitivity reaction	DICT	dose-intensive chemotherapy
DHS	Department of Human Services	DID	death(s) from intercurrent disease
	duration of hospital stay		delayed ischemia deficit
	dynamic hip screw		dissociative identity disorder
DHST	delayed hypersensitivity test		drug-induced disease
DHT	dihydrotachysterol (Hytakeral;	di,di	dichorionic, diamniotic
	DHT®)	DIE	died in emergency department
	dihydrotestosterone		drug-induced esophagitis
	dissociated hypertropia	DIED	died in emergency department
	Dobhoff tube	DIEP	deep inferior epigastric perforator
DHTF	Dobhoff tube feeding	DIF	differentiation-inducing factor
DI	(Beck) Depression Inventory	DIFF	differential blood count
	date of injury	DIG	digoxin (this is a dangerous
	Debrix Index		abbreviation)
	detrusor instability	DIH	died in hospital
	diabetes insipidus	DIHS	drug-induced hypersensitivity
	diagnostic imaging		syndrome
	Disability Index	DIJOA	dominantly inherited juvenile optic
	dorsal interossei		atrophy
	drug interactions	DIL	daughter-in-law
D&I	debridement and irrigation		dilute
	dry and intact		drug-induced lupus
DIA	drug-induced agranulocytosis		drug information leaflet
	drug-induced amenorrhea	DILC	dose-intensity limiting criterium
	Drug Information Association	DILD	diffuse infiltrative lung disease
diag.	diagnosis		drug-induced liver disease
DIAM	drug-induced aseptic meningitis	DILE	drug-induced lupus erythematosus
DIAP-	(causes of transient	DILS	drug-induced lupus syndrome
PERS	incontinence) delirium/confusion,	DIM	diminish
	infection, (urinary), atrophic	D5IMB	Ionosol MB with 5% dextrose
	urethritis/ vaginitis, pharmaceuti-		injection
	cals, psychological, excessive	DIMD	drug-induced movement disorders
	excretion (e.g., CHF,	DIMOAD	diabetes insipidus, diabetes mellitus,
	hyperglycemia) restricted		optic atrophy, and deafness
	mobility, and stool impaction	DIMS	disorders of initiating and
DIAS	diastolic		maintaining sleep
DIAS BP	diastolic blood pressure	DIND	delayed ischemic neurologic deficit
Diath SW	diathermy short wave	DIOS	distal ileal obstruction syndrome
DIAZ	diazepam (Valium)		distal intestinal obstruction syndrome

DIP	desquamative interstitial pneumonia	D$_L$	maximal diffusing capacity
	diphtheria toxoid vaccine	DLB	dementia with Lewy bodies
	diplopia		direct laryngoscopy and
	distal interphalangeal		bronchoscopy
	drip infusion pyelogram	DLBCL	diffuse large B-cell lymphoma
	drug-induced parkinsonism	DLBD	diffuse Lewy body disease
DIP$_{ant}$	diphtheria antitoxin	DLBL	diffuse large B-cell lymphoma
DIPC	dynamic infusion	DLC	double lumen catheter
	pharmacocavemosometry	DLCL	diffuse large cell lymphoma
DIPJ	distal interphalangeal joint	DLCO sb	diffusion capacity of carbon
DIR	directions		monoxide, single breath
DIRD	drug-induced renal disease	DLD	date of last drink
DIS	Diagnostic Interview Schedule	DLE	decrement-load exercise
	(questionnaire)		discoid lupus erythematosus
	digital imaging spectrophotometer		disseminated lupus erythematosis
	dislocation	DLF	digitalis-like factor
DISC	disabled infectious single cycle		ductal lavage fluid
	(virus)	DLI	donor leukocyte
	dynamic integrated stabilization		infusions
	chair	DLIF	digoxin-like immunoreactive factors
disch.	discharge	DLIS	digoxin-like immunoreactive
DISCUS	Dyskinesia Indentification System		substance
	Condensed User Scale	DLMP	date of last menstrual period
DISH	diffuse idiopathic skeletal hyperostosis	DLNG	dl-norgestrel
DISI	dorsal intercalated segmental	DLNMP	date of last normal menstrual period
	(segment) instability	DLNs	distant lymph nodes
DISIDA	diisopropyl iminodiacetic acid	DLP	dislocation of patella
D$_5$ISOM	5% Dextrose and Isolyte M		double-limb progression
D$_5$ISOP	5% Dextrose and Isolyte P	DLPD	diffuse lymphocytic poorly
DISR	drug-induced skin reactions		differentiated
DIST	distal	DLPFC	dorsolateral prefrontal cortex
	distilled	DLQI	Dermatology Life Quality Index
DIT	diiodotyrosine	D5LR	dextrose 5% in lactated Ringer
	drug-induced thrombocytopenia		injection
DIU	death in utero	DLROW	a test used in mental status
	diuretic(s)		examinations (patient is asked to
DIV	double-inlet ventricle		spell WORLD backwards)
DIVA	digital intravenous angiography	DLRT	dogleg radiotherapy
Div ex	divergence excess	DLS	daily living skills
DIVP	dilute intravenous Pitocin		digitalis-like substances
DJD	degenerative joint disease		dynamic light scattering
DK	dark	DLSC	double-lumen subclavian catheter
	diabetic ketoacidosis	DLST	drug-induced lymphocyte stimulation
	diseased kidney		test
DKA	diabetic ketoacidosis	DLT	dose-limiting toxicity
	didn't keep appointment		double-lung transplant
DKB	deep knee bends	DLTT	dosing least toxic time
DKC	double knee to chest	DLU	diffused lung uptake
	dyskeratosis congenita	DLV	delavirdine (Rescriptor)
D-K-S	Damus-Kaye-Stansel	DLW	doubly labeled water
	(operation/procedure)	DM	dehydrated and malnourished
DL	danger list		dermatomyositis
	deciliter (dL; 100 mL)		dextromethorphan
	diagnostic laparoscopy		diabetes mellitus
	direct laryngoscopy		diabetic mother
	drug level		diastolic murmur
	dual lumen		disease management
dL	deciliter (100 mL)	DM-1	diabetes mellitus type 1

DM-2	diabetes mellitus type 2
DMA	Director of Medical Affairs
DMAC	disseminated *Mycobacterium avium* complex
DMAD	disease-modifying antirheumatic drug
DMAE	dimethylaminoethanol
DMAIC	disseminated *Mycobacterium avium-intracellulare* complex
DMARD	disease modifying antirheumatic drug
DMAS	Drug Management and Authorization Section
DMAT	disaster medical assistance team
DMB	data monitoring board
DMBA	dimethylbenzanthracene
DMC	dactinomycin, methotrexate, and cyclophosphamide
	data monitoring committee
	diabetes management center
DMD	Descemet membrane detachment
	disciform macular degeneration
	Doctor of Dental Medicine
	drowsiness monitoring device
	Duchenne muscular dystrophy
DMD w/ SRNM	disciform macular degeneration with subretinal neovascular membrane
DME	diabetic macular edema
	Director of Medical Education
	durable medical equipment
DMEC	data-monitoring and ethics committee
DMEM	Dulbecco Modified Eagle Medium
DMEPOS	durable medical equipment, prosthetics, orthotics, and supplies
DMERC	Durable Medical Equipment Regional Carrier
DMEs	drug-metabolizing enzymes
DMETS	Division of Medication Errors and Technical Support (FDA)
DMF	decayed, missing, or filled
	dimethylformamide
	distant metastases-free
	Drug Master File
DMFI	distant metastases free interval
DMFS	decayed, missing, or filled surfaces
	distant metastases free survival
DMFT	decayed, missing, and filled teeth
DMH	Department of Mental Health
DMI	desipramine (Norpramin)
	diabetic muscle infarction
	diaphragmatic myocardial infarction
DM Isch	diaphragmatic myocardial ischemia
DMKA	diabetes mellitus ketoacidosis
DMN	dysplastic melanocytic nevus
DMO	dimethadone
DMOADs	disease-modifying osteoarthritis drugs

DMOOC	diabetes mellitus out of control
DMORTs	Disaster Mortuary Operational Response Teams
DMP	data monitoring plan
	dimethyl phthalate
DMPA	depot-medroxypro-gesterone acetate
DMPC	dimyristoylphosphatidyl choline
DMPG	dimyristoylphosphatidyl glycerol
d-MPH	dexmethylphenidate (Focalin)
DMPK	drug metabolism and pharmacokinetics
DMPM	diffuse malignant peritoneal mesothelioma
DMPS	dimercaptopropane-sulfonic acid
D-MRI	dynamic magnetic resonance imaging
DMS	dimethylsulfide
DMSA	succimer (dimercaptosuccinic acid; Chemet)
DMSO	dimethyl sulfoxide
DMT	dimethyltryptamine
DMTU	dimethylthiourea
DMV	disk, macula, and vessels
	Doctor of Veterinary Medicine
DMVP	disc, macula, vessel, periphery
DMX	diathermy, massage, and exercise
DN	denuded
	diabetic nephropathy
	dicrotic notch
	down
	dysplastic nevus (nevi)
D & N	distance and near (vision)
DNA	deoxyribonucleic acid
	did not answer
	did not attend
	does not apply
DNA ds	deoxyribonucleic acid double-stranded
DNA ss	deoxyribonucleic acid single-stranded
DNCB	dinitrochlorobenzene
DNC	Dermatology Nurse, Certified
	did not come
	dilatation and curettage (usually written as D&C)
DND	died a natural death
DNE	diabetes nurse educator
DNEPTE	did not exist prior to enlistment
DNET	dysembryoplastic neuroepithelial tumor
DNFB	Discharged, No Final Bill (report)
DNFC	does not follow commands
DNI	do not intubate
DNIC	diffuse noxious inhibitory control
DNIF	duties not including flying
DNKA	did not keep appointment
DNMT	DNA (desoxyribonucleic acid) methyltransferase

DNN	did not nurse		drug overdose
DNP	did not pay	DODD	demand oxygen delivery device
	dinitrophenylhydrazine	DOE	date of examination
	do not publish		disease-oriented evidence
DNR	daunorubicin		dyspnea on exertion
	did not respond	DOES	disorders of excessive somnolence
	do not report	DOH	Department of Health
	do not resuscitate	DOI	date of implant (pacemaker)
	dorsal nerve root		date of injury
DNS	deviated nasal septum		digital object identifier
	Director of Nursing Services	DO₂I	oxygen delivery index
	Doctorate, Nursing Science	DOJ	Department of Justice
	doctor did not see patient	DOL	days of life
	do not show	DOL #2	second day of life
	dysplastic nevus syndrome	DOLV	double-outlet left ventricle
D₅ 1/4 NS	dextrose 5% in 1/4 normal saline	DOM	Doctor of Oriental Medicine
	(0.225% sodium chloride)		domiciliary
	injection		domiciliary care
D₅ 1/2NS	dextrose 5% in 0.45% sodium	DOMS	delayed-onset muscle soreness
	chloride injection	DON	Director of Nursing
D₅NS	5% dextrose in normal saline (0.9%		donepezil HCl (Aricept)
	sodium chloride) injection	DONFL	dissociated optic nerve fiber layer
DNT	did not test	DOOC	diabetes out of control
	dysembryoplastic neuroepithelial	DOP	degenerate oligonucleotide-primed
	tumor		dopamine
DO	detrusor overactivity	DOPS	diffuse obstructive pulmonary
	diet order		syndrome
	dissolved oxygen		dihydroxyphenylserine
	distocclusal		Director of Pharmacy Service(s)
	distraction osteogenesis	DOR	date of release
	Doctor of Osteopathy	DORV	double-outlet right ventricle
	doctor's order	DORx	date of treatment
D/O	disorder	DOS	date of surgery
✓DO	check doctor's order		dead on scene
DO₂	oxygen delivery		doctor's order sheet
DOA	date of admission	DOSA	day of surgery admission
	dead on arrival	DOSAK	Central Tumor Registry operated by
	dominant optic atrophy		the German-Austrian-Swiss
	driver of automobile		Association for Head and Neck
	duration of action		Tumors
DOA-DRA	dead on arrival despite resuscitative	DOSS	docusate sodium (dioctyl sodium
	attempts		sulfosuccinate)
DOB	dangle out of bed	DOT	date of transcription
	date of birth		date of transfer
	Dobrava hantavirus		died on table
	dobutamine		directly observed therapy
	doctor's order book		Directory of Occupational Titles
DOC	date of conception		Doppler ophthalmic test
	diabetes out of control	DOTS	directly observed treatment, short
	died of other causes		course
	diet of choice	DOV	date of visit
	docetaxel (Taxotere)		distribution of ventilation
	drug of choice	DOX	doxepin
DOCA	desoxycorticosterone acetate		doxorubicin (Adriamycin)
DOCP	desoxycorticosterone pivalate	doz	dozen
DOD	date of death	DP	dental prosthesis
	dead of disease		depersonalization
	Department of Defense		diastolic pressure

D

	disability pension
	discharge planning
	dorsalis pedis (pulse)
D/P	dialysate-to-plasma ratio
DPA	Department of Public Assistance
	dipropylacetic acid
	D-penicillamine (penicillamine; Cuprimine)
	dual photon absorptiometry
	durable power of attorney
DPAP	diastolic pulmonary artery pressure
DPB	days postburn
	diffuse panbronchiolitis
DPBS	Dulbecco phosphate-buffered saline
DPC	delayed primary closure
	discharge planning coordinator
	distal palmar crease
DPCP	diphenylcyclopropenone (diphencyprone)
DPD	dihydropyrimidine dehydrogenase
DPDL	diffuse poorly differentiated lymphocytic lymphoma
DPEJ	direct percutaneous endoscopic jejunostomy
DPF	docetaxel, cisplatin, (Platinol) and fluorouracil
2,3-DPG	2,3-diphosphoglyceric acid
DPH	Department of Public Health
	diphenhydramine (Benadryl)
	Doctor of Public Health
	phenytoin (diphenylhydantoin; Dilantin)
DPI	dietary protein intake
	Doppler perfusion index
	dry powder inhaler
	dry powder for inhalation
DPIL	dextrose (percentage), protein (grams per kilogram) Intralipid® (grams per kilogram)
DPJ	dislocation of prosthetic joint
DPL	diagnostic peritoneal lavage
D5PLM	dextrose 5% and Plasmalyte M® injection
DPM	distintegrations per minute (dpm)
	Doctor of Podiatric Medicine
	drops per minute
DPN	^{11}C-diprenorphine
	deep peroneal nerve
	diabetic peripheral neuropathy
DPNP	diabetic peripheral neuropathic pain
DPOA	durable power of attorney
DPOAE	distortion-product otoacoustic emission
DPOAHC	durable power of attorney for health care
DPP	dentine phosphoproteins
	dorsalis pedal pulse
	duration of positive pressure
DPP-4	dipeptidyl peptidase 4

DPPC	colfosceril palmitate (dipalmitoylphosphatidylcholine)
DPPE	tesmilifene (diethyl phenylmethyl phenoxy ethanamine)
DPR	Department of Professional Regulation
	diagnostic procedure room
DPS	disintegration per second
DPSS	Department of Public Social Service
DPsy	Doctor of Psychology
DPT	Demerol, Phenergan, and Thorazine (this is a dangerous abbreviation)
	diphtheria, pertussis, and tetanus (immunization)
	Driver Performance Test
DPTPM	diphtheria, pertussis, tetanus, poliomyelitis, and measles
DPU	delayed pressure urticaria
DPUD	duodenal peptic ulcer disease
DPVSs	dilated perivascular spaces
DPXA	dual-photon x-ray absorptiometry
DQ	developmental quotients
D/Q	deep quiet
D&Q	deep and quiet
DQA	Data Quality Audit
DQM	data quality manager
DQOL	diabetes quality of life
DQOLS	Dermatology Quality of Life Scales
Dr	doctor
DR	delivery room
	diabetic retinopathy
	diagnostic radiology
	dining room
	diurnal rhythm
	drug resistant
DRA	distal rectal adenocarcinoma
	drug-related admissions
DRAPE	drug-related adverse patient event
DRC	dose-response curve
DRE	digital rectal examination
	Drug Recognition Expert (for detection of impaired drivers)
DREAM	downstream regulatory element antagonistic modulator (gene)
DRESS	depth resolved surface coil spectroscopy
	drug rash with eosinophilia and systemic symptoms
DREZ	dorsal root entry zone
DRG	diagnosis-related groups
	dorsal root ganglia
DRGE	drainage
DRI	defibrillation response interval
	Dietary Reference Intakes
	Discharge Readiness Index
	dopamine reuptake inhibitor
DRIL	distal revascularization internal ligation

DRM   drug-related morbidity
DRN   dorsal raphe nucleus
      drug-related neutropenia
DRP   data review plan
      drug-related problem
DRPLA   dentatorubral-pallidolluysian atrophy
DRPn   drug-resistant *Streptococcus pneumoniae*
DRR   drug regimen review
DRS   designated record set
      Disability Rating Scale
      disease-related symptoms
      Duane retraction syndrome
DRSG   dressing
DRSI   disease-related symptom improvement
DRSP   drug-resistant *Streptococcus pneumoniae*
DRT   drug-related thrombocytopenia
DrTPar   diphtheria toxoid (reduced antigen quantity for adults), tetanus toxoid, and acellular pertussis (reduced antigen quantity for adults) vaccine, for adult use
DRUB   drug screen-blood
DRUJ   distal or radial ulnar joint
dRVVT   diluted Russell viper venom time
DS   deep sleep
      Dextrostix
      dietary supplement
      discharge summary
      disoriented
      distant supervision
      double strength
      Down syndrome
      drug screen
D/S   5% dextrose and 0.9% sodium chloride (saline) injection
%DS   percent diameter stenosis
D&S   diagnostic and surgical
      dilation and suction
D5S   dextrose 5% in 0.9% sodium chloride (saline) injection
D$_5$-1/2S   5% dextrose in 0.45% sodium chloride (saline) injection
18Ds   Special Operations Forces medics
DSA   digital subtraction angiography (angiocardiography)
DSAP   disseminated superficial actinic porokeratosis
DSB   drug-seeking behavior
DSBs   double-strand (DNA) breaks
DSC   differential scanning calorimeter
      Down syndrome child
      dynamic susceptibility contrast
DSD   degenerative spinal disease
      detrusor sphincter dyssynergia
      digital selenium drum (radiology)

      discharge summary dictated
      dry sterile dressing
DSDB   direct self-destructive behavior
ds DNA   double-stranded desoxyribonucleic acid
DSF   doxorubicin, streptozocin, and fluorouracil
DSG   desogestrel
      dressing
DSG   deoxyspergulin
DSHEA   Dietary Supplement Health and Education Act of 1994
DSHR   delayed skin hypersensitivity reaction
DSHS   Department of Social and Health Services
DSI   deep shock insulin
      Depression Status Inventory
DSIAR   double-stapled ileoanal reservoir
DSM   disease state management
      drink skim milk
DSM-IV   Diagnostic and Statistical Manual of Mental Disorders, 4th edition
dSMA   distal spinal muscular atrophy
DSMB   Data and Safety Management Board
      Data and Safety Monitoring Board
DSMC   Data Safety and Monitoring Committee
DSMO   Designated Standard Maintenance Organization
DSO   distal subungual onychomycosis
DSP   diabetic sensorimotor polyneuropathy
      digital signal processor
      distal symmetrical polyneuropathy
DSPC   distearoylphosphatidyl choline
DSPD   dangerous severe personality disorder
D-SPINE   dorsal spine
DSPN   distal symmetric polyneuropathy
DSPS   delayed sleep phase syndrome
DSRCT   desmoplastic small round cell tumor
DSRF   drainage subretinal fluid
DSS   dengue shock syndrome
      Department of Social Services
      Disability Status Scale
      discharge summary sheet
      disease-specific survival
      distal splenorenal shunt
      docusate sodium (dioctyl sodium sulfosuccinate)
DSSLR   double, seated straight leg raise
DSSN   distal symmetric sensory neuropathy
DSSP   distal symmetric sensory polyneuropathy
DSST   Digit-Symbol Substitution Test
DST   daylight saving time
      dexamethasone suppression test
      digit substitution test
      donor-specific (blood) transfusion

DSU	day stay unit	DTPA	pentetic acid (diethylenetriaminepen-taacetic acid)
	day surgery unit		
DSUH	direct suggestion under hypnosis	DTP$_a$	diphtheria, tetanus toxoids, acellular
D/Sum	discharge summary		pertussis vaccine, for pediatric use
DSV	digital subtraction ventriculography	DTPa-HIB	diphtheria toxoid, tetanus toxoid,
DSVP	Dietary Supplement Verification		acellular pertussis, and
	Program (United States		*Haemophilus influenzae* type b
	Pharmacopeia Purity Compliance)		conjugate vaccine
DSW	Doctorate in Social Work	DTPa-HIB-	diphtheria toxoid, tetanus
DSWI	deep sternal wound infection	IPV	toxoid, acellular pertussis,
	deep surgical wound infection		*Haemophilus influenzae* type b
DSX	dysmetabolic syndrome X		conjugate, and poliovirus
DT	delirium tremens		inactivated vaccine
	dietary thermogenesis	DTP$_w$	diphtheria, tetanus toxoids, whole-cell pertussis vaccine
	dietetic technician		
	diphtheria and tetanus toxoids, adsorbed, pediatric strength	DTR	Dance Therapist, Registered
			deep tendon reflexes
	discharge tomorrow		Dietetic Technician Registered
	docetaxel (Taxotere)	dtr	daughter
D/T	date/time	DTs	delirium tremens
	due to	DTS	danger to self
d/t	due to		donor specific transfusion
d4T	stavudine (Zerit)	3D TSE	three-dimensional turbo-spin echo (images)
D & T	diagnosis and treatment		
	dictated and typed	DTT	diphtheria tetanus toxoid
DTaP	diphtheria and tetanus toxoids with acellular pertussis vaccine		dithiothreitol
		DTUS	diathermy, traction, and ultrasound
DTBC	tubocurarine (D-tubocurarine)	DVG	double vein graft
DTBE	Division of Tuberculosis Elimination	DTV	due to void
DTC	day treatment center	DTVP	Developmental Test of Visual Perception
	differentiated thyroid cancer		
	direct-to-consumer (advertising)	DTwP	diphtheria and tetanus toxoids with whole-cell pertussis vaccine
	diticarb (diethyldiothio-carbamate)		
	tubocurarine (D-tubocurarine)	DTX	detoxification
DTCA	direct-to-consumer advertising	DU	decubitus ulcer
DTD	diastropic dysplasia		depleted uranium
DTD #30	dispense 30 such doses		developmental unit
DTF	deep transverse friction		diabetic urine
DTH	delayed-type hypersensitivity		diagnosis undetermined
DTI	Department of Trade and Industry (United Kingdom)		duodenal ulcer
			duroxide uptake
	diffusion-tensor imaging	DUB	Dubowitz (score)
	Doppler tissue imaging		dysfunctional uterine bleeding
DTIC	dacarbazine (DTIC-Dome)	DUBI	dysfunctional urinary bladder instability
D TIME	dream time		
DTIs	direct thrombin inhibitors	DUCL	dorsal ulnocarpal ligament
DTM	deep tissue massage	DUD	dihydrouracil dehydrogenase
	dermatophyte test medium	DUE	drug use evaluation
DTMS	drug therapy management service	D&UE	dilation and uterine evacuation
DTO	danger to others	DUF	Doppler ultrasonic flowmeter
	deodorized tincture of opium (warning: this is *NOT* paregoric)	DUI	driving under the influence
		DUID	driving under the influence of drugs
DTOGV	dextral-transposition of great vessels	DUII	driving under the influence of intoxicants
DTP	differential time to positivity		
	diphtheria, tetanus toxoids, pertussis (antigens unspecified) vaccine	DUIL	driving under the influence of liquor
		DUKM	dialysate urea kinetic modeling
	distal tingling on percussion (+Tinel sign)	DUM	drug use monitoring
		DUN	dialysate urea nitrogen

DUNHL	diffuse undifferentiated non-Hodgkins lymphoma	D/W	dextrose in water discussed with
DUO	Duotube®	D-W	Dandy-Walker
DUR	drug utilization review duration		(deformity/malformation) Danis-Weber (classification for ankle fractures)
DUS	digital ultrasound distal urethral stenosis	D₅W	5% dextrose (in water) injection
	Doppler ultrasound stethoscope	D10W	10% dextrose (in water) injection
	duplex ultrasonography	D20W	20% dextrose (in water) injection
3DUS	three-dimensional ultrasound	D50W	50% dextrose (in water) injection
DUSN	diffuse unilateral subacute	D70W	70% dextrose (in water) injection
	neuroretinitis	5 DW	5% dextrose (in water) injection
DV	distance vision	DWDL	diffuse well-differentiated
	domestic violence		lymphocytic lymphoma
	double vision	DWI	diffusion-weighted (magnetic
D&V	diarrhea and vomiting		resonance) imaging
	disc and vessels		driving while intoxicated
DVA	Department of Veterans Affairs		driving while impaired
	directional vacuum-assisted (biopsy)	DWI/PI	diffusion-weighted imaging/
	distance visual acuity		perfusion imaging
	vindesine (Eldisine; desacetyl	DWMRI	diffusion-weighted magnetic
	vinblastine amide sulfate)		resonance imaging
DVAB	directional vacuum-assisted biopsy	DWR	deep water running
DVC	direct visualization of vocal cords	DWRT	delayed work recall test
D V®	dienestrol vaginal cream	DWSCL	daily-wear soft contact lens
Cream		DWV	Dandy-Walker variant (a congenital
DVD	dissociated vertical deviation		anomaly)
	double-vessel disease	DWW	dynamic wall walk
DVH	dose-volume histogram	Dx	diagnosis
DVI	atrioventricular sequential pacing		disease
	digital vascular imaging	DXA	dual-energy x-ray absorptiometry
	direct visual inspection	DXG	dioxalane guanine
DVIU	direct vision internal urethrotomy	DxLS	diagnosis responsible for length of
DVLA	Driver and Vehicle Licensing Agency		stay
	(United Kingdom)	DXM	dexamethasone
DVPX	divalproex sodium (Depakote)		dextromethorphan
DVM	Doctor of Veterinary Medicine	DXR	delayed xenograft rejection
DVMP	disc, vessels, and macula periphery	DXT	deep x-ray therapy
DVP	digital volume pulse	DXRT	deep x-ray therapy
DVPA	daunorubicin, vincristine,	DXS	Dextrostix®
	prednisone, and asparaginase	DY	dusky (infant color)
DVR	Division of Vocational Rehabilitation		dysprosium
	dose-volume relationship	DYF	drag your feet (author's note: see
	double-valve replacement		you in court)
DVSA	digital venous subtraction	DYFS	Division of Youth and Family
	angiography		Services
DVT	deep vein thrombosis	DysD	dysthymic disorder
	digital volume tomography	DYTRO	dynamic tone-reducing orthosis
DVTS	deep venous thromboscintigram	DZ	diazepam (valium)
DVVC	direct visualization of vocal cords		disease
DW	daily weight		dizygotic
	deionized water		dozen
	detention warrant	DZP	diazepam (Valium)
	dextrose in water	DZT	dizygotic twins
	diffusion-weighted (imaging)	DZX	dexrazoxane (Zinecard)
	distilled water		
	doing well		
	double wrap		

D

E

E   East (as in the location e.g., 2E,
      would be second floor, East wing)
    edema
    effective
    eloper
    enema
    engorged
    eosinophil
    Escherichia
    esophoria for distance
    ethambutol [part of tuberculosis
      regimen, see RHZ(E/S)/HR]
    evaluation
    evening
    expired
    eye
    methylenedioxy-methamphetamine
      (MDMA; Ecstasy)

E' elbow
    esophoria for near

E_1 estrone
E_2 estradiol
E_3 estriol
4E   4 plus edema
E11   Echovirus 11
    embryonic day 11 (11-day-old
      embryo)
E20   Enfamil 20®
E → A   say E,E,E, comes out as A,A,A upon
      auscultation of lung showing
      consolidation
EA   early amniocentesis
    elbow aspiration
    electroacoustic analysis
    electroacupuncture
    enteral alimentation
    epidural anesthesia
    episodic ataxia
    esophageal atresia
E/A   ratio of peak mitral early diastolic
      and atrial contraction velocity
    European American
E&A   evaluate and advise
EAA   electrothermal atomic absorption
    essential amino acids
    extrinsic allergic alveolitis
EAB   elective abortion
    Ethical Advisory Board
EAC   erythema annulare centrifugum
    esophageal adenocarcinoma
    external auditory canal
EACA   aminocaproic acid (epsilon-
      aminocaproic acid)
    esophageal adenocarcinoma

EADL   extended activities of daily living
EADs   early after-depolarizations
EAE   experimental allergic
      encephalomyelitis
    experimental autoimmune
      encephalomyelitis
EAEC   enteroaggregative *Escherichia coli*
EAggEC   enteroaggregative *Escherichia coli*
EAHF   eczema, allergy, and hay fever
EAL   electronic artificial larynx
EAM   external auditory meatus
EAP   Early Access Program (premarketing
      use of drug)
    Employment (Employee) Assistance
      Programs
    erythrocyte acid phosphatase
    etoposide, doxorubicin
      (Adriamycin), and cisplatin
      (Platinol)
EAR   estimated average requirement
    excess absolute risk
EARLIES   early decelerations
EART   extended abdominal radiation
      therapy
EAR OX   ear oximetry
EAS   external anal sphincter
EASC   endoscopic ambulatory surgery
      center
EASE   Estimation and Assessment of
      Substance Exposure (model)
EAST   external rotation, abduction stress
      test
EAT   Eating Attitudes Test
    ectopic atrial tachycardia
EATL   enteropathy-associated T-cell
      lymphoma
EAU   experimental autoimmune uveitis
EB   eosinophilic bronchitis
    epidermolysis bullosa
    Epstein-Barr (virus)
EBA   epidermolysis bullosa acquisita
EBB   electron beam boosts
    equal breath bilaterally
EBBS   equal bilateral breath sounds
EBC   early (stage) breast cancer
    endoscopic brush cytology
    esophageal balloon catheter
EBCPGs   evidence-based clinical practice
      guidelines
EBCT   electron-beam computed tomography
EBCTCG   Early Breast Cancer Trialists'
      Collaborative Group
EBD   endocardial border delineation
    endoscopic balloon dilation
    evidence-based decision (making)
EBE   equal bilateral expansion
EBEA   Epstein-Barr (virus) early antigen
EBF   erythroblastosis fetalis

E

EBL	endoscopic band ligation
	estimated blood loss
EBL-1	European bat lyssavirus 1
EBLV	European bat lyssavirus
EBM	evidence-based medicine
	expressed breast milk
EBMT	European Bone Marrow Transplant
	(registry group)
EBNA	Epstein-Barr (virus) nuclear antigen
EBO	evidence-based outcomes
EBOS	early-onset benign occipital seizure
EBOV	Ebola virus
EBO-Z	Ebola Zaire virus
EBP	epidural blood patch
EBR	external beam radiotherapy
	eye-blink rate
EBRs	evidence-based recommendations
EBRT	external beam radiation therapy
EBS	empiric Bayesian screening
	epidermolysis bullosa simplex
EBSB	equal breath sounds bilaterally
EBT	electron beam tomography
	erythromycin breath test
EBV	Epstein-Barr virus
EBVCA	Epstein-Barr viral capsid antigen
EBVEA	Epstein-Barr virus, early antigen
EBVNA	Epstein-Barr virus, nuclear antigen
EC	ejection click
	electrical cardioversion
	electrocautery
	emergency contraception
	endocervical
	enteric coated
	Escherichia coli
	esophageal candidiasis
	etopside and carboplatin
	European Community
	extracellular
	eye care
	eyes closed
E$_2$C	estradiol cypionate
E & C	education and counseling
ECA	enteric coated aspirin (tablets)
	Epidemiological Catchment Area
	ethacrynic acid
	external carotid artery
ECAD	extracorporeal albumin dialysis
e-CAM	electronic Compilation of Analytical
	Methods
ECASA	enteric coated aspirin (tablets)
ECBD	exploration of common bile duct
ECBO	enterocytopathogenic bovine orphan
	(virus)
ECC	early childhood caries
	edema, clubbing, and cyanosis
	embryonal cell cancer
	emergency cardiac care
	Emergency Communications Center

	endocervical curettage
	estimated creatinine clearance
	external cardiac compression
	extracorporeal circulation
ECCE	extracapsular cataract extraction
ECD	electron capture dissociation
	endocardial cushion defect
	equivalent current dipole
	Erdheim-Chester disease
	expanded criteria donor
E-CD	E-cadherin
ECDB	encourage to cough and deep breathe
ECDC	European Centre for Disease
	Prevention and Control
ECDPC	European Centre for Disease
	Prevention and Control (EDCD is
	used)
ECE	endothelin-converting enzyme
	extracapsular extension
ECEMG	evoked compound electromyography
ECF	epirubicin, cisplatin, and fluorouracil
	extended care facility
	extracardiac Fontan (procedure)
	extracellular fluid
ECF-A	eosinophil chemotactic factors of
	anaphylaxis
ECFV	extracellular fluid volume
ECG	electrocardiogram
ECGE	extracorporeal gas exchange
ECHINO	echinocyte
ECHO	echocardiogram
	enterocytopathogenic human orphan
	(virus)
	etoposide, cyclophosphamide,
	doxorubicin
	(hydroxydaunomycin), and
	vincristine (Oncovin)
ECHO (2D)	echocardiogram (2-dimensional)
EChoG	electrocochleography
ECHO/RV	echocardiography/
	radionuclide ventriculography
ECI	extracorporeal irradiation
ECIB	extracorporeal irradiation of blood
ECIC	external carotid and internal carotid
	extracranial to intracranial
	(anastamosis)
EC/IC	extracranial/intracranial
ECID	European Centre for Infectious
	Disease
ECK1	*Escherichia coli* K1
ECL	electrochemiluminescence
	enterochromaffin-like
	extend of cerebral lesion
	extracapillary lesions
ECLA	extracorporeal lung assist
ECLP	extracorporeal liver perfusion
ECM	erythema chronicum migrans
	esophagocardiomyotomy

	extracellular mass
	extracellular matrix
ECM/BCM	extracellular mass, body cell mass ratio
ECMO	enterocytopathogenic monkey orphan (virus)
	extracorporeal circulation membrane oxygenation (oxygenator)
ECN	extended care nursery
ecNOS	endothelial constitutive nitric oxide synthetase
ECochG	electrocochleography
ECOG	Eastern Cooperative Oncology Group
ECoG	electrocochleography
	electrocorticogram
E coli	*Escherichia coli*
ECO~tox~	*Escherichia coli* (heat-labile toxin) vaccine
ECP	emergency care provider
	emergency contraceptive pills
	eosinophil cationic protein
	extracorporeal photochemotherapy
	extracorporeal photopheresis
ECPL	endocavitary pelvic lymphadenectomy
ECPD	external counterpressure device
ECPP	extracorporeal photophoresis
ECR	emergency chemical restraint
	extensor carpi radialis
ECRB	extensor carpi radialis brevis
ECRL	extensor carpi radialis longus
ECS	elective cosmetic surgery
	electrocerebral silence
	endometrial-cancer-specific
ECT	electroconvulsive therapy
	emission computed tomography
	enhanced computed tomography
ECTb	Emory Cardiac Toolbox
ECTR	endoscopic carpal tunnel release
ECU	electrocautery unit
	emergency care unit
	emotional care units
	environmental control unit
	extensor carpi ulnaris
ECV	emergency center visits
	external cephalic version (obstetrics)
ECVD	extracellular volume depletion
ECVE	extracellular volume expansion
ECVP	extracellular volume depletion (dehydration)
ECW	extracellular water
ED	eating disorder(s)
	education
	effective dose
	elbow disarticulation
	emergency department
	emotional disorder

	epidural
	erectile dysfunction
	ethynodiol diacetate
	every day (this is a dangerous abbreviation)
	extensive disease
	extensor digitorum
ED~50~	median effective dose
EDA	elbow disarticulation
EDAM	edatrexate
EDAP	Emergency Department Approved for Pediatrics
	etoposide, dexamethasone, cytarabine, (Ara-C and cisplatin (Platinol)
EDAS	encephalodural arterio-synangiosis
EDAT	Emergency Department Alert Team
EDAX	energy-dispersive analysis of x-rays
EDB	ethylene dibromide
	extensor digitorum brevis
EDC	effective dynamic compliance
	electrodesiccation and curettage
	end diastolic counts
	estimated date of conception
	estimated date of confinement
	estramustine, docetaxel, and carboplatin
	extensor digitorum communis
EDCF	endothelium-derived constricting factor
EDCP	eccentric dynamic compression plates
EDCTP	European and Developing Countries Clinical Trials Partnership
EDD	endothelium-dependent dilation
	esophageal detector device
	expected date of delivery
EdD	Doctor of Education
EDENT	edentulous
EDF	elongation, derotation, and flexion
EDH	epidural hematoma
	extradural hematoma
EDHF	endothelium-derived hyperpolarizing factor
EDI	Eating Disorders Inventory
	electrodeionization
EDITAR	extended-duration topical arthropod repellent
EDL	extensor digitorum longus
ED/LD	emotionally disturbed and learning disabled
EDLF	endogenous digitalis-like factors
EDLS	endogenous digitalis-like substance
EDM	early diastolic murmur
	esophageal Doppler monitor
	extensor digiti minimi
EDMD-AD	autosomal dominate Emery-Dreifuss muscular dystrophy

EDNO	endothelium-related nitric oxide	EEP	end expiratory pressure
ED-OU	emergency department/observation unit	EER	extended endocardial resection extraesophageal reflux
EDP	emergency department physician end-diastolic pressure	EES®	erythromycin ethylsuccinate
		EET	early exercise testing
EDQ	extensor digiti quinti (tendon)	EEUS-NA	endoscopic esophageal ultrasound-guided needle aspiration
EDQM	European Directorate for the Quality of Medicines	EEV	encircling endocardial ventriculotomy
EDQV	extensor digiti quinti five	EF	eccentric fixation
EDR	edrophonium (Tensilon) escalating dose regimen extreme drug resistance		ejection fraction endurance factor erythroblastosis fetalis
EDRF	endothelium derived relaxing factor (nitric oxide)		extended-field (radiotherapy)
EDS	Ehlers-Danlos syndrome excessive daytime somnolence	EFA	essential fatty acid estimated fetal age
EDSS	Expanded Disability Status Scale (Score)	EFAD	essential fatty acid deficiency
		E-FAP	Emory Functional Ambulation Profile
EDT	exposure duration threshold	EFBW	estimate fetal body weight
EDTA	edetic acid (ethylenedi-aminetetraacetic acid)	EFD	episode free day
		EFE	endocardial fibroelastosis epidemic fatal encephalopathy
EDTU	emergency diagnostic and treatment unit	EFF	effacement
EDU	eating disorder unit	EFI	extended-field irradiation
EDV	end-diastolic volume epidermal dysplastic verruciformis	EFHBM	eosinophilic fibrohistiocytic lesion of bone marrow
EDW	estimated dry weight	EFM	electronic fetal monitor(ing) external fetal monitoring
EDX	edatrexate electrodiagnostic energy-dispersive X-ray (analysis)	EFMM	external fetal maternal monitor
		EFMT	electric field mediated transfer
EDXRF	energy-dispersive x-ray fluorescence	EFN	effusion
EE	emetic episodes emotional exhaustion end to end energy expenditure equine encephalitis erosive esophagitis esophageal endoscopy ethinyl estradiol exchange efficiency (units) expressed emotion external ear	EFPIA	European Federation of Pharmaceutical Industries and Associations
		EFR	effective filtration rate
		EFS	event-free survival
		EFV	efavirenz (Sustiva)
		EFW	estimated fetal weight
		EF/WM	ejection fraction/wall motion
		e.g.	for example
		EGA	esophageal gastric (tube) airway estimated gestational age
E & E	eyes and ears	EGB	endoscopic grasp biopsy
EEA	electroencephalic audiometry elemental enteral alimentation end-to-end anastomosis energy expended with activity	EGb	extract of Ginkgo biloba
		EGBUS	external genitalia, Bartholin, urethral, and Skene glands
EEC	ectrodactyly-ectodermal dysplasia (cleft syndrome) endogenous erythroid colony	EGC	early gastric carcinoma
		EGCG	epigallocatechin gallate
		EGFR	epidermal growth factor receptor
EECP	enhanced external counter-pulsation	EGD	esophagogastroduodeno-scopy
EEE	eastern equine encephalomyelitis edema, erythema, and exudate external eye examination	EGDT	esophagogastric devascularization and transection
		EGF	epidermal growth factor
EEG	electroencephalogram	EGF-R	epidermal growth factor receptor
EELS	electron energy loss spectrometry	EGG	electrogastrography
EEN	estimated energy needs	EGJ	esophagogastric junction
EENT	eyes, ears, nose, and throat	EGL	eosinophilic granuloma of the lung

EGS	ethylene glycol succinate
EGSs	external guide sequences
EGTA	esophageal gastric tube airway
	ethyleneglycoltetracetic acid
EH	eccentric hypertrophy
	educationally handicapped
	enlarged heart
	essential hypertension
	extramedullary hematopoiesis
Eh	*Entamoeba histolytica*
EHB	elevate head of bed
	extensor hallucis brevis
EHBA	extrahepatic biliary atresia
EHBF	extrahepatic blood flow
EHC	enterohepatic circulation
EHD	electronic home detention
EHDA	etidronate sodium
EHDP	etidronate disodium (Didronel)
EHE	epithelioid hemangioendothelioma
EHEC	enterohemorrhagic *Escherichia coli*
EHF	epidemic hemorrhagic fever
	extremely high frequency
EHH	episodic hypothermia with hyperhidrosis
	esophageal hiatal hernia
EHI	exertional heat illness
EHL	electrohydraulic lithotripsy
	extensor hallucis longus
EHN	ethotoin
EHO	extrahepatic obstruction
EHPH	extrahepatic portal hypertension
EHR	electronic health record
2EHRZ/ 6HE	daily ethambutol, isoniazid, rifampicin, and pyrazinamide for 2 months, followed by isoniazid and ethambutol for 6 months
2[EHRZ]₃/ 6HE	the same as 2EHRZ/6HE but given three times weekly in the initial intensive phase
2EHRZ/ 4HR	The same as 2EHRZ/6HE, followed by 4 months of daily isoniazid and rifampicin
EHS	Early Head Start (program)
	electrical hypersensitivity
	employee health service
	Engelbreth-Holm-Swarm (tumor)
	exertional heat stroke
EHT	electrohydrothermosation
	essential hypertension
EI	entry inhibitor
	environmental illness
	enzyme immunoassay
	extensor indicis
E/I	expiratory to inspiratory (ratio)
E & I	endocrine and infertility
EIA	enzyme immunoassay
	exercise-induced asthma

EIAB	extracranial-intracranial arterial bypass
EIAC	enzyme-inducing anticonvulsants
EIACD	enzyme-inducing anticonvulsant drug
EIAD	extended-interval aminoglycoside dosing
EIAV	equine infectious anemia virus
EIB	exercise-induced bronchospasm
EIC	early ischemic change(s)
	electrical impedance cardiography
	endometrial intraepithelial carcinoma
	epidermal inclusion cyst
	extensive intraductal component
EICA	extra-intracranial artery (bypass)
EID	electroimmunodiffusion
	electronic infusion device
EIDC	extreme intervertebral disk collapse
EIEC	enteroinvasive *Escherichia coli*
EIL	elective induction of labor
EIN	Employer Identification Number
eIND	Electronic Investigational New Drug (application)
EIOA	excessive intake of alcohol
EIP	elective interruption of pregnancy
	end-inspiratory pressure
	extensor indicis proprius
eIPV	enhanced inactivated polio vaccine
EIR	entomological inoculation rate
EIS	electrical impedance scanning
	endoscopic injection scleropathy
EISR	expanded international search report
EIT	electrical impedance tomography
EITB	enzyme-linked immuno-electrotransfer blot
EIV	external iliac vein
EJ	ejection
	elbow jerk
	external jugular
EJB	ectopic junctional beat
EJN	extended jaundice of newborn
EJP	excitatory junction potential
EJV	external jugular vein
EK	Ektachem 400 (see page 298)
	erythrokinase
EKC	epidemic keratoconjunctivitis
EKG	electrocardiogram
EKO	echoencephalogram
EKY	electrokymogram
EL	exercise limit
	exploratory laparotomy
E-L	external lids
ELA	Establishment License Application
ELAD	extracorporeal liver-assist device
ELAFF	extended lateral arm free flap
ELAM	endothelial leukocyte adhesion molecule
ELAMS	Electronic Laboratory Animal Monitoring System

ELB	early light breakfast
	elbow
ELBW	extremely low birth weight (less than 1000 g)
ELC	earlobe creases
ELCA	excimer laser coronary angioplasty
ELD	end-of-life decision(s)
ELDs	end-of-life decisions
ELDU	extralabel drug use
ELEC	elective
ELF	elective low forceps
	endoscopic laser foraminotomy
	epithelial lining fluid
	etoposide, leucovorin, and fluorouracil
	extremely low frequency
ELFA	enzyme-linked fluorescent immunoassay
ELG	endolumenal gastroplication
	endoluminal graft
ELH	endolymphatic hydrops
ELI	endomyocardial lymphocytic infiltrates
ELIG	eligible
ELIOT	electron intraoperative treatment
ELISA	enzyme-linked immunosorbent assay
ELISPOT	enzyme-linked immunospot
ELITT	endometrial laser intrauterine thermal therapy
Elix	elixir
ELLIP	ellipotocytosis
ELM	epiluminescent microscopy
	external laryngeal manipulation
ELM scale-2	Early Language Milestone Scale - second edition
ELND	elective lymph node dissection
ELOP	estimated length of program
ELOS	estimated length of stay
ELP	electrophoresis
	eruptive lingual papillitis
ELPS	excessive lateral pressure syndrome
ELR	elevating leg rests (wheelchair description)
ELS	Eaton-Lambert syndrome
	Editor in the Life Sciences
	endolymphatic sac
ELSD	evaporative light scattering detection
ELSI	ethical, legal, and social implications
ELSS	emergency life support system
ELST	endolymphatic sac tumor
ELT	endoscopic laser therapy
	euglobulin lysis time
ELTR	European Liver Transplant Registry
ELVIS™	Enzyme Linked Virus Inducible System
EM	early memory
	ejection murmur
	electron microscope
	emergency medicine
	emmetropia
	eosinophilia-myalgia (syndrome)
	erythema migrans
	erythema multiforme
	erythromelalgia
	esophageal manometry
	estramustine (Emcyt)
	extensive metabolizers
	external monitor
E & M	Evaluation and Management (coding system)
EMA	early morning awakening
	endomysial antibody
EMA-CO	etoposide, methotrexate, dactinomycin (actinomycin-D), cyclophosphamide, and vincristine (Oncovin)
EMB	endometrial biopsy
	endomyocardial biopsy
	eosin-methylene blue (agar)
	ethambutol (Myambutol)
	Explanation of Medicare Benefits
EMBx	endomyocardial biopsy
EMC	encephalomyocarditis
	endometrial currettage
	essential mixed cryoglobulinemia
	extraskeletal myxoid chondrosarcoma
EMD	electromechanical dissociation
EMDA	electromotive drug administration
EMDR	eye movement desensitization and reprocessing
EME	extreme medical emergency
EMEA	European Medicines Evaluation Agency
EMF	elective midforceps
	electromagnetic field(s)
	electromagnetic flow
	electromotive forces
	endomyocardial fibrosis
	erythrocyte maturation factor
	evaporated milk formula
EMG	electromyograph
	emergency
	essential monoclonal gammopathy
EMI	educably mentally impaired
	elderly and mentally infirm
	electromagnetic interference
EMIC	emergency maternity and infant care
E-MICR	electron microscopy
EMIT	enzyme-multiplied immunoassay technique (test)
EML	essential medicines lists (World Health Organization)
EMLA®	eutectic mixture of local anesthetics (lidocaine and prilocaine in an emulsion base)

E

EMLB	erythromycin lactobionate
EMMA	eye-movement measuring apparatus
EMMV	extended mandatory minute ventilation
EMo	ear mold
EMP	electromolecular propulsion
	estramustine phosphate (Emcyt)
EMPD	extramammary Paget disease
EMPI	enterprise master patient index
EMR	educable mentally retarded
	electrical muscle stimulation
	electronic medical record
	emergency mechanical restraint
	empty, measure, and record
	endoscopic mucosal resection
	eye-movement recording
EMS	early morning specimen
	early morning stiffness
	electrical muscle stimulation
	emergency medical services
	eosinophilia myalgia syndrome
EMSA	electrophoretic mobility shift assay
EMSU	early morning specimen of urine
EMT	emergency medical technician
	epithelial-mesenchymal transformation
	estramustine (Emcyt)
EMTA	Emergency Medical Technician, Advanced
EMTALA	Emergency Medical Treatment and Labor Act
EMTC	emergency medical trauma center
EMT-D	emergency medical technician-defibrillation
EMTP	Emergency Medical Technician, Paramedic
EMU	early morning urine
	electromagnetic unit
	epilepsy monitoring unit
EMV	equine morbilli virus
	eye, motor, verbal (grading for Glasgow Coma Scale)
EMVC	early mitral valve closure
EMW	electromagnetic waves
EMZL	extranodal marginal-zone (B-cell) lymphoma
EN	enema
	enteral nutrition
	erythema nodosum
E/N	eggnog
E 50% N	extension 50% of normal
ENA	extractable nuclear antigen
ENB	esthesioneuroblastoma
ENC	encourage
eNDA	Electronic New Drug Application
ENDO	endodontia
	endodontics

	endoscopy
	endotracheal
EndoCAB	plasma antiendotoxin core antibody
ENF	Enfamil
ENF c Fe	Enfamil with iron
ENG	electronystagmogram
	engorged
ENL	enlarged
	erythema nodosum leprosum
ENMG	electroneuromyography
ENMT	ears, nose, mouth, and throat
ENOG	electroneurography
eNOS	endothelial nitric oxide synthase
ENP	extractable nucleoprotein
ENRD	endoscopy-negative reflux disease
ENS	enteric nervous system
	exogenous natural surfactant
ENT	ears, nose, throat
ENTIS	European Network of Teratology Information Services
ENTV	enzootic nasal tumor virus
ENVD	elevated new vessels on the disk
ENVE	elevated new vessels elsewhere
ENVT	environment
ENZ	enzastaurin
EO	elbow orthosis
	embolic occlusion
	eosinophilia
	ethylene oxide
	eyes open
E & O	errors and omissions
EOA	erosive osteoarthritis
	esophageal obturator airway
	examine, opinion, and advice
	external oblique aponeurosis
EOAE	evoked otoacoustic emissions
EOB	edge of bed
	end of bed
	explanation of benefits
EOC	Emergency Operations Center
	enema of choice
	epithelial ovarian cancer
EOD	early-onset disease
	end of day
	end organ damage
	every other day (this is a dangerous abbreviation)
	extent of disease
EOE	Equal Opportunity Employer
	extraosseous Ewing sarcoma
EOFAD	early-onset form of familial Alzheimer disease
E of I	evidence of insurability
EOG	electro-oculogram
	electro-olfactogram
	Ethrane, oxygen, and gas (nitrous oxide)

EOGBS	early-onset group B streptococcal (sepsis)	
EOL	end of file	
EOLC	end-of-life-care	
EOM	error of measurement external otitis media extraocular movement extraocular muscles	
EOMB	explanation of Medicare benefits	
EOMG	early-onset myasthenia gravis	
EOMI	extraocular muscles intact	
EOO	external oculomotor ophthalmoplegia	
EOP1	end-of-phase 1	
EOP2	end-of-phase 2	
EOR	emergency operating room end of range	
EORA	elderly onset rheumatoid arthritis	
EORTC	European Organization for Research and the Treatment of Cancer	
EOS	end of study eosinophil	
EP	ectopic pregnancy electrophysiologic elopement precaution endogenous pyrogen Episcopalian esophageal pressure etoposide and cisplatin (Platinol) evoked potentials	
E&P	estrogen and progesterone	
EPA	eicosapentaenoic acid Environmental Protection Agency	
EPAB	extracorporeal pneumoperititoneal access bubble	
E-Panel	electrolyte panel (See page 298)	
EPAP	expiratory positive airway pressure	
EPB	extensor pollicis brevis	
EPBD	endoscopic papillary balloon dilatation	
EPC	erosive prephloric changes external pneumatic compression	
EPCs	endothelial progenitor cells	
EPCV	engineering, procurement, construction, and validation	
EPD	electrode placement device equilibrium peritoneal dialysis	
EPEC	enteropathogenic *Escherichia coli*	
EPEG	etoposide (VePesid)	
EPEs	extrapyramidal effects	
EPF	endoscopic plantar fasciotomy Enfamil Premature Formula® extrapyramidal features	
EPG	electronic pupillography Episodic Payment Group	
EPHI	electronic protected health information	
EPI	echoplanar imaging epinephrine	

	epirubicin (Ellence) epitheloid cells exercise pressure index exocrine pancreatic insufficiency Expanded Program of Immunizations, (World Health Organization) Eysenck Personality Inventory
EPIC	etoposide, prednisolone, ifosfamide, and cisplatin
EPID	epidural
epiDX	epirubicin (4′-epidoxorubicin; Ellence)
EPIG	epigastric
EPIS	epileptic postictal sleep episiotomy
epith.	epithelial
EPL	effective patent life extensor pollicis longus (tendon)
EPM	electronic pacemaker
EPMR	electronic patient medical record
EPN	emphysematous pyelonephritis ependymoma estimated protein needs
EPO	epoetin alfa (erythropoietin; Epogen) evening primrose oil exclusive provider organization
EPOCH	etoposide, prednisone, vincristine (Oncovin), cyclophosphamide, doxorubicin (hydroxydaunorubicin)
EPP	erythropoietic protoporphyria extrapleural pneumonectomy
EPPK	epidermolytic palmoplantar keratoderma
EPPROM	extremely preterm premature rupture of the membranes (less than or equal to 24 weeks)
EPQ	Exercise Participation Questionnaire
EPQ-R	Eysenck Personality Questionnaire— Revised
EPR	electronic prescription record electron paramagnetic (spin) resonance electrophrenic respiration emergency physical restraint epirubicin (Ellence) estimated protein requirement
EPS	electrolyte-polyethyleneglycol solution electrophysiologic study expressed prostatic secretions extrapulmonary shunt extrapyramidal syndrome (symptom)
EPSA	evoked potential signal averaging
EPSCCA	extrapulmonary small cell carcinoma
EPSDT	early periodic screening, diagnosis, and treatment

E

EPSE	extrapyramidal side effects		endocardial resection procedure
EPSP	excitatory postsynaptic potential		endoscopic retrograde
EPSS	E point septal separation		pancreatography
EPT	electroporation therapy		event-related potentials
	endpoint temperature		estrogen receptor protein
EPT®	early pregnancy test		exposure and ritual prevention
EPTE	existed prior to enlistment	ERPF	effective renal plasma flow
EPTS	existed prior to service	ER/PR	estrogen receptor/progesterone
EQC	equivalent quality control		receptor
ER	emergency room	ERS	endoscopic retrograde
	end range		sphincterotomy
	estrogen receptors		evacuation of retained secundines
	extended release		(afterbirth)
	extended external rotation	ERSR	Electronic Regulatory Submission
	external resistance		and Review
E & R	equal and reactive	ERS-TM	Event Reporting System -
	examination and report		Transfusion Medicine
ER+	estrogen receptor-positive	ERT	estrogen replacement therapy
ER−	estrogen receptor-negative		external radiotherapy
ERA	estrogen receptor assay	ERTD	emergency room triage
	evoked response audiometry		documentation
%ERAD	eradication rates	ERUS	endorectal ultrasound
ERAS	Electronic Residency Application	ERV	early revascularization
	Service		expiratory reserve volume
erbB1	estrogen receptor (tyrosine kinase	e-Rx	electronic prescription
	family) type B1	Er:YAG	Erbium: yttrium aluminum garnet
ERBD	endoscopic retrograde biliary		(laser)
	drainage	ERYTH	erythromycin
ER by ICA	estrogen receptor	ES	electrical stimulation
	immunocytochemistry assay		*Eleutherococcus senticosus* (Siberian
ERC	endoscopic retrograde		Ginseng)
	cholangiography		embryonic stem (cells)
ERCP	endoscopic retrograde		emergency service
	cholangiopancreatography		endoscopic sclerotherapy
ERCT	emergency room computerized		endoscopic sphincterotomy
	tomography		end-to-side
ERD	early retirement with disability		ever-smokers
	erectile dysfunction		Ewing sarcoma
ERE	external rotation in extension		ex-smoker
ERF	external rotation in flexion		extra strength
ERFC	erythrocyte rosette forming cells	ESA	early systolic acceleration
ERG	electroretinogram		end-to-side anastomosis
ERI	elective replacement indicator		ethmoid sinus adenocarcinoma
ERIG	equine-rabies immune globulin	ESADDI	estimated safe and adequate daily
ERL	effective refractory length		dietary intake
ERLND	elective regional lymph node	ESAP	evoked sensory (nerve) action
	dissection		potential
ERM	epiretinal membrane	ESAS	Edmonton System Assessment
ERMBT	erythromycin breath testing		System
ERMS	exacerbating-remitting multiple	ESAT	extrasystolic atrial tachycardia
	sclerosis	ESBL	extended-spectrum beta-lactamases
ERN	error-related negativity (signal)	ESBLKP	extended-spectrum beta-lactamase-
ERNA	equilibrium radionuclide		producing *Klebsiella pneumoniae*
	angiocardiography	ESC	embryonic stem cells
ERO	effective regurgitant orifice		end systolic counts
	(cardiology)	ESCC	esophageal squamous cell carcinoma
ERP	effective refractory period	ESCOP	European Scientific Cooperative on
	emergency room physician		Phytotherapy

E

ESCS	electrical spinal cord stimulation		established patient
ESD	early supported discharge		estimated
	Emergency Services Department		exercise stress test
	esophagus, stomach, and duodenum		expressed sequence tag
ESE	exon splice enhancer	E-stim	electrical stimulation
eSET	elective single embryo transfer	ESTs	expressed sequence tags
ESF	external skeletal fixation	ESU	electrosurgical unit
ESFT	Ewing sarcoma family of tumors	ESWL	extracorporeal shock wave lithotripsy
ESHAP	etopside, methylprednisolone (Solu-Medrol), high-dose cytarabine (ara-C), and cisplatin (Platinol)	ESWT	extracorporeal shockwave therapy
		ET	ejection time
			embryo transfer
ESI	electrospray ionization		endocrine therapy
	epidural steroid injection		endometrial thickness
ESI-MS	electrospray ionization-mass spectrometry		endothelin
			endotoxin
ESIN	elastic stable intramedullary nailing		endotracheal
ESKD	end-stage kidney disease		endotracheal tube
ESL	English as a second language		enterostomal therapy (therapist)
ESLD	end-stage liver disease		epirubicin and paclitaxel (Taxol)
	end-stage lung disease		esotropia
ESM	ejection systolic murmur		essential thrombocythemia
	endolymphatic stromal myosis		essential tremor
	ethosuximide (Zarontin)		eustachian tube
ESMO	European Society of Medical Oncology		Ewing tumor
			exchange transfusion
ESN	educationally subnormal		exercise treadmill
ESN(M)	educationally subnormal-moderate		exposure time
ESN(S)	educationally subnormal-severe	et	and
ESO	esophagus	ET′	esotropia at near
	esotropia	E(T)	intermittent esotropia at infinity
ESO/D	esotropia at distance	E(T′)	intermittent esotropia at near
ESO/N	estropia at near	ET-1	endothelin-1
ESP	endometritis, salpingitis, and peritonitis	2ET	two embryo transfer
		ET @ 20′	esotropia at 6 meters (infinity)
	end-systolic pressure	ETA	endotracheal airway
	especially		ethionamide (Trecator-SC)
	extrasensory perception	ETAC	early treatment of the allergic child
ESPAC	European Study Group for Pancreatic Cancers	et al	and others
		ETBD	etiology to be determined
ES/PNET	Ewing sarcomas and peripheral neuroectodermal tumor	EtBr	ethidium bromide
		ETC	and so forth
ESR	early sheath removal		electrothermal capsulorrhaphy
	electron spin resonance		Emergency and Trauma Center
	erythrocyte sedimentation rate		endoscopic tissue culture
ESRD	end-stage renal disease		epirubicin, paclitaxel (Taxol), and cyclophosphamide
ESRF	end-stage renal failure		
ESRS	Extrapyramidal Symptom Rating Scale		estimated time of conception
		ETCH-C	Evaluation Tool of Children's Handwriting-Cursive
ESS	emotional, spiritual, and social		
	endometrial stromal sarcoma	ETCO$_2$	end-tidal carbon dioxide
	endoscopic sinus surgery	ETD	electron transfer dissociation
	Epworth Sleepiness Scale		endoscopic transformational diskectomy
	essential		
	euthyroid sick syndrome		eustachian tube dysfunction
EST	Eastern Standard Time		eye-tracking dysfunction
	endoscopic spincterotomy	ETDLA	esophageal-tracheal double lumen airway
	electroshock therapy		
	electrostimulation therapy	ETE	end-to-end

ETEC	enterotoxigenic *Escherichia coli*	EUG	extrauterine gestation
ETF	early treatment failure	EUL	extra uterine life
	eustachian tubal function	EUM	external urethral meatus
ETFN	empiric therapy in a febrile neutropenic (patient)	EUP	Experimental Use Permit extrauterine pregnancy
ETG	Episodic Treatment Group	EUS	endoscopic ultrasonography
ETGT	equal to or greater than		esophageal ultrasound
ETH	elixir terpin hydrate		external urethral sphincter
	ethanol	EUS-FNA	endoscopic ultrasonography with
	Ethrane		fine-needle aspiration
ETHc̄C	elixir terpin hydrate with codeine	EUTH	euthanasia
ETI	ejective time index	EV	epidermodysplasia verruciformis
	endotracheal intubation		esophageal varices
ETKTM	every test known to man		etoposide and vincristine
ETL	echo train length (radiology)		eversion
ETLE	extratemporal lobe epilepsy	eV	electron volt (unit of radiation
ETLT	equal to or less than		energy)
ETO	estimated time of ovulation	EV71	enterovirus-71
	ethylene oxide	EVA	Entry and Validation Application
	etoposide (VePesid)		ethylene vinyl acetate
	eustachian tube obstruction		etoposide, vinblastine, and
EtOH	alcohol (ethyl alcohol)		doxorubicin (Adriamycin)
	alcoholic	EVAC	evacuation
ETOP	elective termination of pregnancy	EVAc	ethylene-vinyl acetate copolymer
ETP	elective termination of pregnancy	eval	evaluate
	electronic transmission of prescriptions	EVAR	endovascular aneurysm repair
		EVC	Ellis-van Creveld (syndrome)
ETS	elevated toilet seat	EVG	endovascular grafting
	endoscopic transthoracic sympathectomy	EWB	emotional well-being
		EWBH	extracorporeal whole body hyperthermia
	endotracheal suction		
	end-to-side	EXC	excision
	environmental tobacco smoke	EVD	external ventricular (ventriculostomy) drain
	erythromycin topical solution		
ETT	endotracheal tube	EVE	endoscopic vascular examination
	endurance treadmill test		evening
	esophageal transit time	EVER	eversion
	exercise tolerance test	EVG	endovascular grafting
	exercise treadmill test (time)	EVH	endoscopic (saphenous) vein
	extrathyroidal thyroxine		harvesting
ETT-Tl	exercise treadmill test with thallium	EVI	Exposure to Violence Interview
		EVL	endoscopic variceal ligation
ETU	emergency and trauma unit	EVLT	endovenous laser therapy
	emergency treatment unit	EVS	endoscopic variceal sclerosis
ETV	endoscopic third ventriculostomy	EW	expiratory wheeze
ETX	edatrexate		elsewhere
ETYA	eicosatetraynoic acid	EWB	estrogen withdrawal bleeding
EU	Ehrlich units	EWCL	extended-wear contact lens
	endotoxin units	EWE	Eastern and Western
	equivalent units		encephalomyelitis vaccine
	esophageal ulcer	EWHO	elbow-wrist-hand orthosis
	etiology unknown	EWL	estimated weight loss
	European Union	EWS	Early Warning Score
	excretory urography		Ewing sarcoma
EUA	examine under anesthesia	EWSCLs	extended-wear soft contact lenses
EUCD	emotionally unstable character disorder	EWT	erupted wisdom teeth
		ex	examined
EUD	external urinary device		example

	excision
	exercise
exam.	examination
ExB	excisional biopsy
EXE	exemestane (Aromasin)
EXEC 22	Executive 22 chemistry profile (see page 298)
EXECHO	exercise echocardiography
EXEF	exercise ejection fraction
EXGBUS	external genitalia, Bartholin (glands), urethral (glands), and Skene (glands)
EXH VT	exhaled tidal volume
EXIT	Ex-Utero Intrapartum Treatment
EXIT 25	Executive Interview (cognitive impairment test)
EXL	elixir
EXOPH	exophthalmos
EXP	experienced
	expired
	exploration
	expose
expect	expectorant
exp. lap.	exploratory laparotomy
EXT	extension
	extensor (tendon)
	external
	extract
	extraction
	extremities
	extremity
Ext mon	external monitor
extrav	extravasation
ext. rot.	external rotation
EXTUB	extubation
EX U	excretory urogram
EZ	Edmonston-Zagreb (vaccine)
EZ-IIT	Edmonston-Zagreb high-titer (vaccine)

F	facial
	Fahrenheit
	fair
	false
	fasting
	father
	feces
	female
	finger
	firm
	flow
	fluoride
	French
	Friday
	fundi
	fundus
F/	full upper denture
/F	full lower denture
(F)	final
°F	degrees Fahrenheit
F=	firm and equal
F_1	offspring from the first generation
F_2	offspring from the second generation
F_3	Fluothane
14 F	14-hour fast required
F II-F XIII	factor 2 through 13
FA	Fanconi anemia
	fatty acid
	femoral artery
	fetus active
	fibroadenoma
	first aid
	fludarabine (Fludara)
	fluorescein angiogram
	fluorescent antibody
	folic acid
	folinic acid (leucovorin calcium) (this is a dangerous abbreviation)
	forearm
	Friedreich ataxia
	functional activities
FAA	febrile antigen agglutination
	folic acid antagonist
FAAD	Fellow American Academy of Dermatology
FAAH	fatty acid amide hydrolase
FAAN	Food Allergy and Anaphylaxis Network
FAAP	family assessment adjustment pass
FAAPM	Fellow, American Academy of Pain Management
FAA SOL	formalin, acetic, and alcohol solution
FAAN	Fellow of the American Academy of Nursing

FAAP	Fellow of the American Academy of Pediatrics	FACOS	Fellow of the American College of Orthopedic Surgeons
FAB	digoxin immune Fab (Digibind)	FACP	Fellow of the American College of Physicians
	French-American-British Cooperative group	FACPRM	Fellow of the American College of Preventive Medicine
	functional arm brace		
FABACs	fatty acid bile acid conjugates	FACR	Fellow of the American College of Radiology
FABER	flexion, abduction, and external rotation	FACS	Fellow of the American College of Surgeons
FABF	femoral artery blood flow		
FAC	ferrite ammonium citrate		fluorescent-activated cell sorter
	fluorouracil, doxorubicin (Adriamycin), and cyclophosphamide	FACSM	Fellow of the American College of Sports Medicine
	fractional area change	FACT	focused appendix computed tomography
	fractional area concentration	FACT-An	Functional Assessment of Cancer Therapy-Anemia
	functional aerobic capacity		
FACA	Fellow of the American College of Anaesthetists	FACT-B	....-Breast
		FACT-F	....-Fatigue
FACAG	Fellow of the American College of Angiology	FACT-G	....-General
		FACT-L	.....-Lung
FACAL	Fellow of the American College of Allergists	FACT-O	....-Ovarian
		FACT-P	....-Prostate
FACAN	Fellow of the American College of Anesthesiologists	FAD	familial Alzheimer disease
			Family Assessment Device
FACAS	Fellow of the American College of Abdominal Surgeons		fetal abdominal diameter
			fetal activity determination
FACC	Fellow of the American College of Cardiology		flavin adenine dinucleotide
		FAE	fetal alcohol effect
FACCP	Fellow of the American College of Chest Physicians	FAEE	fatty acid ethyl ester
		FAF	frequency-altered feedback
FACCPC	Fellow of the American College of Clinical Pharmacology & Chemotherapy	FAFSA	Free Application for Federal Student Aid
		FAGA	full-term appropriate for gestational age
FACD	Fellow of the American College of Dentists		
		FAH	fumarylacetoacetase hydrolase
FACEM	Fellow of the American College of Emergency Medicine	FAI	Functional Assessment Inventory
		FAK	focal adhesion kinase
FACEP	Fellow of the American College of Emergency Physicians	FAL	femoral arterial line
		FALL	fallopian
FACES	pain scale for assessing pain intensity	FALS	familial amyotrophic lateral sclerosis
		FAM	family
FACG	Fellow of the American College of Gastroenterology		fluorouracil, doxorubicin (Adriamycin), and mitomycin
FACH	forceps to after-coming head		full allosteric modulators
FACIT-F	Functional Assessment of Chronic Illness Therapy Fatigue Subscale	FAMA	fluorescent antibody to membrane antigen
		FAME	fluorouracil, doxorubicin (Adriamycin), and semustin (methyl CCNU)
FACLM	Fellow of the American College of Legal Medicine		
FACN	Fellow of the American College of Nutrition	FAMMM	familial atypical multiple mole melanoma
FACNP	Fellow of the American College of Neuropsychopharmacology	FAM-S	fluorouracil, doxorubicin (Adriamycin), mitomycin, and streptozotocin
FACO	Fellow of the American College of Otolaryngology	FAMTX	fluorouracil, doxorubicin (Adriamycin), and methotrexate
FACOG	Fellow of the American College of Obstetricians & Gynecologists	FANA	fluorescent antinuclear antibody

FANG	fluorescent angiography	FBM	felbamate (Felbatol)
FANSS&M	fundus anterior, normal size and shape and mobile		fetal breathing motion
			foreign body, metallic
FAO	fatty acid oxidation	FBP	frontal bite plane (dental)
	Food and Agriculture Organization	FBRCM	fingerbreadth below right costal margin
FAP	Facility Admission Profile		
	familial adenomatous polyposis	FBS	failed back syndrome
	familial amyloid polyneuropathy		fasting blood sugar
	femoral artery pressure		fetal bovine serum
	fibrillating action potential		foreign body sensation (eye)
	functional ambulation profile	FBSS	failed back surgery syndrome
FAQ	frequently asked question(s)	FBU	fingers below umbilicus
FAR	frontal arousal rhythm	FBW	fasting blood work
F-ara-A	fludarabine phosphate (Fludara)	FC	family conference
f-ARPV	fosamprenavir (Lexiva)		febrile convulsion
FARS	Fatality Analysis Reporting System		female child
FAS	fetal alcohol syndrome		fever, chills
FASAY	functional analysis of separated alleles in yeast		film coated (tablets)
			financial class
FASC	fluorescent-activated substrate conversion (assay)		finger clubbing
			finger counting
	fasciculations		flexion contractor
FASHP	Fellow of the American Society of Health-System Pharmacists		flow compensation (radiology)
			flucytosine (Ancobon)
FASPS	familial advanced sleep-phase syndrome		foam cuffed (tracheal or endotracheal tube)
			Foley catheter
FAST	fetal acoustic stimulation testing		follows commands
	flow assisted short-term		foster care
	fluorescent allergosorbent technique		French Canadian
	focused assessment with sonography for trauma		functional capacity
			functional class
FAT	Fetal Activity Test	F/C	film coated (tablet)
	fluorescent antibody test	F + C	flare and cells
	food awareness training	F & C	foam and condom
FAV	facio-auricular vertebral	5FC	flucytosine (this is a dangerous abbreviation as it can be seen as 5FU)
FAZ	foveal avascular zone		
FB	fasting blood (sugar)		
	finger breadth		
	flexible bronchoscope	FCA	Federal False Claims Act
	foreign body		femoral cortical allograft
F/B	followed by	FCAS	familial cold autoinflammatory syndrome
	forward/backward		
	forward bending	F. cath.	Foley catheter
FBC	full (complete) blood count	FCBD	fibrocystic breast disease
FBCOD	foreign body, cornea, right eye	FCC	familial cerebral cavernoma
FBCOS	foreign body, cornea, left eye		familial colonic cancer
FBD	familial British dementia		family centered care
	fibrocystic breast disease		femoral cerebral catheter
	functional bowel disease		follicular center cells
FBF	forearm blood flow		fracture compound comminuted
FBG	fasting blood glucose	FCCA	Final Comprehensive Consensus Assessment
	foreign-body-type granulomata		
FBH	hydroxybutyric dehydrogenase	FCCC	fracture complete, compound, and comminuted
FBHH	familial benign hypocalciuric hypercalcemia		
		FCCL	follicular center cell lymphoma
FBI	flossing, brushing, and irrigation	FCCM	Fellow, American College of Critical Care Medicine
	full bony impaction		
FBL	fecal blood loss	FCCU	family centered care unit

F

FCD	feces collection device
	fibrocystic disease
FCDB	fibrocystic disease of the breast
FCE	fluorouracil, cisplatin, and etoposide
	functional capacity evaluation
FCFD	fluorescence capillary-fill device
FCH	familial combined hyperlipidemia
	fibrosing cholestatic hepatitis
FCHL	familial combined hyperlipemia
FCI	flow cytometric immunophenotyping
FCL	fibular collateral ligament
F-CL	fluorouracil and calcium leucovorin
FCM	facial choreic movements
	flow cytometry
FCMC	family centered maternity care
FCMD	Fukiyama congenital muscular dystrophy
FCMN	family centered maternity nursing
FCNV	fever, cough, nausea, and vomiting
FCOU	finger count, both eyes
FCP	formocresol pulpotomu
FCR	flexor carpi radialis
	fractional catabolic rate
FCRB	flexor carpi radialis brevis
FCRT	fetal cardiac reactivity test
	focal cranial radiation therapy
FCS	fever, chills, and sweating
FCSNVD	fever, chills, sweating, nausea, vomiting, and diarrhea
FCSRT	Free and Cued Selective Reminding Test
FCT	fever-clearance time
FCU	flexor carpi ulnaris (tendon)
FCV	feline calicivirus
FD	familial dysautonomia
	fetal demise
	fetal distress
	focal distance
	food diary
	forceps delivery
	Forestier Disease
	free drain
	full denture
	fully dilated
	functional deficits
F & D	fixed and dilated
FDA	Food and Drug Administration
	fronto-dextra anterior
FDB	first-degree burn
	flexor digitorum brevis
FDBL	fecal daily blood loss
FDC	familial dilated cardiomyopathy
	fixed-dose combination (preparations)
FDCA	Food, Drug, and Cosmetic Act
FDCs	follicular dendritic cells
FDE	fixed-drug eruption
FDF	flexor digitorum profundus (tendon)

FDG	feeding
	fluorine-18-labeled deoxyglucose ([18]fluorodeoxyglucose)
FDGB	fall down, go boom
FDG-PET	positron emission tomography with [18]fluorodeoxyglucose
FDGS	feedings
FDI	first dorsal interosseous
	food-drug interaction
	Functional Disability Index
FDIU	fetal death in utero
FDL	flexor digitorum longus
FDLMP	first day of last menstrual period
FDM	fetus of diabetic mother
	flexor digiti minimi
FDP	fibrin-degradation products
	fixed-dose procedure
	flexor digitorum profundus
FDPCA	fixed-dose patient-controlled analgesia
FD-PET	fluorodopa-positron emission tomography
FDQB	flexor digiti quinti brevis
FDR	first-dose reaction
FDS	flexor digitorum superficialis
	for duration of stay
FDT	frequency-doubling technology (perimetry for visual field screening)
	fronto-dextra transversa (right frontotransverse)
	Functional Dexterity Test
FE	field echo (radiology)
	frequency encode (radiology)
Fe	female
	iron
F & E	full and equal
FEB	febrile
FEC	fluorouracil, epirubicin, and cyclophosphamide
	fluorouracil, etoposide, and cisplatin
	forced expiratory capacity
FECG	fetal electrocardiogram
FeCh	ferrochelatase
FECP	free erythrocyte coproporphyrin
FeCrNi	iron-chromium-nickel alloy
FECT	fibroelastic connective tissue
FED	fish eye disease
FEE	Far-Eastern equine encephalitis
FEES	fiberoptic endoscopic evaluation (examination) of swallowing
FEESST	flexible endoscopic evaluation of swallowing with sensory testing
FEF	forced expiratory flow rate
$FEF_{25\%-75\%}$	forced expiratory flow during the middle half of the forced vital capacity

FEF$_{x-y}$	forced expiratory flow between two designated volume points in the forced vital capacity
FEHBP	Federal Employee Health Benefits Plan
FEL	familial erythrophagocytic lymphohistiocytosis
FeLV	feline leukemia virus
FEM	femoral
FEMA	Federal Emergency Management Agency
FEM-FEM	femoral femoral (bypass)
FEM-POP	femoral popliteal (bypass)
FEM-TIB	femoral tibial (bypass)
FERGs	focal electroretinograms
FEN	fluid, electrolytes, and nutrition
FENa	fractional extraction of sodium
FENIB	familial encephalopathies with neuroserpin inclusion bodies
FEN-PHEN	fenfluramine and phentermine
FENS	field-electrical neural stimulation
FEOM	full extraocular movements
FEP	free erythrocyte porphyrins
	free erythrocyte protoporphorin
	functional exercise program
FER	flexion, extension, and rotation
FERPA	Family Educational Rights and Privacy Act
FERR	serum ferritin
FES	fat embolism syndrome
	floppy eyelid syndrome
	forced expiratory spirogram
	functional electrical stimulation
FeSO$_4$	ferrous sulfate
FESS	functional endonasal sinus surgery
	functional endoscopic sinus surgery
FET	familial essential tremor
	fixed erythrocyte turnover
	frozen embryo transfer
FETI	fluorescence (fluorescent) energy transfer immunoassay
FEUO	for external use only
FEV	familial exudative vitreoretinopathy
FEV$_1$	forced expiratory volume in one second
FEVC	forced expiratory vital capacity
FEV$_{1\%VC}$	forced expiratory volume in one second as percent of forced vital capacity
FEVR	familial exudative vitreoretinopathy
FF	fat free
	fecal frequency
	filtration fraction
	finger-to-finger
	five-minute format
	flat feet
	force fluids
	formula fed
	forward flexion
	foster father
	Fox-Fordyce (disease)
	fundus firm
	further flexion
F/F	face-to-face
F&F	filiform and follower
	fixes and follows
F→F	finger to finger
FF1/U	fundus firm 1 cm above umbilicus
FF2/U	fundus firm 2 cm above umbilicus
FF@u	fundus firm at umbilicus
FFA	free fatty acid
	fundus fluorescein angiogram
	fusiform face area
FFAT	Free Floating Anxiety Test
FFB	flexible fiberoptic bronchoscopy
FFCD	French Foundation for Digestive Cancerology
FFD	fat-free diet
	focal-film distance
FFDM	freedom from distant metastases
	full-field digital mammography
FFE	free-flow electrophoresis
FFF	field-flow fractionation
	freedom from (biochemical and/or clinical) failure
FFI	fast food intake
	fatal familial insomnia
FFM	fat-free mass
	Five-Factor Model (of personality)
	five-finger movement
	freedom from metastases
FFN	fetal fibronectin
FFP	free from progression
	fresh frozen plasma
FFPE	formalin-fixed, paraffin-embedded
FFQ	food frequency questionnaire
FFR	freedom from relapse
	Forward Functional Reach (test)
FFROM	full, free range of motion
FFS	failure-free survival
	fee-for-service
	Fight For Sight
	flexible fiberoptic sigmoidoscopy
FFT	fast-Fourier transforms
	flicker fusion threshold
FFTC	fast-Fourier Transform Convolution
FFTDWB	flat foot touchdown weight bearing
FFTP	first full-term pregnancy
FFU/1	fundus firm 1 cm below umbilicus
FFU/2	fundus firm 2 cm below umbilicus
FG	fibrin glue
	fusiform gyrus
FGAs	first-generation antihistamines
	first-generation antipsychotics
FGC	familial gigantiform cementoma
	full gold crown

FGF	fibroblast growth factor
FGID	functional gastrointestinal disorder(s)
FGM	female genital mutilation
FGP	fundic gland polyps
FGR	fetal growth restriction
FGS	fibrogastroscopy
	focal glomerulosclerosis
FH	familial hypercholesterolemia
	family history
	favorable histology
	fetal head
	fetal heart
	fundal height
FH+	family history positive
FH−	family history negative
FHA	filamentous hemagglutinin
FHB	flexor hallucis brevis
FHC	familial hypertrophic cardiomyopathy
	family health center
FHCIC	Fuchs heterochromic iridocyclitis
FHD	family history of diabetes
FHF	fulminant hepatic failure
FHH	familial hypocalciuric hypercalcemia
	fetal heart heard
FHI	frontal horn index
	Fuchs heterochromic iridocyclitis
FHL	flexor hallucis longus
	functional hallux limitus
FHM	familial hemiplegic migraine
FHN	family history negative
FHNH	fetal heart not heard
FHO	family history of obesity
FHP	family history positive
FHR	fetal heart rate
FHRB	fetal heart rate baseline
FHRV	fetal heart rate variability
FHS	fetal heart sounds
	fetal hydantoin syndrome
FHT	fetal heart tone
FHVP	free hepatic vein pressure
FHX	fluorouracil, hydroxyurea, and radiotherapy
FHx	family history
FI	fecal incontinence
	fiscal intermediary
FIA	familial intracranial aneurysms
	Family Independence Agency (formerly Department of Social Services)
FIAC	fiacitabine
FIAU	fialuridine
FIB	fibrillation
	fibula
	focused ion-beam
FICA	Federal Insurance Contributions Act (Social Security)
$FiCO_2$	fraction of inspired carbon dioxide
FICS	Fellow of the International College of Surgeons
FID	father in delivery
	free induction decay
FIF	forced inspiratory flow
FiF	Functional Intact Fibrinogen (test)
FIGE	field inversion gel electrophoresis
FIGLU	formiminoglutamic acid
FIGO	International Federation of Gynecology and Obstetrics
FIH	first-in-human (trial)
FIL	father-in-law
	Filipino
FIM	functional independence measure
FIN	flexible intramedullary nail
FIND	follow-up intervention for normal development
FiO_2	fraction of inspired oxygen
FIP	feline infectious peritonitis
	flatus in progress
FIRI	fasting insulin resistance index
FISH	fluorescent (fluorescence) *in situ* hybridization
FISP	fast imaging with steady state precision
FITC	fluorescein isothiocyanate conjugated
FIV	feline immunodeficiency virus
	in vitro fertilization (French)
FIVC	forced inspiratory vital capacity
FIX	factor IX (nine)
FJB	facet joint block
FJN	familial juvenile nephrophthisis
FJP	familial juvenile polyposis
FJROM	full joint range of motion
FJS	finger joint size
FJV	first jejunal vein
FK506	tacrolimus (Prograf)
FKA	failed to keep appointment
	formally known as
FKBP	FK-506 binding protein (tacrolimus; Prograf)
FKD	Kinetic Family Drawing
FKE	full-knee extension
FKGL	Flesh-Kincaid Grade Level (score)
FL	fatty liver
	femur length
	fetal length
	fluid
	fluorescein
	fluorouracil and leucovorin
	flutamide and leuprolide acetate
	focal laser
	focal length
	follicular lymphoma
	full liquids
	functional limitations
fL	femtoliter (10^{-15} liter)

F/L	father-in-law
FLA	free-living amebic (ameba)
	low-friction arthroplasty
FLAG	**fl**udarabine, **a**ra-C (cytarabine), and
	G-CSF (filgrastim)
FLAIR	fluid-attenuated inversion recovery
FLAP	fluorouracil, leucovorin, doxorubicin
	(Adriamycin), and cisplatin
	(Platinol)
	5-lipoxygenase activating protein
FLASH	fast low-angle shot
FLAVO	flavopiridol
FLB	funny looking beat
FLBS	funny looking baby syndrome (see
	note under FLK)
FLC	follicular large cell lymphoma
	fuzzy logic control
FLD	fatty liver disease
	fluid
	flutamide and leuprolide acetate
	depot
	full lower denture
FL Dtr	full lower denture
FLE	frontal lobe epilepsy
FLe	fluorouracil and levamisole
flcxsig	flexible sigmoidoscopy
FLF	funny looking facies (see note under
	FLK)
FLGA	full-term, large for gestational age
FLIC	Functional Living Index– Cancer
FLIE	Functional Living Index– Emesis
FLK	funny looking kid (should never be
	used: unusual facial features, is a
	better expression)
FLM	fetal lung maturity
fl. oz.	fluid ounce
FLP	fasting lipid profile
	Functional Limitations Profile
FL REST	fluid restriction
FLS	fibroblast-like synoviocytes
	flashing lights and/or scotoma
	flu-like symptoms
FLT	fluorothymidine
FLU	fluconazole (Diflucan)
	fludarabine (Fludara)
	flunisolide (Aero Bid)
	fluoxetine (Prozac)
	fluticasone propionate (Flonase)
	influenza
FLU A	influenza A virus
FLUO	Fluothane
fluoro	fluoroscopy
FLUT	flutamide (Eulexin)
FLV	Friend leukemia virus
FLW	fasting laboratory work
FLZ	flurazepam (Dalmane)
FM	face mask
	fat mass

	fetal movements
	fibromyalgia (syndrome)
	fine motor
	floor manager
	fluorescent microscopy
	foster mother
F & M	firm and midline (uterus)
F-MACHOP	fluorouracil, methotrexate, cytarabine
	(ara-C), cyclophosphamide,
	doxorubicin
	(hydroxydaunorubicin), vincristine
	(Oncovin), and prednisone
FMC	fetal movement count
FMD	family medical doctor
	fibromuscular dysplasia
	flow-mediated dilatation
	foot-and-mouth disease
FMDV	foot-and-mouth disease virus
FME	Frühsommer-meningoenzephalitis
	vaccine
	full-mouth extraction
FMEA	failure mode effects analysis
FMEN-1	familial multiple endocrine
	neoplasia, type 1
FMF	familial Mediterranean fever
	fetal movement felt
	forced midexpiratory flow
FMG	fine mesh gauze
	foreign medical graduate
FMH	family medical history
	fibromuscular hyperplasia
FM 100-hue	Farnsworth-Munsell 100-hue test
FmHx	family history
FML(r)	fluorometholone
FMLA	Family and Medical Leave Act of
	1993
FMN	first malignant neoplasm
	flavin mononucleotide
FMOA	full-mouth odontectomy and
	alveoloplasty
FMOL	femtomole (10^{-15} mole)
FMP	fasting metabolic panel
	first menstrual period
	functional maintenance program
FMPA	full-mouth periapicals
FMR	fetal movement record
	focused medical review
	functional magnetic resonance
	(imaging)
	functional mitral regurgitation
FMR1	fragile X mental retardation 1
FMRD	full-mouth restorative dentistry
fMRI	functional magnetic resonance
	imaging
FMRP	fragile X mental retardation protein(s)
FMS	fibromyalgia syndrome
	fluorouracil, mitomycin, and
	streptozocin

F

	full-mouth series
F & MS	frontal and maxillary sinuses
FMT	fluorescein meniscus time (dry-eye test)
	functional muscle test
FMTC	familial medullary thyroid carcinoma
FMU	first morning urine
FMV	flow-mediated vasodilation
	fluorouracil, semustine (methyl-CCNU), and vincristine
FMX	full-mouth x-ray
FMZ	flumazenil (Romazicon)
FN	facial nerve
	false negative
	febrile neutropenia
	femoral neck
	finger-to-nose (test)
	flight nurse
F/N	fluids and nutrition
F to N	finger-to-nose
FNA	femoral neck anteversion
	fine-needle aspiration
FNa	filtered sodium
FNAB	fine-needle aspiration biopsy
FNAC	fine-needle aspiratory cytology
FNB	femoral nerve block
FNC	Family Nurse Clinician
FNCJ	fine-needle catheter jejunostomy
FND	fludarabine, mitoxantrone (Novantrone), and dexamethasone
	focal neurological deficit
FNF	femoral-neck fracture
	finger-nose-finger (test)
FNH	focal nodular hyperplasia
FNHL	follicular non-Hodgkin lymphoma
FNMTC	familial nonmedullary thyroid carcinoma
FNP	Family Nurse Practitioner
FNR	false-negative rate
FNS	food and nutrition services
	functional neuromuscular stimulation
F/NS	fever and night sweats
FNT	finger-to-nose (test)
FNTC	fine-needle transhepatic cholangiography
FO	foot orthosis
	foramen ovale
	foreign object
	fronto-occipital
FOB	father of baby
	fecal occult blood
	feet out of bed
	fiberoptic bronchoscope
	foot of bed
FOBT	fecal occult blood test
FOC	father of child
	fluid of choice
	fronto-occipital circumference

FOCF	first observation carried forward
FOD	fixing right eye
	free of disease
FOEB	feet over edge of bed
FOF	fell on floor
FOG	Fluothane, oxygen and gas (nitrous oxide)
	full-on gain
FOH	family ocular history
FOI	fiberoptic intubation
	flight of ideas
FOIA	Freedom of Information Act
FOID	fear of impending doom
FOL	fiberoptic laryngoscopy
FOLFIRI	leucovorin, (folinic acid) fluorouracil, and irinotecan
FOLFOX	leucovorin calcium (folinic acid), fluorouracil, and oxaliplatin
FOM	floor of mouth
FOMi	fluorouracil, Oncovin, (vincristine), and mitomycin
FONSI	finding of no significant impact
FOO	family of origin
FOOB	fell out of bed
FOOSH	fell on outstretched hand
FOP	fasting office profile
	fibrodysplasia ossificans progressiva
FOPS	fiberoptic proctosigmoidoscopy
FORMIL	foreign military
FOS	fiberoptic sigmoidoscopy
	fixing left eye
	force of stream (urology)
	fosphenytoin (Cerebyx)
	fructooligosaccharides
	future order screen
FOSC	freestanding outpatient surgery center
FOT	forced oscillation technique
	form of thought
	frontal outflow tract
FOV	field of view
FOVI	field of vision intact
FOW	fenestration of oval window
FOZ	functional optical zone
FP	fall precautions
	false positive
	familial porencephaly
	family planning
	family practice
	family practitioner
	family presence
	fibrous proliferation
	flat plate
	fluorescence polarization
	fluticasone propionate
	food poisoning
	frozen plasma
F/P	fluid/plasma (ratio)

F-P	femoral popliteal	FRACTS	fractional urines
fpA	fibrinopeptide A	FRAG	fragment
FPAL	full term, premature, abortion, living	FRAG-X	Fragile X Syndrome
FPB	femoral-popliteal bypass	FRAP	family risk assessment program
	flexor pollicis brevis		fluorescence recovery after
FPC	familial polyposis coli		photobleaching
	family practice center	FRC	frozen red cells
FPD	feto-pelvic disproportion		functional residual capacity
	fixed partial denture	FRCPC	Fellow of the Royal College of
FPDL	flashlamp-pumped pulsed dye laser		Physicians of Canada
FPE	first-pass effect	FRCPE	Fellow of the Royal College of
FPG	fasting plasma glucose		Physicians of Edinburgh
FPHx	family psychiatric history	FRCSC	Fellow of the Royal College of
FPIA	fluorescence-polarization		Surgeons of Canada
	immunoassay	FRCSE	Fellow of the Royal College of
FPIES	food protein-induced enterocolitis		Surgeons of Edinburgh
	syndrome	FRCSI	Fellow of the Royal College of
FPL	federal poverty level		Surgeons of Ireland
	final printed labeling (FDA	FRE	flow-related enhancement
	document)	FRET	fluoresence resonance energy
	flexor pollicis longus (tendon)		transfer
	final printed labeling	FRF	filtration replacement fluid
FPLD	familial partial lipodystrophy	FRG	Functional Related Groups
FPLV	feline panleucopenia virus	FRH	febrile-range hyperthermia
FPM	full passive movements	FRJM	full range of joint movement
FPN	ferroportin	FRN	fetal rhabdomyomatous
FPNA	first-pass nuclear angiocardiography		nephroblastoma
FPNP	Family Planning Nurse Practitioner	FRNT	focus-reduction neutralization test
FPO	fetal pulse oximetry	FROA	full range of affect
FPOR	follicle puncture for oocyte retrieval	FROM	full range of motion
FPU	family participation unit	FROMAJE	functioning, reasoning, orientation,
FPV	fosamprenavir (Lexiva)		memory, arithmetic, judgment,
FPZ	fluphenazine (Prolixin; Permitil)		and emotion (mental status
FPZ-D	fluphenazine decanoate (Prolixin		evaluation)
	Decanoate)	FRP	follicle regulatory protein
FQ	fluoroquinolones		functional refractory period
	frequency	FRS	Functional Rating Scale
FR	fair	FRSN	fluoroquinolone-resistant
	father		*Streptococcus pneumoniae*
	Father (priest)	FRSS	forward resuscitative surgery system
	Federal Register	FS	fetoscope
	first responder		fibromyalgia syndrome
	flow rate		fingerstick
	fluid restriction		flexible sigmoidoscopy
	fluid retention		foreskin
	fractional reabsorption		fractional shortenings
	freestyle, no head or lower-extremity		frozen section
	fixation (aquatic therapy)		full strength
	frequent relapses		functional status
	Friends	F & S	full and soft
	frothy	FSA	Family Services Association
	full range	FSAD	female sexual arousal disorder(s)
Fr	French (catheter gauge)	FSALO	Fletcher suite after loading ovoids
F/R	fire/rescue	FSALT	Fletcher suite after loading tandem
F & R	force and rhythm (pulse)	FSB	fetal scalp blood
FRA	fall risk assessment		full spine board
	fluorescent rabies antibody	FSBG	fingerstick blood glucose
FRAC	fracture	FSBM	full-strength breast milk

FSBS	fingerstick blood sugar		flexor tendon
FSC	Fatigue Symptom Checklist		fluidotherapy
	flexible sigmoidoscopy		follow through
	Forensic Science Center		foot (ft)
	fracture, simple, and comminuted		Fourier transform (radiology)
	fracture, simple, and complete		free testosterone
FSCC	fracture, simple, complete, and		full-term
	comminuted	F_3T	trifluridine (Viroptic)
FSD	female sexual dysfunction	FT_3	free triiodothyronine
	focal-skin distance	FT_4	free thyroxine
	fracture, simple, and depressed	FT_4I	free thyroxine index
FSE	fast spin-echo	FTA	fluorescent titer antibody
	fetal scalp electrode		fluorescent treponemal antibody
FSF	fibrin stabilizing factor	FTA-ABS	fluorescent treponemal antibody
FSG	fasting serum glucose		absorption
	focal and segmental	FTAGA	full-term average gestational age
	glomerulosclerosis	FTB	fingertip blood
FSGA	full-term, small for gestational age	FTBD	full-term born dead
FSGN	focal segmental glomerulonephritis	FTBI	fractionated total body irradiation
FSGS	focal segmental glomerulosclerosis	FTC	emtricitabine (Emtriva)
FSH	facioscapulohumeral		fallopian tube carcinoma
	follicle-stimulating hormone		Federal Trade Commission
FSHMD	facioscapulohumeral muscular		frames to come
	dystrophy		full to confrontation
FSIQ	Full-Scale Intelligence Quotient (part	FTD	failure to descend
	of Wechsler test)		frontotemporal degeneration
FSL	fasting serum level		frontotemporal dementia
FSM	functional status measures		full-term delivery
F-SM/C	fungus, smear and culture	FTE	failure to engraft
FSME	Frühsommer-meningoencephalitis	FTEs	full-time equivalents
FSO	for screws only (prosthetic cups)	FTF	finger-to-finger
FSOP	French Society of Pediatric		free thyroxine fraction
	Oncology	FTFTN	finger-to-finger-to-nose
FSP	fibrin split products	FTG	full-thickness graft
FSR	fractionated stereotactic radiosurgery	FTI	farnesyltransferase inhibitor
	fusiform skin revision		force-time integral
FSRP	Framingham Stroke Risk Profile		free thyroxine index
FSRS	fractionated stereotactic radiosurgery	FTICR-MS	Fourier-transform ion cyclotron
FSRT	fractionated stereotactic radiotherapy		resonance-mass spectrometry
FSS	Fatigue Severity Scale	F TIP	finger tip
	federal supply schedule (cost source)	FTIR	Fourier-transform infrared
	fetal scalp sampling		spectroscopy
	fetal scalp stimulation	FTIUP	full-term intrauterine pregnancy
	Flinders Symptom Score	FTKA	failed to keep appointment
	Forensic Science Service (United	FTLB	full-term living birth
	Kingdom)	FTLD	frontotemporal lobar degeneration
	French steel sound (dilated to	FTLFC	full-term living female child
	#24FSS)	FTLMC	full-term living male child
	frequency-selective saturation	FTM	female-to-male (transmission)
	full-scale score		fluid thioglycollate medium
FST	forward surgical team(s)	FTMH	full-thickness macular hole(s)
FSW	feet of sea water (pressure)	FTMS	Fourier-transform mass
	field service worker		spectrometer
FT	family therapy	FTN	finger-to-nose
	fast-twitch		full-term nursery
	feeding tube	FTNB	full-term newborn
	filling time	FTND	Fagerstrom Test for Nicotine
	finger tip		Dependence

	full-term normal delivery	FUNG-S	fungus smear
FTNSD	full-term, normal, spontaneous delivery	FUO	fever of undetermined origin
		FUOV	follow-up office visit
FTO	full-time occlusion (eye patch)	FU/LP	full upper denture, partial lower denture
FTOZ	frontotemporal orbitozygomatic		
FTOZ1	one-piece frontotemporal orbitozygomatic	FUP	follow-up
		FUS	fusion
FTP	failure to progress	FUT	fibrinogen update test
	full-term pregnancy	FUV	follow-up visit
FTR	father	FV	femoral vein
	failed to report	F & V	fruits and vegetables
	failed to respond	FVC	false vocal cord(s)
	for the record		forced vital capacity
FTRAM	free transverse rectus abdominis myocutaneous (flap)	FVD	fever, vomiting, and diarrhea
		FVFR	filled voiding flow rate
FTSD	full-term spontaneous delivery	FVH	focal vascular headache
FTSG	full-thickness skin graft	F VIII	factor VIII (factor eight; antihemophilic factor)
FTT	failure to thrive		
	fetal tissue transplant	FVL	factor V-Leiden (mutation)
	Finger-Tapping Test		femoral vein ligation
Ftube	feeding tube		flow volume loop
FTUPLD	full-term uncomplicated pregnancy, labor, and delivery		functional visual loss
		FVP	foot venous pressure
FTV	Fortovase (saquinavir, soft gel cap)	FVR	feline viral rhinotracheitis
	functional trial visit		forearm vascular resistance
FTW	failure to wean	FW	fetal weight
FU	fraction unbound	F/W	followed with
	fluorouracil	F waves	fibrillatory waves
F & U	flanks and upper quadrants		flutter waves
F/U	follow-up	FVWs	flow-velocity waveforms (umbilical artery Doppler)
	fundus at umbilicus		
F↑U	fingers above umbilicus	FWB	fetal well-being
F↓U	fingers below umbilicus		full-weight bearing
5 FU	fluorouracil		functional well-being
FUA	flat and upright (x-ray of the) abdomen	FWCA	functional work capacity assessment
		FWD	fairly well developed
FUB	functional uterine bleeding	FWHM	full-width at half maximum (radiology)
FUCO	fractional uptake of carbon monoxide		
		FWS	fetal warfarin syndrome
FUD	fear, uncertainty, and doubt	FWW	front-wheel walker
	frequency, urgency, and dysuria	Fx	fractional urine
	full upper denture		fracture
FUDR(r)	floxuridine	Fx-BB	fracture both bones
FU Dtr	full upper denture	Fx-dis	fracture-dislocation
FUFA	fluorouracil and leucovorin (folinic acid)	F XI	Factor XI (eleven)
		FXN	function
FU/FL	full upper denture, full lower denture	FXR	fracture
FUFOL	fluorouracil and leucovorin calcium (folinic acid)	FXS	fragile X syndrome
		FXTAS	fragile X associated tremor/ataxia syndrome
Fugl	Fugl-Meyer Assessment of Motor Recovery After Stroke		
		FY	fiscal year
FUL	federal upper limit (price list)	FYC	facultative yeast carrier
FULG	fulguration	FYI	for your information
5FU/LV	fluorouracil and leucovorin	FZ	flutamide and goserelin acetate (Zoladex)
FUN	follow-up note		
FUNASA	Fundão Naçional de Sade (Brazil's national health agency)	FZRC	frozen red (blood) cells
FUNG-C	fungus culture		

F

G

G   gallop
     gastrostomy
     gauge
     gauss (a unit of magnetic flux density in radiology)
     gavage feeding
     gingiva
     good
     grade
     gram (g) (28.35 g = 1 ounce)
     gravida
     guaiac
     guanosine
G +   gram-positive
     guaiac positive
G −   gram-negative
     guaiac negative
↑g   increasing
↓g   decreasing
G1-4   grade 1-4
G-11   hexachlorophene
GA   Gamblers Anonymous
     gastric analysis
     general anesthesia
     general appearance
     gestational age
     ginger ale
     glycyrrhetinic acid
     granuloma annulare
     glucose/acetone
Ga   gallium
^{67}Ga   gallium citrate Ga 67
GAA   alpha-glucosidase (gene)
     glacial acetic acid
GABA   gamma-aminobutyric acid
GABHS   group A beta hemolytic streptococci
GABS   group A beta (hemolytic) streptococci
GAD   generalized anxiety disorder
     glutamic acid decarboxylase
GAE   granulomatous amebic encephalitis
GAEB   good air entry bilaterally
GAF   geographic adjustment factors
     Global Assessment of Functioning (scale)
GAG   glycosaminoglycan
GAGS   global acne grading system
GAHM   genioglossus advancement and hyoid myotomy
GAGPS   glycosaminoglycan polysulfate
GAGS   global acne grading system
GAHM   genioglossus advancement and hyoid myotomy

GAL   galanthamine hydrobromide (Razadyne)
     gallon
G'ale   ginger ale
GALI-PUT   galactose-1-phosphate uridye transferase enzyme
GALT   galactose-1-phosphate uridyltransferase (gene)
     gut-associated lymphoid tissue
GAM   Gamma Knife
     gene-activated matrices
GAMT   guanidinoacetate methyltransferase
GAN   giant axonal neuropathy
GAO   General Accounting Office
GAP   GTPase activating protein
GAP-43   growth-associated protein-43
GAR   gonnococcal antibody reaction
GARFT   glycinamide ribonucleotide formyl transferase
GAS   general adaption syndrome
     ginseng-abuse syndrome
     Glasgow Assessment Schedule
     Global Assessment Scale
     group A streptococcal (*Streptococcus pyogenes*) disease vaccine
     group *A* streptococci
Gas Anal F&T   gastric analysis, free and total
Ga scan   gallium scan
Gastroc   gastrocnemius
GAT   geriatric assessment team
     Goldmann applanation tonometry
     group adjustment therapy
GATB   General Aptitude Test Battery
GAU   geriatric assessment unit
GAVE   gastric antral vascular ectasia
Gaw   airway conductance
GB   gallbladder
     gingival bleeding
     Ginkgo biloba
     Guillain-Barré (syndrome)
G & B   good and bad
GBA   gingivobuccoaxial
     ganglionic-blocking agent
GBBS   group B beta hemolytic streptococcus
GBD   global burden of disease
GBE   *Ginkgo biloba* extract
GBEF   gallbladder ejection fraction
GBG   gonadal-steroid binding globulin
GBH   gamma benzene hexachloride (lindane)
GBIA   Guthrie bacterial inhibition assay
GBL   gamma butyrolactone
GBM   glioblastoma multiforme
     glomerular basement membrane
GBMI   guilty but mentally ill
GBP   gabapentin (Neurontin)

	gastric bypass	G-CSF	filgrastim (granulocyte colony-stimulating factor)
	gated blood pool (imaging)		
GBPS	gated blood pool scan	GCST	Gibson-Cooke sweat test
GBR	gamma band response (audiology)	GCT	general care and treatment
	good blood return		germ-cell tumor
	guided bone regeneration		giant-cell tumor
GBS	gallbladder series		granulosa cell tumor
	gastric bypass surgery	GCU	gonococcal urethritis
	group B streptococcal (*Streptococcus agalactiae*) disease vaccine	GCV	ganciclovir (Cytovene)
			great cardiac vein
	group B streptococci	GCVF	great cardiac vein flow
	Guillain-Barré syndrome	GD	gastric distension
GBV-C	GB virus type C (also known as hepatitis G virus)		Gaucher disease
			generalized delays
GBW	generalized body weakness		gestational diabetes
GBX	gall bladder extraction (cholecystectomy)		good
			gravely disabled
GC	gas chromatography		Graves disease
	gastric cancer	Gd	gadolinium
	geriatric chair (Gerichair)	G & D	growth and development
	gingival curettage	GDA	gastroduodenal artery
	gliomatosis cerebri	GDB	Guide Dogs for the Blind
	gonococci (gonorrhea)	Gd-BOPTA	gadolinium benzyloxypropionic tetra acetate
	good condition		
	graham crackers	GDC	Guglielmi detachable coil
G−C	gram-negative cocci	GDD	glaucoma drainage devices
G+C	gram-positive cocci	Gd-DTPA	gadopentetate (Magnevist)
GCA	ghost cell ameloblastoma	Gd-DTPA-BMA	gadodiamide (Omniscan)
	giant cell arteritis		
GCBP	gated cardiac blood pool	GD FA	grandfather
GCC	glassy cell carcinoma	GDH	glutamic dehydrogenase
	guanylyl cyclase C	Gd-HPD03A	gadoteridol
GCE	general conditioning exercise		
GCDFP	gross cystic disease fluid protein	GDJ	gastroduodenal junction
GCF	giant cell fibroblastoma	g/dl	grams per deciliter
	gingival crevicular fluid	GDM	gestational diabetes mellitus
GCI	General Cognitive Index	GDM A-1	gestational diabetes mellitus, insulin controlled, Type I
GCIIS	glucose control insulin infusion system		
		GDM A-2	gestational diabetes mellitus, diet controlled, Type II
GCL	generalized congenital lipodystrophy		
GCM	giant cell myocarditis	GD MO	grandmother
	good central maintained	Gd-MRI	gadolinium-enhanced magnetic resonance imaging
GCMD	generalized cardiovascular metabolic disease		
		GDNF	glial (cell line) derived neurotrophic factor
GCMN	giant congenital melanocytic nevus		
GC-MS	gas chromatography-mass spectroscopy	GDP	gamma-detecting probe
			gel diffusion precipitin
GC-O	gas chromatography-olfactometry	GDPs	general dental practitioners
GCP	gentamicin, clindamycin, and polymyxin topical preparation	GDR	glucose disposal rate
		GDS	Geriatric Depression Scale
	good clinical practice		Global Deterioration Scale
GCR	gastrocolonic response	GDx®	a scanning laser polarimeter
	glucocerebrosidase	GE	gainfully employed
GCS	Glasgow Coma Scale		gastric emptying
	glucocorticosteroid(s)		gastroenteritis
	graduated compression stockings		gastroesophageal
GCSE	generalized convulsive status epilepticus		group exercise
		GEA	gastroepiploic artery

G

GEC	galactose elimination capacity	
GED	General Educational Development (Test)	
GEE	gait energy expenditure	
	generalized estimating equations (statistics)	
	Global Evaluation of Efficacy	
	glycine ethyl ester	
	graft-enteric erosion	
GEF	graft-enteric fistula	
GEH	generalized eruptive histiocytosis	
GEJ	gastroesophageal junction	
GEL	giant esophageal leiomyoma	
GEM	gemcitabine (Gemzar)	
	gemfibrozil (Lopid)	
	generalized erythema multiforme	
GEMOX	gemcitabine and oxaliplatin	
GEMU	geriatric evaluation and management unit	
GEN	genital	
GenD	genetic doping	
GEN/ ENDO	general anesthesia with endotracheal intubation	
GENT	gentamicin	
GENTA/P	gentamicin-peak	
GENTA/T	gentamicin-trough	
GEP	gastroenteropancreatic	
	gene expression profiles	
GEQ	generic equiavalent	
GER	gastroesophageal reflux	
GERD	gastroesophageal reflux disease	
GES	gastric emptying scintigraphy	
GEST	gestational	
GET	gastric emptying time	
	graded exercise test	
GET 1/2	gastric emptying half-time	
GETA	general endotracheal anesthesia	
GETS	Glasgow and Edinburgh Throat Scale	
GETV	gadolinium-enhancing tumor volume	
GEU	geriatric evaluation unit	
GF	gastric fistula	
	gluten free	
	grandfather	
GFAAS	graphite furnace atomic absorption spectrometry	
GFAP	glial fibrillary acidic protein	
GF-BAO	gastric fluid, basal acid output	
GFCL	Goldmann fundus contact lens	
GFD	gluten-free diet	
GFFF	gravitational field-flow fractionation	
GFJ	grapefruit juice	
GFM	good fetal movement	
GFP	green fluorscent protein	
GFR	glomerular filtration rate	
	grunting, flaring, and retractions	
GFS	glaucoma filtering surgery	
GG	gamma globulin	
	Gates-Glidden (dental drills)	

	guaifenesin (glyceryl guaiacolate)
G=G	grips equal and good
GGDS	global genome damage score
GGE	Gastrografin enema
	generalized glandular enlargement
GGF	great grandfather
GGM	great grandmother
GGO	ground-glass opacity
GGS	glands, goiter, and stiffness
	group G streptococci
GGT	gamma-glutamyl-transferase
GGTP	gamma-glutamyl-transpeptidase
GH	general health
	genetic hemochromatosis
	gingival hyperplasia
	glenohumeral
	good health
	growth hormone
GH₃	Gerovital
GHAA	Group Health Association of America
GHB	gamma hydroxybutyrate (sodium oxybate; Xyrem)
GHb	glycosylated hemoglobin
GHD	growth hormone deficiency
GHDA	growth hormone deficiency (syndrome) in adults
GHG	greenhouse gases
GHI	growth hormone insufficiency
GHJ	glenohumeral joint
G-H jt	glenohumeral joint
GHLC	glenohumeral ligament complex
GHP(S)	gated heart pool (scan)
GHQ	General Health Questionnaire
GHQ-30	General Health Questionnaire
GHRF	growth hormone releasing factor
GI	gastrointestinal
	gingival index (dental)
	glycemic index
	granuloma inguinale
GIA	gastrointestinal anastomosis
GIB	gastric ileal bypass
	gastrointestinal bleeding
GIC	general immunocompetence
	Global Impression of Change
GID	gastrointestinal distress
	gender identity disorder
GIDA	Gastrointestinal Diagnostic Area
GIFD #3	colonoscope
GIFT	gamete intrafallopian (tube) transfer
GIH	gastrointestinal hemorrhage
GIK	glucose-insulin-potassium
GIL	gastrointestinal (tract) lymphoma
GING	gingiva
	gingivectomy
G1K	greater than one thousand
GIO	glucocorticoid-induced osteoporosis
GIOP	glucocorticoid-induced osteoporosis

G

GIP	gastric inhibitory peptide	GLYCOS Hb	glycosylated hemoglobin
	giant cell interstitial pneumonia		
	glucose-dependent insulinotropic polypeptide	GM	gastric mucosa
			general medicine
GIPU	gastrointestinal procedure unit		genetically modified
GIR	glucose infusion rate		geometric mean
GIRDCA	Gruppo Italiano Ricerca Dermatiti da Contatto e Ambientali (patch test series)		gram (g)
			grand mal
			grandmother
			gray matter
GIS	gas in stomach	G-M	Geiger-Müller (counter)
	gastrointestinal series	GM +	gram-positive
GISA	glycopeptide intermediate-resistant *Staphylococcus aureus*	GM −	gram-negative
		gm %	grams per 100 milliliters
GIST	gastrointestinal stromal tumor	GmbH	*Gesellschaft mit beschränkter Haftung* (a corporation with restricted liability or a private limited liability company)
GIT	gastrointestinal tract		
GITS	gastrointestinal therapeutic system		
	gut-derived infectious toxic shock		
GITSG	Gastrointestinal Tumor Study Group	GMC	general medical clinic
			general medical condition
GITT	glucose insulin tolerance test		geometric mean concentration
GIWU	gastrointestinal work-up	GMCD	grand mal convulsive disorder
giv	given	GM-CSF	sargramostim (granulocyte-macrophage colony-stimulating factor; Leukine)
GJ	gastrojejunostomy		
	grapefruit juice		
GJH	generalized joint hypermobility	GME	gaseous microemboli
GJIC	gap junction intercellular communication		graduate medical education
GJT	gastrojejunostomy tube	GMF	general medical floor
G1K	greater than one thousand	GMFCS	Gross Motor Function Classification System
GK	Gamma Knife		
GKRS	gamma-knife radiosurgery	GMFM	gross motor function measure
GKS	gamma-knife surgery	GMH	germinal matrix hemorrhage
GKT	gamma-knife thalamotomy	GML	gingival margin levels (dental)
GL	gastric lavage	GMLOS	geometric mean length of stay
	glaucoma	GMOs	genetically modified organisms
	greatest length	GMP	general medical panel (see page 298)
GLA	gamolenic acid		Good Manufacturing Practices
	gingivolinguoaxial		guanosine monophosphate
	glucose-lowering agents	GMR	gallop, murmur or rub
GLB	Graham-Leach-Bliley Act of 1999	GMS	galvanic muscle stimulation
GLC	gas-liquid chromatography		general medical services
GLD	Glanders (*Actinobacillus mallei*) vaccine		general medicine and surgery
			Gomori methenamine silver (stain)
GLF	ground-level fall	GM&S	general medicine and surgery
GLIO	glioblastoma	GMSPS	Glasgow Meningococcal Septicemia Prognostic Score
GLM	general linear model		
GLN	glomerulonephritis	GMTs	geometric mean antibody titers
GLOC	gravity-induced loss of consciousness	GN	glomerulonephritis
			graduate nurse
GLP	Gambro Liendia Plate		gram-negative
	Good Laboratory Practice (Principles of)	GNA	*Galanthus nivalis* agglutinin
		GNB	ganglioneuroblastoma
	group-living program		gram-negative bacilli
GLP-1	glucagon-like peptide-1		gram-negative bacteremia
GLR	gravity lumbar reduction	GNBM	gram-negative bacillary meningitis
GLU	glucose		
GLU 5	five-hour glucose tolerance test	GNC	gram-negative cocci
GLUC	glucose	GND	gram-negative diplococci

G

GNID	gram-negative intracellular diplococci	G/P	gravida/para
GNP	Gerontological Nurse Practitioner	G_4P_{3104}	four pregnancies (gravid), 3 went to term, one premature, no abortion (or miscarriage), and 4 living children (p = para)
GNR	gram-negative rods		
GnRH	gonadotropin-releasing hormone		
GNS	gram-negative sepsis oblimersen sodium (Genasense)		
		GPA	gelatin particle agglutination
GnSAF	gonadotropin surge attenuating factor		global program on AIDS
		G#P#A#	gravida (number of pregnancies) para (number of live births) abortion (number of abortions)
GNT	Graduate Nurse Technician		
GNYHA	Greater New York Hospital Association	GPB	gram-positive bacilli
		GPC	gel-permeation chromatography
GO	Graves ophthalmopathy Greek Orthodox		giant papillary conjunctivitis glycerophosphorylcholine
GOAT	Galveston Orientation and Amnesia Test		G-protein coupled gram-positive cocci
GOBI	growth monitoring, *o*ral rehydration, *b*reast feeding, and *i*mmunization	GPCL	gas-permeable contact lens
		GPCR	G protein-coupled receptors
GOCS	Global Obsessive-Compulsive Scale	GPC/TP	glycerylphosphorylcholine to total phosphate
GOD	glucose oxidase	G6PD	glucose-6-phosphate dehydrogenase
GOG	Gynecologic Oncology Group		
GOJ	gastro-oesophageal junction (UK and other countries)	GPGL	gamma probe guided lymphoscintigraphy
GOK	God only knows	GPI	general paralysis of the insane
GOLD	Global Initiative for Chronic Obstructive Lung Disease (guidelines)		glucose-6-phosphate isomerase glycoprotein IIb/IIIa receptor inhibitor(s)
		GPi	globus pallidus interna
GOM	granular osmiophilic material	G-PLT	giant platelets
GOMER	get out of my emergency room	GPMAL	gravida, para, multiple births, abortions, and live births
GON	gonococcal ophthalmia neonatorum		
		GPN	General Pediatric Nurse
	greater occipital neuritis		glossopharyngeal neuralgia
GONA	glaucomatous optic nerve atrophy		graduate practical nurse
GONIO	gonioscopy	GPO	group purchasing organization
GOO	gastric outlet obstruction	GPP	Good Programming Practice
GOR	gastro-oesophageal reflux (United Kingdom)	GPRD	General Practice Research Database (United Kingdom)
	general operating room	GPS	Goodpasture syndrome
GORD	gastro-oesophageal reflux disease (United Kingdom)	GPS™	Gravitational Platelet Separation (System)
GOS	gadolinium oxyorthosilicate	GPT	glutamic pyruvic transaminase
	galactose oxidase and Schiff reagent (test)		Grooved Pegboard Test (of hand function)
	Glasgow Outcome Scale	GPVP	good pharmacovigilance process
GOT	glucose oxidase test		
	glutamic-oxaloacetic transaminase (aspartate aminotransferase)	GPX	glutathione peroxidase
		GPx-1	glutathione peroxidase-1
	goals of treatment	GR	gastric resection
GOX	glucose oxidation		growth rate
GP	gabapentin (Neurontin)	gr	grain (approximately 65 mg) (this is a dangerous abbreviation)
	general practitioner		
	globus pallidus	G−R	gram-negative rods
	glucose polymers	G+R	gram-positive rods
	glycoprotein	GRA	granisetron (Kytril)
	gram-positive		glucocorticoid remediable aldosteronism
	grandparent		
	gutta percha		

G

gravida 6,	6 pregnancies		glucogen storage disease
para 4-	resulting in 4-full term	GSD-1	glycogen storage disease, type 1
0-2-3	deliveries with 0 premature births	GSE	genital self-examination
	and 2 abortions or miscarriages		gluten sensitive enteropathy
	and 3 living children		grip strong and equal
GRAS	generally recognized as safe	GSH	glutathione
GRASE	Generally Recognized as Safe and	GSI	genuine stress incontinence
	Effective	GSIS	glucose-stimulated insulin secretion
GRASS	gradient recalled acquisition in a	GSK	GlaxoSmithKline
	steady state	GSM	Global System of Mobile
Grav.	gravid (pregnant)		Communication
GRC	gastric remnant cancers		grey-scale median
GRD	gastroesophageal reflux disease	GSMD	gestational sack and maternal date
GRD DTR	granddaughter	GSP	generalized social phobia
GRD SON	grandson		general survey panel
GRE	glycopeptide-resistant enterococci		Good Statistical Practice
	graded resistive exercise	GSPN	greater superficial petrosal
	gradient-recalled echo		neurectomy
	gradient refocused echo	GSR	galvanic skin resistance (response)
GR-FR	grandfather		gastrosalivary reflex
GRKP	gentamicin-resistant *Klebsiella*	GSS	Gerstmann-Sträussler-Scheinker
	pneumoniae		(syndrome)
GR-MO	grandmother	GST	glutathione S-transferase
GRN	granules		gold sodium thiomalate
	green		(Myochrysine)
GRO	growth-related oncogene	GSTM	gold sodium thiomalate
GRP	Good Regulatory Practice		(Myochrysine)
	group	GSUI	genuine stress urinary incontinence
$Gr_1P_0AB_1$	one pregnancy, no births, and one	GSV	greater saphenous vein
	abortion	GSW	gunshot wound
GRP HM	group home	GSWA	gunshot wound to abdomen
GRR	gross reproduction rate	GT	gait
GRT	gastric residence time		gait training
	glandular replacement therapy		gastrostomy
	Graduate Respiratory Therapist		gastrotomy tube
	grasp and release test		gene therapy
	group-randomized trial		glucose tolerance
GRTT	Graduate Respiratory Therapist		great toe
	Technician		greater trochanter
GRV	gastric residual volume		green tea
GS	gallstone		group therapy
	generalized seizure	GTA	glutaraldehyde
	general surgery	GTB	gastrointestinal tract bleeding
	Gleason score	GTC	generalized tonic-clonic (seizure)
	gliosarcoma	GTCS	generalized tonic-clonic seizure
	glucosamine sulfate	GTD	gestational trophoblastic disease
	gluteal scts	GTE	general therapeutic exercise
	Gram stain		Green tea extract
	grip strength	GTF	gastrostomy tube feedings
G/S	5% dextrose (glucose) and 0.9%		glucose tolerence factor
	sodium chloride (saline) injection	GTH	gonadotropic hormone
G & S	gait and stance	GTN	gestational trophoblastic neoplasms
GSAP	greatest single allergen present		glomerulo-tubulo-nephritis
G-SAS	Gambling Symptom Assessment		glyceryl trinitrate (name for
	Scale		nitroglycerin in the United
GS-Cbl	glutathionylcobalamin		Kingdom)
GSCU	geriatric skilled care unit	GTO	Golgi tendon organ(s)
GSD	gallstone disease	GTP	glutamyl transpeptidase

G

	green tea polyphenols
	guanosine triphosphate
GTPAL	gestation, term, preterm, abortion and living
GTR	granulocyte turnover rate
	gross total resection
	guided tissue regeneration
GTS	Gilles de la Tourette syndrome
gtt.	drops
GTT	gestational trophoblastic tumor
	glucose tolerance test
GTT agar	gelatin-tellurite-taurocholate agar
GTT3H	glucose tolerence test, 3 hours (oral)
gtts.	drops
G-tube	gastrostomy tube
GU	gastric upset
	genitourinary
	gonococcal urethritis
GUAR	guarantor
GUD	genital ulcer disease
GUI	genitourinary infection
GUM	Genitourinary Medicine (clinics)
GUS	genitourinary sphincter
	genitourinary system
GUSTO	Global Utilization of Streptokinase and TPA for Occluded Arteries
GV	gentian violet
	growth velocity
GVF	Goldmann visual fields
	good visual fields
GVG	vigabatrin (gamma-vinyl GABA)
GVH	generalized visceral hypersensitivity
GVHD	graft-versus-host disease
GVL	graft-versus leukemia
GVM	Graft-versus malignancy
GVN	gentamicin, vancomycin, and nystatin
GVS	gastric vertical stapling
GVSDS	growth velocity standard deviation score
GVT	graft-versus-tumor
G/W	dextrose (glucose) in water
G&W	glycerin and water (enema)
GWA	gunshot wound of the abdomen
GWBI	General Well-Being Index
GWD	Guinea-worm disease
GWMFT	Graded Wolf Motor Function Test
GWS	Gulf-war syndrome
GWT	gunshot wound of the throat
GWTG	Get With The Guidelines (American Heart Association program)
GWX	guide-wire exchange
GXP	graded exercise program
GXT	graded exercise test
Gy	gray (radiation unit)
GYN	gynecology
GZTS	Guilford-Zimmerman Temperament Survey

H	*Haemophilis*
	head
	heart
	height
	Helicobacter
	heroin
	Hispanic
	hour
	husband
	hydrogen
	hyperopia
	hypermetropia
	hyperphoria
	hypodermic
	isoniazid [part of tuberculosis regimen, see RHZ(E/S)/HR]
	objective angle
	trastuzumab (Herceptin)
H′	hip
Ⓗ	hypodermic injection
H²	hiatal hernia
H₂	hydrogen
3H	high, hot, and a helluva lot
H24	24 hour
HA	headache
	hearing aid
	heart attack
	hemadsorption
	hemagglutination
	hemolytic anemia
	Hispanic American
	hospital-acquired
	hospital admission
	hyaluronan
	hyaluronic acid
	hyperalimentation
	hypermetropic astigmatism
	hypothalmic amenorrhea
H/A	head-to-abdomen (ratio)
	holding area
HA-1A®	nebacumab
HAA	haloacetic acid
	hepatitis-associated antigen
HAAB	hepatitis A antibody
HAAF	hypoglycemia-associated autonomic failure
HAART	highly active antiretroviral treatment
HABF	hepatic artery blood flow
HAC	hydroxyapatite cement
HAc	acetic acid
HACA	human antichimeric antibodies
HACCP	Hazard Analysis Critical Control Point(s)

G

HACE	hepatic artery chemoembolization		human albumin microspheres
	high-altitude cerebral edema	HAMA	human antimurine antibody
HACEK	*Haemophilus*	HAM-A	Hamilton Anxiety (scale)
group	*parainfluenzae, H. aphrophilus,*	HAM D	Hamilton Depression (scale)
	and *H. paraphrophilus,*	HAMS	hamstrings
	Actinobacillus	HAN	heroin-associated nephropathy
	actinomycetemcomitans,	HANE	hereditary angioneurotic edema
	Cardiobacterium hominis,	HAO	hearing aid orientation
	Eikenella corrodens, and *Kingella*	HAP	hearing aid problem
	kingae		heredopathia atactica
HACS	hyperactive child syndrome		polyneuritiformis
HAD	HIV (human immunodeficiency		hospital-acquired pneumonia
	virus)-associated dementia		hydroxyapatite
	human adjuvant disease	HAPC	hospital-acquired penetration contact
	hypertonic acetate dextran	HAPD	home-automated peritoneal dialysis
HADH	the reduced form of nicotinamide-	HAPE	high-altitude pulmonary edema
	adenine dinucleotide (hydride	HapMap	A catalog of common genetic
	donors in biochemical redox		variants that occur in human
	reactions)		beings. It describes what these
HADS	Hospital Anxiety and Depression		variants are, where they occur in
	Scale		our DNA, and how they are
HAE	hearing aid evaluation		distributed among people within
	hepatic artery embolization		populations and among
	herb-related adverse event		populations in different parts of
	hereditary angioedema		the world. (The International
HAEC	Hirschprung associated enterocolitis		Haplotype Map Project)
HAF	hyperalimentation fluid		(www.hapmap.org)
HAFM	hospital-acquired *Plasmodium*	HAPS	hepatic arterial perfusion
	falciparum malaria		scintigraphy
HAGG	hyperimmune antivariola gamma	HAPTO	haptoglobin
	globulin	HAQ	Headache Assessment Questionnaire
HAGHL	humeral avulsion of the		Health Assessment Questionnaire
	glenohumeral ligament	HAR	high-altitude retinopathy
HAGL	humeral avulsion of the		hyperacute rejection
	glenohumeral ligament	HARDI	high-angular resolution diffusion-
HAH	high-altitude headache		weighted imaging
HAI	hemagglutination inhibition assay	HARH	high-altitude retinal hemorrhage
	hepatic arterial infusion	HARP	hypoprebetalipoproteinemia,
HAIC	hepatic arterial infusional		acanthocytosis, retinitis
	chemotherapy		pigmentosa, and pallidale
HAK	hyperalimentation kit		degeneration (syndrome)
HAL	hemorrhoidal artery ligation	HARS	Hamilton Anxiety Rating Scale
	hip axis length		HIV-associated adipose redistribution
	hyperalimentation		syndrome
HALE	health-adjusted life expectancy	HAS	Hamilton Anxiety (Rating) Scale
HALN	hand-assisted laparoscopic (radical)		headache associated with sexual
	nephrectomy		activity
HALO	halothane (Fluothane)		Holmes-Adie syndrome
	hours after light onset		home assessment service
HALRI	hospital-acquired lower respiratory		hyperalimentation solution
	infections	HASCI	head and spinal cord injury
HALRN	hand-assisted laparoscopic radical	HASCVD	hypertensive arteriosclerotic
	nephrectomy		cardiovascular disease
HALS	hand-assisted laparoscopic surgery	HASHD	hypertensive arteriosclerotic heart
HAM	Haldol, Ativan, and morphine		disease
	high-dose cytarabine (ara-C) and	HAT	head, arms, and trunk
	mitoxantrone		heterophile antibody titer
	HTLV-1-associated myelopathy		histone acetyltransferase

H

	hormone ablative therapy	HBID	hereditary benign intraepithelial
	hospital arrival time		dyskeratosis
	human African trypanosomiasis	HBIG	hepatitis B immune globulin
	(sleeping sickness)	Hb	mutant hemoglobin with a
HAV	hallux abducto valgus	Kansas	low affinity for oxygen
	hepatitis A vaccine	HBLs	hemangioblastomas
	hepatitis A virus	HBLV	B-lymphotropic virus human
HAV-HBV	hepatitis A virus, and hepatitis B	HBM	Health Belief Model
	virus vaccine		human bone marrow
HAZWO	Hazardous Waste	HBNK	heparin-binding neurotrophic factor
PER	Operations and Emergency	hBNP	human B-type natriuretic peptide
	Response		(nesiritide [Natrecor])
HB	heart-beating (donor)	HBO	hyperbaric oxygen (HBO_2 preferred)
	heart block	HBO_2	hyperbaric oxygen
	heel-to-buttock	HbO_2	hemoglobin, oxygenated
	hemoglobin (Hb)		hyperbaric oxygen (HBO_2 preferred)
	hepatitis B	HBOC	hemoglobin-based oxygen carrier
	high calorie		hereditary breast and ovarian cancer
	hold breakfast	HBOT	hyperbaric oxygen treatment/therapy
	housebound		(HBO_2T preferred)
	hydrocodone bitartrate	HBO_2T	hyperbaric oxygen treatment
1^0HB	first degree heart block	HBP	high blood pressure
HB1°	first degree heart block	HBPM	home blood pressure monitoring
HB2°	second degree heart block	HBr	hydrobromide
HB3°	third degree heart block	HBS	Health Behavior Scale
HBAB	hepatitis B antibody	HbS	sickle cell hemoglobin
Hb A_{1c}	glycosylated hemoglobin	HBsAg	hepatitis B surface antigen
HBAC	hyperdynamic beta-adrenergic	HbSC	sickle cell hemoglobin C
	circulatory	HBSS	Hank balanced salt solution
HbAS	sickle cell trait	HbSS	sickle cell anemia
HBBW	hold breakfast for blood work	HBT	hydrogen breath test
HBC	health and beauty care		hypertrophy of the base of the
	hereditary breast cancer		tongue
	hit by car	HBV	hepatitis B vaccine
HBcAb	hepatitis B core antibody (antigen)		hepatitis B virus
HBc AB	hepatitis B core antibody		honey-bee venom
HBc Ag	hepatitis B core antigen	HBVig	hepatitis B virus immune globulin
HbCO	carboxyhemoglobin	HBVP	high biological value protein
HB core	hepatitis B core antigen	HBW	high birth weight
HbCV	*Haemophilus* b conjugate vaccine	H/BW	heart-to-body weight (ratio)
HBD	has been drinking	HBEX	home-based exercise
	hydroxybutyrate dehydrogenase	HC	hair count
HBDH	hydroxybutyrate dehydrogenase		hairy cell
HBE	hepatitis B epsilon		handicapped
	human bronchial epithelial (cells)		head circumference
	hypopharyngoscopy, bronchoscopy,		healthy controls
	and esophagoscopy		heart catheterization
HBeAb	hepatitis Be antibody (antigen)		heel cords
HBED	hydroxybenzylethylene-diamine		Hickman catheter
	diacetic acid		home care
HbF	fetal hemoglobin		hot compress
HBF	hepatic blood flow		housecall
HBGA	had it before, got it again		Huntington chorea
HBGM	home blood glucose monitoring		hydrocephalus
HBH	Health Belief Model		hydrocortisone
HBHC	hospital based home care	4-HC	4-hydroperoxycyclo-phosphamide
HBI	Harvey-Bradshaw Index	H & C	hot and cold
	hemibody irradiation	HCA	health care aide

H

	heterocyclic antidepressant	HCT	head computerized (axial)
	hypercalcemia		tomography
	hypothermic circulatory arrest		hematopoietic cell transplantation
HCAO	hepatitis C-associated osteosclerosis		hematocrit
H-CAP	altretamine (hexamethyl-melamine),		histamine challenge test
	cyclophosphamide, doxorubicin		human chorionic thyrotropin
	(Adriamycin), and cisplatin		hydrochlorothiazide (this is a
	(Platinol)		dangerous abbreviation)
HCB	hexachlorobenzene		hydrocortisone
HCBR	human carbonyl reductase	HCTU	home cervical traction unit
HCC	hepatocellular carcinoma	HCTZ	hydrochlorothiazide (this is a
HCD	herniate cervical disk		dangerous abbreviation)
	hydrocolloid dressing	HCV	hepatitis C vaccine
HCFA	Health Care Financing Administration		hepatitis C virus
HCFC	hydrochlorofluorocarbon	HCVD	hypertensive cardiovascular disease
HCFU	1-hexylcarbamoyl-5-fluorouracil	HCWs	healthcare workers
	(Camofur)	HCY	homocysteine
hCG	human chorionic gonadotropin	HCYS	homocysteine
HCH	hexachlorocyclohexane	HD	haloperidol decanoate
	hygroscopic condenser humidifier		Hansen disease
HCI	home care instructions		hearing distance
HCL	hairy cell leukemia		heart disease
HCl	hydrochloric acid (when it appears		Heller-Dor (procedure)
	separately [not as part of a drug		heloma durum
	name])		hemodialysis
	hydrochloride (when part of a drug		herniated disk
	name, as in thiamine HCl		high dose
	[thiamine hydrochloride])		hip disarticulation
HCLF	high carbohydrate, low fiber (diet)		Hirschsprung disease
HCLs	hard contact lenses		Hodgkin disease
HCLV	hairy cell leukemia variant		hospital day
HCM	health care maintenance		hospital discharge
	heterogeneous cation-exchange		house dust
	membrane		Huntington disease
	hypercalcemia of malignancy	HDA	heteroduplex analysis
	hypertrophic cardiomyopathy		high-dose arm
HCMV	human cytomegalovirus	HDAC	histone deacetylase
HCO₃	bicarbonate	HD-AC	high-dose cytarabine
HCP	handicapped	HDAC2	histone deacetylase 2
	healthcare provider	HD-ara-C	high-dose cytarabine (ara-C)
	hearing conservation programs	HDBQ	Hilton Drinking Behavior
	hereditary coporphyria		Questionnaire
	hexachlorophene	HD-Bu	high-dose busulfan
	home chemotherapy program	HDC	habilitative day care
	hospital chemistry profile		high-dose chemotherapy
	hydrocephalus		histamine dihydrochloride
HCPCS	HCFA (Health Care Financing	HDC-ASCS	high-dose chemotherapy with
	Administration) Common		autologous stem cell support
	Procedural Coding System	HDCC	high-dose combination chemotherapy
HCQ	hydroxychloroquine (Plaquenil)	HD-CPA	high-dose cyclophosphamide
HCR	health care review	HDCPT	high-dose cyclophosphamide therapy
HCS	heel-cord stretches	HDC-SCR	high-dose chemotherapy with stem-
	human chorionic		cell rescue
	somatomammotropin	HDCT	high-dose chemotherapy
	hypercoagulable states	HDCV	rabies virus vaccine, human diploid
17-HCS	17-hydroxycorticosteroids		(human diploid cell vaccine)
HCSE	horse chestnut seed extract	HDE	Humanitarian Device Exemption
HCSS	hypersensitive carotid sinus syndrome		(FDA)

H

HDF	hemodiafiltration	HEA	health
HDG	hydrogel (dressing)	HEAR	hospital emergency ambulance radio
HDGC	hereditary diffuse gastric cancer	HEAT	human erythrocyte agglutination test
HDH	high-density humidity	HEB	hydrophilic emollient base
HDI	high-definition image	HEC	Health Education Center
HDIs	histone deacetylase inhibitors	HeCOG	Hellenic Cooperative Oncology
HDK	high-dose ketoconazole		Group
HDL	high-density lipoprotein	HEDIS	Health Employer Data and
HDL-C	high-density lipoprotein cholesterol		Information Set
HDLW	hearing distance for watch to be	HEENT	head, eyes, ears, nose, and throat
	heard in left ear	HeFH	heterozygous familial
HDM	home-delivered meals		hypercholesterolemia
	house dust mite	HEI	Health Eating Index (US Department
HDMEC	human dermal microvascular		of Agriculture)
	endothelial cells	HEICS	Hospital Emergency Incident
HDMP	high-dose methylprednisolone		Command System
HD-MTX	high-dose methotrexate	HEK	human embryonic kidney
HD-MTX-	high-dose methotrexate	HEL	*Helicobacter pylori* vaccine
CF	and leucovorin (citrovorum factor)		human embryonic lung
HD-MTX/	high-dose methotrexate	HeLa	Helen Lake (tumor cells)
LV	and leucovorin	HELLP	hemolysis, elevated liver
HDN	hemolytic disease of the newborn	Syn-	enzymes, and low
	heparin dosing nomogram	drome	platelet count
	high-density nebulizer	HEM	hypertensive emergency
HDNS	Hodgkin disease, nodular sclerosis	HEMA	hydroxyethylmethacrylate
HDP	high-density polyethylene	HEMI	hemiplegia
	hydroxymethyline diphosphonate	HEMOSID	hemosiderin
HDPA	high-dose pulse administration	HEMPAS	hereditary erythrocytic
HDPAA	heparin-dependent platelet-associated		multinuclearity with positive
	antibody		acidified serum test
HDPC	hand piece	HEMS	helicopter emergency medical
HDPE	high-density polyethylene		services
HDR	heparin dose response	HEN	hemorrhages, exudates, and nicking
	high-dose rituximab		home enteral nutrition
	husband to delivery room	He-Ne	helium-neon
HDRA	histoculture drug response assay	HEP	hemoglobin electrophoresis
HDRB	high-dose rate brachytherapy		hemorrhage, exudates, and
HDRS	Hamilton Depression Rating Scale		papilledemaa
HDRW	hearing distance for watch to be		heparin
	heard in right ear		hepatic
HDS	Hamilton Depression (Rating) Scale		hepatoerythropoietic porphyria
	herniated disk syndrome		hepatoma
HDSCR	health deviation self-care requisite		histamine equivalent prick
HDT	habilitative day treatment		home exercise program
	hearing distraction test	HEPA	hamster egg penetration assay
HDU	hemodialysis unit		high-efficiency particulate air (filter)
	high-dependency unit (an intensive	hep cap	heparin cap
	care unit)	HER2	human epidermal growth factor 2
HDV	hepatitis D virus	HERP	human exposure (dose)/ rodent
HDW	hearing distance (with) watch		potency (dose)
HDYF	how do you feel	HES	hetastarch (hydroxyethyl starch;
HE	hard events		Hespan)
	hard exudate		hypereosinophilic syndrome
	health educator	HEs	hypertensive emergencies
	hepatic encephalopathy	hES	human embryonic stem
H&E	hematoxylin and eosin	20-HETE	20-hydroxyeico-satetraenoic acid
	hemorrhage and exudate	HETF	home enteral tube feeding
	heredity and environment	HEV	hepatitis E vaccine

	hepatitis E virus	HFV	high-frequency ventilation
	high-endothelial venule		high-fruit/vegetable (diet)
Hex	altretamine	HFX RT	hyperfractionated radiation therapy
	(hexamethylmelamine; Hexalen)	HG	handgrasp
Hexa-CAF	altretamine (hexamethylmelamine),		handgrip
	cyclophosphamide, methotrexate		hemoglobin
	(amethopterin), and fluorouracil		hyperemesis gravidarum
HF	Hageman factor	Hg	mercury
	hard feces	HGA	high-grade astrocytomas
	hay fever	Hgb	hemoglobin
	head of fetus	Hgb	hemoglobin
	heart failure	ELECT	electrophoresis
	high frequency	Hgb F	fetal hemoglobin
	Hispanic female	Hgb S	sickle cell hemoglobin
	hot flashes	HGD	high grade dysplasia
	house formula	HGE	human granulocytic ehrlichiosis
HFA	health facility administrator	HGES	handgrasp equal and strong
	high-functioning autism	HGF	hepatocyte growth factor
	hydrofluoroalkane-134a		hereditary gingival fibromatosis
HFAS	hereditary flat adenoma syndrome	HGG	high-grade glioma
HFB	high-frequency band		human gamma globulin
HFC	hydrofluorocarbon	HGH	human growth hormone
HFCB	horizontal flow clean bench	HGI	Human Genome Initiative
HFCC	high-frequency chest compression	HGM	home glucose monitoring
HFD	high-fiber diet	HGN	hypogastric nerve
	high-forceps delivery	HGNT	high-grade neuroendocrine tumors
	high-frequency discharges	HGO	hepatic glucose output
HFE	hemochromatosis gene		hip guidance orthosis
hFH	heterozygous familial	HGP	Human Genome Project
	hypercholesterolemia	HGPIN	high-grade prostatic intraepithelial
HFHL	high-frequence hearing loss		neoplasia
HFI	hereditary fructose intolerance	HGPRT	hypoxanthine-guanine
HFIP	hexafluoro-isopropranolol		phosphoribosyl-transferase
HFJV	high-frequency jet ventilation	HGS	hand-grip strength
H flu	*Haemophilus influenzae*		human genome sequence
HFM	hand-foot-and-mouth (disease) (often	HGSIL	high-grade squamous intraepithelial
	caused by coxsackievirus A16)		lesion
	hemifacial microsomia	HGV	hepatitis G vaccine
HFMD	hand-foot-and-mouth disease (often		hepatitis G virus
	caused by coxsackievirus A16)	HH	hard of hearing
HFO	high-frequency oscillation		head hood
HFOV	high-frequency oscillatory ventilation		hereditary hemochromatosis
HFP	hepatic function panel (see page 298)		hiatal hernia
	Hoffa fat pad		home health
HFPPV	high-frequency positive pressure		homonymous hemiopia
	ventilation		household
HFR	hemorrhagic fever with renal		hyperhomocystinemia
	syndrome vaccine		hypogonadotropic hypogonadism
HFRS	hemorrhagic fever with renal		hypoeninemic hypoaldosteronism
	syndrome	H/H	hemoglobin/hematocrit
HFRT	hyperfractionated radiotherapy	H&H	hematocrit and hemoglobin
HFS	hand-foot skin (reaction)	HHA	health hazard appraisal
	hand-foot syndrome		hereditary hemolytic anemia
	hemifacial spasm		home health agency
	hot flash score		home health aid
HFSH	human follicle-stimulating hormone	HH Assist	hand-held assist
HFST	hearing-for-speech test	HHC	home health care
HFUPR	hourly fetal urine production rate	HHCA	home health care agency

	hypothermic hypokalemic cardioplegic arrest	HIB$_{PRP-OMP}$	*haemophilus influenzae* type b vaccine, PRP-OMP conjugate vaccine
HHcy	hyperhomocystinemia		
HHD	Doctor of Holistic Health	HIB$_{PRP-T}$	*haemophilus influenzae* type b vaccine, PRP-T conjugate vaccine
	hand-held dynamometer		
	home hemodialysis	HIB$_{ps}$	*haemophilus influenzae* type b polysaccharide vaccine
	household distance (physical therapy goal of mobility)		
		HIC	Human Investigation Committee
	hypertensive heart disease		Humphriss immediate contrast (astigmatism test)
HHFM	high-humidity face mask		
HHH	hypermethionemia, hyperammonemia, and homocitrolinemia (syndrome)	hi-cal	high caloric
		HICF	high-information-content fingerprinting
HHHQ	Health Habits and History Questionnaire (Block-National Cancer Institute)	HICPAC	Hospital Infection Control Practices Advisory Committee (Centers for Disease Control and Prevention guidelines)
HHIE-S	hearing handicap inventory for the elderly-short form		
		HID	headache, insomnia, and depression
HHM	high-humidity mask		herniated intervertebral disk
	humoral hypercalcemia of malignancy	HIDA	hepato-iminodiacetic acid (lidofenin)
HHN	hand-held nebulizer	HiDAC	high-dose cytarabine (ara-C)
HHNC	hyperosmolar hyperglycemic nonketotic coma	HIDS	hyperimmunoglobulinemia D syndrome
HHNK	hyperglycemic hyperosmolar nonketotic (coma)	HIE	hyperimmunoglobulinemia E
			hypoxic-ischemic encephalopathy
HHNS	hyperosmolar-hyperglycemic nonketotic syndrome	HIF	*Haemophilus influenzae*
			higher integrative functions
HHRG	Home Health Resource Group (reimbursement categories for home health)	HIFU	high-intensity focused ultrasonography
		HIHA	high impulsiveness, high anxiety
		HIHARS	hyperventilation-induced high-amplitude rhythmic slowing
HHS	Health and Human Service (US Department of)		
		HII	hepatic-iron index
HHT	hereditary hemorrhagic telangiectasis	HIIC	heated intraoperative intraperitoneal chemotherapy
HHTC	high-humidity trach collar		
HHTM	high-humidity trach mask	HIL	hypoxic-ischemic lesion
HHTS	high-humidity tracheostomy shield	HILA	high impulsiveness, low anxiety
HHV-8	human herpesvirus 8	HILIC	hydrophilic interaction chromatography
HI	*Haemophilus influenzae*		
	head injury	HILP	hyperthermic isolated limb perfusion
	health insurance	HIM	health information management
	hearing impaired		hexyl-insulin monoconjugate
	hemagglutination inhibition	HIN	*haemophilus influenzae* nontypable strain(s) vaccine
	homicidal ideation		
	hospital insurance	HINI	hypoxic-ischemic neuronal injury
	human insulin	HINN	Hospital-issued Notice of Noncoverage
HIA	hemagglutination inhibition antibody		
		HIO	health insuring organization
HIAA	hydroxyindoleacetic acid		hepatic iron overload
5-HIAA	5-hydroxyindoleacetic acid	HIP	health insurance plan
HIAP	human intracisternal A-type particle	HIPA	heparin-induced platelet aggregation
HIB	*Haemophilus influenzae* type b (vaccine)	HIPAA	Health Insurance Portability and Accountability Act of 1996
		HIPC	hormone-independent prostate cancer
HIB$_{cn}$	*haemophilus influenzae* type b conjugate vaccine	HIPPS	Health Insurance Prospective Payment System
HIB$_{HbOC}$	*haemophilus influenzae* type b vaccine, HbOC conjugate vaccine		
		hi-pro	high-protein
HIB$_{PRP-D}$	*haemophilus influenzae* type b vaccine, PRP-D conjugate vaccine	HIR	head injury routine

H

HIS	Hanover Intensive Score		hepatic lipase
	Health Intention Scale		Hickman line
	high-intermittent suction		hyperlipidemia
	histidine	H&L	heart and lung
	Home Incapacity Scale	HLA	human leukocyte antigen
	hospital (healthcare) information		human lymphocyte antigen
	system	HLADR	human leukocyte antigen, type DR
HISMS	How I See Myself Scale	HLA nega-	heart, lungs, and
HISTO	histoplasmin skin test	tive	abdomen negative
	histoplasmosis	HLB	head, limbs, and body
HIT	heparin-induced thrombocytopenia	HLD	haloperidol decanoate (Haldol)
	histamine-inhalation test		herniated lumbar disk
	home infusion therapy		high-level disinfection
HITS	high-intensity transient signals		high-lipid disorder
HITTS	heparin-induced thrombotic	HLDP	hypoglossia-limb deficiency
	thrombocytopenia syndrome		phenotype
HIU	head injury unit	HLES	hypertensive lower esophageal
HIV	human immunodeficiency virus		sphincter
	human immunodeficiency virus	HLGR	high-level gentamicin resistance
	vaccine	HLH	hemophagocytic lymphohistiocytosis
HIV-1	human immunodeficiency virus		human luteinizing hormone
	type 1	HLHS	hypoplastic left-heart syndrome
HIV-2	human immunodeficiency virus	HLI	head lice infestation
	type 2	HLK	heart, liver, and kidneys
HIVAN	human immunodeficiency virus-	HLM	heart-lung machine
	associated nephropathy		hemosiderin-laden macrophages
HIVAT	home intravenous antibiotic therapy	HLOS	hypertensive lower oesophageal
HIVD	herniated intervertebral disk		sphincter (United Kingdom and
HIV-D	human immunodeficiency virus-		other countries)
	related dementia	HLP	hyperlipoproteinemia
hi-vit	high-vitamin	hLS	human lung surfactant
HIVMP	high-dose intravenous	HLT	heart-lung transplantation
	methylprednisolone		(transplant)
HIVN	human immunodeficiency virus	HLV	herpes-like virus
	nephropathy		hypoplastic left ventricle
HJB	Howell-Jolly bodies	HM	hand motion
HJR	hepatojugular reflux		head movement
HK	hand-to-knee		heart murmur
	heel-to-knee		heavily muscled
	hexokinase		heloma molle
hK6	human kallikrein 6		Hispanic male
HKAFO	hip-knee-ankle-foot orthosis		Holter monitor
HKAO	hip-knee-ankle orthosis		home
HKD	hyperkinetic disorder		human milk
HKMN	Hickman (catheter)		human semisynthetic insulin
HKO	hip-knee orthosis		humidity mask
HKS	heel-knee-shin (test)	HMA	hemorrhages and microaneurysms
HKT	heterotopic kidney transplant		heteroduplex mobility assay
HL	hairline	HMB	beta-hydroxy-beta methylbutyrate (a
	half-life		leucine metabolite)
	hallux limitus		homatropine methylbromide
	haloperidol		hypersensitivity to mosquito bites
	harelip	HMBA	hexamethylene bisacetamide
	hearing level	HMD	hyaline membrane disease
	hearing loss	HMDP	hydroxymethyline diphosphonate
	heavy lifting	HME	heat and moisture exchanger
	hemilaryngectomy		heat, massage, and exercise
	heparin lock		hereditary multiple exostoses

H

	home medical equipment
	human monocytic ehrlichiosis
HMEF	heat moisture exchanging filter
HMETSC	heavy metal screen
HMF	human milk fortifier
HMG	human menopausal gonadotropin
HMG CoA	hydroxymethyl glutaryl coenzyme A
HMI	healed myocardial infarction
	history of medical illness
HMIS	hospital medical information system
HMK	homemaking
HM & LP	hand motion and light perception
HMM	altretamine (hexamethyl-melamine; Hexalen)
HMO	Health Maintenance Organization
	hypothetical mean organism
HMP	health maintenance plan
	hereditary metabolic profile
	hexose monophosphate
	hot moist packs
HMPAO	hexylmethylpropylene amineoxine
HMPC	Committee on Herbal Medicinal Products (EMEA)
HMPV	human metapneumovirus
HMR	histocytic medullary reticulosis
	Hoechst Marion Roussel
¹H-MRS	proton magnetic resonance spectroscopy
HMS	hyper-reactive malarial splenomegaly
	hypodermic morphine sulfate (this is a dangerous abbreviation)
HMS®	medrysone
hMSCs	human mesenchymal stem cells
HMSN I	hereditary motor and sensory neuropathy type I
HMSR	high medical-social risk
HMSS	hyperactive malarial splenomegaly syndrome
HMV	home mechanical ventilation
HMWK	high-molecular weight kininogen
HMX	heat massage exercise
HN	head and neck
	head nurse
	high nitrogen
	home nursing
H&N	head and neck
HN2	mechlorethamine HCl (Mustargen)
HNC	head and neck cancer
	Holistic Nurse, Certified
	human neutrophil collagenase
	hyperosmolar nonketotic coma
HNCa	head and neck cancer
HNCCG	Head and Neck Cancer Cooperative Group
HNE	human neutrophil elastase
HNI	hospitalization not indicated
HNKDC	hyperosomolar nonketotic diabetic coma

HNKDS	hyperosmolar nonketotic diabetic state
HNLN	hospitalization no longer necessary
HNMM	mucosal melanomas of the head and neck
¹H-NMR	proton nuclear magnetic resonance (spectroscopy)
HNN	hybrid neural network
HNP	herniated nucleus pulposus
HNPCC	heredity nonpolyposis colorectal cancer
HNPP	hereditary neuropathy with liability to pressure palsies
HNRNA	heterogeneous nuclear ribonucleic acid
HNS	0.45% sodium chloride injection (half-normal saline)
	head and neck surgery
	head, neck, and shaft
HNSCC	squamous cell carcinoma of the head and neck
HNSN	home, no services needed
HNT	hantaan (hantavirus) vaccine
HNV	has not voided
HNWG	has not worn glasses
HO	hand orthosis
	heme oxygenase
	Hemotology-Oncology
	heterotropic ossification
	hip orthosis
	house officer
H/O	history of
+HO	hemoccult positive
H₂O	water
H₂O₂	hydrogen peroxide
HOA	hip osteoarthritis
	hypertropic osteoarthropathy
HOB	head of bed
HOB UPSOB	head of bed up for shortness of breath
HOC	Health Officer Certificate
HOCM	high-osmolality contrast media
	hypertrophic obstructive cardiomyopathy
HOD	heroin overdose
HOG	halothane, oxygen, and gas (nitrous oxide)
	Hoosier Oncology Group
HOH	hand-over-hand (rehabilitation term)
	hard of hearing
HOI	hospital onset of infection
HOM	high-osmolar contrast media
HOMA	homeostatic assessment model algorithm (index)
	homeostatic model assessment
HOME	Home Observation for Measurement of the Environment
HONC	Hooked on Nicotine Checklist
	hyperosmolar, nonketotic coma

HONK	hyperosmolar nonketotic (coma)	HPET	*Helicobacter pylori* eradication therapy
HOP	hourly output		
HOPI	history of present illness	HPF	high-power field
Hopkins-25	Hopkins Symptom Checklist-25	HPFH	hereditary persistence of fetal hemoglobin
HOR	higher-order repeat		
HORF	high-output renal failure	HPG	human pituitary gonadotropin
HORS	Hemiballism/Hemichorea Outcome Rating Score	HPI	history of present illness
		HPIP	history, physical, impression, and plan
HOS	Health Outcomes Survey		
	hybrid orthosis system	HPK	hyperkeratosis
HOSP	hospital	HPL	human placenta lactogen
	hospitalization		hyperlipidemia
HOT	home oxygen therapy		hyperplexia
HOTV	letter symbols used in pediatric visual acuity testing	HPLC	high-performance (pressure) liquid chromatography
HOVT	letter symbols used in pediatric visual acuity testing	HPM	hemiplegic migraine
		HPMC	high-performance membrane chromatography
Ho:YAG	holmium: yttrium-aluminum-garnet		hydroxypropyl methylcellulose
HP	hard palate	HPN	home parenteral nutrition
	Harvard pump	HPNI	hemodialysis prognostic nutrition index
	Helicobacter pylori		
	hemipelvectomy	HPNS	high-pressure nervous syndrome
	hemiplegia	HPO	hydrophilic ointment
	herbal products		hypertrophic pulmonary osteoarthropathy
	high-protein (supplement)		
	hot packs	HPOA	hypertrophic pulmonary osteoarthropathy
	house physician		
	hydrogen peroxide	2HPP	2-hour postprandial (blood sugar)
	hydrophilic petrolatum	2HPPBS	2-hour postprandial blood sugar
Hp	*Helicobacter pylori*	HPPM	hyperplastic persistent pupillary membrane
H&P	history and physical		
HPA	hybridization protection assay	hPRL	prolactin, human
	hypothalamic-pituitary-adrenal (axis)	HPS	hantavirus pulmonary syndrome
HPAE-PAD	high-pH anion exchange chromatography coupled with pulsed amperometric detection		hepatopulmonary syndrome
			Helicobacter pylori serology
			hypertrophic pyloric stenosis
HPAI	highly pathogenic avian influenza A virus	HpSA	*Helicobacter pylori* stool antigen
		HPT	heparin protamine titration
HPAT	home parenteral antibiotic therapy		histamine provocation test
HPB	Health Protection Branch (the Canadian equivalent of the U.S. Food and Drug Administration)		home pregnancy test
			hyperparathyroidism
		HPTD	highly permeable transparent dressing
HPC	hemangiopericytoma	hPTH	human parathyroid hormone I_{34} (teriparatide)
	hereditary prostate cancer		
	history of present condition (complaint)	HPTM	home prothrombin time monitoring
		HPTX	hemopneumothorax
HPCE	high-performance capillary electrophoresis	HPV	human papilloma virus
			human papilloma virus vaccine
HPD	high-protein diet		human parvovirus
	home peritoneal dialysis	*H pylori*	*Helicobacter pylori*
	hours post dose	HPZ	high-pressure zone
HpD	hematoporphyrin derivative	HQC	hydroquinone cream
HP&D	hemoprofile and differential	HQL	health-related quality of life
HPDP	health promotion and disease prevention	HR	hallux rigidus
			Harrington rod
HPE	hemorrhage, papilledema, exudate		hazard ratio
	history and physical examination		
	holoprosencephaly		

	health related	HRST	heat, reddening, swelling, or
	heart rate		tenderness
	hemorrhagic retinopathy		heavy-resistance strength training
	histamine release	HRT	heart rate
	hospital record		heart rate turbulence
	hour		Heidelberg retina tomograph
Hr 0	zero hour (when treatment starts)		heparin-response test
Hr -2	minus two hours (two hours prior to		high-risk transfer
	treatment)		hormone replacement therapy
H & R	hysterectomy and radiation		hyperfractioned radiotherapy
HRA	high-right atrium	HRV	heart rate variability
	histamine-releasing activity		heterogeneous resistance to
H2RA	histamine$_2$-receptor antagonist		vancomycin
HRC	Human Rights Committee	HS	bedtime
HRCT	high-resolution computed		half-strength
	tomography		hamstrings
HRD	hazard ratios of death		hamstring sets
	human retroviral disease		Harmonic scalpel
	hypertension renal disease		Hartman solution (lactated Ringers)
	hypoparathyroidism, retardation, and		heart size
	dysmorphism (syndrome)		heart sounds
HRE	high-resolution electrocardiography		heavy smoker
HRECG	high-resolution electrocardiography		heel spur
HRF	Harris return flow		heel stick
	health-related facility		hereditary spherocytosis
	histamine-releasing factor		herpes simplex
	hypertensive renal failure		hidradenitis suppurativa
	hypoxic respiratory failure		high school
HRI	HMG-CoA (3-hydroxy-		hippocampal sclerosis
	3-methylglutaryl-coenzyme A)		Hurler syndrome
	reductase inhibitors	H → S	heel-to-shin
HRIF	histamine inhibitory releasing factor	H&S	hearing and speech
HRIG	human rabies immune globulin		hemorrhage and shock
HRL	head rotated left		hysterectomy and sterilization
HRLA	human reovirus-like agent	HSA	Health Services Administration
HRLM	high-resolution light microscopy		(Administrator)
hRLX-2	synthetic human relaxin		Health Systems Agency
HRMPC	hormone-refractory metastatic		human serum albumin
	prostate cancer		hypersomnia-sleep apnea
HRMS	high-resolution mass spectrometry	HSAN	hereditary sensory and autonomic
HRNB	Halstead-Reitan Neuropsychological		neuropathy (types I-IV)
	Battery	HSB	husband
HROs	high-reliability organizations	HSBS	evening blood sugar
HRP	high-risk pregnancy	HSBG	heel-stick blood gas
	horseradish peroxidase	HSC	hematopoietic stem cell
HRP-2	histidine-rich protein-2	HSCL	Hopkins Symptom-Check List
HRPC	hormone-refractory prostate cancer	HSCR	Hirschsprung disease
HRQL	health-related quality of life	hs-CRP	high-sensitivity C-reactive protein
HRQOL	health-related quality of life	HSCSS	hypersensitive carotid sinus
HRR	head rotated right		syndrome
HRRC	Human Research Review Committee	HSCT	hematopoietic stem cell transplant
HRS	Haw River syndrome	HSD	Honestly Significant Difference (test)
	hepatorenal syndrome		(Turkey)
	Hodgkin-Reed-Sternberg (cells)		hypoactive sexual desire (disorder)
HRSD	Hamilton Rating Scale for	HSDD	hypoactive sexual desire disorder
	Depression	HSE	herpes simplex encephalitis
HRSEM	high-resolution scanning electron		human skin equivalent
	microscopy		hypertonic saline-epinephrine

H

HSEES	Hazardous Substances Emergency Events Surveillance		hypermetropia
			hyperopia
HSES	hemorrhagic shock and encephalopathy		hypertension
			hyperthermia
HSG	herpes simplex genitalis		hyperthyroid
	hysterosalpingogram	H/T	heel and toe (walking)
HSGYV	heat, steam, gum, yawn, and Valsalva maneuver (for otitis media)	H&T	hospitalization and treatment
		H(T)	intermittent hypertropia
		HT-1	hereditary tyrosinemia type 1
H-SIL	high-grade squamous intraepithelial lesions	5-HT$_1$	serotonin (5-hydroxytryptamine)
		HTA	Health Technology Assessment (Program)
HSJ	hepatic schistosomiasis japonica		hydrothermal ablation
HSK	herpes simplex keratitis		hypertension (French)
HSL	herpes simplex labialis	ht. aer.	heated aerosol
	hormone-sensitive lipase	HTAT	human tetanus antitoxin
HSM	hepatosplenomegaly	HTB	hot tub bath
	holosystolic murmur	HTC	heated tracheostomy collar
HSN	Hansen-Street nail		high-throughput (protein) crystallization
	heart sounds normal		
	hereditary sensory neuropathy		hypertensive crisis
HSOs	health services organizations	HTDS	high-throughput drug screening
HSP	heat shock protein	HTE	highly-treatment experienced (patients)
	Henoch-Schönlein purpura		
	hereditary spastic paraplegia	hTERT	human telomerase reverse transcriptase
	hysterosalpingography		
HSPC	hydrogenated soy phosphatidyl choline	HTF	house tube feeding
		HTGL	hepatic triglyceride lipase
HSPE	high-strength pancreatic enzymes	HTK	heel-to-knee (test)
HSQ	Health Status Questionnaire	HTL	hearing threshold level
HSR	heated serum reagin		honey-thick liquid (diet consistency)
	hypersensitivity reaction		human T-cell leukemia
	hypofractionated stereotactic radiotherapy		human thymic leukemia
		HTLV III	human T-cell lymphotrophic virus type III
HSS	half-strength saline (0.45% Sodium Chloride)		
		HTM	Haemophilus test medium
HSSE	high soap-suds enema		high threshold mechanoceptors
HS-tk	herpes simplex thymidine kinase	HTML	hypertext markup language
HSV	herpes simplex virus	HTN	hypertension
	highly selective vagotomy	HTO	high tibial osteotomy
HSV-1	herpes simplex virus type 1	HTP	House-Tree-Person-test
	herpes simplex virus type 1 vaccine	5-HTP	serotonin (5-hydroxytryptophan)
HSV$_2$	herpes simplex virus type 2 vaccine	HTR	hard tissue replacement
HSV$_{12}$	herpes simplex virus types 1, 2 vaccine	hTRT	human telomerase reverse transcriptase
HSV-2	herpes simplex virus type 2	HTS	head traumatic syndrome
HSVE	herpes simplex virus encephalitis		heel-to-shin (test)
HT	hammertoe		Hematest(r) stools
	head trauma		high-throughput screening
	healing time	HTSCA	human tumor stem cell assay
	hearing test	HtSDS	height standard deviation score
	heart	H-TSH	human thyroid-stimulating hormone
	heart transplant	HTT	hand thrust test
	height		hyalinizing trabecular tumor
	heparin trap (hep-trap; heparin lock; a venous access device)	HTV	herpes-type virus
		HTVD	hypertensive vascular disease
	high temperature	HTX	hemothorax
	hormonotherapy	HTx	heart transplant
	Hubbard tank		

H

HU	head unit		HVPG	hepatic venous pressure gradient
	hydroxyurea		HYPT	hyperventilation provocation test
	hypertensive urgencies		HVR	hypoxic ventilatory response
Hu	Hounsfield units		HVS	hyperventilation syndrome
HUAEC	human umbilical endothelial cells		HVS-TK	herpes simplex virus thymidine kinase
HUCB	human umbilical cord blood		HW	hemiwalker
HUH	Humana Hospital			heparin well
HUI	Health Utilities Index			homework
HUI2	Health Utilities Index Mark 2			housewife
HUIFM	human leukocyte interferon meloy		HWB	hot water bottle
HUK	human urinary kallikrein		HWFE	housewife
HUM	heat, ultrasound, and massage		HWG	has worn glasses
HUM 70/30	human insulin, regular 30 units/mL with human insulin isophane suspension 70 units/mL (Humulin® 70/30 insulin)		HWH	halfway house
			HWP	hot wet pack
			HWPG	has worn prescription glasses
			Hx	history
HUMARA	human androgen receptor assay			hospitalization
HUM L	human insulin zinc suspension (Humulin® L Insulin)		HXM	altretamine (hexamethylmelamine; Hexalen)
HUM N	human insulin isophane suspension (Humulin® N Insulin)		Hx & Px	history and physical (examination)
			Hy	hypermetropia
HUM R	human insulin, regular (Humulin® R Insulin)		HyCoSy	hysterosalpingo-contrast sonography
			HYDRO	hydronephrosis
HUR	hydroxyurea			hydrotherapy
HUS	head ultrasound		HYG	hygiene
	hemolytic uremic syndrome		HYPER	above
	husband			higher than
husb	husband		Hyper Al	hyperalimentation
HUT	head-upright tilt (test)		Hyper K	hyperkalemia
	hyperplasia of usual type		HYPER T & A	hypertrophic tonsils and adenoids
HUTT	head-up tilt-table testing			
HUVEC	human umbilical vein endothelial cells		HYPO	below
				hypodermic injection
HV	hallux valgus			lower than
	Hantavirus		Hypo K	hypokalemia
	has voided		hypopit	hypopituitarism
	healthy volunteers		HYs	healthy years of life
	Hemovac®		Hyst	hysterectomy
	hepatic vein		Hz	Hertz
	herpesvirus		HZ	herpes zoster
	home visit		HZD	herpes zoster dermatitis
	hypervariable		HZO	herpes zoster ophthalmicus
H&V	hemigastrecotomy and vagotomy		HZV	herpes zoster virus
HVII	hypervariable segment II			
HVA	homovanillic acid			
HVD	hypertensive vascular disease			
HVDO	hypovitaminosis D osteopathy			
HVE	high-voltage electrophoresis			
HVES	high-voltage electrical stimulation			
HVF	Humphrey visual field			
HVFD	homonymous visual field defects			
HVGS	high-voltage galvanic stimulation			
HVI	hollow viscus injury			
HVL	half-value layer			
	hippocampal volume loss			
HVOD	hepatic veno-occlusive disease			
HVOO	hepatic venous outflow obstruction			
HVPC	high-voltage pulsed current			

H

I

I impression
incisal
incontinent
independent
initial
inspiration
intact (bag of waters)
intermediate
iris
one
I_2 iodine
I^{131} radioactive iodine
I-3+7 idarubicin and cytarabine
IA ideational apraxia
idiopathic anaphylaxis
incidental appendectomy
incurred accidentally
indigenous Australian(s)
intra-amniotic
intra-arterial
invasive aspergillosis
I & A irrigation and aspiration
IAA ileoanal anastomosis
insulin autoantibodies
interrupted aortic arch
intra-abdominal abscess
intra-arterial angiography
IAAA inflammatory abdominal aortic
aneurysms
IAAT intra-abdominal adipose tissue
IAB incomplete abortion
induced abortion
intermittent androgen blockade
IABC intra-aortic balloon counterpulsation
IABCP intra-aortic balloon counterpulsation
IABP intra-aortic balloon pump
intra-arterial blood pressure
IAC internal auditory canal
intra-arterial chemotherapy
isolated adrenal cell
IACC intra-arterial cytoreductive
chemotherapy
IAC-CPR interposed abdominal
compressions—cardiopulmonary
resuscitation
IACG intermittent angle-closure glaucoma
IACNS isolated angiitis of central nervous
system
IACP intra-aortic counterpulsation
IAD implantable atrial defibrillator
intermittent androgen deprivation
intractable atopic dermatitis
intraoperative autologous (blood)
donation

IADHS inappropriate antidiuretic hormone
syndrome
IADL Instrumental Activities of Daily
Living
IA DSA intra-arterial digital subtraction
arteriography
IAEA International Atomic Energy Agency
IAET International Association for
Enterostomal Therapy (Standards
of Care Dermal Wounds: Pressure
Ulcers)—see WOCN
IAF intra-abdominal fat
IAG indolyl-3-acryloylglycine
IAGT indirect antiglobulin test
IAHA immune adherence hemagglutination
IAHC intra-arterial hepatic chemotherapy
IAHD idiopathic acquired hemolytic disease
IAI intra-abdominal infection
intra-abdominal injury
intra-amniotic infection
IALD instrumental activities of daily living
IAM internal auditory meatus
IAN indinavir (Crixivan) associated
nephrolithiasis
inferior alveolar nerve
intern's admission note
IAO immediately after onset
IAP independent adjudicating panel
intermittent acute porphyria
intra-abdominal pressure
intracarotid amobarbital procedure
IAPP islet amyloid polypeptide
IAQ indoor air quality
IARC International Agency for Research
on Cancer
IART intra-atrial reentrant tachycardia
IAS idiopathic ankylosing spondylitis
intermittent androgen suppression
internal anal sphincter
Interpersonal Adjective Scales
IASD interatrial septal defect
IAT immunoaugmentive therapy
indirect antiglobulin test
intracarotid amobarbital test
intraoperative autologous transfusion
IATT intra-arterial thrombolytic therapy
IAV infraclavicular axillary vein
intermittent assist ventilation
IAVC intrinsic atrioventricular conduction
IB ileal bypass
insulin-receptor binding test
isolation bed
investigator's brochure
IB1A interferon beta-1a (Avonex)
IBAM idiopathic bile acid malabsorption
IBBB intra-blood-brain barrier
IBBBB incomplete bilateral bundle branch
block

IBC	Institutional Biosafety Committee		intracerebral
	invasive bladder cancer		intracranial
	iron binding capacity		intraincisional
IBCLC	International Board-Certified		ion chromatography
	Lactation Consultant		irritable colon
IBD	infectious bursal disease	I/C	imipenem-cilastatin (Primaxin)
	inflammatory bowel disease	ICA	ileocolic anastomosis
	isosulfan blue dye		intermediate care area
IBDQ	Inflammatory Bowel Disease		internal carotid artery
	Questionnaire		intracranial abscess
IBE	individual bioequivalence		intracranial aneurysm
IBG	iliac bone graft		islet-cell antibody
IBI	intermittent bladder irrigation	ICa	calcium, ionized
ibid	at the same place	ICAAC	Interscience Conference on
IBILI	indirect bilirubin		Antimicrobial Agents and
IBM	ideal body mass		Chemotherapy
	inclusion body myositis	ICAD	intracranial atherosclerotic disease
IBMI	initial body mass index	ICAM	intracellular adhesion molecule
IBMTR	International Bone Marrow Transplant	ICAM-1	intercellular adhesion molecule-1
	Registry	ICAO	internal carotid artery occlusion
IBNR	incurred but not reported	ICAS	intermediate coronary artery
IBOW	intact bag of waters		syndrome
IBP	ibuprofen	ICAT	infant cardiac arrest tray
	intrableb pigmentation		isotope-coded affinity tag
IBPB	interscalene brachial plexus block	ICB	intracranial bleeding
IBPS	Insall-Burstein posterior stabilizer	ICBG	iliac crest bone graft
IBR	immediate breast reconstruction	ICBT	intercostobronchial trunk
	infectious bovine rhinotracheitis	ICC	idiopathic chronic cough
IBRS	Inpatient Behavior Rating Scale		immunocytochemistry
IBS	irritable bowel syndrome		Indian childhood cirrhosis
IBS-D	Irritable Bowel Syndrome– Diarrhea		Infection Control Committee
	Type		intracluster correlation coefficient
IBT	ink blot test (Rorschach test)		intraclass correlation coefficient
	interblinking time		invasive cervical carcinoma
	immune-based therapy		islet cell carcinoma
IBTR	intrabreast-tumor recurrence	ICCD	intensified charge-coupled device
	ipsilateral breast tumor recurrence	ICCE	intracapsular cataract extraction
IBU	ibuprofen	ICCU	intensive coronary care unit
IBW	ideal body weight		intermediate coronary care unit
IC	between meals	ICD	implantable cardioverter
	iliac crest		defibrillator
	immune complex		indigocarmine dye
	immunocompromised		informed consent document
	incipient cataract (grade 1+ to 4+)		instantaneous cardiac death
	incomplete		intercusp distance (dental)
	indirect calorimetry		isocitrate dehydrogenase
	indirect Coombs (test)		irritant contact dermatitis
	individual counseling	ICDA	International Classification of
	informed consent		Disease, Adapted
	inspiratory capacity	ICDB	incomplete database
	intensive care	ICDC	implantable cardioverter defibrillator
	intercostal		catheter
	intercourse	ICD 9 CM	International Statistical Classification
	intermediate care		of Diseases, 9th Revision, Clinical
	intermittent catheterization		Modification
	intermittent claudication	ICD-10	International Classification of
	interstitial changes		Diseases and Related Health
	interstitial cystitis		Problems, 10th revision

ICD-10-PCS	International Statistical Classification of Diseases, 10th Revision, Procedure Coding Classification System
ICDO	International Classification of Diseases for Oncology
ICE	ice, compression, and elevation
	ifosfamide, carboplatin, and etoposide
	individual career exploration
	interleukin-1 alpha converting enzyme
	interleukin-1 beta converting enzyme
	intracardiac echocardiography
+ ice	add ice
ICECI	International Classification of External Causes of Injuries
ICER	incremental cost-effectiveness ratio
ICES	ice, compression, elevation, and support
ICF	intermediate care facility
	intracellular fluid
ICFDH	International Classification of Functioning, Disability, and Health
ICG	indocyanine green
ICGA	indocyanine green angiography
ICH	immunocompromised host
	International Conference on Harmonization (of Technical Requirements for Registration of Pharmaceuticals for Human Use)
	intracerebral hemorrhage
	intracranial hemorrhage
ICHD-II	International Classification of Headache Disorders, 2nd Edition
ICHI	International Classification of Health Interventions
ICI	intracranial injury
ICIQ-SF	International Consultation on Incontinence Questionnaire
ICIT	intensified conventional insulin therapy
ICL	intracorneal lens
	isocitrate lyase
ICLE	intracapsular lens extraction
ICM	intercostal margin
	intercostal muscle
	ischemic cardiomyopathy
ICN	infection control nurse
	intensive care nursery
ICN2	neonatal intensive care unit level II
ICP	inductively coupled plasma
	intercostal position (for chest lead)
	intracranial pressure
	intrahepatic cholestasis of pregnancy
ICPC	International Classification of Primary Care
ICPC-2	International Classification of Primary Care, 2nd revision
ICP-MS	inductively-coupled plasma—mass spectrometer
ICP-OES	inductively-coupled plasma—optical emission spectrometry
ICPP	intubated continuous positive pressure
ICR	intercaudate nucleus ratio
	intercostal retractions
	intrastromal corneal ring
ICRC	International Committee of the Red Cross
ICRF-159	razoxane
ICRP	International Commission on Radiological Protection
ICRS	intrastromal corneal ring segments
ICS	ileocecal sphincter
	inhaled corticosteroid(s)
	intercostal space
ICSC	idiopathic central serous choroidopathy
ICSH	interstitial cell-stimulating hormone
ICSI	intracytoplasmic sperm injection
ICSR	Individual Case Safety Reports
	intercostal space retractions
ICT	icterus
	indirect Coombs test
	inflammation of connective tissue
	intensive conventional therapy
	intermittent cervical traction
	intracranial tumor
	intracutaneous test
	islet cell transplant
ICTP	C-terminal telopeptide of type I collagen
ICTX	intermittent cervical traction
ICU	intensive care unit
	intermediate care unit
ICV	intracerebroventricular
ICVH	ischemic cerebrovascular headache
ICW	in connection with
	intact canal wall
	intercellular water
ID	identification
	identify
	idiotype
	ifosfamide, mesna uroprotection, and doxorubicin
	immunodiffusion
	induction delivery
	infectious disease (physician or department)
	initial diagnosis
	initial dose
	intellectual disability
	internal derangement
	intradermal

I

id	the same	IDU	idoxuridine
I & D	incision and debridement		infectious disease unit
	incision and drainage		injecting drug user
	irrigation and debridement	IDV	indinavir (Crixivan)
IDA	idarubicin (Idamycin)		intermittent demand ventilation
	iron deficiency anemia	IDVC	indwelling venous catheter
IDAM	infant of drug abusing mother	IE	ifosfamide, and etoposide with
IDB	incomplete database		mesna
IDC	idiopathic dilated cardiomyopathy		immunoelectrophoresis
	invasive ductal cancer		induced emesis
IDCF	immunodiffusion complement		infectious enteritis
	fixation		infective endocarditis
IDCM	idiopathic dilated cardiomyopathy		inner ear
IDD	insulin-dependent diabetes		internal/external (rotation)
	intervertebral disk disease		international unit (European
	iodine-deficiency disorders		abbreviation)
I/DD	intellectual and developmental	I & E	ingress and egress (tubes)
	disabilities		internal and external
IDDD	Interview for Deterioration in Daily	*i.e.*	that is
	Life in Dementia	IEC	independent ethics committee
IDDM	insulin-dependent diabetes mellitus		inpatient exercise center
IDDS	implantable drug delivery system		intradiskal electrothermal
IDE	Investigational Device Exemption		coagulation
IDEA	Individuals with Disabilities	IED	immune-enhancing diet
	Education Act		improvised explosive device
IDET	intradiskal electrothermal therapy		intermittent explosive disorder
IDFC	immature dead female child	IEED	involuntary emotional expression
IDH	isocitric dehydrogenase		disorder
IDI	Interpersonal Dependency Inventory	IEF	isoelectric focusing
	intrathecal drug infusion	IEI	idiopathic environmental intolerance
IDK	internal derangement of knee	IEL	internal elastic lamina
IDL	intermediate-density lipoprotein		intestinal-intraepithelial lymphocyte
	ischemic digital loss	IELT	Intravaginal Ejaculatory Latency
IDLH	immediately dangerous to life or		Time
	health	IEM	immune electron microscopy
IDM	infant of a diabetic mother		inborn errors of metabolism
IDMC	immature dead male child	iEMG	integrated electromyography
	Independent Data Monitoring	IEMR	integrated electronic medical records
	Committee	IEN	intraepithelial neoplasia
IDNA	iron-deficient, not anemic	IEP	idiopathic eosinophilic pneumonia
IDO	idiopathic detrusor overactivity		immunoelectrophoresis
IDP	initiate discharge planning		Individualized Education Plan
	inosine diphosphate	IEPA	immunoelectrophoresis analysis
IDPN	intradialytic parenteral nutrition	I:E ratio	inspiratory to expiratory time ratio
IDR	idarubicin (Zavedos)	IES	Impact of Event Scale
	idiosyncratic drug reaction	IET	infantile estropia
	intradermal reaction	IF	idiopathic flushing
IDS	infectious disease service		ifosfamide (Ifex)
	integrated delivery system		immunofluorescence
	intradermal smears		index finger
IDSA	Infectious Disease Society of		injury factor
	America (guidelines)		interferon
IDT	intensive diabetes treatment		interfrontal
	interdisciplinary team		intermaxillary fixation
	intradermal test		internal fixation
IDTF	independent diagnostic testing		intrinsic factor
	facility		involved field (radiotherapy)
IDTP	immunodiffusion tube precipitin	IFA	immunofluorescent assay

	imported fire ants
	indirect fluorescent antibody
IFAT	immunofluorescence antibody test (technique)
IFC	interferential current
IFE	immunofixation electrophoresis
	in-flight emergency
IFG	impaired fasting glucose
IFI	invasive fungal infection
IFL	indolent follicular lymphoma
	irinotecan, fluorouracil, and leucovorin
IFM	internal fetal monitoring
IFN	interferon
IFN α-1	interferon alfa-1
IFNB	interferon beta-1 b (Betaseron)
IFO	ifosfamide (Ifex)
	in front of
iFOBT	immunochemical fecal occult blood tests
IFOP	infrared fiber-optic probe
IFOS	ifosfamide (Ifex)
IFP	inflammatory fibroid polyps
IFPMA	International Federation of Pharmaceutical Manufacturers Associations
IFSAC	Inventory of Functional Status After Childbirth
IFSE	internal fetal scalp electrode
IFSP	individualized family service plan
IgA	immunoglobulin A
IGCS	inpatient geriatric consultation services
IgD	immunoglobulin D
IGDE	idiopathic gait disorders of the elderly
IGDM	infant of gestational diabetic mother
IgE	immunoglobulin E
IGF-I	insulin-like growth factor I
IGFA	indocyanine-green fundus angiography
IGFBP-3	insulin-like growth factor-binding protein 3
IgG	immunoglobulin G
IGHL	inferior glenohumeral ligament
IGI	image guided implantology
IGIM	immune globulin intramuscular
IGIV	immune globulin intravenous
IgM	immunoglobulin M
IGP	interstitial glycoprotein
IGR	intrauterine growth retardation
IGT	impaired glucose tolerance
IGTN	impaired glucose tolerance and neuropathy
	ingrown toenail
IH	indirect hemagglutination
	infectious hepatitis
	inguinal hernia

	inhaled (this is a dangerous abbreviation)
	in-house
IHA	immune hemolytic anemia
	indirect hemagglutination
	infusion hepatic arteriography
	intrahepatic arterial
IHC	idiopathic hypercalciuria
	immobilization hypercalcemia
	immunohistochemistry
	inner hair cell (in cochlea)
IHD	intermittent hemodialysis
	intraheptic duct (ule)
	ischemic heart disease
IHDN	integrated health delivery network
IHES	idiopathic hypereosinophilic syndrome
IHH	idiopathic hypogonadotrophic hypogonadism
IHHE	infantile hepatic hemangioendothelioma
IHO	idiopathic hypertrophic osteoarthropathy
IHP	idiopathic hypoparathyroidism
	inferior hypogastric plexus
	isolated hepatic perfusion
IHPH	intrahepatic portal hypertension
IHPS	infantile hypertrophic pyloric stenosis
IHR	inguinal hernia repair
	intrinsic heart rate
IHS	Indian Health Service
	integrated healthcare system
	International Headache Society (criteria)
	Idiopathic Headache Score
IHs	iris hamartomas
IHSA	iodinated human serum albumin
IHSS	idiopathic hypertrophic subaortic stenosis
IHT	insulin hypoglycemia test
IHU	inpatient hospice unit
IHW	inner-heel wedge
II	internal iliac (artery)
IIA	internal iliac artery
IICP	increased intracranial pressure
IICU	infant intensive care unit
IID	infectious intestinal disease
IIDD	idiopathic inflammatory demyelinating diseases
IIEF	International Index of Erectile Function
IIF	indirect immunofluorescence
IIH	idiopathic infantile hypercalcemia
	iodine-induced hyperthyroidism
IIHT	iodide-induced hyperthyroidism
IIM	idiopathic inflammatory myopathies
	intracortical interaction mapping

IINB	iliohypogastric ilioinguinal nerve block	ILS	intralabyrinthine schwannomas
IIP	idiopathic interstitial pneumonitis	ILT	interstitial laser therapy
IIPF	idiopathic interstitial pulmonary fibrosis	ILVEN	inflammatory linear verrucal epidermal nevus
IJ	ileojejunal	IM	ice massage

IINB   iliohypogastric ilioinguinal nerve block
IIP   idiopathic interstitial pneumonitis
IIPF   idiopathic interstitial pulmonary fibrosis
IJ   ileojejunal
     internal jugular
I&J   insight and judgment
IJC   internal jugular catheter
IJD   inflammatory joint disease
IJO   idiopathic juvenile osteoporosis
IJP   internal jugular pressure
IJR   idiojunctional rhythm
IJT   idiojunctional tachycardia
IJV   internal jugular vein
IK   immobilized knee
     interstitial keratitis
IKDC   International Knee Documentation Committee (evaluation; score; form)
IL   immature lungs
     interleukin (1, 2, etc.)
     intralesional
     Intralipid®
IL-2   aldesleukin (Proleukin; interleukin-2)
IL-11   oprelvekin (Neumega; interleukin-11)
ILA   inferior lateral angle
     insulin-like activity
ILB   incidental Lewy body
ILBBB   incomplete left bundle branch block
ILBW   infant, low birth weight (less than 2,500 g)
ILC   interstitial laser coagulation
     invasive lobular cancer
ILCOR   International Liaison Committee on Resuscitation
ILD   immature lung disease
     indentation load deflection
     interlaminar distance in flexion
     intermediate density lipoproteins
     interstitial lung disease
     ischemic leg disease
ILE   infantile lobar emphysema
     involutional lateral entropion
ILF   indicated low forceps
ILFC   immature living female child
ILHP   ipsilateral hemidiaphragmatic paresis
ILI   influenza-like illness
     isolated limb infusion
ILM   internal limiting membrane
ILMC   immature living male child
ILMI   inferolateral myocardial infarct
ILP   interstitial laser photocoagulation
     isolated limb perfusion
ILQTS   idiopathic long QT (interval) syndrome
ILR   implantable loop recorder

ILS   intralabyrinthine schwannomas
ILT   interstitial laser therapy
ILVEN   inflammatory linear verrucal epidermal nevus
IM   ice massage
     imatinib mesylate (Gleevec) (This is a very dangerous abbreviation)
     infectious mononucleosis
     intermetatarsal
     internal medicine
     intramedullary
     intramuscular
IMA   inferior mesenteric artery
     internal mammary artery
IMAC   ifosfamide, mesna uroprotection, doxorubicin (Adriamycin), and cisplatin
     immobilized metal affinity chromatography
IMAE   internal maxillary artery embolization
IMAG   internal mammary artery graft
IMARD   immunomodulating antirheumatic drugs
IMAT   intensity-modulated arc therapy
IMB   intermenstrual bleeding
IMBP   immobilized mismatch binding protein
IMC   intermittent catheterization
     intramedullary catheter
IMCI   Integrated Management of Childhood Illness
IMCU   intermediate care unit
IME   important medical event
     independent medical examination (evaluation)
     isometric exercise
IMF   idiopathic myelofibrosis
     ifosfamide, mesna uroprotection, methotrexate, and fluorouracil
     immobilization mandibular fracture
     inframammary fold
     intermaxillary fixation
IMG   internal medicine group
IMGU   insulin-mediated glucose uptake
IMH   idiopathic myocardial hypertrophy
     intramural hematoma
IMH   indirect microhemagglutination (test)
IMI   imipramine
     impending myocardial infarction
     inferior myocardial infarction
     intramuscular injection
^{131}I-MIBG   iodine^{131}-metaiodobenzyl-guanidine (iobenguane ^{131}I)
IMIG   intramuscular immunoglobulin
IMLC   incomplete mitral leaflet closure
IMM   immunizations
IMN   idiopathic membranous nephropathy

I

	immune modulating nutrition (immunonutrition)	INDO	indomethacin
	internal mammary (lymph) node	^{111}In-DTPA	indium pentetate
IMP	impacted	INE	infantile necrotizing encephalomyelopathy
	important		
	impression	INEX	inexperienced
	improved	INF	infant
	inosine monophoshate		infarction
IMPX	impaction		infected
IMQ	Infant/Child Monitoring Questionnaires		infection
			inferior
IMR	infant mortality rate		influenza virus vaccine, not otherwise specified
IMRA	immunoradiometric assay		information
IMRS	intensity-modulated radiosurgery		infused
IMRT	intensity-modulated radiation therapy		infusion
IMS	immunosuppressants		intravenous nutritional fluid
	incurred in military service	INF$_a$	influenza virus, attenuated live vaccine
	involuntary movements		
	ion mobility spectrometry	INFas	influenza virus attenuated live vaccine, intranasal
IMT	inspiratory muscle training		
	intimal medial thickness	INFC	infected
IMU	intermediate medicine unit		infection
IMV	inferior mesenteric vein	INFi	influenza virus inactivated vaccine
	intermittent mandatory ventilation	INFs	influenza virus vaccine, split viron
	intermittent mechanical ventilation	INFs-AB3	influenza virus inactivated vaccine, split virion, types A and B, trivalent
IMVP-16	ifosfamide, mesna uroprotection, methotrexate, and ctoposide		
IN	insulin	INF$_w$	influenza virus vaccine, whole viron
	intranasal (this is a dangerous abbreviation as it can be read as IV [intravenous] or IM [intramuscular]; use nasally or intranasal)	ING	inguinal
		✓ing	checking
		INH	inhalation
			isoniazid (isonicotinic acid hydrazide)
In	indium		
in.	inch	INI	intranuclear inclusion
INAD	in no apparent distress	inj	injection
	Investigational New Animal Drug		injury
INB	intercostal nerve blockade	INK	injury not known
INC	incisal	INN	International Nonproprietary Name
	incision	INO	inhaled nitrous oxide
	incomplete		internuclear ophthalmoplegia
	incontinent	INOP	internodal ophthalmoplegia
	increase	iNOS	inducible nitric oxide synthase
	inside-the-needle catheter	inpt	inpatient
INCC	Institut National du Cancer du Canada	INQ	inferior nasal quadrant
		INR	international normalized ratio (for anticoagulant monitoring)
INCMNSZ	Instituto Nacional de Ciencias Médicas y Nutrición (Mexico)		
		INS	idiopathic nephrotic syndrome
Inc Spir	incentive spirometer		inspection
IND	indinavir (Crixivan)		insurance
	induced	INSS	International Neuroblastoma Staging System
	Investigational New Drug (application)		
		INST	instrumental delivery
INDA	Investigational New Drug Application	INT	intermittent needle therapy
			internal
INDIGO	interstitial laser ablation of the prostate	Int mon	internal monitor
		INTERP	interpretation
INDM	infant of nondiabetic mother	Int Med	internal medicine

intol	intolerance		incubation period
int-rot	internal rotation		individualized plan
int trx	intermittent traction		Infrapatellar
intub	intubation		inpatient
INV	Invirase (saquinavir, hard gel cap)		in plaster
inver	inversion		interphalangeal
INVOS	in vivo optical spectroscopy		interstitial pneumonia
IO	inferior oblique		intestinal permeability
	initial opening		intraperitoneal
	intestinal obstruction		invasive procedures
	intraocular pressure		inverted (inverting) papilloma
	intra-Ommaya	I/P	iris/pupil
	intraoperative	IP3	inositol triphosphate
	intraosseous	IPA	independent practice association
I&O	intake and output		interpleural analgesia
IOA	intact on admission		invasive pulmonary aspergillosis
IOC	intern on call		isopropyl alcohol
	intraoperative cholangiogram	IPAA	ileo-pouch anal anastamosis
IOCG	intraoperative cholangiogram	IPAH	idiopathic pulmonary arterial
IOD	implant-supported overdenture		hypertension
	interorbital distance	IPAP	inspiratory positive airway pressure
IODM	infant of diabetic mother	IPB	infrapopliteal bypass
IOF	intraocular fluid	IPC	indirect pulp cavity
IOFB	intraocular foreign body		intermittent pneumatic compression
IOFNA	intraoperative fine needle aspiration		(boots)
IOH	idiopathic orthostatic hypotension		intraperitoneal chemotherapy
IO-HDRBT	intraoperative high-dose-rate	IPCD	idiopathic paroxysmal cerebral
	brachytherapy		dysrhythmia
IOI	idiopathic orbital inflammation		infantile polycystic disease
	intraosseous infusion	IPCK	infantile polycystic kidney (disease)
IOL	induction of labor	IPCT	intraperitoneal chemotherapy
	intraocular lens	IPD	idiopathic Parkinson disease
	intraocular lymphoma		immediate pigment darkening
IOLI	intraocular lens implantation		inflammatory pelvic disease
IOLM	intraoperative lymphatic mapping		intermittent peritoneal dialysis
IOM	Institute of Medicine		interpupillary distance
ION	ischemic optic neuropathy		invasive pneumococcal disease
IONIS	indirect optic nerve injury syndrome	IPEX	immune dysregulation,
IONTO	iontophoresis		polyendocrinopathy, enteropathy,
IOOA	inferior oblique overaction		X-linked (syndrome)
IOP	intraocular pressure	IPF	idiopathic pulmonary fibrosis
	intraosseous puncture		inpatient psychiatric facility
IOR	ideas of reference		interstitial pulmonary fibrosis
	immature oocyte retrieval	IPFD	intrapartum fetal distress
	inferior oblique recession	IPG	immobilized pH gradient
IO-RB	intraocular retinoblastoma		impedance plethysmography
IORT	intraoperative radiation therapy		individually polymerized grass
IOS	intraoperative sonography	IPH	idiopathic pulmonary hemosiderosis
IOSH	Institute for Occupational Safety and		interphalangeal
	Health		intraparenchymal hemorrhage
IOT	intraocular tension		intraperitoneal hemorrhage
IOTEE	intraoperative transesophageal	IPHC	intraperitoneal hyperthermic
	echocardiography		chemotherapy
IOTT	intensification-of-treatment trigger	IPHEP	independent progressive home
	(criteria)		exercise program
IOUS	intraocular ultrasound	IPHP	intraperitoneal hyperthermic
IOV	initial office visit		chemotherapy
IP	ice pack	IPI	International Prognostic Index

IPJ	interphalangeal joint	IQR	interquartile range
IPK	intractable plantar keratosis	IQWiG	Leiter des Institus für Qualität and
IPL	intense pulsed light		Wirtschaftlichkeit im
IPM	intranodal-palisaded		Gesundheitswesen (Institute for
	myofibroblastoma		Quality and Economy in
	intrauterine pressure monitor		Healthcare)
	interventional pain management	IR	immediate-release (tablets)
IPMI	inferoposterior myocardial infarct		immunoreactive
IPMN	intraductal papillary mucinous		inferior rectus
	neoplasm		infrared
IPN	infantile periarteritis nodosa		insulin resistance
	intern's progress note		internal reduction
	interstitial pneumonia		internal resistance
IPOF	immediate postoperative fitting		internal rotation
IPOM	intraperitoneal onlay mesh		intraoral radiography (dental)
IPOP	immediate postoperative prosthesis	I&R	insertion and removal
IPP	inflatable penile prosthesis	IRA	infarct-related artery
	intrapleural pressure	IRAAF	intraoperative radiofrequency
	intravesical protrusion of the prostate		ablation for chronic atrial
	isolated pelvic perfusion		fibrillation
IPPA	inspection, palpation, percussion,	IRA-EEA	ileorectal anastomoses with end-to-
	and auscultation		end anastomosis
IPPB	intermittent positive-pressure	IRAP	interleukin-1 receptor antagonist
	breathing		protein
IP-PDT	intraperitoneal photodynamic therapy	IRB	Institutional Review Board
IPPE	initial preventive physical	IRBBB	incomplete right bundle branch block
	examination	IRBC	immature red blood cell
IPPF	immediate postoperative prosthetic		irradiated red blood cells
	fitting	iRBCs	*Plasmodium falciparum* infected red
IPPI	interruption of pregnancy for		blood cells
	psychiatric indication	IRBP	implantable rotary blood pump
IPPV	intermittent positive pressure		interphotoreceptor retinoid-binding
	ventilation		protein
IPS	idiopathic pneumonia syndrome	IRC	indirect radionuclide cystography
	infundibular pulmonic stenosis		infrared coagulation
	initial prognostic score		Institutional Review Committee
	intermittent photic stimulation		(Board)
IPSCs	islet-producing stem cells	IRCU	intensive respiratory care unit
IPSF	immediate postsurgical fitting	IRD	immune renal disease(s)
IPSID	immunoproliferative small intestinal	IRDA	intermittent rhythmic delta activity
	disease	IRDM	insulin-requiring diabetes mellitus
IPSP	inhibitory postsynaptic potential		insulin-resistant diabetes mellitus
IPSS	inferior petrosal sinus sampling	IR-DRGs	International Refined Diagnosis
I-PSS	International Prostate Symptom		Related Groups
	Score	IRDS	idiopathic respiratory distress
IPST	intraprocedural stent thrombosis		syndrome
I PSY	intermediate psychiatry		infant respiratory distress syndrome
IPT	intended primary treatment	IRE	internal rotation in extension
	intermittent pelvic traction	IRED	infrared-emission detection
iPTH	parathyroid hormone by	IRF	inpatient rehabilitation facilities
	radioimmunoassay		internal rotation in flexion
IPTX	intermittent pelvic traction	IRH	intraretinal hemorrhage
IPV	inactivated poliovirus vaccine	IRI	immunoreactive insulin
	intimate partner violence		irinotecan (Camptosar)
IPVC	interpolated premature ventricular	IRIV	immunopotentiating reconstituted
	contraction		influenza virosomes
IPW	interphalangeal width	IRM	magnetic resonance imaging
IQ	intelligence quotient		(French)

IRMA	immediate response mobile analysis (blood analysis system)		infant skin control
			intermittent self-catheterization
	immunoradiometric assay		intermittent straight catheterization
	intraretinal microvascular abnormalities		isolette servo-control
		ISCM	intramedullary spinal cord metastases
IRMS	isotope-ratio mass spectrometry		
IRN	iterated rippled noise	I/SCN	urinary iodine/thiocyanate ratio
IRNS	intercostal repetitive nerve stimulation	ISCOM	immunostimulating complex
		ISCP	infection surveillance and control program
IROS	ipsilateral routing of signals		
IROX	irinotecan and oxaliplatin	ISCs	irreversible sickle cells
IRP	intellectual property rights	ISCU	infant special care unit
IRR	infrared radiation	ISD	inhibited sexual desire
	intrarenal reflux		initial sleep disturbance
	irregular rate and rhythm		intrinsic (urethral) sphincter deficiency
IRRC	Institutional Research Review Committee		
			isosorbide dinitrate (Isordol)
irreg	irregular	ISDN	isosorbide dinitrate (Isordol)
IRR HYDRO	irreversible hydrocolloid	ISE	internal scalp electrode
			ion-sensitive electrode
IRRs	incidence rate ratios	ISEL	*in situ* end labeling
IRS	Information and Referral Society	ISF	interstitial fluid
	insulin receptor substrate	ISFET	ion-selective field effect transistor
	insulin-resistance syndrome	ISG	immune serum globulin (immune globulin)
IRSB	intravenous regional sympathetic block		
		ISH	isolated systolic hypertension
IRSG	Intergroup Rhabdomyosarcoma Study Group	ISHH	*in situ* hybridization histochemistry
		ISHLT	International Society for Heart and Lung Transplantation
IRT	immunoreactive trypsin		
	incident response team	ISHT	isolated systolic hypertension
IRV	inspiratory reserve volume	ISI	International Sensitivity Index
	inverse ratio ventilation	ISK	isokinetic
IS	incentive spirometer	ISMA	infantile spinal muscular atrophy
	induced sputum	ISMN	isosorbide mononitrate
	Information Services (Department)	ISMO®	isosorbide mononitrate
	in situ	ISMP	Institute for Safe Medication Practices
	intercostal space		
	inventory of systems	ISNA	iron-sufficient, not anemic
	ipecac syrup	ISO	International Organization for Standardization
I-S	Ionescu-Shiley (prosthetic heart valve)		
			isodose
I & S	intact and symmetrical		isolette
I/S	instruct/supervise		isoproterenol
ISA	ileosigmoid anastomosis	ISOE	isoetharine
	Incest Survivors Anonymous	ISOF	isoflurane (Florane)
	intrinsic sympathomimetic activity	ISOK	isokinetic
ISAAC	International Study of Asthma and Allergies in Childhood (questionnaire; protocol)	ISOM	isometric
		ISOs	isoenzymes
		ISP	inferior spermatic plexus
ISADH	inappropriate secretion of antidiuretic hormone		interspace
		ISPP	individualized sleep promotion plan
ISAM	infant of substance abusing mother	*ISQ*	as before; continue on (*in status quo*)
ISB	incentive spirometry breathing		
ISBN	International Standard Book Number	ISR	injection site reaction
ISBP	interscalen brachial plexus		in-stent restenosis
ISC	carcinoma *in situ* (also CIS)		integrated secretory response
	indwelling subclavian catheter	ISRCTN	International Standard Randomized Controlled Trial Number
	infant servo-control		

I

ISS	idiopathic short stature	ITMTX	intrathecal methotrexate
	Individual Self-Rating Scale	ITN	irinotecan (Camptosar)
	Injury Severity Score	ITNs	insecticide treated nets
	irritable stomach syndrome	ITOC	intratracheal oxygen catheter
	Integrated Summary of Safety	ITOP	intentional termination of pregnancy
IS10S	10% invert sugar in 0.9% sodium	ITOU	intensive therapy observation unit
	chloride (saline) injection	ITP	idiopathic thrombocytopenic
ISSP	Infant Support Services Program		purpura
IST	immunosuppressive therapy		interim treatment plan
	injection sclerotherapy	ITPA	Illinois Test of Psycholinguistic
	insulin sensitivity test		Ability
	insulin shock therapy	ITQ	inferior temporal quadrant
ISU	intermediate surgical unit	ITR	isotretinoin (Accutane)
ISW	interstitial water	ITRA	itraconazole (Sporanox)
IS10W	10% invert sugar injection (in water)	ITS	internal transcribed spacer
ISWI	incisional surgical wound infection		isometric trunk stabilization
IT	incentive therapy	ITSCU	infant-toddler special care unit
	individual therapy	ITT	identical twins (raised) together
	inferior-temporal		incremental treadmill test
	inferior turbinate		insulin tolerance test
	information technology		intention-to-treat (analysis)
	Information Technology	ITU	infant-toddler unit
	(Department)		intensive therapy unit
	Inhalation Therapist		intensive treatment unit
	inhalation therapy	ITVAD	indwelling transcutaneous vascular
	inspiratory time		access device
	intensive therapy	ITX	immunotoxin(s)
	intermittent traction	ITx	intestinal transplantation
	interpreted	ITZ	itraconazole (Sporanox)
	intertrochanteric	IU	international unit (this is a dangerous
	intertuberous		abbreviation as it is read as
	intrathecal (dangerous abbreviation)		intravenous; use "units")
	intratracheal (dangerous, could be	IUC	intrauterine catheter
	interupted as intrathecal)	IUCD	intrauterine contraceptive device
	intratumoral	IUD	intrauterine death
ITA	individual treatment assessment		intrauterine device
	inferior temporal artery	IUDE	intrauterine drug exposure
	itasetron		intravenous drug exposure
ITAG	internal thoracic artery graft	IUDR	idoxuridine (Herplex)
ITAL	intrathoracic artificial lung	IUFB	intrauterine foreign body
ITB	iliotibial band	IUFD	intrauterine fetal death (demise)
	intrathecal baclofen		intrauterine fetal distress
ITBC	intraluminal typical bronchial	IUFT	intrauterine fetal transfusion
	carcinoid	IUGR	intrauterine growth retardation
ITBS	iliotibial band syndrome		(restriction)
	Iowa Tests of Basic Skills	IUI	intrauterine insemination
ITC	Incontinence Treatment Center	IULN	institutional upper limit of normal
	in-the-canal (hearing aid)	IUMR	intrauterine myelomeningocele repair
	isothermal titration calorimetry	IUP	intrauterine pregnancy
ITCP	idiopathic thrombocytopenic purpura	IUPB	infected units per billion
ITCU	intensive thoracic cardiovascular unit	IUPC	intrauterine pressure catheter
ITE	insufficient therapeutic effect	IUPD	intrauterine pregnancy delivered
	in-the-ear (hearing aid)	IUP,TBCS	intrauterine pregnancy, term birth,
ITF	inpatient treatment facility		cesarean section
ITFF	intertrochanteric femoral fracture	IUP,TBLC	intrauterine pregnancy, term birth,
ITGV	intrathoracic gas volume		living child
ITM	Institute of Tropical Medicine,	IUR	intrauterine retardation
	(Antwerp, Belgium)	IUS	intrauterine system

IUT	intrauterine transfusion		methylprednisolone
IUTD	immunizations up to date	IVNC	isolated ventricular noncompaction
IV	four	IVO	intraoral vertical osteotomy
	interview	IVOX	intravascular oxygenator
	intravenous (i.v.)		(oxygenation)
	intravertebral	IVP	intravenous push (this is a dangerous
	invasive		meaning as it is read as intravenous
	inversion		pyelogram)
	symbol for class 4 controlled		intravenous pyelogram
	substances	IVPB	intravenous piggyback
IVA	Intervir-A	IVPF	isovolume pressure flow
IVAD	implantable venous access device	IVPU	intravenous push
	implantable vascular access device	IVR	idioventricular rhythm
IVBAT	intravascular bronchoalveolar tumor		interactive voice-response (system)
IVC	inferior vena cava		intravaginal ring
	inspiratory vital capacity		intravenous retrograde
	intravenous chemotherapy		intravenous rider (this is a dangerous
	intravenous cholangiogram		abbreviation as it has been read as
	intraventricular catheter		IVP-intravenous push)
	intraventricular conduction		isovolumic relaxation (time)
IVCCM	in-vivo corneal confocal microscopy	IVRA	intravenous regional anesthesia
IVCD	intraventricular conduction defect	IVRAP	intravenous retrograde access port
	(delay)	IVRG	intravenous retrograde
IVCF	inferior vena cava filter	IV-RNV	intravenous radionuclide venography
IVCI	intravenous continuous infusion	IVRO	intraoral vertical ramus osteotomy
IVCP	inferior vena cava pressure	IVRS	interactive voice response system
IVCV	inferior venacavography	IVRT	isovolumic relation time
IVD	instrumental vaginal delivery	IVS	intraventricular septum
	intervertebral disk		irritable voiding syndrome
	intravenous drip	IVSD	intraventricular septal defect
	in vitro diagnostic	IVSE	interventricular septal excursion
	ischemic vascular dementia	IVSO	intraoral vertical segmental
IVDA	intravenous drug abuse		osteotomy
IVDSA	intravenous digital subtraction	IVSS	intravenous Soluset®
	angiography	IVST	interventricular septum thickness
IVDU	intravenous drug user	IVT	intravenous transfusion
IVET	in vivo expression technology		intraventricular
IVF	intervertebral foramina	IVTTT	intravenous tolbutamide tolerance
	intravenous fluid(s)		test
	in vitro fertilization	IVU	intravenous urography (urogram)
IVFA	intravenous fluorescein angiography	IVUC	intravenous ultrasound catheter
IVFE	intravenous fat emulsion	IVUS	intravascular ultrasound
IVF-ET	in vitro fertilization-	IW	inspiratory wheeze
	embryo transfer	IWD	individual with a disability
IVFT	intravenous fetal transfusion	IWI	inferior wall infarction
IVGG	intravenous gamma globulin	IWL	insensible water loss
IVGTT	intravenous glucose tolerance test		involuntary weight loss
IVH	intravenous hyperalimentation	IWMI	inferior wall myocardial infarct
	intraventricular hemorrhage	IWML	idiopathic white matter lesion
IVID	intravenous iron dextran (INFeD;	IWT	ice-water test
	DexFerrum)		impacted wisdom teeth
IVIG	intravenous immunoglobulin	Ixa	ixabepilone
IVJC	intervertebral joint complex		
IVL	intravascular lymphomatosis		
	intravenous lock		
IVLBW	infant of very low birth weight (less		
	than 1,500 g)		
IVMP	intravenously administered		

I

J

J   Jaeger measure of near vision with
20/20 about equal to J1
    jejunostomy
    Jewish
    joint
    joule
    juice

J 1-16   Jaeger near acuity notation (1 to 16
scale)

JA   joint aspiration

Jack   jackknife position

JAFAR   Juvenile Arthritis Functional
Assessment Report

JAMA   *Journal of the American Medical
Association*

JAMG   juvenile autoimmune myasthenia
gravis

JAN   Japanese Accepted Name

JAR   junior assistant resident

JARAN   junior assistant resident admission
note

JBE   Japanese B encephalitis

JBS   Johanson Blizzard syndrome

JC   junior clinicians (medical students)

JCA   juvenile chronic arthritis

JCAHO   Joint Commission on Accreditation
of Healthcare Organizations

JCC   Jackson cross cylinder (astigmatism
test)

JCO   Journal of Clinical Oncology

JCOG   Japanese Clinical Oncology Group

JCQ   Job Content Questionnaire

JD   Doctor of Jurisprudence (a law
degree)
    jaundice

JDG   jugulodigastric

JDM   juvenile diabetes mellitus

JDMS   juvenile dermatomyositis

JE   Japanese encephalitis

JEB   junctional escape beat

JEJ   jejunum

JEN   Japanese encephalitis vaccine

JER   junctional escape rhythm

JET   jejunal extension tube
    junctional ectopic tachycardia

JEV   Japanese encephalitis virus

JF   joint fluid

JFS   Jewish Family Service

JGCT   juvenile granulosa cell tumor

JGI   jejunogastric intussusception

JHR   Jarisch-Herxheimer reaction

JI   jejunoileal

JIA   juvenile idiopathic arthritis

JIB   jejunoileal bypass

JIS   juvenile idiopathic scoliosis

JJ   jaw jerk

J & J   Johnson & Johnson Health Care
Systems, Inc.

JLO   Judgment of Line Orientation (test)

JLP   juvenile laryngeal papillomatosis

JM-9   iproplatin

JME   juvenile myoclonic epilepsy

JMS   junior medical student

JNA   juvenile nasopharyngeal
angiofibroma

JNB   jaundice of newborn

JNCL   juvenile-onset neuronal ceroid
lipofuscinosis

JND   just noticeable difference

JNT   joint

JNVD   jugular neck vein distention

JODM   juvenile-onset diabetes
mellitus

JOF   juvenile ossifying fibroma

JOMAC   judgment, orientation, memory,
abstraction, and calculation

JOMACI   judgment, orientation, memory,
abstraction, and calculation intact

JOR   jaw-opening reflex

JORRP   juvenile-onset recurrent respiratory
papillomatosis

JP   Jackson-Pratt (drain)
    Jobst pump
    joint protection

JPB   junctional premature beats

JP BS   Jackson-Pratt to bulb suction

JPC   junctional premature contraction

JPOF   juvenile psammomatoid ossifying
fibroma

JPS   joint position sense

JPT   Japanese from Tokyo (populations
included in HapMap - see
HapMap)

JR   junctional rhythm

JRA   juvenile rheumatoid arthritis

JRAN   junior resident admission note

Jr BF   junior baby food

JRC   joint replacement center

JSF   Japanese spotted fever

JSRV   jaagziekte sheep retrovirus

JSW   joint space width

JT   jejunostomy tube
    joint
    junctional tachycardia

JTF   jejunostomy tube feeding

JTH   Jebsen Test of Hand (Function)

JTJ   jaw-to-jaw (position)

JTP   joint projection

JTPS   juvenile tropical pancreatitis
syndrome

J-Tube   jejunostomy tube

JUV   juvenile

J

JV	jugular vein
JVC	jugular venous catheter
JVD	jugular venous distention
JVI	jugular-valve incompetencce
JVP	jugular venous pressure
	jugular venous pulsation
	jugular venous pulse
JVPT	jugular venous pulse tracing
JW	Jehovah's Witness
Jx	joint
JXG	juvenile xanthogranuloma

K

K	cornea
	kelvin
	ketamine (Ketalar, Vitamin K, Special K, and Super K)
	kilodalton
	Kosher
	potassium
	thousand
	vitamin K
K′	knee
K$^+$	potassium
K$_1$	phytonadione (AquaMETHYTON)
K$_2$	menatetrenone
K$_3$	menadione
K$_4$	menadiol sodium diphosphate
17K	17-ketosteroids
510(k)	Medical Device Premarket Notification
KA	kainic acid
	kala-azar
	keratoacanthoma
	ketoacidosis
Ka	first order absorption constant in hr.$^{-1}$
KAB	knowledge, attitude, and behavior
K-ABC	Kaufman Assessment Battery for Children
KABINS	knowledge, attitude, behavior, and improvement in nutritional status
KACT	kaolin-activated clotting time
KAFO	knee-ankle-foot orthosis
KAO	knee-ankle orthosis
KAS	Katz Adjustment Scale
KASH	knowledge, abilities, skills, and habits
kat	katal
K-A units	King-Armstrong units
KB	ketone bodies
	knee-bearing
Kb	kilobase (genetics; 1,000 base pairs)
KBD	Kashin-Beck disease
KC	kangaroo care
	keratoconjunctivitis
	keratoconus
	knees-to-chest
	Korean conflict
kcal	kilocalorie
KCCT	kaolin cephalin clotting time
KChIPs	potassium channel-interacting proteins
kCi	kilocurie
KCl	potassium chloride
KCS	keratoconjunctivitis sicca
KCZ	ketoconazole (Nizoral)

J

KD	Kawasaki disease	KK	knee kick
	Keto Diastix®		knock-knee
	ketogenic diet	KKS	kallikrein-kinin system
	kidney donors	K & L	Kellgren and Lawrence (scale for
	knee disarticulation		osteoarthritis assessment)
	knowledge deficit	KLB	klebsiella vaccine
kd	kilodalton	KL-BET	Kleihauer-Betke
KDA	known drug allergies	Kleb	*Klebsiella*
kDa	kilodalton	KLH	keyhole limpet hemocyanin
KDC®	brand name of infant warmer	K-Lor®	potassium chloride tablets
KDQ	Kidney Disease Questionnaire	KLS	kidneys, liver, and spleen
KDU	Kidney Dialysis Unit		Kleine-Levin syndrome
KE	first order elimination rate constant	KM	kanamycin
	in hr.$^{-1}$	KMC	kangaroo-mother care
KED	Kendrick extrication device	KMnO$_4$	potassium permanganate
k$_{el}$	elimination rate constant	KMO	Kaiser-Meyer-Olkin (measure of
KET	ketamine (Ketalar)		statistical sampling adequacy)
	ketoconazole (Nizoral)	KMV	killed measles vaccine
	ketones	KN	knee
KETO	ketoconazole (Nizoral)	KNO	keep needle open
17 Keto	17 ketosteroids	KNSA	Kron Nutritive Sucking Apparatus
keV	kilo-electron volts	KO	keep open
KEVD	Krupin eye valve with disc		knee orthosis
KF	kidney function		knocked out
KFA	kinetic fibrinogen assay	KOH	potassium hydroxide
KFAB	kidney-fixing antibodies	KOL	key opinion leader
KFAO	knee-foot-ankle orthosis	KOR	keep open rate
KFD	Kyasanur Forrest disease	KP	hot pack
KFE	knee flexion and extension		keratoprecipitate
KFR	Kayser-Fleischer ring		kinetic perimetry
KFS	Klippel-Feil syndrome	kPa	kilopascal
kg	kilogram (1 kg = 2.2 pounds)	KPD	kidney paired donation
K-G	Kimray-Greenfield (filter)	KPE	Kelman phacoemulsification
KGD	ketogenic diet	KPM	kilopounds per minute
KGF	keratinocyte growth factor	KPS	Karnofsky performance status
KGC	Keflin, gentamicin, and carbenicillin		(scores) (scale)
17-KGS	17-ketogenic steroids	KQI	key quality indicators
KGy	kiloGray	Kr	krypton
K24H	potassium, urine 24-hour	K-rod	Küntscher rod
KHF	Korean hemorrhagic fever	KS	Kawasaki syndrome
KHQ	King's Health Questionnaire		Kaposi sarcoma
kHz	kilohertz		kidney stone
KI	karyopyknotic index		Klinefelter syndrome
	knee immobilizer	17-KS	17-ketogenic steroids
	potassium iodide		17-ketosteroids
KID	keratitis, ichthyosis, and deafness	KSA	knowledge, skills, and abilities
	(syndrome)	K-SADS	Kiddie Schedule for Affective
	kidney		Disorders and Schizophrenia
kilo	kilogram	KSE	knee sling exercises
	thousand	KSHV	Kaposi sarcoma-associated
KIN	kinetic		herpesvirus
KISS	saturated solution of potassium	KS/OI	Kaposi sarcoma and opportunistic
	iodide		infections
KIT	Kahn Intelligence Test	KSP	Karolinska Scales of Personality
KIU	kallikrein inhibitor units	KSR	potassium chloride sustained release
KJ	kilojoule		(tablets)
	knee jerk	KSS	Kearns-Sayre syndrome
KJR	knee-jerk reflex	KSW	knife stab wound

K

KT	kidney transplant
	kinesiotherapy
	known to
KTC	knee-to-chest
KTP	potassium-titanyl-phosphate (laser)
KTS	Klippel-Trenaunay syndrome
KTU	kidney transplant unit
	known to us
KTx	kidney transplantation
KTZ	ketoconazole (Nizoral)
KUB	kidney(s), ureter(s), and bladder
	kidney ultrasound biopsy
KUS	kidney(s), ureter(s), and spleen
KV	kilovolt
KVO	keep vein open
KVP	kilovolt peak
KW	Keith-Wagener (ophthalmoscopic finding, graded I-IV)
	Kimmelstiel-Wilson
KWB	Keith, Wagener, Barker
KWIC	keywork in context
K-wire	Kirschner wire

L

L	fifty
	Laribacter
	left (this is a dangerous abbreviation; spell out "left" to avoid surgical errors)
	lente insulin (this is a dangerous abbreviation, since there is also a Lantus insulin available)
	levorotatory
	lingual
	Listeria
	liter (1 L = 1,000 mL = 1 quart plus about 2 ounces)
	liver
	lumbar
	lung
l	levorotatory
L′	lumbar
Ⓛ	left (this is a dangerous abbreviation; spell out "left" to avoid surgical errors)
$L_1...L_5$	lumbar nerve 1 through 5
	lumbar vertebra 1 through 5
L1-2	lumbar spine, between first and second vertebrae (the disk space)
LA	language age
	laryngeal amyloid
	latex agglutination
	Latin American
	left arm
	left atrial
	left atrium
	leukoaraiosis (a radiologic finding)
	light adaptation
	linguoaxial
	linoleic acid
	lives alone
	local anesthesia
	long acting
	lupus anticoagulant
L + A	light and accommodation
	living and active
LAA	large artery atherosclerosis
	left atrium and its appendage
LAAM	levomethadyl acetate (L-alpha acetylmeth-adol, Orlaam)
LAAs	leukemia-associated antigens
LAB	laboratory
	left abdomen (LAb)
LABA	laser-assisted balloon angioplasty
	long-acting beta-2 agonist
LABBB	left anterior bundle branch block
LABC	locally advanced breast cancer

K

LABD	linear immunoglobulin A bullous dermatosis
LABR	laparoscopic-assisted bowel resection
LAC	laceration
	lactobacillus acidophilus vaccine
	laparoscopic-assisted colectomy
	left antecubital
	left atrial catheter
	locally advanced cancer
	long arm cast
	lupus anticoagulant
LAc	Licensed Acupuncturist
LACC	locally advanced cervical carcinoma
LACI	lacunar circulation infarct
	lipoprotein-associated coagulation inhibitor
LACS	laser-assisted capsular shrinkage
LACT-ART	lactate arterial
LAD	laser anesthesia device
	left anterior descending
	left atrial dimension
	left axis deviation
	leukocyte adhesion deficiency
	ligament augmentation device
LADA	left anterior descending (coronary) artery
LADCA	left anterior descending coronary artery
LADD	left anterior descending diagonal
LAD-MIN	left axis deviation minimal
LADPG	laparoscopically assisted distal partial gastrectomy
LAE	left atrial enlargement
	long above elbow
LAEC	locally advanced esophageal cancer
LAF	laminar air flow
	Latin-American female
	low animal fat
	lymphocyte-activating factor
LAFB	left anterior fascicular block
LAFF	lateral arm free flap
LAFM	locally acquired *Plasmodium falciparum* malaria
LAFR	laminar airflow room
LAG	lymphangiogram
LAGB	laparoscopic-adjustable gastric banding
LAH	left anterior hemiblock
	left atrial hypertrophy
LAHB	left anterior hemiblock
LAI	left atrial isomerism
LAIT	latex agglutination inhibition test
LAIV	live, attenuated influenza vaccine
LAK	lymphokine-activated killer
LAL	left axillary line
	limulus amebocyte lysate
LALLS	low-angle laser light scattering

LALT	larynx-associated lymphoid tissue
	low-air loss therapy (mattress)
LAM	lactational anovulatory method (birth control)
	laminectomy
	laminogram
	laparoscopic-assisted myomectomy
	laser-assisted myringotomy
	Latin-American male
	lymphangioleiomyomatosis
lam✓	laminectomy check
LAMA	laser-assisted microanastomosis
LAMB	mucocutaneous lentigines, atrial myxoma, and blue nevus (syndrome)
L-AMB	liposomal amphotericin B
LAMMA	laser microprobe mass analysis
LAN	lymphadenopathy
LANC	long arm navicular cast
LA-NSCLC	locally-advanced nonsmall-cell lung cancer
LAO	left anterior oblique
LAP	laparoscopy
	laparotomy
	left abdominal pain
	left atrial pressure
	leucine amino peptidase
	leukocyte alkaline phosphatase
	lower abdominal pain
LAPA	locally-advanced pancreatic adenocarcinoma
lap-appy	laparoscopic appendectomy
LAPC	locally advanced pancreatic cancer
	locally-advanced prostate cancer
lap chole	laparoscopic cholecystectomy
LAPMS	long arm posterior molded splint
LAPW	left atrial posterior wall
LAQ	long arc quad
LAR	laryngeal adductor reflex
	left arm, reclining
	long-acting release
	low anterior resection
LARC	Locally-advanced rectal cancer
LARM	left arm
LARS	laparoscopic antireflux surgery
LARSI	lumbar anterior-root stimulator implants
LAS	lactic acidosis syndrome
	laxative abuse syndrome
	left arm, sitting
	leucine acetylsalicylate
	long arm splint
	low-amplitude signal
	lymphadenopathy syndrome
	lymphangioscintigraphy
	lysine acetylsalicylate

L

LASA	Linear Analogue Self-Assessment (scales)	LBBB	left bundle branch block
	lipid-associated sialic acid	LBBx	left breast biopsy
LASCC	locally advanced squamous cell carcinoma	LBC	liquid-based cytology
		LBCD	left border of cardiac dullness
LASEC	left atrial spontaneous echo contrast	L/B/Cr	electrolytes, blood urea nitrogen, and serum creatinine (see page 298)
LASER	light amplification by stimulated emission of radiation	LBD	large bile duct
LASGB	laparoscopic-adjustable silicone gastric banding		left border dullness
			left brain-damaged
LASIK	laser *in situ* keratomileusis		Lewy body dementia
L-ASP	asparaginase (Elspar)		ligand-binding domain
LAST	left anterior small thoracotomy		low back disability
LASW	Licensed Advanced Social Worker		low bone density
LAT	lateral	LBE	long below elbow
	latex agglutination test	LBG	Landry-Guillain-Barré (syndrome)
	left anterior thigh	LBH	length, breadth, and height
	lidocaine, epinephrine, (Adrenalin) and tetracaine	LBI	Lewy body-like inclusions
			low back injury
LATCH	literature attached to chart	LBM	last bowel movement
lat.men.	lateral meniscectomy		lean body mass
LATS	long-acting thyroid stimulator		loose bowel movement
LAUP	laser-assisted uvula-palatoplasty	LBMI	last body mass index
LAV	left atrial volume	LBNA	lysis bladder neck adhesions
	live attenuated flavivirus	LBNP	lower-body negative pressure
	lymphadenopathy associated virus	LBO	large bowel obstruction
LAVA	laser-assisted vasal anastomosis	LBOTC	laryngeal and base-of-tongue carcinomas
LAVH	laparoscopically assisted vaginal hysterectomy	LBP	low back pain
			low blood pressure
LAVHLSO	laparoscopically assisted vaginal hysterectomy, left salpingo-oophorectomy	LBQC	large base quad cane
		LBRF	louse-borne relapsing fever
LAVHRSO	laparoscopically assisted vaginal hysterectomy, right salpingo-oophorectomy	LBS	low back syndrome
			pounds
		LBT	low back tenderness
LAVM	laparoscopic-assisted vaginal myomectomy		low back trouble
		LBV	left brachial vein
LAW	left atrial wall		Lewy body variant
LAWER	life-terminating acts without the explicit request		low biological value
		LBVO	left brachial vein occlusion
LAX	laxative	LBW	lean body weight
LB	large bowel		low birth weight (less than 2,500 g)
	lateral bend	LBWI	low birth weight infant
	left breast	LC	Laënnec cirrhosis
	left buttock		laparoscopic cholecystectomy
	live births		lethal concentration
	low back		left circumflex
	lung biopsy		leisure counseling
	lymphoid body		level of consciousness
lb	pound (1 lb = 0.454 Kg)		levocarnitine (Carnitor)
L&B	left and below		living children
LB3	colonoscope		low calorie
4LB	four-layer bandages		lung cancer
LBA	laser balloon angioplasty	L & C	lids and conjunctivae
	lower-body adiposity	3LC	triple-lumen catheter
	lymphocyte blastogenesis assay	LC50	median lethal concentration
LBB	left breast biopsy	LCA	Leber congenital amaurosis
	long-back board		left circumflex artery
			left coronary artery

L

	leukocyte common antigen		late cortical response
	life cycle assessment		late cutaneous reaction
	light contact assist		ligase chain reaction
LCAD	long-chain acyl-coenzyme A		locus control region
	dehydrogenase	LCRS	Living Conditions Rating Scale
LCAH	life-care at home	LCS	Leydig cell stimulation
LCAL	large-cell anaplastic lymphoma		lids, conjunctiva, and sclera
LCAR	L-carnitine		low constant suction
LCAT	lecithin cholesterol acyltransferase		low continuous suction
LCB	left costal border		Lung Cancer Subscale
LCCA	left circumflex coronary artery	LCSG	left cardiac sympathetic
	left common carotid artery		ganglionectomy
	leukocytoclastic angiitis		lost child support group
LCCE	Lamaze-Certified Childbirth	LCSS	Lung Cancer Symptom Score
	Educator	LCSW	Licensed Clinical Social Worker
LCCS	low cervical cesarean section		low continuous wall suction
LCD	coal tar solution (*liquor carbonis*	LCT	long-chain triglyceride
	detergens)		low cervical transverse
	localized collagen dystrophy		lymphocytotoxicity
	low-calcium diet	LCTA	lungs clear to auscultation
LCDC	Laboratory Centre for Disease	LCTCS	low cervical transverse cesarean
	Control (Canada)		section
LCDCP	low-contact dynamic compression	LCTD	low-calcium test diet
	plate	LCV	leucovorin
LCDE	laparoscopic common duct		leukocytoclastic vasculitis
	exploration		low cervical vertical
LCE	laparoscopic cholecystectomy	LCX	left circumflex coronary artery
	left carotid endarterectomy	LD	lactic dehydrogenase (formerly
	leukocyte esterase		LDH)
LCF	late clinical failure		laser Doppler
	left circumflex		last dose
LCFA	long-chain fatty acid		latissimus dorsi
LCFM	left circumflex marginal		learning disability
LCGU	local cerebral glucose utilization		learning disorder
LCH	Langerhans cell histiocytosis		left deltoid
	local city hospital		Legionnaires disease
LCINS	lung cancer in never-smokers		lethal dose
LCIS	lobular cancer *in situ*		levodopa
LCL	lateral collateral ligament		Licensed Dietician
	localized cutaneous leishmaniasis		liver disease
LCLC	large-cell lung carcinoma		living donor
LCM	laser-capture microdissection		loading dose
	left costal margin		long dwell
	lower costal margin		low density
	lymphocytic choriomeningitis		low dosage
LCMI	left ventricular mass index		Lyme disease
LC-MS-	liquid chromatography	L&D	labor and deliver
MS	coupled to tandem mass	L/D	labor and delivery
	spectrometry		light to dark (ratio)
LCN	lidocaine	LD-1	lactic dehydrogenase 1
LCNB	large-core needle biopsy	LD-5	lactic dehydrogenase 5
LCNEC	large-cell neuroendocrine carcinoma	LD$_{50}$	median lethal dose
LCO	low cardiac output	LDA	laser-Doppler anemometry
LCP	long, closed, posterior (cervix)		low density areas
LCPD	Legg-Calvé-Perthes disease		low-dose arm
LCPUFAs	long-chain polyunsaturated fatty	LDB	Legionnaires disease bacterium
	acids	LDCOC	low-dose combination oral
LCR	cerebrospinal fluid (French)		contraceptive

LD-CT	low-dose (spiral) computed tomography
LDD	laser disk decompression
	Lee and Desu D (test)
	light-dark discrimination
	lumbar disk disease
LDDS	local dentist
LDEA	left deviation of electrical axis
LDEI	large-dose extended-interval (dosing)
LDF	laser-Doppler flowmetry
LDH	lactic dehydrogenase
LDIH	left direct inguinal hernia
LDIR	low-dose of ionizing radiation
LDI-TOF-MS	laser desorption/ionization time-of-flight-mass spectrometer
LDK	low-dose ketoconazole
LDL	limitation of daily life
	low-density lipoprotein
LDL-C	low-density lipoprotein cholesterol
LDLT	living donor liver transplantation
LDM	lorazepam, dexamethasone, and metoclopramide
	low-dose metronomic (chemotherapy)
LDMRT	low-dose mediastinal radiation therapy
LDN	laparoscopic donor nephrectomy
	living-donor nephrectomy
LDNF	lung-derived neurotrophic factor
LDO	Licensed Dispensing Optician
l-dopa	levodopa
LDP	laparoscopic distal pancreatectomy
LD-PCR	limiting dilution polymerase chain reaction
LDPM	laser Doppler perfusion monitoring
LDR	labor, delivery, and recovery
	length-to-diameter ratio
	long-duration response
LDR/P	labor, delivery, recovery, and postpartum
LDS	Language Development Survey
LDT	left dorsotransverse
LD-T	lactic dehydrogenase total
LDUB	long double upright brace
LDUH	low-dose unfractionated heparin
LDV	laser-Doppler velocimetry
LE	labor epidural
	lateral epicondylitis (tennis elbow)
	left ear
	left eye
	lens extraction
	leptin
	live embryo
	local excision
	lower extremities
	lupus erythematosus
LEA	lower extremity amputation
	lumbar epidural anesthesia
LEAD	lower extremity arterial disease

LEAP	Lower Extremity Amputation Prevention (program)
LEB	lumbar epidural block
LEC	lens epithelial cell
	low-emetogenic chemotherapy
LECBD	laparoscopic exploration of the common bile duct
LE-CEMRA	lower extremity contrast-enhanced magnetic resonance angiography
LED	liposomal encapsulated doxorubicin (Doxil)
	lowest effective dose
	lupus erythematosus disseminatus
LEE	lower extremity edema
LEEP	loop electrosurgical excision procedure
LEF	lower extremity fracture
LEH	liposome-encapsulated hemoglobin
LEHPZ	lower esophageal high pressure zone
LEJ	ligation of the esophagogastric junction
LEL	low-energy laser
LEM	lateral eye movements
	light electron microscope
LEMS	Lambert-Eaton myasthenic syndrome
LENT-SOMA	Late Effect of Normal Tissue—Subjective Objective Management Analytic (toxicity table)
LEP	leptospirosis
	limited English proficiency
	liposome-encapsulated paclitaxel
	lower esophageal pressure
LEP 2	leptospirosis 2
LE prep	lupus erythematosus preparation
L-ERX	leukoerythroblastic reaction
LES	local excitatory state
	lower esophageal sphincter
	lumbar epidural steroids
	lupus erythematosus systemic
LESEP	lower extremity somatosensory evoked potential
LESG	Late Effects Study Group
LESI	lumbar epidural steroid injection
LESP	lower esophageal sphincter pressure
LET	lateral elbow tendinopathy
	left esotropia
	leukocyte esterase test
	lidocaine, epinephrine and tetracaine gel
	linear energy transfer
LEU	leucine
LEV	levamisole (Ergamisol)
	levator muscle
LEVA	levamisole (Ergamisol)
LeY	Lewis Y (antigen)
LF	laparoscopic fundoplications

	Lassa fever	LGL	large granular lymphocyte
	left foot		low-grade lymphoma(s)
	left frontal		Lown-Ganong-Levine (syndrome)
	living female	LGLS	Lown-Ganong-Levine syndrome
	low fat	LGM	left gluteus medius (maximus)
	low forceps	LGN	lateral geniculate leaflet
	low frequency		lobular glomerulonephritis
	lymphatic filariasis	LGNET	low grade neuroendocrine carcinoma
LFA	left femoral artery	LG-NHL	low-grade non-Hodgkin lymphoma
	left forearm	LGS	Lennox-Gastaut syndrome
	left fronto-anterior		low-Gomco suction
	leukocyte function-associated antigen	LGSIL	low-grade squamous intraepithelial
	low-friction arthroplasty		lesion
	lymphocyte function-associated	LGV	lymphogranuloma venerum
	antigen	LH	learning handicap
LFA-1	leukocyte function-associated		left hand
	antigen-1		left hemisphere
LFB	low-frequency band		left hyperphoria
LFC	living female child		luteinizing hormone
	low-fat and cholesterol		lymphoid hyperplasia
LFCS	low-flap cesarean section	LHA	left hepatic artery
LFD	lactose-free diet	LHC	left heart catheterization
	low-fat diet	LHD	left-hand dominant
	low-fiber diet	LHF	left heart failure
	low-forceps delivery	LHG	left hand grip
	lunate fossa depression	LHH	left homonymous hemianopsia
LFGNR	lactose fermenting gram-negative rod	LHI	Labor Health Institute
LFI	local-field irradiation	LHL	left hemisphere lesions
LFL	left frontolateral		left hepatic lobe
LFM	lateral force microscopy	LHON	Leber hereditary optic neuropathy
LFP	left frontoposterior	LHP	left hemiparesis
LFS	leukemia-free survival	LHR	legal health record
	Li-Fraumeni syndrome		leukocyte histamine release
	liver function series	LHRH	luteinizing hormone-releasing
LFT	latex flocculation test		hormone
	left fronto-transverse	LHRH-A	luteinizing hormone-releasing
	liver function tests		hormone analogue
	low-flap transverse	LHRT	leukocyte histamine release test
LFU	limit flocculation unit	LHS	left hand side
	lost to follow-up		long-handled sponge
LG	large	LHSH	long-handled shoe horn
	laryngectomy	LHT	left hypertropia
	left gluteal	LI	lactose intolerance
	linguogingival		lamellar ichthyosis
	lymphography		large intestine
L-G	Lich-Gregoire		laser iridotomy
	(ureteroneocystostomy)		learning impaired
LGA	large for gestational age		linguoincisal
	left gastric artery		liver involvement
	localized granuloma annulare	Li	lithium
LGBP/LC	laparoscopic gastric bypass with	LIA	laser interference acuity
	simultaneous cholecystectomy		left iliac artery
LGBT	lesbian, gay, bisexual, and transsexual	LIB	left in bottle
LGG	low-grade gliomas		local in breast
L-GG	*Lactobacillus rhamnosus* strain GG	LIC	left iliac crest
LGI	lower gastrointestinal (series)		left internal carotid
LGIOS	low-grade intraosseous-type		leisure interest class
	osteosarcoma	LICA	left internal carotid artery

L

LICD	lower intestinal Crohn disease	LITA	left internal thoracic artery
LICM	left intercostal margin	LITH	lithotomy
Li₂CO₃	lithium carbonate	LITHO	lithotripsy
LICS	left intercostal space	LITT	laser-induced thermotherapy
LID	levodopa-induced dyskinesia	LIV	left innominate vein
Lido	lidocaine	L-IVP	limited intravenous pyelogram
LIF	laser-induced fluorescence	LIVB	live birth
	left iliac fossa	LIVC	left inferior vena cava
	left index finger	LIVPRO	liver profile (see page 298)
	leukemia-inhibiting factor	LIWS	low intermittent wall suction
	liver (migration) inhibitory factor	LJ	left jugular
LIFE	laser-induced fluorescence emission		lockable joints
	lung imaging fluorescence	LJL	lateral joint line
	endoscopy	LJM	limited joint mobility
LIG	ligament	LK	lamellar keratoplasty
	lymphocyte immune globulin		left kidney
LIGHTS	phototherapy lights	LKA	Lazare-Klerman-Armour (Personality
LIH	laparoscopic inguinal herniorrhaphy		Inventory)
	left inguinal hernia	LKM-3	liver-kidney microsomal antibodies
LIHA	low impulsiveness, high anxiety		type 3
LIJ	left internal jugular	LKS	Landau-Kleffner syndrome
LILA	low impulsiveness, low anxiety		liver, kidneys, spleen
LILT	low-intensity laser therapy	LKSB	liver, kidneys, spleen, and bladder
LIM	limited toxicology screening	LKSNP	liver, kidneys, and spleen not
LIMA	left internal mammary artery (graft)		palpable
LIMS	laboratory information management	LL	large lymphocyte
	system(s)		left lateral
LIN	liquid nitrogen		left leg
LINAC	linear accelerator		left lower
LINCL	late-infantile neuronal ceroid		left lung
	lipofuscinosis		lepromatous leprosy
LINDI	lithium-induced nephrogenic		lid lag
	diabetes insipidus		long leg (brace or cast)
LING	lingual		lower lid
LIO	laser-indirect ophthalmoscope		lower limb
	left inferior oblique (muscle)		lower lip
LIOU	laparoscopic intraoperative		lower lobe
	ultrasound		lumbar laminectomy
LIP	lithium-induced polydipsia		lumbar length
	lymphocytic interstitial pneumonia		lymphocytic leukemia
LIPV	left inferior pulmonary vein		lymphoblastic lymphoma
LIQ	liquid	L&L	lids and lashes
	liquor	LL2	limb lead two
	lower inner quadrant	LLA	lids, lashes, and adnexa
LIR	left iliac region		limulus lysate assay
	left inferior rectus	LLAs	lipid-lowering agents
LIR-1	leucocyte immunoglobulin-like	LLAT	left lateral
	receptor-1	LLB	last living breath
LIS	late-onset idiopathic scoliosis		left lateral bending
	lateral internal sphincterotomy		left lateral border
	left intercostal space		long leg brace
	locked-in syndrome	LLC	laparoscopic laser cholecystectomy
	low intermittent suction		Lewis lung carcinoma
	lung injury score		limited liability corporation
LISS	low ionic strength saline		long leg cast
LISW	Licensed Independent Social Worker	LLBCD	left lower border of cardiac dullness
LIT	literature	LLCH	localized Langerhans' cell
	liver injury test		histiocytosis

L

LLD	late-life depressions	LME	left mediolateral episiotomy
	left lateral decubitus	LMEE	left middle ear exploration
	left length discrepancy	LMF	left middle finger
	leg length differential		melphalan (L-PAM), methotrexate,
LLE	left lower extremity		and fluorouracil
	little league elbow	LMFT	Licensed Marriage and Family
LLETZ	large-loop excision of the		Therapist
	transformation zone	LMHC	Licensed Mental Health Counselor
LLFG	long leg fiberglas (cast)	LMI	large multivalent immunogen
LLG	left lateral gaze	L/min	liters per minute
LL-GXT	low-level graded exercise test	LML	left medial lateral
LLI	leg-length inequality		left middle lobe
LLL	left lower lid	LMLE	left mediolateral episiotomy
	left lower lobe (lung)	LMM	lentigo maligna melanoma
LLLE	lower lid, left eye	LMN	letter of medical necessity
LLLNR	left lower lobe, no rales		lower motor neuron
LLLT	low-level laser therapy	LMNL	lower motor neuron lesion
LLN	lower limit of normal	LMP	last menstrual period
LLO	Legionella-like organism		left mentoposterior
LLOD	lower lid, right eye		low malignant potential
	lower limit of detection	LMP1	latent membrane protein 1
LLOS	lower lid, left eye	LMPC	laser microdissection and pressure
LLP	Limited Liability Partnership		catapulting
	long leg plaster	LMR	left medial rectus
LLPDD	late luteal phase dysphoric disorder	LMRM	left modified radical mastectomy
LLPS	low-load prolonged stress	LMRP	Local Medical Review Policy
LLQ	left lower quadrant (abdomen)	LMS	lateral medullary syndrome
LLR	left lateral rectus		leiomyosarcomas
LLRE	lower lid, right eye	LMT	left main trunk
LLS	lazy leukocyte syndrome		left mentotransverse
LLSB	left lower sternal border		Licensed Massage Therapist
LLSD	laser light scattering detector		light moving touch
LLT	left lateral thigh	LMW	low molecular weight
	lowest level term	LMWD	low molecular weight dextran
LLWC	long leg walking cast	LMWH	low molecular weight heparins
LLX	left lower extremity	LN	latent nystagmus
LM	landmarks		left nostril (nare)
	left main		lymph nodes
	light microscopy	LN₂	liquid nitrogen
	linguomesial	LNA	alpha-linolenic acid
	living male	LNB	lymph node biopsy
	lung metastases	LNC	Legal Nurse Consultant
L/M	liters per minute	LNCaP	lymph node carcinoma of the
LMA	laryngeal mask airway		prostate
	left mentoanterior	LNCC	Legal Nurse Consultant, Certified
	liver membrane autoantibody	LNCs	lymph node cells
LMAM	left message on answering	LND	light-near dissociation
	machine		lonidamine
LMB	Laurence-Moon-Biedl syndrome		lymph node dissection
	left main bronchus	LNE	lymph node enlargement
LMC	living male child		lymph node excision
LMCA	left main coronary artery	LNF	laparoscopic Nissen fundoplication
	left middle cerebral artery	LNG	levonorgestrel
LMCAT	left middle cerebral artery	LNM	lymph node metastases
	thrombosis	LNMC	lymph node mononuclear cells
LMCL	left midclavicular line	LNMP	last normal menstrual period
LMD	local medical doctor	LNNB	Luria-Nebraska Neuropsychological
	low molecular weight dextran		Battery

L

LNS	lymph node sampling		low-osmolar (contrast) media
LNT	late neurological toxicity	LOMSA	left otitis media, suppurative, acute
LNU	laparoscopic nephroureterectomy	LOMSC	left otitis media, suppurative, chronic
	learned nonuse (splint)	LoNa	low sodium
LO	lateral oblique (x-ray view)	LOO	length of operation
	linguo-occlusal	LOOCV	leave-one-out cross-validation
	lumbar orthosis	LOP	laparoscopic orchiopexy
5-LO	5-lipoxygenase		leave on pass
LOA	late-onset agammaglobulinemia		left occiput posterior
	leave of absence		level of pain
	left occiput anterior	LOQ	limit(s) of quantitation
	long-acting opioid		lower outer quadrant
	looseness of associations	LOR	loss of resistance
	lysis of adhesions	LORS-I	Level of Rehabilitation Scale-I
LOAD	late-onset Alzheimer disease	LOS	length of stay
LOAEL	lowest observed adverse effect level		loss of sight
LOB	loss of balance		lower oesophageal sphincter (United
LOC	laxative of choice		Kingdom and other countries)
	level of care		low-output syndrome
	level of comfort	lo-SES	lower socioeconomic status
	level of concern	LOT	left occiput transverse
	level of consciousness		Licensed Occupational Therapist
	local	LOV	loss of vision
	loss of consciousness	LOVA	loss of visual acuity
LOCF	last observation carried forward	LOX	lipid oxidation
	(used for inputting data missing	LOZ	lozenge
	due to dropouts in longitudinal	LP	laparoscopic pyeloplasty
	clinical trials)		Licensed Psychologist
LOCM	low-osmolality contrast media		light perception
LOD	limit of detection		linguopulpal
	line of duty		lipid panel (see page 298)
	log of odds		lipoprotein
LOE	lack of efficacy		low protein
	left otitis externa		lumbar puncture
LOEL	lowest-observed-effect level	L/P	lactate-pyruvate ratio
LOF	leaking of fluids		lidocaine and prilocaine
	leave on floor	LP5	Life-Pak 5
LOFD	low-outlet forceps delivery	LPA	left pulmonary artery
LOG	Logmar chart	Lp(a)	lipoprotein (a)
logMAR	logarithm of the minimum angle of	LPA%	left pulmonary artery oxygen
	resolution		saturation
LOH	loss of heterozygosity	L-PAM	melphalan (Alkeran)
LOHF	late-onset hepatic failure	LPC	laser photocoagulation
LOHP	oxaliplatin (Eloxatin)		Licensed Professional Counselor
LOIH	left oblique inguinal hernia	LPCC	Licensed Professional Certified
LOI	level of injury		Counselor
	Leyton Obsessional Inventory	LPC-L	lymphoplasmacytoid lymphoma
	loss of imprinting	LPcP	light perception with projection
LOINC	Logical Observation Identifier	LPD	leiomyomatosis peritonealis
	Names and Codes		disseminata
LOL	laughing out loud		low-potassium dextran
	left occipitolateral		low-protein diet
	little old lady		luteal phase defect
LOLINAD	little old lady in no apparent distress		luteal phase deficiency
LOM	left otitis media		lymphoproliferative disease
	limitation of motion	LPDA	left posterior descending artery
	little old man	LPEP	left pre-ejection period
	loss of motion	LPF	late parasitological failure

L

	liver plasma flow	LR1A	labor room 1A
	low-power field	LRA	left radial artery
	lymphocytosis-promoting factor		left renal artery
LPFB	left posterior fascicular block	LRC	locoregional control
LPH	left posterior hemiblock		lower rib cage
	lumbar puncture headache	LRCP	Licentiate of the Royal College of
LPHB	left posterior hemiblock		Physicians
LPI	laser peripheral iridectomy	LRCS	Licentiate of the Royal College of
	last patient in		Surgeons
	leukotriene pathway inhibitor	LRD	limb reduction defects
LPICA	left posterior internal carotid artery		living-related donor
LPIH	left-posterior-inferior hemiblock		living renal donor
LPL	laparoscopic pelvic	LRDT	living-related donor transplant
	lymphadenectomy	LRE	localization-related epilepsy
	left posterolateral	LREH	low-renin essential hypertension
	lipoprotein lipase	LRF	left rectus femoris
	lymphoplasmacytic lymphoma		left ring finger
LPLC	low-pressure liquid chromatography		local-regional failure
LPLND	laparoscopic pelvic lymph node	L&R gtt	Levophed and Regitine drip
	dissection		(infusion)
LPM	latent primary malignancy	LRHT	living-related hepatic transplantation
	liters per minute	LRI	lower respiratory infection
LPME	liquid-phase microextraction	LRLT	living-related liver transplantation
LPN	laparoscopic partial nephrectomy	LRM	left radical mastectomy
	Licensed Practical Nurse		local regional metastases
LPO	left posterior oblique	LRMP	last regular menstrual period
	light perception only	LRN	laparoscopic radical nephrectomy
LPPC	leukocyte-poor packed cells	LRND	left radical neck dissection
LPPH	late postpartum hemorrhage	LRO	long-range objective
LPR	laryngopharyngeal reflux	Lrot	left rotation
	leprosy (Hansen disease) vaccine	LRP	laparoscopic radical prostatectomy
LPS	last Pap smear		lung-resistance protein
	lipopolysaccharide	LRQ	lower right quadrant
LPSDT	laryngopharyngeal sensory	LROU	lateral rectus, both eyes
	discrimination testing	LRR	light reflection rheography
LP	lumboperitoneal shunt		locoregional recurrences
SHUNT		LRRT	locoregional radiotherapy
LPsP	light perception without projection	LRS	lactated Ringer solution
LPT	leptospirosis (Leptospira-Leptospires		lumbosacral radicular syndrome
	sp.) vaccine	LRT	living renal transplant
	Licensed Physical Therapist		local radiation therapy
LPTN	Licensed Psychiatric Technical		lower respiratory tract
	Nurse	LRTD	living relative transplant donor
LPV	left portal vein	LRTI	ligament reconstruction with tendon
	left pulmonary vein		interposition
	lopinavir (Kaletra)		lower respiratory tract infection
LQTS	long QT (interval) syndrome	LRV	left renal vein
LR	labor room		log reduction value
	lactated Ringer (injection)	LRW	LAL (Limulus amebocyte lysate)
	laser resection		reagent water
	lateral rectus	LRZ	lorazepam (Ativan)
	late relapse	LS	left side
	left-right		legally separated
	light reflex		Leigh syndrome
	likelihood ratios		liver scan
	local recurrence		liver-spleen
L&R	left and right		low salt
L → R	left to right		lumbosacral

	lung sounds	LSO	left salpingo-oophorectomy
L/S	lecithin-sphingomyelin ratio		left superior oblique
L&S	ligation and stripping		lumbosacral orthosis
	liver and spleen	LSP	left sacrum posterior
L5-S1	lumbar fifth vertebra to sacral first vertebra (where the lumbar and sacral spines join)		liver-specific (membrane) lipoprotein
		L–Spar	Elspar (asparaginase)
		L-spine	lumbar spine
LSA	left sacrum anterior	LSQ	Life Situation Questionnaire
	lipid-bound sialic acid	LSR	left superior rectus
	lymphosarcoma	L/S ratio	lecithin/sphingomyelin ratio
LSAs	low-sedating antihistamines	LSS	limb-sparing surgery
LSB	left scapular border		liver-spleen scan
	left sternal border		lumbar spinal stenosis
	local standby	LSSS	large, simple safety study
	lumbar spinal block		Liverpool Seizure Severity Scale
	lumbar sympathetic block	LST	left sacrum transverse
LS BPS	laparoscopic bilateral partial salpingectomy	LSTAT	life support for trauma and transport
		LSTC	laparoscopic tubal coagulation
LSC	laser-scanning cytometry	LSTL	laparoscopic tubal ligation
	last sexual contact	LSTM	lean soft tissue mass
	late systolic click	L's & T's	lines and tubes
	least significant change	LSU	life support unit
	left subclavian (artery) (vein)	LSV	left subclavian vein
	lichen simplex chronicus		lesser saphenous vein
	liquid scintillation counting	LSVC	left superior vena cava
LSCA	left scapuloanterior	LSW	left-side weakness
LSCC	laryngeal squamous cell carcinoma		Licensed Social Worker
LSCCB	limited-state small-cell cancer of the bladder	LT	laboratory technician
			left
LSCM	laser-scanning confocal microscopy		left thigh
LSCP	left scapuloposterior		left triceps
LSCS	lower segment cesarean section		leukotrienes
LSD	least significant difference		Levin tube
	low-salt diet		light
	lumbosacral derangement		light touch
	lysergide		low transverse
LSE	local side effects		lumbar traction
LSed	level of sedation		lung transplantation
LSF	low-saturated fat		lunotriquetral
LSFA	low-saturated fatty acid (diet)		lymphotoxin
LSH	laparoscopic supracervical hysterectomy	L&T	lettuce and tomato
		LT3	liothyronine sodium (Cytomel)
	leishmaniasis vaccine	LT4	levothyroxine
LSI	levonorgestrel subdermal implant	LTA	laryngotracheal applicator
L-SIL	low-grade squamous intraepithelial lesions		laryngeal tracheal anesthesia
			lateral thoracic arteries
LSK	liver, spleen, and kidneys		local tracheal anesthesia
LSKM	liver-spleen-kidney-megalgia	LTAC	long-term acute care
LSL	left sacrolateral	LTAS	left transatrial septal
	left short leg (brace)	LTB	laparoscopic tubal banding
LSLF	low sodium, low fat (diet)		laryngotracheobronchitis
LSM	laser scanning microscope	LTB$_4$	leukotriene B$_4$
	late systolic murmur	LTBI	latent tuberculosis infection
	least squares mean	LTC	left to count
	limited sampling model		long-term care
	liver, spleen masses		long thick closed
LSMFT	liposclerosing myxofibrous tumor	LTC$_4$	leukotriene C$_4$
LSMT	life-sustaining medical treatment	LTC-101	long-term care form-101

L

LTCBDE	laparoscopic transcystic common bile duct exploration	LTx	liver transplant lung transplantation
LTCCS	low-transverse cervical cesarean section	LTZ	letrozole (Femara)
		LU	left upper
LTCF	long-term care facility		left ureteral
LTCH	long-term care hospital (average length of stay greater than 25 days)		living unit Lutheran
		L & U	lower and upper
LTC-IC	long-term culture-initiating cells	LUA	left upper arm
LTCR	long-term complete remission(s)	LUD	left uterine displacement
LTCS	low-transverse cesarean section	LUE	left upper extremity
LTD	largest tumor dimension	Lues I	primary syphilis
	leg transfer device	Lues II	secondary syphilis
	line, tube, and drain (incident)	Lues III	tertiary syphilis
	lipid tear deficiency	LUFF	lateral upper arm free flap (reconstruction of pharyngeal defect)
	long-term depression		
	long-term disability		
LTD_4	leukotriene D_4	LUL	left upper lid
LTE	less than effective		left upper lobe (lung)
LTE_4	leukotriene E_4	LUM	laparoscopic-ultraminilaparotomic myomectomy
LTED	long-term estrogen deprivation		
LTF	lost to follow-up	LUNA	laparoscopic uterosacral nerve ablation
LTFU	long-term follow-up		
LTG	lamotrigine (Lamictal)	LUOB	left upper outer buttock
	long-term goal	LUOQ	left upper outer quadrant
	low-tension glaucoma	LUQ	left upper quadrant
LTGA	left transposition of great artery	LURD	living-unrelated donor
LTH	left total hip (arthroplasty)	LUS	laparoscopic ultrasonography
	luteotropic hormone		lower uterine segment
LTK	laser thermal keratoplasty	LUSB	left upper scapular border
	left total knee (arthroplasty)		left upper sternal border
LTL	laparoscopic tubal ligation	LUST	lower uterine segment transverse
	left temporal lobectomy	LUT	lower urinary tract
LTM	long-term memory	LUTD	lower urinary tract dysfunction
	long-term monitoring	LUTS	lower urinary tract symptoms
LTNPs	long-term nonprogressors (AIDS patients)	LUTT	lower urinary tract tumor
		LUW	lungworm vaccine
LTOT	long-term oxygen therapy	LUX	left upper extremity
LTP	laser trabeculoplasty	LV	leave
	long-term plan		left ventricle
	long-term potentiation		leucovorin
LTPA	leisure-time physical activity		live virus
LTR	long terminal repeats	LVA	left ventricular aneurysm
	lower trunk rotation	LVC	laser vision correction
LTRA	leukotriene receptor antagonist		low-viscosity cement
LTS	laparoscopic tubal sterilization		low-vision clinic
	long-term survivors	LVAD	left ventricular assist device
LTT	lactose tolerance test	LV Angio	left ventricular angiogram
	lymphocyte transformation test	L-VAM	leuprolide acetate, vinblastine, doxorubicin (Adriamycin), and mitomycin
LTUI	low transverse uterine incision		
LTV	long-term variability		
	long-term ventilation	LVAS	left ventricular assist system
	Luche tumor virus	LVAT	left ventricular activation time
LTV+	long-term variability– average to moderate	LVBP	left ventricle bypass pump
		LVD	left ventricular dimension
LTV 0	long-term variability–absent		left ventricular dysfunction
LTVC	long-term venous catheter	LVDd	left ventricular end-diastolic diameter
LTWN	long-term low-level white noise		

L

LVDP	left ventricular diastolic pressure	LVSWI	left ventricular stroke work index
LVDs	left ventricular systolic diameter	LVT	levetiracetam (Keppra)
LVDT	linear variable differential transformer	LVV	left ventricular volume
			live varicella vaccine
LVDV	left ventricular diastolic volume	LVW	left ventricular wall
LVE	left ventricular enlargement	LVWI	left ventricular work index
LVEDD	left ventricular end-diastolic diameter	LVWMA	left ventricular wall motion abnormality
LVEDP	left ventricular end diastolic pressure	LVWMI	left ventricular wall motion index
LVEDV	left ventricular end-diastolic volume	LVWT	left ventricular wall thickness
LVEF	left ventricular ejection fraction	LW	lacerating wound
LVEP	left ventricular end pressure		living will
LVESD	left ventricular end-systolic dimension	L & W	Lee and White (coagulation)
			living and well
LVESV	left-ventricular end-systolic volumes	LWAQ	Living with Asthma Questionnaire
LVESVI	left ventricular end-systolic volume index	LWCT	Lee-White clotting time
		LWBS	left without being seen
LVET	left ventricular ejection time	LWC	leave without consent
LVF	left ventricular failure	LWCT	left without completing treatment
	left visual field	LWOP	leave without pay
LVFP	left ventricular filling pressure	LWOT	left without treatment
LVFU	leucovorin and fluorouracil	LWP	large whirlpool
LVFWR	left ventricular free wall rupture	LX	larynx local irradiation
LVG	left ventrogluteal		lower extremity
LVH	left ventricular hypertrophy	LXC	laxative of choice
LVHR	laparoscopic ventral hernia repair	LXT	left exotropia
LVID	left ventricular internal diameter	LYCD	live-yeast cell derivative
LVIDd	left ventricle internal diameter at end-diastole	LYEL	lost-years of expected life
		LYG	lymphomatoid granulomatosis
LVIDs	left ventricle internal dimension systole	LYM	Lyme disease vaccine
			lymphocytes
LVL	large volume leukapheresis	lymphs	lymphocytes
	left vastus lateralis	LYS	large yellow soft (stools)
LVM	left ventricular mass		life-year saved (cost of)
LVMI	left ventricular mass index		lysine
LVMM	left ventricular muscle mass	lytes	electrolytes (Na, K, Cl, etc.)
LVN	Licensed Visiting Nurse		electrolyte panel (see page 298)
	Licensed Vocational Nurse	LZ	landing zone
LVO	left ventricular overactivity	LZP	lorazepam (Ativan)
LVOT	left ventricular outflow tract		
LVOTO	left ventricular outflow tract obstruction		
LVP	large volume parenteral		
	left ventricular pressure		
LVPW	left ventricular posterior wall		
LVR	leucovorin		
LVRS	lung-volume reduction surgery		
LVRT	liver-volume replaced by tumor		
LVS	laryngeal videostroboscopy		
	left ventricular strain		
LVS EMI	left ventricular subendocardial myocardial ischemia		
LVSF	left ventricular systolic function		
LVSI	lymph-vascular space invasion (involvement)		
LVSP	left ventricular systolic pressure		
LVSW	left ventricular stroke work		

L

M

M	male
	manual
	marital
	married
	masked (audiology)
	mass
	medial
	memory
	mesial
	meta
	meter (m)
	mild
	million
	minimum
	molar
	Monday
	monocytes
	mother
	mouth
	murmur
	muscle
	Mycobacterium
	Mycoplasma
	myopia
	myopic
	thousand
Ⓜ	murmur
M₁	first mitral sound
M1	left mastoid
	tropicamide 1% ophthalmic solution (Mydriacyl)
M1 to M7	categories of acute nonlymphoblastic leukemia
M₂	second mitral sound
m²	square meters (body surface)
M2	right mastoid
M-2	vincristine, carmustine, cyclophosphamide, melphalan, and prednisone
M₃	third mitral sound
M-3	medical student 3rd year
3M	mitomycin, mitoxantrone, and methotrexate
M-3+7	mitoxantrone and cytarabine
M-4	medical student 4th year
M200	volociximab
MA	machine
	Master of Arts
	mean arterial (blood pressure)
	medical assistance
	medical authorization
	megestrol acetate
	menstrual age
	mental age
	meter angle
	Mexican American
	microalbuminuria
	metabolic acidosis
	microaneurysms
	Miller-Abbott (tube)
	milliamps
	monoclonal antibodies
	motorcycle accident
M/A	mood and/or affect
MA-1	Bennett volume ventilator
MAA	macroaggregates of albumin
	Marketing Authorization Application (European Union)
MAARI	medically attended acute respiratory illness
MAAS	Motor Activity Assessment Scale
MAB	Massachusetts Biologic Laboratories
	maximum androgen blockade
Mab	monoclonal antibody
MABC	Movement Assessment Battery for Children
MABM	mandibular alveolar bone mass
MABP	mean arterial blood pressure
MAC	macrocytic erythrocytes
	macrophage
	macula
	maximal allowable concentration
	medial arterial calcification
	membrane attack complex
	Mental Adjustment to Cancer (scale)
	methotrexate, dactinomycin (Actinomycin D), and cyclophosphamide
	mid-arm circumference
	minimum alveolar concentration
	monitored anesthesia care
	multi-access catheter
	Mycobacterium avium complex
MACC	methotrexate, doxorubicin, (Adriamycin) cyclophosphamide, and lomustine (Cee Nu)
MACCC	Master Arts, Certified Clinical Competence
MACE	major adverse cardiac (cardiovascular) event(s)
	Malon antegrade continence (colonic) enema
MACOP-B	methotrexate, doxorubicin, (Adriamycin) cyclophosphamide, vincristine (Oncovin), prednisone, and bleomycin with leucovorin rescue
MACRO	macrocytes
MACS	magnetic activated cell sorting
MACs	malignancy-associated changes

M

MACTAR	McMaster-Toronto Arthritis Patient Reference (Disability Questionnaire)	MALT	mucosa-associated lymphoid tissue
		MALToma	lymphoma of mucosa-associated lymphoid tissue
MAD	major affective disorder	MAM	mammogram
	mandibular advancement device		Mexican-American male
	mind altering drugs		monitored administration of medication
	moderate atopic dermatitis		
MADD	Mothers Against Drunk Driving	MAMC	mid-arm muscle circumference
	multiple acyl-CoA dehydrogenase deficiency	Mammo	mammography
		MAMP	milliampere
MADL	mobility activities of daily living	m-AMSA	amsacrine
MADRS	Montgomery-Åsburg Depression Rating Scale	MAMTT	minimal active muscle tendon tension
MAE	medical air evacuation	MAN	malignancy associated neutropenia
	moves all extremities		massive aspiration of newborn
MAES	moves all extremities slowly	MAND	McCarron Assessment of Neuromuscular Development
MAEEW	moves all extremities equally well		
MAEW	moves all extremities well	Mand	mandibular
MAF	malignant ascites fluid	MANE	Morrow Assessment of Nausea and Emesis
	metabolic activity factor		
	Mexican-American female	MANOVA	multivariate analysis of variance
MAFAs	movement-associated fetal (heart rate) accelerations	MAO	maximum acid output
			methylaminolevulinate
MAFO	molded ankle/foot orthosis	MAO-A	monoamine oxidase type A
MAFP	maternal alpha-fetoprotein	MAO-B	monoamine oxidase type B
MAG	medication administration guideline (record)	MAOI	monoamine oxidase inhibitor
		MAOP	Mid-Atlantic Oncology Program
mag cit	magnesium citrate	MAP	magnesium, ammonium, and phosphate (Struvite stones)
MAGIC	mouth and genital ulcers with inflamed cartilage (syndrome)		
			malignant atrophic papulosis
MAGP	meatal advancement glandulophaleoplasty		mean airway pressure
			mean arterial pressure
mag sulf	magnesium sulfate		Medical Assistance Program
MAHA	macroangiopathic hemolytic anemia		megaloblastic anemia of pregnancy
MAHS	malignancy-associated hemophagocytic syndrome		Miller Assessment for Preschoolers (test for developmental delays)
MAI	maximal aggregation index		mitogen-activated protein
	Medication Appropriateness Index		mitomycin, doxorubicin (Adriamycin), and cisplatin (Platinol)
	minor acute illness		
	Mycobacterium avium-intracellulare		
MAID	mesna, doxorubicin (Adriamycin), ifosfamide, and dacarbazine		morning after pill (oral contraceptives)
			muscle-action potential
	monofocal acute inflammatory demyelinating (lesions)		*Mycobacterium avium* subspecies *paratuberculosis*
MAIR	metabolic acidosis-induced retinopathy		*MYH* (MutY homolog) - associated polyposis
MAL	malaria vaccine	MAPC	multipotent adult progenitor cell
	malignant	MA-PD	Medicare Part C prescription drug plan
	methyl aminolevulinate		
	midaxillary line	MAPI	Millon Adolescent Personality Inventory
	Motor Activity Log		
MALDI	matrix-assisted laser desorption ionization	MAPS	Make a Picture Story
		MAR	marital
MALDI-TOFMS	matrix-assisted laser desorption ionization-time-of-flight mass spectrometry		medication administration record
			melanoma-associated retinopathy
			mineral apposition rates
MALG	Minnesota antilymphoblast globulin		
malig	malignant	MARE	manual active-resistive exercise

M

MARSA	methicillin-aminoglycoside-resistant *Staphylococcus aureus*	MBC	male breast cancer
MARV	Marburg virus		maximum bladder capacity
MAS	macrophage activation syndrome		maximum breathing capacity
	McClune-Albright syndrome		metastatic breast cancer
	meconium aspiration syndrome		methotrexate, bleomycin, and cisplatin
	Memory Assessment Scale		minimal bactericidal concentration
	minimum-access surgery	MB-CK	a creatinine kinase isoenzyme
	mobile arm support	MBD	metabolic bone disease
	Modified Ashworth Scale		metastatic bone disease
MASA	mutant allele-specific amplification		methylene blue dye
MASDA^SM	Multiple-Allele-Specific Diagnostic Assay		minimal brain damage
			minimal brain dysfunction
MASER	microwave amplification (application) by stimulated emission of radiation	MBE	may be elevated
			medium below elbow
		MBF	meat-base formula
MASH	mobile Army surgical hospital		myocardial blood flow
MASHPOT	mashed potatoes	MBFC	medial brachial fascial compartment
MAST	mastectomy	MBEST	modulus blipped echo-planar single-pulse technique
	medical antishock trousers		
	Michigan Alcoholism Screening Test	MBHI	Millon Behavioral Health Inventory
	military antishock trousers	MBI	Maslach Burnout Inventory
MAT	manual arts therapy		methylene blue installation
	maternal		Modified Barthel Index
	maternity	MBL	mannose-binding lectin
	mature		menstrual blood loss
	medication administration team		metallo-bcta-lactamases
	metabolic activation therapy	MBL-D	mannan-binding lectin deficiency
	microscopic agglutination test	MBM	mind-body medicine
	Miller-Abbott tube		mother's breast milk
	Miller Analogies Test	MBNW	multiple-breath nitrogen washout
	multifocal atrial tachycardia	MBO	malignant bowel obstruction
MATHS	muscle pain, allergy, tachycardia and tiredness, and headache syndrome		mesiobuccal occulsion
		MBOT	mucinous borderline ovarian tumors
MAU	microalbuminuria		
MAVR	mitral and aortic valve replacement	MBP	malignant brachial plexopathy
max	maxillary		mannan-binding protein
	maximal		mannosc-binding protein
MAX A	maximum assistance (assist)		mechanical bowel preparation
MAXCONT	maximum contrast method		medullary bone pain
MAxL	midaxillary line		mesiobuccopulpal
MAYO	mayonnaise		myelin basic protein
MB	buccal margin	MBq	megabecquerels
	mandible	MBR	major breakpoint region
	Mallory body	MBS	modified barium swallow
	Medical Board	MBT	maternal blood type
	medulloblastoma		multiple blunt trauma
	mesiobuccal	MBTS	modified Blalock-Taussig shunt
	methylene blue	MC	male child
	myocardial bands		medium-chain (triglycerides)
M/B	mother/baby		metacarpal
MBA	Master of Business Administration		metatarso - cuneiform
	Mini Battery of Achievement		microcalcifications (breast)
M-BACOD	methotrexate (high-dose), bleomycin, doxorubicin (Adriamycin), cyclophosphamide, vincristine (Oncovin), and dexamethasone with leucovorin rescue		mini-laparotomy cholecystectomy
			mitoxantrone and cytarabine
			mitral commissurotomy
			mixed cellularity
			molluscum contagiosum

M

	monocomponent highly purified pork insulin	mcg	microgram (1,000 mcg = 1 milligram) (do not hand write μg, as it is mistakenly read as milligram [mg])
	Moraxella catarrhalis		
	mouth care		
	multicenter (study)	MCG	magnetocardiogram
	myocarditis		magnetocardiography
m + c	morphine and cocaine	MCGN	minimal-change glomerular nephritis
MC3	third metacarpal	MCH	mean corpuscular hemoglobin
MCA	Medicines Control Agency (United Kingdom)		microfibrillar collagen hemostat
			muscle contraction headache
	megestrol, cyclophosphamide, and doxorubicin (Adriamycin)	MCHC	mean corpuscular hemoglobin concentration
	metacarpal amputation	MCHL	medial head of the coracohumeral ligament
	micrometastases clonogenic assay		
	middle cerebral aneurysm	MCI	mild cognitive impairment
	middle cerebral artery	mCi	millicurie
	monoclonal antibodies	MCID	minimum clinically important difference(s)
	motorcycle accident		
	multichannel analyzer	mckat	microkatal (1 millionth [10^{-6}] of a katal)
	multiple congenital anomalies		
2-MCA	2-methyl citric acid	MCL	mantle cell lymphoma
MCAD	medium-chain acyl-CoA dehydrogenase		maximum comfort level
			medial collateral ligament
MCAF	monocyte chemoattractant and activity factor		midclavicular line
			midcostal line
MCAO	middle cerebral artery occlusion		modified chest lead
MCAP	middle cerebral artery pressure		most comfortable level
McAS	McCune-Albright syndrome	mcL	microliter (1/1,000 of an mL)
MCAT	Medical College Admission Test	MCLL	most comfortable listening level
MCB	Medicines Control Board (United Kingdom's equivalent to the United States Food and Drug Administration)	MCLNS	mucocutaneous lymph node syndrome
		MCMI	Millon Clinical Multiaxial Inventory
		mcmol	micromoles (one millionth [10^{-6}] of a mole)
	midcycle bleeding	MCN	minimal change nephropathy
	middle chamber bubbling	MCNS	minimal change nephrotic syndrome
MCBDD	National Center on Birth Defects and Developmental Disabilities	MCO	managed care organization
			mupirocin calcium ointment (Bactroban Nasal)
McB pt	McBurney point		
MCBS	Medicare Current Beneficiary Survey	MCP	mean carotid pressure
MCC	meningococcal serogroup C conjugate		metacarpophalangeal joint
			metoclopramide (Reglan)
	Merkel cell carcinoma		monocyte chemotactic protein
	microcrystalline cellulose	MCR	Medicare
	midstream clean-catch		metabolic clearance rate
MCCU	mobile coronary care unit		minor cluster region
MCD	malformation of cortical development		myocardial revascularization
		MC=R	moderately constricted and equally reactive
	mean cell diameter		
	Medicaid	MCRC	metastatic colorectal cancer
	minimal-change disease	MCS	manufacturer cannot supply
	multicystic dysplasia		mental component summary
MCDK	multicystic dysplasia of the kidney		microculture and sensitivity
MCDT	mast cell degranulation test		moderate constant suction
MCE	major coronary event		multiple chemical sensitivity
	myocardial contrast echocardiography		myocardial contractile state
		MCSA	minimal cross-sectional area
MCF	multicentric foci	M-CSF	macrophage colony-stimulating factor
MCFA	medium-chain fatty acid		

M

MC-SR	moderately constricted and slightly reactive	MDCT	multidetector-row computed tomography
MCT	manual cervical traction	MDD	major depressive disorder
	mean circulation time		manic-depressive disorder
	medial canthal tendon	MDE	major depressive episode
	medium chain triglyceride	MDF	myocardial depressant factor
	medullary carcinoma of the thyroid	MDGF	macrophage-derived growth factor
	microwave coagulation therapy	MDGs	Millennium Development Goals
MCTC	metrizamide computed tomography cisternogram	MDI	manic-depressive illness
			mental developmental index
MCTD	mixed connective tissue disease		metered-dose inhaler
MCTZ	methyclothiazide (Enduron)		methylenedioxyindenes
MCU	micturating cystourethrogram		multi-directional instability
MCV	mean corpuscular volume		multiple daily injection
MCVRI	minimal coronary vascular resistance index		multiple dosage insulin
		MDIA	Mental Development Index, Adjusted
MCYLS	marginal cost per year of life saved	MDII	multiple daily insulin injection
MD	macula degeneration	MDIS	metered-dose inhaler-spacer (device)
	maintenance dialysis	MDiv	Master of Divinity
	maintenance dose	MDM	mid-diastolic murmur
	major depression		minor determinant mix (of penicillin)
	mammary dysplasia		
	manic depression	MDMA	methylenedioxy-methamphetamine (ecstasy)
	mean deviation		
	medical doctor	MDNT	midnight
	mediodorsal	MDO	mentally disordered offender
	Menière disease	MDOT	modified directly observed therapy
	mental deficiency	MDP	methylene diphosphonate
	mesiodistal	MDPH	Michigan Department of Public Health
	microdialysis		
	movement disorder		
	multiple dose	MDPI	maximum daily permissible intake
	muscular dystrophy	MDR	Medical Device Reporting (regulation)
	myocardial damage		
MD-50®	diatrizoate sodium injection 50%		minimum daily requirement
MDA	malondialdehyde		multidrug resistance
	manual dilation of the anus	MD=R	moderately dilated and equally reactive
	mass drug administrations (diethylcarbamazine plus albendazole to stop transmission of filariasis)	MDR-1	multidrug resistance gene
		MDRD	Modification of Diet in Renal Disease
		MDRE	multiple-drug-resistant enterococci
	Medical Devises Agency (United Kingdom)	MDREF	multidrug resistant enteric fever
	methylenedioxyamphetamine	MDRO	multidrug resistant organism
	micrometastases detection assay	MDRS I/P	Mattis Dementia Rating Scale-Initiation/Perseveration subscale
	motor discriminative acuity		
	Multichannel Discrete Analyzer	MDRSP	multidrug resistant Streptococcus pneumoniae
MDAC	multiple-dose activated charcoal		
MDACC	MD Anderson Cancer Center	MDRT	multiple-drug rescue therapy
MDA LDL	malondialdehydeconjugated low-density lipoprotein	MDRTB	multidrug resistant tuberculosis
		MDS	maternal deprivation syndrome
MDASI	MD Anderson Symptom Inventory		Miller-Dieker syndrome
MDASI-BT	MD Anderson Symptom Inventory-Brain Tumor Module		Minimum Data Set
			myelodysplastic syndromes
MDC	Major Diagnostic Category	MD-SR	moderately dilated and slightly reactive
	medial dorsal cutaneous (nerve)		
MDCM	mildly dilated congestive cardiomyopathy	MDTS®	Metered Dose Transdermal Spray system

M

MDSU	medical day stay unit
MDT	maggot debridement therapy
	Mechanical Diagnostic Therapist
	motion detection threshold
	multidisciplinary team
	multidrug therapy
MDTM	multidisciplinary team meeting
MDTP	multidisciplinary treatment plan
MDU	maintenance dialysis unit
	microvascular Doppler
	ultrasonography
MDUO	myocardial disease of unknown
	origin
MDV	Marek disease virus
	multiple dose vial
MDY	month, date, and year
ME	macular edema
	manic episode
	medical events
	medical evidence
	medical examiner
	mestranol
	Methodist
	middle ear
	myalgic encephalomyelitis
M/E	metabolic/endocrine
	monitor and evaluate
	myeloid-erythroid (ratio)
M&E	Mecholyl and Eserine
	mucositis and enteritis
MEA	microwave endometrial ablation
	measles virus vaccine
MEA-I	multiple endocrine adenomatosis
	type I
MEB	Medical Evaluation Board
	methylene blue
MEC	meconium
	middle ear canal(s)
	mitoxantrone, etoposide, and
	cytarabine
	moderately emetogenic
	chemotherapy
MeCCNU	semustine
MECG	maternal electrocardiogram
MeCP	semustine (methyl CCNU)
	cyclophosphamide, and prednisone
MED	male erectile dysfunction
	maximal (maximum) economic dose
	medial
	median erythrocyte diameter
	medical
	medication
	medicine
	medium
	medulloblastoma
	minimal erythema dose
	minimum effective dose
	multiple epiphyseal dysplasia

MEd	Master of Education
MEDAC	multiple endocrine deficiency
	Addison disease (autoimmune)
	candidiasis
MEDCO	Medcosonolator
MedDRA	Medical Dictionary for Regulatory
	Activities
MEDEX	medication administration record
MED-LARS	Medical Literature
	Analysis and Retrieval System
MEDLINE	National Library of Medicine
	medical database
MED NEC	medically necessary
MedPAR	Medicare Provider Analysis Review
	File
MEDS	medications
MEE	maintenance energy expenditure
	measured energy expenditure
	middle ear effusion
MEE/OC	middle ear exploration with ossicular
	chain reconstruction
MEF	maximum expired flow rate
	middle ear fluid
MEFR	mid expiratory flow rate
MEFV	maximum expiratory flow-volume
MEG	magnetoencephalogram
	magnetoencephalography
Meg-CSF	megakaryocytic colony-stimulating
	factor
MEGX	monoethylglycinexylidide
MeHg	methylmercury
MEI	magnetic endoscope imaging
	medical economic index
MEIA	microparticle enzyme immunoassay
MEKC	micellar electrokinetic
	chromatography
MEL	maximum exposure limit
	melatonin
MELAS	mitochondrial encephalomyopathy
	with lactic acidosis, and stroke-
	like episodes (syndrome)
MEL B	melarsoprol (Arsobal)
MELD	Model for End-Stage Liver Disease
	(score)
MEM	memory
	monocular estimate method (near
	retinoscopy)
MEMB	modified eosin-methylene blue
	(agar)
MEN	medically-enhanced normality
	meningeal
	meninges
	meningitis
	meningococcal (*Neisseria*
	meningitidis) (serogroups
	unspecified) vaccine
MEN (II)	multiple endocrine neoplasia (type
	II)

M

MEN$_{cn-AC}$ meningococcal (*Neisseria meningitidis*) serogroups A, C conjugate vaccine

MEN$_{cn-B}$ meningococcal (*Neisseria meningitidis*) serogroup B conjugate vaccine

MEN$_{ps}$ meningococcal (*Neisseria meningitidis*) polysaccharide vaccine, not otherwise specified

MEN$_{ps-ACYW}$ meningococcal (*Neisseria meningitidis*) serogroups A, C, Y, W-135 polysaccharide vaccine

MEN$_{ps-B}$ meningococcal (*Neisseria meningitidis*) serogroup B polysaccharide vaccine

MENS   microcurrent electrical neuromuscular stimulation
mini-electrical nerve stimulator

MEO   malignant external otitis
Medical Examiner's Office

MeOH   methyl alcohol

MEOS   microsomal ethanol oxidizing system

MEP   maximal expiratory pressure
meperidine (Demerol)
motor-evoked potential
multimodality-evoked potential

MEPA   Medication Error Prevention Analysis (FDA)

MEPS   Medical Expenditure Panel Survey

mEq   milliequivalent

mEq/24 H   millequivalents per 24 hours

mEq/L   milliequivalents per liter

MER   medical evidence of record
methanol-extracted residue (of phenol-treated BCG)

M/E ratio   myeloid/erythroid ratio

MERRF   myoclonic epilepsy and ragged red fibers

MERS-TM   Medical Event Reporting System - Transfusion Medicine

MES   maximal electroshock
mesial

MESA   microsurgical epididymal sperm aspiration

MESCC   metastatic epidural spinal cord compression

MeSH   Medical Subject Headings of the National Library of Medicine

MESS   Mangled Extremity Severe Score

MEST   mesodermal specific transcript (gene)

MET   medical emergency team
medical emergency treatment
metabolic
metamyelocytes
metastasis
metronidazole

meT   methyltestosterone

META   metamyelocytes

METH   methamphetamine
methicillin

MetHb   methemoglobin
methemoglobinemia

methyl CCNU   semustine

methyl G   mitroguazone dihydrochloride (Zyrkamine)

methyl GAG   mitroguazone dihydrochloride (Zyrkamine)

METS   metabolic equivalents (multiples of resting oxygen uptake)
metastases

METT   maximum exercise tolerance test

MEV   million electron volts

MEWDS   multifocal evanescent white dot syndrome

MEX   Mexican

MF   Malassezia folliculitis
Malassezia furfur
masculinity/femininity
meat-free
median frequency (anesthesia-depth monitor)
mesial facial
methotrexate and fluorouracil
midcavity forceps
middle finger
midforceps
mother and father
mycosis fungoides
myelofibrosis
myocardial fibrosis

M/F   male-female ratio

M & F   male and female
mother and father

MFA   malaise, fatigue, and anorexia

MFAT   multifocal atrial tachycardia

MFB   metallic foreign body
multiple-frequency bioimpedance

MFC   medial femoral condyle

MfC   *Medicines for Children*

MFCU   Medicaid Fraud Control Unit

MFD   Memory for Designs
midforceps delivery
milk-free diet
multiple fractions per day

MFEM   maximal forced expiratory maneuver

mfERG   multifocal electroretinography

MFFT   Matching Familiar Figures Test

MFH   malignant fibrous histiocytoma

MFI   mean fluorescent intensity
Multidimensional Fatigue Inventory

M-FISH   multicolor fluorescence in situ hybridization

MFM   maternal fetal medicine
multifidus muscle

M

MFNS	mometasone furoate nasal spray (Nasonex)	MGP	Marcus Gunn pupil
			medical group practice
MFPS	myofascial pain syndrome	MGPS	Multi-item Gamma Poisson Shrinker
MFR	mid-forceps rotation	MGR	murmurs, gallops, or rubs
	myofascial release	MGS	magnetic guidance system
MFS	Marfan syndrome		malignant glandular schwannoma
	maternal-fetal surgery	$MgSO_4$	magnesium sulfate (Epsom salt) (this
	Medicare Fee Schedule		is dangerous terminology as it can
	metastases free survival		be interpreted as morphine sulfate)
	Miller-Fisher syndrome	MGT	management
	mitral first sound	*mgtt*	minidrop (60 minidrops = 1 mL)
	monofixation syndrome	MGUS	monoclonal gammopathy of
MFT	muscle function test		undetermined significance
MFU	medical follow-up	MGW	multiple gunshot wound
MFVNS	middle fossa vestibular nerve	MGW	magnesium sulfate,
	section	enema	glycerin, and water enema
MFVPT	Motor Free Visual Perception Test	M-GXT	multistage graded exercise test
MFVR	minimal forearm vascular resistance	mGy	milligray (radiation unit)
MG	Marcus Gunn	MH	macular hemorrhage
	Michaelis-Gutmann (bodies)		macular hole
	milligram (mg)		malignant hyperthermia
	myasthenia gravis		marital history
mg	milligram (1,000 mg = 1 gram)		medical history
Mg	magnesium		menstrual history
mG	milligauss		mental health
μg	microgram (1/1000 of a milligram)		moist heat
	(This is a dangerous abbreviation	MHA	Mental Health Assistant
	when hand written, as it is read as		methotrexate, hydrocortisone, and
	mg. Use mcg)		cytarabine (ara-C)
M&G	myringotomy and grommets		microangiopathic hemolytic anemia
mg%	milligrams per 100 milliliters		microhemagglutination
MGBG	mitoguazone (Zyrkamine)		migraine headache
MGCT	malignant glandular cell tumor	MHA-TP	microhemagglutination-*Treponema*
MGD	mammography-detected (breast		*pallidum*
	cancer)	MHB	maximum hospital benefits
	meibomian gland dysfunction	MHb	methemoglobin
MGd	motexafin gadolinium (Xcytrin)	MHBSS	modified Hank balanced salt solution
MGDF	megakaryocyte growth and	MHC	major histocompatibility complex
	development factor		mental health center (clinic)
mg/dl	milligrams per 100 milliliters		mental health counselor
MGF	macrophage growth factor	M/hct	microhematocrit
	mast cell growth factor	MHD	10-hydroxycarbazepine
	maternal grandfather		(oxcarbazepine metabolite)
MGG	May-Grünwald-Giemsa (stain)		maintenance hemodialysis
MGGM	maternal great grandmother		maximum heart distance (radiation
MGHL	middle glenohumeral ligament		therapy)
mg/kg	milligram per kilogram	mHg	millimeters of mercury
mg/kg/d	milligram per kilogram per day	MHH	mental health hold
mg/kg/hr	milligram per kilogram per hour	MHI	Mental Health Index (information)
MGM	maternal grandmother	MHL	maximum heart length (radiation
	milligram (mg is correct)		therapy)
MGMA	Medical Group Management		mesenchymal hamartoma of the liver
	Association	MHIP	mental health inpatient
MGN	membranous glomerulonephritis	MH/MR	mental health and mental
MGO	methylglyoxal		retardation
MgO	magnesium oxide	MHN	massive hepatic necrosis
MG/OL	molecular genetics/oncology	MHO	medical house officer
	laboratory	MHP	moist heat packs

M

MHRA	Medicines and Healthcare Products Regulatory Agency (United Kingdom)	MID	mesioincisodistal
			microvillus inclusion disease
			minimal ineffective dose
MHRI	Mental Health Research Institute		multi-infarct dementia
MHS	major histocompatibility system	MIDAS	migraine disability assessment scale
	malignant hyperthermia susceptible	MIDCAB	minimally invasive direct coronary artery bypass
	monomethyl hydrogen sulfate		
	multihospital system	MIDD	maternally inherited diabetes and deafness
MHsFHF	malarial hepatitis-simulating fulminant-hepatic failure		
		MID EPIS	midline episiotomy
MHSI	medical hyperspectral imaging	Mid I	middle insomnia
MHT	malignant hypertension	MIE	maximim inspiratory effort
	mental health team		meconium ileus equivalent (cystic fibrosis)
	Mental Health Technician		
MHTAP	microhemagglutination assay for antibody to *Treponema pallidum*		medical improvement expected
		MIEI	medication-induced esophageal injury
MHV	mechanical heart valves		
	middle hepatic vein	MIF	Merthiolate, iodine, and formalin
MHW	medial heel wedge		mifepristone (RU 486; Mifeprex)
	mental health worker		migration inhibitory factor
MHX	methohexital sodium	MIFR	midinspiratory flow rate
MHx	medical history	MIF 50% VC	midinspiratory flow at 50% of vital capacity
MHxR	medical history review		
MHz	megahertz	MIG	measles immune globulin
MI	membrane intact	MIGET	multiple inert gas elimination technique
	mental illness		
	mental institution	MIH	medication-induced headache
	mesial incisal		migraine with interparoxysmal headache
	mitral insufficiency		
	myocardial infarction		myointimal hyperplasia
MIA	medically indigent adult	MII	multichannel intraluminal impedance
	missing in action	MIL	military
MIBE	measles inclusion body encephalitis		mesial incisal lingual (surface)
MIBI	technetium Tc99m sestamibi (a myocardial perfusion agent; Cardiolite)		mother-in-law
		MIMCU	medical intermediate care unit
		MIN	mammary intraepithelial neoplasia
MIBG	iobenguane sulfate I 123 (meta-iodobenzyl guanidine I 123)		melanocytic intraepidermal neoplasia
			mineral
MIBK	methylisobutylketone		minimum
MIC	maternal and infant care		minor
	methacholine inhalation challenge		minute (min)
	medical intensive care	MIN A	minimal assistance (assist)
	microscope	MIME	mitoguazone, ifosfamide, methotrexate, and etoposide with mesna
	microcytic erythrocytes		
	minimum inhibitory concentration		
MICA	mentally ill, chemical abuser	MINE	Medical Information Network of Europe
MICAR	Mortality Medical Indexing, Classification, and Retrieval		
			mesna, ifosfamide, mitoxantrone (Novantrone), and etoposide
MICE	mesna, ifosfamide, carboplatin, and etoposide		medical improvement not expected
MICN	Mobile Intensive Care Nurse	MINI	Mini International Neuropsychiatric Interview
MICR	methacholine inhalation challenge response		
		MIO	minimum identifiable odor
MICRO	microcytes		monocular indirect ophthalmoscopy
MICROG	microgram	MIP	macrophage inflammatory protein
MICS	minimally invasive cardiac surgery		maximum inspiratory pressure
MICU	medical intensive care unit		maximum-intensity projection (radiology)
	mobile intensive care unit		

M

	mean intrathoracic pressure		mediolateral
	mean intravascular pressure		middle lobe
	medical improvement possible		midline
	metacarpointerphalangeal		mucosal leishmaniasis
	Michigan Biologic Products Institute	mL	milliliter (1,000 mL = 1 liter)
MIRD	medical internal radiation dose	M/L	monocyte to lymphocyte (ratio)
MIRP	myocardial infarction rehabilitation		mother-in-law
	program	MLA	medical laboratory assay
MIRS	Medical Improvement Review		mento-laeva anterior
	Standard	MLAC	minimum local analgesic
MIS	management information systems		concentration
	minimally invasive surgery	MLAP	mean left atrial pressure
	mitral insufficiency	MLBW	moderately low birth weight
	moderate intermittent suction	MLC	metastatic liver cancer
MISA	mentally ill and substance abusing		minimal lethal concentration
MISC	miscarriage		mixed lymphocyte culture
	miscellaneous		multilevel care
M Isch	myocardial ischemia		multilumen catheter
MISH	multiple *in situ* hybridization		myelomonocytic leukemia, chronic
MISO	misonidazole	MLD	manual lymph drainage
MISS	minimally invasive spine surgery		masking level difference
	Modified Injury Severity Score		melioidosis (*Pseudomonas*
	(Scale)		*pseudomallei*) vaccine
	Mothers in Sympathy and Support		metachromatic leukodystrophy
MIT	meconium in trachea		microlumbar diskectomy
	miracidia immobilization test		microsurgical lumbar diskectomy
	mono-iodotyrosine		minimal lethal dose
	multiple injection therapy (of		minimal luminal diameter
	insulin)	MLDA	Mutational Load Distribution
MITO-C	mitomycin (Mutamycin)		Analysis
MITOX	mitoxantrone (Novantrone)	MLDT	Manual Lymph Drainage Therapist
MIU	million international units	MLE	maximum likelihood estimation
	minor injury unit		midline (medial) episiotomy
mIU	milli-international unit (one-	MLEE	multilocus enzyme electrophoresis
	thousandth of an International	MLF	median longitudinal fasciculus
	unit)	MLN	manifest latent nystagmus
MIVA	mivacurium (Mivacron)		mediastinal lymph node
MIVE	maximum isometric voluntary		melanoma vaccine
	extension		mesenteric lymph node
MIVF	maximum isometric voluntary	MLNS	minimal lesions nephrotic syndrome
	flexion		mucocutaneous lymph node
MIW	mental inquest warrant		syndrome (Kawasaki syndrome)
mix mon	mixed monitor	MLO	mesiolinguo-occlusal
MJ	marijuana	MLP	mento-laeva posterior
	megajoule		mesiolinguopulpal
MJD	Machado-Joseph Disease		midlevel provider
MJL	medial joint line	MLPJ	mechanical loosening of prosthetic
MJS	medial joint space		joint
MJT	Mead Johnson tube	MLPN	Medical Licensed Practical Nurse
μkat	microkatal (micro-moles/sec)	MLPP	maximum loose-packed position
MKAB	may keep at bedside	MLR	middle latency response
MKB	married, keeping baby		mixed lymphocyte reaction
MK-CSF	megakaryocyte colony-stimulating		multiple logistic regression
	factor	MLRA	multiple linear-regression analysis
MKI	mitotic-karyorrhectic index	MLS	macrolides, lincosamides, and
MKM	Mehrkoordinaten Manipulator		streptogramins
	microgram per kilogram per minute		Maroteaux-Lamy syndrome
ML	malignant lymphoma		maximum likelihood score

M

	mediastinal B-cell lymphoma with sclerosis
MLST	multi-locus sequence typing
MLT	melatonin
	mento-laeva transversa
MLU	mean length of utterance
MLV	monitored live voice
MLWHF	Minnesota Living with Heart Failure (questionnaire)
MM	major medical (insurance)
	malignant melanoma
	malignant mesothelioma
	Marshall-Marchetti
	medial malleolus
	medication management
	member months
	meningococcic meningitis
	mercaptopurine and methotrexate
	methadone maintenance
	micrometastases
	millimeter (mm)
	mismatch (ing)
	mist mask
	morbidity and mortality
	motor meal
	mucous membrane
	multiple myeloma
	muscle movement
	myelomeningocele
mM.	millimole (mmol)
mm	millimeter
M&M	milk and molasses
	morbidity and mortality
MMA	methylmalonic acid
	methylmethacrylate
	middle meningeal artery
MMC	mitomycin (mitomycin C)
	myelomeningocele
MMCT	mitomycin C trabeculectomy
MMD	malignant metastatic disease
	moyamoya disease
	mucus membranes dry
	myotonic muscular dystrophy
MME	membrane metalloendopeptidase
MMECT	multiple monitor electroconvulsive therapy
MMEFR	maximal mid-expiratory flow rate
MMF	mean maximum flow
	mycophenolate mofetil (CellCept)
MMFR	maximal mid-expiratory flow rate
MMG	mammography
	mechanomyography
mm Hg	millimeters of mercury
MMI	maximal medical improvement
MMK	Marshall-Marchetti-Krantz (cystourethropexy)
MML	minimal masking level (audiology)
MMM	metastatic malignant melanoma

	mitoxantrone, methotrexate, and mitomycin
	mucous membrane moist
	myelofibrosis with myeloid metaplasia
mMMSE	modified version of the mini mental status examination
MMMT	malignant mixed mesodermal tumor
	metastatic mixed müllerian tumor
MMN	mismatch negativity
	multifocal motor neuropathy
MMOA	maxillary mandibular odontectomy alveolectomy
mmol	millimole
μmol	micromole
MMP	matrix metalloproteinase
	mitochondrial myopathy
	mucous membrane pemphigoid
	multiple medical problems
	multiplexed molecular profiling (system)
MMP-8	metalloproteinase-8
MMPI	matrix metalloproteinase inhibitor
	Minnesota Multiphasic Personality Inventory
MMPI-A	Minnesota Multiphasic Personality Inventory - Adolescent version
MMPI-D	Minnesota Multiphasic Personality Inventory-Depression Scale
6-MMPR	6-methylmercaptopurine riboside
MMPs	membership medical practices
MMR	measles, mumps, and rubella
	menometrohaggia
	midline malignant reticulosis
	mild mental retardation
	mismatch repair
MMRISK	a skin cancer mnemonic; **m**oles that are atypical, **m**oles that are many in number, **r**ed hair or freckles, **i**nability to tan, **s**unburn, **k**indred
MMRS	Metropolitan Medical Response System
MMR-VAR	measles virus, mumps virus, rubella virus, and varicella virus vaccine
MMS	Medication Management Standards
	Mini-Mental State (examination)
	Mohs micrographic surgery
MMSE	Mini-Mental State Examination
MMT	malignant mesenchymal tumors
	manual muscle test
	meal-tolerance test
	medial meniscal tear
	methadone maintenance treatment
	Mini Mental Test
	mixed müllerian tumors
MMTP	Methadone Maintenance Treatment Program

MMTV	malignant mesothelioma of the tunica vaginalis		mobilization
			mother of baby
	monomorphic ventricular tachycardia	MOB-PT	mitomycin, vincristine (Oncovin), bleomycin, and cisplatin (Platinol)
	mouse mammary tumor virus		
MMV	mandatory minute volume	MOC	medial olivocochlear
MMWR	*Morbidity and Mortality Weekly Report*		Medical Officer on Call
			metronidazole, omeprazole, and clarithromycin
MN	Master's Degree in Nursing		
	midnight		mother of child
	mononuclear	MOCI	Maudsley Obsessive-Compulsive Inventory
Mn	manganese		
M&N	morning and night	MOD	maturity onset diabetes
	Mydriacyl and Neo-Synephrine		medical officer of the day
MNC	monomicrobial necrotizing cellulitis		mesio-occlusodistal
	mononuclear leukocytes		moderate
MNCV	motor nerve conduction velocity		mode of death
MND	minor neurological dysfunction		moment of death
	modified neck dissection		multiorgan dysfunction
	motor neuron disease	MOD A	moderate assistance (assist)
MNF	myelinated nerve fibers	MODEMS	Musculoskeletal Outcomes Data Evaluation and Management Scale
MNG	multinodular goiter		
MNM	mononeuritis multiplex		
MNMCB	motor neuropathy with multifocal conduction block	MOD I	modified independent (for example, a patient who is independent, but requires a walker)
MNNB	Monas-Nitz Neuropsychological Battery		
		MODM	mature-onset diabetes mellitus
MnP2	mandibular second premolar	MODS	multiple-organ dysfunction syndrome (score)
MNPRT	mixed neutron and photon radiotherapy		
		MODY	maturity-onset diabetes of youth
MNR	marrow neutrophil reserve	MOE	movement of extremities
MNS	mean nocturnal saturation	MOEMs	micro-opto-electro-mechanical systems
MNSc	Master of Nursing Science		
MnSOD	manganese superoxide dismutase	MOF	mesial occlusal facial
Mn SSEPS	median-nerve somatosensory-evoked potentials		methotrexate, vincristine (Oncovin), and fluorouracil
			methoxyflurane (Penthrane)
MNTB	medial nucleus of the trapezoid body		multiple-organ failure
MNX	meniscectomy	MOFS	multiple-organ failure syndrome
MNZ	metronidazole (Flagyl)	MOG	myelin oligodendrocyte glycoprotein
MO	medial oblique (x-ray view)	MOH	medication overuse headache
	menhaden oil		Ministry of Health
	mesio-occlusal	MoH	Ministry of Health (Canada)
	mineral oil	Mohs	Mohs technique; serial excision and microscopic examination of skin cancers
	month (mo)		
	months old		
	morbidly obese	MOI	mechanism of injury
	mother		multiplicity of infection
	myositis ossificans	MoICU	mobile intensive care unit
Mo	molybdenum	MOID	Mammalian Orthologous Intron Database
M/O	morning of		
MOA	mechanism of action	MOJAC	mood orientation, judgement, affect, and content
	metronidazole, omeprazole, and amoxicillin		
		MOL	method of limits
MoAb	monoclonal antibody	MOM	milk of magnesia
MOAHI	mixed obstructive apnea and hypopnea index		mother
			mucoid otitis media
MOB	medical office building	MoM	multiples of the median
	mobility	MOMP	major outer membrane protein

M

MON	maximum observation nursery	MPA	main pulmonary artery
	monitor		Medical Products Agency (Sweden)
MONO	infectious mononucleosis		medroxyprogesterone acetate
	monocyte	MPa	megapascal
	monospot	MPAC	Memorial Pain Assessment Card
mono, di	monochorionic, diamniotic	MPA/E₂C	medroxyprogesterone acetate;
mono,	monochorionic,		estradiol cypionate (Lunelle)
mono	monoamniotic	MPAP	mean pulmonary artery pressure
MOP	medical outpatient	MPAQ	McGill Pain Assessment
8 MOP	methoxsalen (Oxsorlen)		Questionnaire
MOPD II	Majewski osteodysplastic primordial	MPAS	Masters of Physician Assistant
	dwarfism type II		Studies
MOPP	mechlorethamine, vincristine	MPB	male-pattern baldness
	(Oncovin), procarbazine, and		mephobarbital
	prednisone	MPBFV	mean pulmonary-blood-flow velocity
MOPV	monovalent oral poliovirus vaccine	MPBNS	modified Peyronie bladder neck
MOR	morphine (This is a dangerous		suspension
	abbreviation)	MPC	meperidine, promethazine, and
mOR	matched odds ratio		chlorpromazine
MOS	Medical Outcome Study		mucopurulent cervicitis
	mirror optical system	MPCC	Medical Policy Coordinating
	months		Committee
mOS	median overall survival	MPCN	microscopically positive and
MOSES	Multidimensional Observational		culturally negative
	Scale for Elderly Subjects	M-PCR	multiplex polymerase chain reaction
MOSF	multiple-organ system failure	MPCU	medical progressive care unit
MOS sf-20	Medical Outcomes Study, short form	MPD	maximum permissable dose
	20 items		methylphenidate (Ritalin)
MOS sf-36	Medical Outcomes Study, short		moisture permeable dressing
	form, 36 items		multiple personality disorder
mOsm	milliosmole		myeloproliferative disorder
mOsmol	milliosmole		myofascial pain dysfunction
MOT	motility examination		(syndrome)
MOTA	Method Other Than Acceleration	mPD	minimal peripheral dose
MOTS	mucosal oral therapeutic system	MPE	malignant pleural effusion
MOTT	mycobacteria other than tubercle		massive pulmonary embolism
MOU	medical oncology unit		mean prediction error
	memorandum of understanding		multiphoton excitation
MOUS	multiple occurrences of unexplained		myxopapillary ependymoma
	symptoms	MPEC	multipolar electrocoagulation
MOV	minimum obstructive volume	MPEG	methoxypolyethylene glycol
	multiple oral vitamin	MPF	methotrexate, cisplatin (Platinol),
MOW	Meals on Wheels		and fluorouracil
MP	malignant pyoderma		methylparaben free
	melphalan and prednisone	m-PFL	methotrexate, cisplatin (Platinol),
	menstrual period		fluorouracil, and leucovorin
	mercaptopurine (Purinethol)	MPGN	membranoproliferative
	metacarpal phalangeal joint		glomerulonephritis
	mitoxantrone and prednisone	MPH	massive pulmonary hemorrhage
	moist park		Master of Public Health
	monitor pattern		methylphenidate (Ritalin)
	monophasic		miles per hour
	motor potential	MPHD	multiple pituitary hormone
	mouthpiece		deficiencies
	myocardial perfusion	MPI	manufacturer's package insert
M & P	Millipore and phase		master patient index
4 MP	methylpyrazole (fomepizole; Antizol)		Maudsley Personality Inventory
6-MP	mercaptopurine (Purenthol)		milk-product intolerance

M

177

	myocardial perfusion imaging		mitral regurgitation
MPIF-1	myeloid progenitor inhibitory factor-1		moderate resistance
		M&R	measure and record
MPJ	metacarpophalangeal joint	MR × 1	may repeat times one (once)
MPK	milligram per kilogram	MRA	magnetic resonance angiography
MPL	maximum permissable level		main renal artery
	mesiopulpolingual		medical record administrator
MPL®	monophosphoryl lipid A		medical research associate
MPLC	medium pressure liquid chromatography		midright atrium
			multivariate regression analysis
MPM	malignant peritoneal mesothelioma	mrad	millirad
	malignant pleural mesothelioma	MRAN	medical resident admitting note
	Mortality Prediction Model	MRAP	mean right atrial pressure
MPN	monthly progress note	MRAS	main renal artery stenosis
	most probable number	MRC	Master of Rehabilitation Counseling
	multiple primary neoplasms	MRCA	magnetic resonance coronary angiography
MPNST	malignant peripheral nerve sheath tumor	MRCC	metastatic renal cell carcinoma
MPO	male-pattern obesity	MRCP	magnetic resonance cholangiopancreatography
	myeloperoxidase		
MPOA	medial preoptic area		Member of the Royal College of Physicians
MPP	massive periretinal proliferation		
	maximum pressure picture		mental retardation, cerebral palsy
MPP	multiple presentation phenotype	MRCPs	movement-related cortical potentials
MPQ	McGill Pain Questionnaire	MRCS	Member of the Royal College of Surgeons
MPPT	methylprednisolone pulse therapy		
MPR	massive periretinal retraction	MRD	margin reflex distance
	multiplanar reconstruction		Medical Records Department
MPS	Maternal Perinatal Scale		Minimal Record of Disability
	mean particle size		minimal residual disease
	mononuclear phagocyte system	MRDD	maximum recommended daily dose
	mucopolysaccharidosis		Mental Retardation and Development Disabilities
	multiphasic screening		
MPS-1	mucopolysaccharidosis I		mentally retarded and developmentally disabled
MPS-II	mucopolysaccharidosis II (Hunter syndrome)		
		MRDM	malnutrition-related diabetes mellitus
MPSS	massively parallel signature sequencing	MRDSA	magnetic resonance digital subtraction angiography
	methylprednisolone sodium succinate	MRE	manual resistance exercise
MPT	melphalan, prednisone, and thalidomide		most recent episode
		MRFC	mouse rosette-forming cells
	multiple parameter telemetry	MR FIT	Multiple Risk Factor Intervention Trial
MPTRD	motor, pain, touch, and reflex deficit		
MPU	maternal pediatric unit	MRG	mortality reference group
MPV	mean platelet volume		murmurs, rubs, and gallops
MQ	mefloquine (Lariam)	MRH	Maddox rod hyperphoria
	memory quotient	MRHD	maximum recommended human dose
MQOL	McGill Quality of Life Questionnaire	MRHT	modified rhyme hearing test
		MRI	magnetic resonance imaging
MR	Maddox rod	M & R I & O	measure and record input and output
	magnetic resonance		
	manifest refraction	MRK	Merck & Co., Inc.
	may repeat	MRKH	Mayer-Rokitansky-Kuster-Hauser (syndrome)
	measles-rubella		
	medial rectus	MRL	minimal response level
	medical record		moderate rubra lochia
	mental retardation	MRLVD	maximum residue limits of veterinary drugs
	milliroentgen		

M

MRLT	mesalamine-related lung toxicity		musculoskeletal
MRM	modified radical mastectomy	M & S	microculture and sensitivity
MRN	magnetic resonance neurography	3MS	Modified Mini-Mental Status
	malignant renal neoplasm		(examination)
	medical record number	MS III	third-year medical student
	medical resident's note	MSA	Medical Savings Accounts
mRNA	messenger ribonucleic acid		membrane-stabilizing activity
MRO	multidrug resistant organism(s)		methane sulfonic acid
MROU	medial rectus, both eyes		metropolitan statistical area
MRP	multidrug resistance-associated		microsomal autoantibodies
	protein		multiple system atrophy
MP-RAGE	magnetization prepared rapid	MSAF	meconium-stained amniotic fluid
	acquisition gradient-echo	MSAFP	maternal serum alpha-fetoprotein
MRPN	medical resident progress note	MSAP	mean systemic arterial pressure
MRPs	medication-related problems	MSAS	Mandel Social Adjustment Scale
MRR	medical record review	MSAS-SF	Memorial Symptom Assessment
MRS	magnetic resonance spectroscopy		Scale–short form
	mental retardation syndrome	MSB	mainstem bronchus
	methicillin-resistant *Staphylococcus*	MSBOS	maximum surgical blood order
	aureus		schedule
MRSA	methicillin-resistant *Staphylococcus*	MSBP	Munchausen syndrome by proxy
	aureus	MSC	major symptom complex
MRSE	methicillin-resistant *Staphylococcus*		Medical Service Corps
	epidermidis		mesenchymal stromal cells
MRSI	magnetic resonance spectroscopic		midsystolic click
	imaging		MS Contin®
MRSS	methicillin-resistant *Staphylococcus*	MSCA	McCarthy Scales of Children's
	species		Abilities
	modified Rodnan skin-thickness	MSCC	malignant spinal cord compression
	score		metastatic spinal cord compression
MRT	magnetic resonance tomography		midstream clean-catch (urine culture)
	malignant rhabdoid tumor	MSCCC	Master Sciences, Certified Clinical
	mean response time		Competence
	modified rhyme test	MSCR-	microbial surface
MRTA	magnetic resonance tomographic	AMMS	component reacting
	angiography		with adhesive matrix
MRU	medical resource utilization		molecules
MRV(r)	mixed respiratory vaccine	MSCs	mesenchymal stem cells
MRX	*Moraxella catarrhalis* vaccine	MSCT	multislice computed tomography
MR × 1	may repeat once	MSCU	medical special care unit
MS	mass spectroscopy	MSCWP	musculoskeletal chest wall pain
	Master of Science	MSD	male sexual dysfunction
	median sternotomy		microsurgical diskectomy
	medical student		midsleep disturbance
	mental status		musculoskeletal disorder
	milk shake	MSDBP	mean sitting diastolic blood
	minimal support		pressure
	mitral sounds	MSDS	material safety data sheet
	mitral stenosis	MSE	mean squared error
	moderately susceptible		Mental Status Examination
	morning stiffness	msec	milliseconds
	morphine sulfate (This is a	MSEL	myasthenic syndrome of Eaton-
	dangerous abbreviation)		Lambert
	motile sperm	MSER	mean systolic ejection rate
	motility study		Mental Status Examination Record
	multiple sclerosis	MSF	meconium-stained fluid
	muscle spasm		Médicins Sans Frontières (Doctors
	muscle strength		Without Borders)

M

	Mediterranean spotted fever
	megakaryocyte stimulating factor
MSG	massage
	methysergide (Sansert)
	monosodium glutamate
MSH	melanocyte-stimulating hormone
MSHA	mannose-sensitive hemagglutinin
MSI	magnetic source imaging
	mass sociogenic illness
	microsatellite instability
	multiple subcortical infarction
	musculoskeletal impairment
MSIA	mass spectrometric immunoassay
MSIR®	morphine sulfate immediate release tablets
MSIS	Multiple Severity of Illness System
MSK	medullary sponge kidney
	musculoskeletal
MSKCC	Memorial Sloan-Kettering Cancer Center
MSL	midsternal line
	multiple symmetrical lipomatosis
MSLT	multiple sleep latency test
MSM	magnetic starch microspheres
	men who have sex with men
	methsuximide (Celontin)
	methylsulfonylmethane
	midsystolic murmur
MSN	Master of Science in Nursing
MSNA	muscle sympathetic nerve activity
MSO	managed services organization
	mentally stable and oriented
	mental status, oriented
	most significant other
MSO$_4$	morphine sulfate (this is a dangerous abbreviation)
MSOD	multisystem organ dysfunction
MSOF	multisystem organ failure
MS-PCR	methylation-specific polymerase chain reaction
MSPN	medical student progress notes
MSPU	medical short procedure unit
MSQ	Mental Status Questionnaire
	meters squared
MSR	muscle stretch reflexes
MSRPP	Multidimensional Scale for Rating Psychiatric Patients
MSS	Marital Satisfaction Scale
	mean sac size
	microsatellite stable
	minor surgery suite
MSSA	methicillin-susceptible *Staphylococcus aureus*
MSS-CR	mean sac size and crown-rump length
MSSP	Maternal Support Services Program
MSSU	midstream specimen of urine

MST	maladies sexuellement transmissibles (French for sexually transmitted diseases)
	mean survival time
	median survival time
	mental stress test
	modified Schirmer test
	multiple subpial transection
MSTA®	mumps skin test antigen
MSTI	multiple soft tissue injuries
MSTS	American Musculoskeletal Tumor Society (functional rating system)
MSU	maple-syrup urine
	midstream urine
	monosodium urate
MSUD	maple-syrup urine disease
MSUS	musculoskeletal ultrasound
MSUs	midstream specimens of urine
mSv	millisievert (radiation unit)
MSW	Master of Social Work
	multiple stab wounds
MT	empty
	macular target
	maggot therapy
	maintenance therapy
	malaria therapy
	malignant teratoma
	Medical Technologist
	metatarsal
	middle turbinate
	monitor technician
	mucosal thickening
	muscles and tendons
	muscle tone
	music therapy (Therapist)
	myringotomy tube(s)
M/T	masses of tenderness
	myringotomy with tubes
M & T	*Monilia* and *Trichomonas*
	muscles and tendons
	myringotomy and tubes
MTA	Medical Technical Assistant
	metatarsal adduction
	multi-targeted antifolate (pemetrexed disodium [Alimta])
MTAD	tympanic membrane of the right ear
MT/AK	music therapy/ audiokinetics
MTAS	tympanic membrane of the left ear
MTAU	tympanic membranes of both ears
MTB	*Mycobacterium tuberculosis*
MTBC	Music Therapist-Board Certified
MTBE	methyl tert-butyl ether
MTBI	mild traumatic brain injury
MTC	magnetization transfer contrast (radiology)
	medullary thyroid carcinoma
	metoclopramide
	mitomycin (Mutamycin)

M

MTCSA	mid-thigh muscle cross-sectional area
MTCT	mother-to-child transmission
MTD	maximum tolerated dose
	metastatic trophoblastic disease
	methadone
	Monroe tidal drainage
	Mycobacterium tuberculosis direct (test)
MTDDA	Minnesota Test for Differential Diagnosis of Aphasia
MTDI	maximum tolerable daily intake
MTDT	*Mycobacterium* tuberculosis direct test
MTE	multiple trace elements
MTE-4®	trace metal elements injection (there is also a #5, #6, and #7)
MTET	modified treadmill exercise testing
MTF	male-to-female (transmission)
	medical treatment facility
MTG	middle temporal gyrus (gyri)
	midthigh girth
MTHFR	methylene tetrahydrofolate reductase
MTI	magnetization transfer imaging
	malignant teratoma intermediate
MTJ	midtarsal joint
MTL	medial temporal lobe
	mediastinal tuberculous lymphadenitis
	Metropolitan Life (Insurance Company) Table (for desirable weight)
MTLE	medial (mesial) temporal-lobe epilepsy
MTLV	midtidal lung volume
MTM	medication therapy management
	modified Thayer-Martin medium
	mouth-to-mouth (resuscitation)
MTNX	methylnaltrexone
mTOR	mammalian target of rapamycin
MTP	master treatment plan
	medical termination of pregnancy
	metatarsophalangeal
	microsomal triglyceride transfer protein
MTPJ	metatarsophalangeal joint
MTR	mother
MTR-O̅	no masses, tenderness, or rebound
MTRS	Licensed Master Therapeutic Recreation Specialist
MTS	mesial temporal sclerosis
MTST	maximal treadmill stress test
MTT	mamillothalamic tract
	mean transit time
	methylthiotetrazole
MTU	malignant teratoma undifferentiated
	methylthiouracil
MTX	methotrexate

MTZ	mirtazapine (Remeron)
	mitoxantrone (Novantrone)
MU	million units
	Murphy unit
mU	milliunits
MUA	manipulation under anesthesia
MUAC	middle upper arm circumference
MUAP	motor unit action potential
MUD	matched-unrelated donor
MUDDLES	miosis, urination, diarrhea, diaphoresis, lacrimation, excitation of central nervous system, and salivation (effects of cholinesterase inhibitors)
MUDPILES	*m*ethanol, metformin; *u*remia; *d*iabetic ketoacidosis; *p*henformin, paraldehyde; *i*ron, isoniazid, ibuprofen; *l*actic acidosis; *e*thanol, ethylene glycol; and *s*alicylates, sepsis (causes of metabolic acidosis)
MUE	medication use evaluation
MUFA	monounsaturated fatty acid
MUG	microgram (mcg is preferred)
MUGA	multigated (radionuclide) angiogram
	multiple gated acquisition (scan)
MUGX	multiple gated acquisition exercise
MUI	mixed urinary incontinence
MULE	microcomputer upper limb exerciser
MULTIP	multipara
MuLV	murine leukemia virus
MUM	mumps virus vaccine
MUNE	motor unit estimates
MUNSH	Memorial University of Newfoundland Scale of Happiness
MUO	metastasis of unknown origin
MUPAT	multiple-site perineal applicator technique
MUPS	melanoma of unknown primary site
MUSE®	Medicated Urethral System for Erection (alprostadil urethral suppository)
mus-lig	musculoligamentous
MUU	mouse uterine units
MV	manual ventilation
	mechanical ventilation
	millivolts
	minute volume
	mitoxantrone and etoposide (VePesid)
	mitral valve
	mixed venous
	multivesicular
MVA	malignant ventricular arrhythmias
	manual vacuum aspiration
	mitral valve area
	modified vaccinia ankara
	motor vehicle accident

M

M-VAC	methotrexate, vinblastine doxorubicin (Adriamycin), and cisplatin
MVB	methotrexate and vinblastine
	mixed venous blood
MVC	maximal voluntary contraction
	motor vehicle collision (crash)
MVc	mitral valve closure
MVD	microvascular decompression
	microvessel density
	mitral valve disease
	multivessel disease
MVE	mitral valve (leaflet) excursion
	Murray Valley encephalitis
MV Grad	mitral valve gradient
MVI	malignant vascular injury
	multiple vitamin injection
MVI®	brand name for parenteral multivitamins
MVI 12®	brand name for parenteral multivitamins
MVIC	maximum voluntary isometric contractions
MVID	microvillus inclusion disease
MVO	mixed venous oxygen saturation
MVO₂	myocardial oxygen consumption
MVP	mean venous pressure
	mitomycin, vinblastine, and cisplatin (Platinol)
	mitral valve prolapse
MVPA	moderate-to-vigorous physical activity
MVPP	mechlorethamine, vinblastine, procarbazine, and prednisone
MVPS	mitral valve prolapse syndrome
MVR	massive vitreous retraction
	micro-vitreoretinal (blade)
	mitral valve regurgitation
	mitral valve replacement
MVRI	mixed vaccine respiratory infections
MVS	mitral valve stenosis
	motor, vascular, and sensory
MVT	movement
	multiform ventricular tachycardia
	multivitamin
MVU	Montevideo units
MVV	maximum ventilatory volume
	maximum voluntary ventilation
	mixed vespid venom
6-MW	6-minute walk (test)
12-MW	12-minute walk (test)
MWB	minimal weight bearing
MWC	major wound complications
MWCO	molecular weight cutoff
MWD	maximum walking distance
	microwave diathermy
6-MWD	6-minute walking distance
M-W-F	Monday-Wednesday-Friday

MWI	Medical Walk-In (Clinic)
MWOA	migraine without aura
MWS	Mickety-Wilson syndrome
MWT	maintenance of wakefulness test
	Mallory-Weiss tear
	malpositioned wisdom teeth
	maximal walking time
6-MWT	6-minute walk test
MWTP	municipal wastewater treatment plants
Mx	manifest refraction
	mastectomy
	maxilla
	movement
	myringotomy
My	myopia
MYD	mydriatic
myelo	myelocytes
	myelogram
MyG	myasthenia gravis
MYOP	myopia
MYR	myringotomy
MYS	medium yellow soft (stools)
MZ	monozygotic
M/Z	mass/charge
MZL	marginal zone lymphocyte
MZT	monozygotic twins

M

N

N	nausea
	negative
	Negro
	Neisseria
	nerve
	neutrophil
	never
	newton
	night
	nipple
	nitrogen
	no
	nodes
	nonalcoholic
	none
	normal
	North (as in the location 2N, would be second floor, North wing)
	not
	notified
	noun
	NPH insulin
	size of sample
N1	study night 1
N I	first through twelfth
N XII	cranial nerves
0.1 N	tenth-normal
N₂	nitrogen
N 2.5	phenylephrine HCl 2.5% ophthalmic solution (Neo-Synephrine)
n-3	omega-3
5'-N	5'-nucleotidase
N-9	nonoxynol 9
NA	Narcotics Anonymous
	Native American
	Negro adult
	new admission
	nicotinic acid
	nonalcoholic
	norethindrone acetate
	normal axis
	not admitted
	not applicable
	not available
	nurse aide
	nurse's aid
	Nurse Anesthetist
	nursing assistant
Na	sodium
Na⁺	sodium
N & A	normal and active
NAA	*N*-acetylaspartate
	National Average Allowance (federal physician office visit cost guide)
	neutron activation analysis
	no apparent abnormalities
	nucleic acid amplification
NAAA	neo-adjuvant androgen ablation
NAAC	no apparent anesthesia complications
NAA/Cr	N-acetylaspartate/creatine ratio
NAAD	neoadjuvant androgen deprivation (therapy)
NAAT	nucleic acid amplification techniques (testing)
NAATPT	not available at the present time
NAB	not at bedside
NABS	normoactive bowel sounds
NAbs	neutralizing antibodies
NABT	normal-appearing brain tissue
NABTC	North American Brain Tumor Consortium
NABX	needle aspiration biopsy
NAC	acetylcysteine (N-acetylcysteine; Mucomyst)
	neoadjuvant chemotherapy
	nipple-areola complex
	no acute changes
	no anesthesia complications
NACD	no anatomical cause of death
NaClO	sodium hypochlorite
NaCl	sodium chloride (salt)
NaCMC	sodium carboxymethyl cellulose
NACS	Neurologic and Adaptive Capacity Score
NACT	neoadjuvant chemotherapy
NAD	nicotinamide adenine dinucleotide
	no active disease
	no acute distress
	no apparent distress
	no appreciable disease
	normal axis deviation
	nothing abnormal detected
NADA	New Animal Drug Application
NADase	nicotinamide adenine dinucleotide glycohydrolase
NADE	New Animal Drug Evaluation
NADPH	nicotinamide adenine dinucleotide phosphate
NADSIC	no apparent disease seen in chest
NaE	exchangeable sodium
NAF	nafcillin
	Native-American female
	Negro adult female
	normal adult female
	Notice of Adverse Findings (FDA post-audit letter)
NaF	sodium fluoride
NAFLD	nonalcoholic fatty liver disease
NAG	narrow angle glaucoma
NaHCO₃	sodium bicarbonate
NAHI	nonaccidental head injury
NAI	no action indicated

N

	no acute inflammation
	nonaccidental injury
	Nuremberg Aging Inventory
NaI	sodium iodide
NAION	nonarteritic ischemic optic neuropathy
NAIT	neonatal alloimmune thrombocytopenia
NAL	nasal angiocentric lymphoma
NAM	nail-apparatus melanoma
	Native-American male
	no abnormal masses
	normal adult male
NAMCS	National Ambulatory Medical Care Survey
nAMD	neovascular age-related macular degeneration
NANB	non-A, non-B (hepatitis) (hepatitis C)
NANBH	non-A, non-B hepatitis (hepatitis C)
NANC	nonadrenergic, noncholinergic
NANDA	North American Nursing Diagnosis Association (taxonomy)
NaNP	sodium nitroprusside (Nipride)
NANSAIDs	nonaspirin, nonsteroidal anti-inflammatory drugs
NANT	New Approaches to Neuroblastoma Therapy (consortium)
NaOCl	sodium hypochlorite
NaOH	sodium hydroxide
NAP	narrative, assessment, and plan
	nosocomial acquired pneumonia
NAPA	N-acetyl procainamide
NAPD	no active pulmonary disease
Na Pent	Pentothal Sodium
NAR	nasal airflow resistance
	no action required
	no adverse reaction
	nonambulatory restraint
	not at risk
	nursing assessment record
NARC	narcotic(s)
NaRI	noradrenaline reuptake inhibitor
NART	National Adult Reading Test (United Kingdom)
NAS	nasal
	neonatal abstinence syndrome
	no abnormality seen
	no added salt
NASBA	nucleic-acid sequencing based amplification
NaSCN	sodium thiocyanate
NASH	nonalcoholic steatohepatitis
NAS-NRC	National Academy of Sciences – National Research Council
NaSSA	noradrenergic and specific serotonergic antidepresssant
NASTT	nonspecific abnormality of ST segment and T wave

NAT	N-acetyltransferase
	no action taken
	no acute trauma
	nonaccidental trauma
	nonspecific abnormality of T wave
	nucleic acid test (testing)
Na^{99m}TcO$_4$$^-$	sodium pertechnetate Tc 99m
NAUC	normalized area under the curve
NAUTI	nosocomially-associated urinary tract infections
NAW	nasal antral window
NAWM	normal-appearing white matter
NB	nail bed
	needle biopsy
	neuroblastomas
	newborn
	nitrogen balance
	note well
NBC	newborn center
	nonbed care
	nuclear, biological, and chemical
NBCCS	nevoid basal-cell carcinoma syndrome
NBD	neurologic bladder dysfunction
	no brain damage
NBF	not breast fed
NBH	new bag (bottle) hung
NBHH	newborn helpful hints
NBI	no bone injury
NBICU	newborn intensive care unit
nBiPAP	nasal bilevel (biphasic) positive airway pressure
NBIs	nosocomial bloodstream infections
NBL/OM	neuroblastoma and opsoclonus-myoclonus
NBM	no bowel movement
	normal bone marrow
	normal bowel movement
	nothing by mouth
NBN	newborn nursery
NBP	needle biopsy of prostate
	no bone pathology
NBQC	narrow base quad cane
NBR	no blood return
NBS	newborn screen (serum thyroxine and phenylketonuria)
	Nijmegen breakage syndrome
	no bacteria seen
	normal bowel sounds
NBT	nitroblue tetrazolium reduction (tests)
	normal breast tissue
NBTE	nonbacterial thrombotic endocarditis
NBTNF	newborn, term, normal female
NBTNM	newborn, term, normal, male
NBW	normal birth weight (2,500–3,999 g)
NC	nasal cannula

N

	Negro child	NCHGR	National Center for Human Genome Research (NIH)
	neurologic check		
	no change	NCHS	National Center for Health Statistics
	no charge	NCICB	National Cancer Institute Center for Bioinformatics
	no complaints		
	noncontributory	NCI	National Cancer Institute
	normocephalic	NCICB	National Cancer Institute Center for Bioinformatics
	nose clamp		
	nose clips	NCIC	National Cancer Institute of Canada
	not classified	NCI-CTC	National Cancer Institute Common Toxicity Criteria
	not completed		
	not cultured	NCIC-CTG	National Cancer Institute of Canada Clinical Trials Group
9 NC	rubitecan (9-nitrocamptothecin; Orathecin)	NCID	National Center for Infectious Diseases (CDC)
NCA	neurocirculatory asthenia	NCIE	nonbullous congenital ichthyosiform erythroderma
	no congenital abnormalities		
N/CAN	nasal cannula	NCIPC	National Center for Injury Prevention and Control (CDC)
NCAP	nasal continuous airway pressure		
NCAS	zinostatin (neocarzinostatin)	NCIS	nursing care information sheet
NC/AT	normocephalic atraumatic	NCIT	Nursing Care Intervention Tool
NCB	natural childbirth	NCJ	needle catheter jejunostomy
	no code blue	NCL	neuronal ceroid lipofuscinosis
NCBI	National Center for Biotechnology Information (NIH)		no cautionary labels
			nuclear cardiology laboratory
NCC	neurocysticercosis	NCKX	sodium-calcium-potassium exchanger
	no concentrated carbohydrates	NCLD	neonatal chronic lung disease
	nursing care card	NCM	nailfold capillary microscope
NCCAM	National Center for Complementary and Alternative Medicine (NIH)		nonclinical manager
		NCNC	normochromic, normocytic
NCCDPHP	National Center for Chronic Disease and Prevention and Health Promotion (CDC)	NCNR	National Center for Nursing Research (NIH)
		NCO	no complaints offered
NCCI	National Correct Coding Initiative		noncommissioned officer
NCCLS	National Committee for Clinical Laboratory Standards	NCOG	North California Oncology Group
		NCP	no caffeine or pepper
NCCN	National Comprehensive Cancer Network		nursing care plan
		NCPAP	nasal continuous positive airway pressure
NCCP	noncardiac chest pain		
NCCTG	North Central Cancer Treatment Group	NCPB	neurolytic celiac plexus block
		NcpPCu	nonceruloplasmin plasma copper
NCCU	neurosurgical continuous care unit	NCPR	no cardiopulmonary resuscitation
NCD	neck-capsule distance	NCQA	National Commission for Quality Assurance
	no congenital deformities		
	normal childhood diseases	NCR	no carbon (paper) required (treated paper which produces a copy of what was written on the paper above)
	not considered disabling		
	not considered disqualifying		
	Nursing-Care Dependency (scale)		
NCDB	National Cancer Data Base	nCR	nodular complete response
NCDR	new case-detection rate	NCRA	National Cancer Registrars Association
NCE	new chemical entity		
NCEH	National Center for Environmental Health (CDC)	NCRC	nonchild-resistant container
		NCRI	National Cancer Research Institute (United Kingdom)
NCEP	National Cholesterol Education Program		
		NCRR	National Center for Research Resources (NIH)
NCF	neurocognitive function		
	neutrophilic chemotactic factor	NCS	nerve conduction studies
	no cold fluids		no concentrated sweets

N

	noncontact supervision	NDM	neonatal diabetes mellitus
	not clinically significant	NDMS	National Disaster Medical System
	zinostatin (neocarzinostatin)	Nd/NT	nondistended, nontender
NCSE	nonconvulsive status epilepticus	NDO	neurogenic detrusor overactivity
NCSN	National Certified School Nurse	NDP	nedaplatin
NCT	neoadjuvant chemotherapy		net dietary protein
	neutron capture therapy		Nurse Discharge Planner
	noncontact tonometry	NDPH	new daily persistent headache
	number connection test	NDR	neurotic depressive reaction
	Nursing Care Technician		normal detrusor reflex
NCTR	National Center for Toxicological	NDRI	norepinephrine and dopamine
	Research		reuptake inhibitor
NCV	nerve conduction velocity	NDS	Neurologic Disability Score
	nuclear venogram		neuropathy disability score
NCVHS	National Committee on Vital and		New Drug Submission
	Health Statistics	NDSC	nasal dermoid sinus cyst
NCX	sodium-calcium exchanger	NDSO	nasolacrimal drainage system
ND	Doctor of Naturopathy (Naturopathic		obstruction
	Physician)	NDST	neurodevelopmental screening test
	nasal deformity	NDT	nasal duodenostomy tube
	nasal discharge		Neurocognitive Driving Test
	nasoduodenal		neurodevelopmental techniques
	natural death		neurodevelopmental treatment
	neck dissection		noise detection threshold
	neonatal death	NDV	Newcastle disease virus
	neurological development	Nd:YAG	neodymium:yttrium-aluminum-garnet
	neurotic depression		(laser)
	Newcastle disease	Nd:YLF	neodymium: yttrium-lithium-fluoride
	no data		(laser)
	no disease	NE	nasoenteric
	nondisabling		nausea and emesis
	nondistended		nephropathica epidemica
	none detectable		neurological examination
	normal delivery		never exposed
	normal development		no effect
	nose drops		no enlargement
	not detected		norethindrone
	not diagnosed		norepinephrine
	not done		not elevated
	nothing done		not examined
	Nursing Doctorate	NEAA	nonessential amino acids
N&D	nodular and diffuse	NEAC	norethindrone acetate
Nd	neodymium	NEAD	nonepileptic attack disorder
NDA	New Drug Application	NEAT	nonexercise activity thermogenesis
	no data available	NEB	hand-held nebulizer
	no demonstrable antibodies	NEC	necrotizing entercolitis
	no detectable activity		noise equivalent counts
NDC	National Drug Code		nonesterified cholesterol
NDD	no dialysis days		not elsewhere classified
NDE	near-death experience	NECT	nonenhanced computed tomography
NDEA	no deviation of electrical axis		(scan)
NDF	neutral density filter (test)	NED	neuroendocrine differentiation
	no disease found		no evidence of disease
NDGA	nordihydroguaiaretic acid	NEDSS	National Electronic Disease
NDI	National Death Index		Surveillance System
	nephrogenic diabetes insipidus	NEE	neonatal epileptic encephalopathy
NDIR	nondispersive infrared	NEEG	normal electroencephalogram
NDIRS	nondispersive infrared spectrometer	NEEP	negative end-expiratory pressure

N

NEF	negative expiratory force		none found
NEFA	nonesterified fatty acid(s)		nonfasting
NEFG	normal external female genitalia		not found
NEFT	nasoenteric feeding tube		nursed fair
NEG	negative		nursing facility
	neglect	Nf	*Naegleria fowleri*
NEI	National Eye Institute (NIH)	NF1	neurofibromatosis type 1
NEJM	*New England Journal of Medicine*	NF2	neurofibromatous type 2
NEM	neurotrophic enhancing molecule	NFA	Nerve Fiber Analyzer®
	no evidence of malignancy	NFALO	Nerve Fiber Analyzer laser
	nucleoside excision mutation		oththalmoscope
NEMD	nonexudative macular degeneration	NFAP	nursing facility-acquired pneumonia
	nonspecific esophageal motility	NFAR	no further action required
	disorder	NFCS	Neonatal Facial Coding System
NENT	nasal endotracheal tube	NFD	no family doctor
NEO	necrotizing external otitis	NFFD	not fit for duty
NEOH	neonatal high risk	NFI	nerve-function impairment
NEOM	neonatal medium risk		no-fault insurance
NEP	needle-exchange program		no further information
	neutral endopeptidase		normal female infant
	no evidence of pathology	NFL	nerve fiber layer
NEPD	no evidence of pulmonary disease		Novantrone (mitoxantrone),
NEPHRO	nephrogram		fluorouracil, and leucovorin
NEPPK	nonepidermolytic palmoplantar	NFLX	norfloxacin (Noroxin)
	keratoderma	NFP	natural family planning
NEQAS	National External Quality Assurance		no family physician
	Scheme (United Kingdom)		not-for-profit
NER	no evidence of recurrence		not for publication
NERD	no evidence of recurrent disease	NFPA	nonfluent progressive aphasia
	nonerosive reflux disease	NFT	no further treatment
NES	nonepileptic seizure	NFTD	normal full-term delivery
	nonstandard electrolyte solution	NFTE	not found this examination
	not elsewhere specified	NFTs	neurofibrillary tangles
NESP	novel erythropoiesis stimulating		neurologic function tests
	protein (darbepoetin [Aranesp])	NFTSD	normal full-term spontaneous
NET	choroidal or subretinal		delivery
	neovascularization	NFTT	nonorganic failure to thrive
	Internet	NFV	nelfinavir (Viracept)
	naso-endotracheal tube	NFW	nursed fairly well
	neuroectodermal tumor	NG	nanogram (ng) (10^{-9} gram)
	neuroendocrine tumors		nasogastric
NETA	norethindrone acetate (Aygestin)		night guard
NETSS	National Electronic		nitroglycerin
	Telecommunications System for		no growth
	Surveillance		norgestrel
NETT	nasal endotracheal tube	ng	nanogram
NEVA	nocturnal electrobioimpedance	NGAL	neutrophil gelatinase-associated
	volumetric assessment (penile		lipocalin
	measurement)	NGB	neurogenic bladder
NEX	nose-to-ear-to-xiphoid	NGF	nerve growth factor
	number of excitations (radiology)	n giv	not given
NETZ	needle (diathermy) excision of the	NGJ	nasogastro-jejunostomy
	transformation zone	NGM	norgestimate
NF	necrotizing fasciitis	NGMAST	*Neisseria gonorrhoeae* multi-antigen
	Negro female		sequence typing
	neurofibromatosis	NGO	nongovernmental organization
	night frequency (of voiding)	NGOs	nongovernmental organizations
	nodular fasciitis	NGR	nasogastric (tube) replacement

N

NGRI	not guilty by reason of insanity	NIADDK	National Institute of Arthritis, Diabetes, and Digestive and Kidney Diseases (NIH)
NGSF	nothing grown so far		
NGT	nasogastric tube		
	normal glucose tolerance	NIAID	National Institute of Allergy and Infectious Diseases (NIH)
NGTD	no growth to date		
NgTD	negative to date	NIAL	not in active labor
NGU	nongonococcal urethritis	NIAMS	National Institute of Arthritis and Musculoskeletal and Skin Diseases (NIH)
NH	normal-hearing nursing home		
NHA	no histologic abnormalities	NIA-RI	National Institute on Aging–Reagan Institute
NHANES III	third National Health and Nutrition Examination Survey		
		NIBP	noninvasive blood pressure
NHB	nonheart-beating (donor)	NIBPM	noninvasive blood pressure measurement
NHBD	nonheart-beating donor		
NHC	neighborhood health center	NIC	Nursing Intervention Classification
	neonatal hypocalcemia	NICC	neonatal intensive care center
	nursing home care		noninfectious chronic cystitis
NH_3	ammonia	NICE	National Institute for Clinical Excellence (United Kingdom)
NH_4Cl	ammonium chloride		
NHCU	nursing home care unit		new, interesting, and challenging experiences
NHD	nocturnal hemodialysis		
	normal hair distribution	NICHD	National Institute of Child Health and Human Development (NIH)
NHE	sodium/hydrogen exchanger		
NHEJ	nonhomologous end-joining	NICO	neuralgia-inducing cavitational osteonecrosis
NHGRI	National Human Genome Research Institute (NIH)		
			noninvasive cardiac output (monitor)
NHIS	National Health Interview Survey		
		NICS	noninvasive carotid studies
NHL	nodular histiocytic lymphoma	NICU	neonatal intensive care unit
	non-Hodgkin lymphomas		neurosurgical intensive care unit
nHL	normalized hearing level	NID	no identifiable disease
NHLBI	National Heart, Lung, and Blood Institute (NIH)		not in distress
		NIDA	National Institute of Drug Abuse (NIH)
NHLPP	hereditary neuropathy with liability for pressure palsy		
		NIDA five	National Institute on Drug Abuse screen for cannabinoids, cocaine metabolite, amphetamine/methamphetamine, opiates, and phencyclidine
NHM	no heroic measures		
NHO	notify house officer		
NHP	Nottingham Health Profile		
	nursing home placement		
NHPs	natural health products	NIDCD	National Institute of Deafness and other Communication Disorders (NIH)
NHPT	nine-hole peg test		
NHS	National Health Service (UK)		
NHT	neoadjuvant hormonal therapy	NIDCR	National Institute of Dental and Craniofacial Research (NIH)
	nursing home transfer		
NHTR	nonhemolytic transfusion reaction	NIDD	noninsulin-dependent diabetes
NHTSA	National Highway Traffic Safety Administration	NIDDK	National Institute of Diabetes and Digestive and Kidney Diseases (NIH)
NHW	nonhealing wound		
NI	neurological improvement	NIDDM	noninsulin-dependent diabetes mellitus
	no improvement		
	no information	NIDR	National Institute of Dental Research (NIH)
	none indicated		
	not identified	NIEHS	National Institute of Environmental Health Sciences (NIH)
	not isolated		
NIA	National Institute on Aging (NIH)	NIF	negative inspiratory force
	no information available		neutrophil inhibitory factor
			not in file
NIAAA	National Institute on Alcohol Abuse and Alcoholism (NIH)	NIFS	noninvasive flow studies

N

NIG	NSAIA (nonsteroidal anti-inflamatory agent) induced gastropathy
NIGMS	National Institute of General Medical Sciences (NIH)
NIH	National Institutes of Health
NIHD	noise-induced hearing damage
NIHL	noise-induced hearing loss
NIHSS	National Institutes of Health Stroke Scale
NIID	neuronal intranuclear inclusion disease
NIL	not in labor
NIMAs	noninherited maternal antigens
NIMH	National Institute of Mental Health (NIH)
NIMHDIS	National Institute for Mental Health Diagnostic Interview Schedule (NIH)
NIMR	National Institute of Medical Research (United Kingdom)
NINDS	National Institute of Neurological Disorders and Stroke (NIH)
NINR	National Institute for Nursing Research (NIH)
NINU	neuro intermediate nursing unit
NINVS	noninvasive neurovascular studies
NIOPCs	no intraoperative complications
NIOSH	National Institute of Occupational Safety and Health (Centers for Disease Control and Prevention)
NIP	catnip
	National Immunization Program
	no infection present
	no inflammation present
NIPAs	noninherited paternal antigens
NIPD	nocturnal intermittent peritoneal dialysis
NIPPV	noninvasive positive-pressure ventilation
NIPS	Neonatal Infant Pain Scale
NIP/S	noninvasive programming stimulation
NIPSV	noninvasive pressure support ventilation
NIR	near infrared
	nitroprusside-induced relaxation
NIRCA	nonisotopic RNase cleavage assay
NISH	nonradioactive *in situ* hybridization
NISS	New Injury Severity Score
NISs	no-impact sports
NIST	National Institute of Standards and Technology
NISV	nonionic surfactant vesicle
NITD	neuroleptic-induced tardive dyskinesia'
Nitro	nitroglycerin (this is a dangerous abbreviation)

	sodium nitroprusside (this is a dangerous abbreviation)
NIV	noninvasive ventilation
NIVLS	noninvasive vascular laboratory studies
NJ	nasojejunal
NJT	nasojejunal tube
NK	natural killer (cells)
	not known
NK$_1$	neurokinin 1
NKA	no known allergies
nkat	nanokatal (nanomole/sec)
NKB	no known basis
	not keeping baby
	neurokinin B
NKC	nonketotic coma
NKD	no known diseases
NKDA	no known drug allergies
NKFA	no known food allergies
NKH	nonketotic hyperglycemia
NKHA	nonketotic hyperosmolar acidosis
NKHHC	nonketotic hyperglycemic-hyperosmolar coma
NKHOC	nonketotic hyperosmolar coma
NKHS	nonketotic hyperosmolar syndrome
NKMA	no known medication (medical) allergies
NKT	natural-killer T (cells)
NL	nasolacrimal
	nonlatex
	normal
	normal libido
nL	nanoliter (if nL was used in the clinical setting it would be dangerous as it could be seen or heard as mL)
NLB	needle liver biopsy
NLC	nocturnal leg cramps
NLC & C	normal libido, coitus, and climax
NLD	nasolacrimal duct
	necrobiosis lipoidica diabeticorum
	no local doctor
NLDO	nasolacrimal duct obstruction
NLE	neonatal lupus erythematosus
	nursing late entry
NLEA	Nutrition Labeling and Education Act of 1990
NLF	nasolabial fold
	nelfinavir (Viracept)
NLFGNR	nonlactose fermenting gram-negative rod
NLM	National Library of Medicine
	no limitation of motion
NLMC	nocturnal leg muscle cramp
NLN	National League for Nursing
	no longer needed
NLNAC	National League for Nursing Accrediting Commission

N

NLO	nasolacrimal occlusion	NMRS	nuclear magnetic resonance spectroscopy
NLP	natural language processing		
	nodular liquifying panniculitis	NMRT (R)	Nuclear Medicine Radiologic Technologist (Registered)
	no light perception		
NLS	neonatal lupus syndrome	NMS	neonatal morphine solution
NLs	neuroimmunophilin ligands		neuroleptic malignant syndrome
NLT	not later than	NMSC	nonmelanoma skin cancer
	not less than	NMSE	normalized mean square root
NLV	nelfinavir (Viracept)	NMSIDS	near-miss sudden infant death syndrome
NM	nanometer (nm) (10^{-9} meters)		
	Negro male	NMT	nebulized mist treatment
	neuromuscular		no more than
	neuronal microdysgenesis	NMTB	neuromuscular transmission blockade
	nodular melanoma	NMTCB	Nuclear Medicine Technology Certification Board
	nonmalignant		
	not measurable	NMT(R)	Nuclear Medicine Technologist Registered
	not measured		
	not mentioned	NMU	nitrosomethylurea
	nuclear medicine	NN	narrative notes
	nurse manager		Navajo neuropathy
N & M	nerves and muscles		neonatal
	night and morning		neural network
NMB	neuromuscular blockade		normal nursery
NMBA	neuromuscular blocking agent		nurses' notes
NMC	no malignant cells	N/N	negative/negative
NMD	Doctor of Naturopathic Medicine	NNB	normal newborn
	neuromuscular disorders		number-needed-to-benefit
	neuronal migration disorders	NNBC	node-negative breast cancer
	Normosol M and 5% Dextrose®	NND	neonatal death
NMDA	N-methyl-D-aspartate		number needed to detain
NMDP	National Marrow Donor Pool	NNDSS	National Notifiable Diseases Surveillance System
NME	new molecular entity		
NMES	neuromuscular electrical stimulation	NNE	neonatal necrotizing enterocolitis
		NNH	number needed to harm
NMF	neuromuscular facilitation	NNIS	National Nosocomial Infections Surveillance
NMH	neurally mediated hypotension		
NMHH	no medical health history	NNM	Nicolle-Novy-MacNeal (media)
NMI	no manifest improvement	NNL	no new laboratory (test orders)
	no mental illness	NNN	normal newborn nursery
	no middle initial	NNO	no new orders
	no more information	NNP	Neonatal Nurse Practitioner
	normal male infant		non-nociceptive pain
NMJ	neuromuscular junction	N:NPK	grams of nitrogen to non-protein kilocalories
NML	normal		
NMKB	not married, keeping baby	NNR	not necessary to return
NMM	nodular malignant melanoma	NNRTI	non-nucleoside reverse transcriptase inhibitor
NMN	no middle name		
NMNKB	not married, not keeping baby	NNS	neonatal screen (hematocrit, total bilirubin, and total protein)
NMO	neuromyelitis optica (Devic syndrome)		
			nicotine nasal spray
nmol	nanomole (one billionth [10^{-9}] of a mole)		non-nutritive sucking
			number needed to screen
NMOH	no medical ocular history	NNT	number needed to treat
NMP	normal menstrual period	NNTB	number needed to treat to benefit
NMPPAS	non-resonant multiphoton photoacoustic spectroscopy	NNTB/ NNTH	number needed to treat, benefit-to-harm ratio
NMR	nuclear magnetic resonance (same as magnetic resonance imaging)	NNTH	number needed to treat to harm
		NNU	net nitrogen utilization

NNWT	noncontact normothermic wound therapy		new-onset seizures
NO	nasal oxygen		nitric oxide synthase
	nitric oxide		no organisms seen
	nitroglycerin ointment		not on staff
	none obtained		not otherwise specified
	nonobese	NOSI	nitric oxide synthase inhibitors
	number (no.)	NOSIE	Nurse's Observation Scale (Schedule) for Inpatient Evaluation
	nursing office		
NO_2	nitrogen dioxide	NOSPECS	categories for classifying eye changes in Graves ophthalmopathy: **n**o signs or symptoms, **o**nly signs, **s**oft tissue involvement with symptoms and signs, **p**roptosis, **e**xtraocular muscle involvement, **c**orneal involvement, and **s**ight loss (visual acuity)
N_2O	nitrous oxide		
NOAA	National Oceanic and Atmospheric Administration		
NOAEL	no observed adverse effect level		
$N_2O:O_2$	nitrous oxide to oxygen ratio		
NOC	nonorgan-confined		
	Nursing Outcome Classification		
noc.	night		
noct	nocturnal	NOT	nocturnal oxygen therapy
NOD	nonobese diabetic	NOTT	nocturnal oxygen therapy trial
	notice of disagreement	NOU	not on unit
	notify of death	NOV	Novartis
NOE	naso-orbitoethmoid	NOV 70/30	human insulin, regular 30 units/mL with human insulin isophane suspension 70 units/mL (Novolin 70/30)
NOED	no observed effect dose		
NOEL	no observable effect level		
NOF	National Osteoporosis Foundation (treatment criteria)		
		NOV L	human insulin zinc suspension (Novolin L)
NOFT	nonorganic failure to thrive		
NOFTT	nonorganic failure to thrive	NOV N	human insulin isophane suspension (Novolin N)
NOGM	nonoxidative glucose metabolism		
NOH	neurogenic orthostatic hypotension	NOV R	human insulin regular (Novolin R)
NOI	nature of illness	NP	nasal polyps
NOK	next of kin		nasal prongs
NOL	not on label		nasopharyngeal
NOM	nonoperative management		near point
	nonsuppurative otitis media		neuropathic pain
NOMI	nonocclusive mesenteric infarction		neurophysin
NOMID	neonatal-onset multisystem inflammatory disease		neuropsychiatric
			neutrogenic precautions
NOMS	not on my shift		newly presented
NO/N_2	nitric oxide; nitrogen		nonpalpable
NONMEM	nonlinear mixed-effects model (modeling)		no pain
			not performed
non pal	not palpable		not pregnant
NonPARs	Nonparticipating Physicians (Medicare)		not present
			nuclear pharmacist
non-REM	nonrapid eye movement (sleep)		nuclear pharmacy
non rep	do not repeat		nursed poorly
NON VIZ	not visualized		nurse practitioner
NOOB	not out of bed	NPA	nasal pharyngeal airway
NOP	not on patient		nasopharyngeal aspirate
NOR	norethynodrel		near point of accommodation
	normal		no previous admission
	nortriptyline	NPAT	nonparoxysmal atrial tachycardia
NOR-EPI	norepinephrine (Levophed)		
norm	normal	NPBC	node-positive breast cancer
NOS	neonatal opium solution (diluted deodorized tincture of opium)	NPC	nasopharyngeal carcinoma
			near-point convergence

N

	Niemann-Pick disease Type C (sphingomyelin lipidosis)	NPPNG	nonpenicillinase-producing *Neisseria gonorrhoeae*
	nodal premature contractions	NPPV	noninvasive positive-pressure ventilation
	nonpatient contact		
	nonproductive cough	NPR	normal pulse rate
	nonprotein calorie		nothing per rectum
	no prenatal care	NPRL	normal pupillary reaction to light
	no previous complaint(s)	NPRM	Notice of Proposed Rulemaking
NP-C	Nurse Practitioner, Certified	NPRS	numerical pain rating scale
NPCC	nonprotein carbohydrate calories	NPS	National Pharmaceutical Stockpile
NPCPAP	nasopharyngeal continuous positive airway pressure		new patient set-up
		NPSA	nonphysician surgical assistant
NPD	narcissistic personality disorder	NPSD	nonpotassium-sparing diuretics
	Niemann-Pick disease	NPSF	National Patient Safety Foundation
	nonprescription drugs	NPSG	National Patient Safety Goal
	no pathological diagnosis		nocturnal polysomnography
NPDL	nodular poorly differentiated lymphocytic	NPSLE	neuropsychiatric systemic lupus erythematosus
NPDR	nonproliferative diabetic retinopathy	NPT	near-patient tests
NPE	neurogenic pulmonary edema		neopyrithiamin hydrochloride
	neuropsychologic examination		nocturnal penile tumescence
	no palpable enlargement		no prior tracings
	normal pelvic examination		normal pressure and temperature
NPEM	nocturnal penile erection monitoring	NPU	net protein utilization
NPF	nasopharyngeal fiberscope	NPV	negative predictive value
	no predisposing factor		nothing per vagina
N-PFMSO₄	nebulized preservative-free morphine sulfate (This is a dangerous abbreviation)	NPWT	negative pressure wound therapy
		NPY	neuropeptide Y
		NPZ	neuropsychologic text z
NPFS	nonpenetrating filtering surgery	NQECN	nonqueratinizing epidermoid carcinoma
NPG	nonpregnant		
	normal-pressure glaucoma	NQMI	non-Q wave myocardial infarction
NPH	isophane insulin (neutral protamine Hagedorn)	NQT	narrow QRS complex tachycardia
		NQW	non-Q-wave
	no previous history	NQWMI	non-Q wave myocardial infarction
	normal-pressure hydrocephalus	NR	do not repeat
NPhx	nasopharynx		newly reformulated
NPI	National Provider Identifier		none reported
	Neuropsychiatric Inventory		nonreactive
	no present illness		nonrebreathing
	Nottingham Prognostic Index		no refills
NPIS	Numeric Pain Intensity Scale		no report
NPJT	nonparoxysmal junctional tachycardia		no response
NPL	insulin lispro protamine suspension		no return
component	neural protamine lispro (insulin)		normal range
NPLSM	neoplasm		normal reaction
NPK	nonprotein kilocalories		not reached
NPM	nothing per mouth		not reacting
NPN	nonprotein nitrogen		not remarkable
NPNC	no prenatal care		not resolved
NPNT	nonpalpable, nontender		number
n.p.o.	nothing by mouth	NRAF	nonrheumatic atrial fibrillation
NPOC	nonpurgeable organic carbon	NRB	Noninstitutional Review Board
NPOD	Neuropsychiatric Officer of the Day		nonrebreather (oxygen mask)
NPP	nonphysician practitioner	NRBC	normal red blood cell
	normal postpartum		nucleated red blood cell
	Nurse Practitioner, Psychiatric	NRBS	nonrebreathing system
NPPI	nonpeptidic protease inhibitor	NRC	National Research Council

	normal retinal correspondence		number of signals averaged
	Nuclear Regulatory Commission		(radiology)
NREH	normal renin essential	NSAA	nonsteroidal antiandrogen
	hypertension	NSABP	National Surgical Adjuvant Breast
NREM	nonrapid eye movement		Project
NREMS	nonrapid eye movement sleep	NSAD	no signs of acute disease
NREMT-P	National Registry of Emergency	NSAIA	nonsteroidal anti-inflammatory agent
	Medical Technicians–Paramedic	NSAID	nonsteroidal anti-inflammatory drug
	level	NSAP	nonspecific abdominal pain
NRF	normal renal function	NSBGP	nonspecific bowel gas pattern
NRI	nerve root involvement	NSC	neural stem cells
	nerve root irritation		no significant change
	no recent illnesses		nonservice-connected
	norepinephrine reuptake inhibitor	NSCC	nonsmall cell carcinoma
NRL	natural rubber latex	NSCD	nonservice-connected disability
N-RLX	nonrelaxed	NSCFPT	no significant change from previous
NRM	nonrebreathing mask		tracing
	no regular medicines	NSCIDRC	National Spinal Cord Injury Data
	normal range of motion		Research Center
	normal retinal movement	NSCLC	nonsmall-cell–lung cancer
NRN	no return necessary	NSCST	nipple stimulation contraction stress
NRNST	nonreassuring-nonstress test		test
NRO	neurology	NSD	nasal septal deviation
NROM	normal range of motion		nominal standard dose
NRP	nonreassuring patterns		nonstructural deterioration
NRPR	nonbreathing pressure relieving		normal spontaneous delivery
NRR	net reproduction rate		no significant disease (difference,
NRS	Neurobehavioral Rating Scale		defect, deviation)
NRSs	nonrandomized studies	NSDA	nonsteroid dependent asthmatic
NRT	neuromuscular reeducation	NSDU	neonatal stepdown unit
	techniques	NSE	neuron-specific enolase
	nicotine-replacement therapy		normal saline enema (0.9% sodium
NRTI	nucleoside reverse transcriptase		chloride)
	inhibitor	N s E	nausea without emesis
NRTs	nitron radical traps	NSEACS	non-ST-elevation acute coronary
NS	nephrotic syndrome		syndromes
	neurological signs	NSF	no significant findings
	neurosurgery	NSFTD	normal spontaneous full-term
	never-smokers		delivery
	nipple stimulation	NSG	nursing
	nodular sclerosis	NSGCT	nonseminomatous germ-cell tumors
	no-show	NSGCTT	nonseminomatous germ-cell tumor
	nonsmoker		of the testis
	normal saline solution (0.9% sodium	NSGI	nonspecific genital infection
	chloride solution)	NSGT	nonseminomatous germ-cell tumor
	normospermic	NSHC	no-self-harm contract
	no sample	NSHD	nodular sclerosing Hodgkin disease
	not seen	NSI	needlestick injury
	not significant		negative self-image
	nuclear sclerosis		no signs of infection
	nursing service		no signs of inflammation
	nutritive sucking	NSICU	neurosurgery intensive care unit
	nylon suture	NSILA	nonsuppressible insulin-like activity
NSA	neck-shaft angle	NSIP	nonspecific interstitial pneumonia
	normal serum albumin (albumin,	NSMMVT	nonsustained monomorphic
	human)		ventricular tachycardia
	no salt added	NSN	Neo-Synephrine
	no significant abnormalities		nephrotoxic serum nephritis

N

NSO	Neosporin® ointment		normal temperature
NSOM	near field scanning optical microscope		normotensive
			nortriptyline
NSOP	no soft organs palpable		not tender
NSP	neck and shoulder pain		not tested
NSPs	needle and syringe exchange programs		nourishment taken
			numbness and tingling
	nonstarch polysaccharides		nursing technician
NSPVT	nonsustained polymorphic	N&T	nose and throat
	ventricular tachycardia		numbness and tingling
NSR	nasoseptal repair	N Tachy	nodal tachycardia
	nonspecific reaction	NT-ANP	N-terminal atrial natriuretic peptide
	normal sinus rhythm	NTBR	not to be resuscitated
	not seen regularly	NTC	neurotrauma center
NSRP	nerve-sparing radical prostatectomy	NTCS	no tumor cells seen
NSS	nephron-sparing surgery	NTD	negative to date
	neurological signs stable		neural-tube defects
	neuropathy symptom score		nitroblue tetrazolium dye (test)
	normal size and shape	NTE	neutral thermal environment
	not statistically significant		not to exceed
	nutritional support service	NTED	neonatal toxic-shock-syndrome-like
	sodium chloride 0.9% (normal saline solution)		exanthematous disease
		NTF	neurotrophic factor
1/2 NSS	sodium chloride 0.45% (1/2 normal saline solution)		normal throat flora
		NTG	nitroglycerin
NSSC	normal size, shape and consistency (uterus)		nontoxic goiter
			nontreatment group
NSSL	normal size, shape, and location		normal tension glaucoma
NSSP	normal size, shape, and position	NTGO	nitroglycerin ointment
NSSTT	nonspecific ST and T-wave	NTI	narrow therapeutic index
NSST-TWCs	nonspecific ST-T wave changes		no treatment indicated
		NTIS	National Technical Information Service (U.S. Department of Commerce)
NST	nonmyeloablative stem-cell transplant		
	Nonsense Syllable Test	NTL	nectar-thick liquid (diet consistency)
	nonstress test		
	normal sphincter tone		nortriptyline (Aventyl; Pamelor)
	not sooner than		no time limit
	nutritional support team	NTLE	neocortical temporal-lobe epilepsy
NSTD	nonsexually transmitted disease	NTM	nocturnal tumescence monitor
NSTEMI	non-ST-segment elevation myocardial infarction		nontuberculous mycobacterium
		NTMB	nontuberculous myobacteria
NSTGCT	nonseminomatous testicular germ cell tumor	NTMI	nontransmural myocardial infarction
		NTND	not tender, not distended
NSTI	necrotizing soft-tissue infection	NTP	narcotic treatment program
NSTT	nonseminomatous testicular tumors		National Toxicology Program
NSU	neurosurgical unit		Nitropaste® (nitroglycerin ointment)
	nonspecific urethritis		nonthrombocytopenic preterm (infant)
NSV	nonspecific vaginitis		
NSVD	nonstructural valve deterioration		normal temperature and pressure
	normal spontaneous vaginal delivery		sodium nitroprusside
NSVT	nonsustained ventricular tachycardia	NTPD	nocturnal tidal peritoneal dialysis
NSX	neurosurgical examination	NT-proBNP	N-terminal pro-brain natriuretic peptide
NSY	nursery		
NT	nasotracheal	NTS	nasotracheal suction
	next time		nicotine transdermal system
	Nordic Track®		nontyphoidal salmonellae
			nucleus tractus solitarii

N

NTSCI	nontraumatic spinal cord injury	NVP	nausea and vomiting of pregnancy
NTT	nasotracheal tube		nevirapine (Viramune)
	near-total thyroidectomy	NVS	neurological vital signs
	nonthrombocytopenic term (infant)		neurovascular status
	nontreponemal test	NVSS	normal variant short stature
NTTP	no tenderness to palpation	NW	naked weight
NTU	nephelometric turbidity units		nasal wash
NTX	naltrexone (ReVia)		normal weight
	neurotoxicity		not weighed
Ntx	N-telopeptide	NWB	nonweight bearing
NTZ	nitazoxanide (Alinia)	NWBL	nonweight bearing, left
NTZ Long-acting®	oxymetazoline nasal spray	NWBR	nonweight bearing, right
		NWC	number of words chosen
NU	name unknown	NWD	neuroleptic withdrawal
NUD	nonulcer dyspepsia		normal well developed
NUG	necrotizing ulcerative gingivitis	NWS	New World screwworm
nullip	nullipara		(*Cochliomyia hominivorax*
NUN	nonurea nitrogen		[Coquerel])
NV	naked vision	NWTS	National Wilms Tumor Study (rating
	nausea and vomiting		scale)
	near vision	NWTSG	National Wilms Tumor Study Group
	negative variation	Nx	nephrectomy
	neovascularization		next
	neurovascular	NX211	liposomal lurtotecan
	new vessel	NYB	New York Blood Center
	next visit	NYD	not yet diagnosed
	nonvenereal	NYHA	New York Heart Association
	nonveteran		(classification of heart disease)
	normal value	NYST	nystagmus
	not vaccinated	NZ	enzyme
	not verified		
N&V	nausea and vomiting		
NVA	near visual acuity		
NVAF	nonvalvular atrial fibrillation		
NVB	Navelbine (vinorelbine tartrate)		
NVBo	oral vinorelbine		
NVC	neurovascular checks		
nvCJD	new-variant Creutzfeldt-Jakob disease		
NVD	nausea, vomiting, and diarrhea		
	neck vein distention		
	neovascularization of the (optic) disc		
	neurovesicle dysfunction		
	normal vaginal delivery		
	no venereal disease		
	no venous distention		
	nonvalvular disease		
NVDC	nausea, vomiting, diarrhea, and constipation		
NVE	native		
	native valve endocarditis		
	neovascularization elsewhere		
NVG	neovascular glaucoma		
	neoviridogrisein		
NVI	neovascularization of the iris		
NVL	neurovascular laboratory		
NVLD	nonverbal learning disability		
NVM	neovascular membrane		

N

O

O	eye
	objective findings
	obvious
	occlusal
	often
	open
	oral
	ortho
	other
	oxygen
	pint
	zero
ō	negative
	no
	none
	pint
	without
O+	blood type O positive
	(O positive is preferred)
O−	blood type O negative
	(O negative is preferred)
Ⓞ	orally (by mouth)
$_1O_2$	singlet oxygen
O_2	both eyes
	oxygen
O_2^-	superoxide
O_3	ozone
O157	*Escherichia coli* O157
OA	occipital artery
	occipitoatlantal
	occiput anterior
	old age
	on admission
	on arrival
	ophthalmic artery
	oral airway
	oral alimentation
	osteoarthritis
	ovarian ablation
	Overeaters Anonymous
O/A	on or about
O & A	observation and assessment
	odontectomy and alveoloplasty
OAA	Old Age Assistance
OAA/S	Observer's Assessment of
	Alertness/Sedation
OAB	overactive bladder
OAC	omeprazole, amoxicillin, and
	clarithromycin
	oral anticoagulant(s)
	overaction
OAD	obliterative airway disease
	obstructive airway disease

	occlusive arterial disease
	overall diameter
OAE	otoacoustic emissions
OAF	oral anal fistula
	osteoclast activating factor
OAG	open angle glaucoma
OAM	omeprazole, amoxicillin, and
	metronidazole
OA/OS	ovarian ablation/suppression
OAP	old age pension
OAR	Ottawa Ankle Rules
OARs	organs at risk (from radiation
	therapy)
OAS	Older Adult Services
	oral allergy syndrome
	organic anxiety syndrome
	outpatient assessment service
	overall survival
	Overt Aggression Scale
OASDHI	Old Age, Survivors, Disability, and
	Health Insurance
OASI	Old Age and Survivors Insurance
OASIS	Outcomes and Assessment
	Information Set
OASO	overactive superior oblique
OASR	overactive superior rectus
OASS	Overt Agitation Severity Scale
OAT	oligoasthenoteratozoospermia
	oral anticoagulant therapy
	ornithine aminotransferase
OATP	organic anion-transporting
	polypeptide
OATS	osteochondral autograft transfer
	system
OAV	oculoauriculovertebral (dysplasia)
OAW	oral airway
OB	obese
	obesity
	obstetrics
	occult blood
	osteoblast
OBA	office-based anesthesia
	Office of Biotechnology Activities
	(NIH)
OB-A	obstetrics-aborted
OBD	obscure digestive bleeding
OB-Del	obstetrics-delivered
OBE	out-of-body experience
OBE-CALP	placebo capsule or tablet
OBF	ocular blood flow
OBG	obstetrics and gynecology
Ob-Gyn	obstetrics and gynecology
Obj	objective
obl	oblique
OB marg	obtuse marginal
OB-ND	obstetrics-not delivered
OBP	office blood pressure

OBRR	obstetric recovery room		oral contraceptive pills
OBS	observed		ova, cysts, parasites
	obstetrical service	OCR	oculocephalic reflex
	organic brain syndrome		optical character recognition
OBT	obtained	OCS	Obsessive-Compulsive Scale
OBTM	omeprazole, bismuth subcitrate,		Office of Child Services
	tetracycline, and metronidazole		(government agency)
OBUS	obstetrical ultrasound		oral cancer screening
OBW	open bed warmer	11-OCS	11-oxycorticosteroid
OC	observed cases	OCT	octreotide (Sandostatin)
	obstetrical conjugate		optical coherence tomograph
	occlusal curvature (dental)		(tomography)
	office call		oral cavity tumors
	on call		ornithine carbamyl transferase
	only child		oxytocin challenge test
	open cholecystectomy	OCU	observation care unit
	open colectomy	OCVM	occult cerebrovascular malformations
	open crib	OCX	oral cancer examination
	optical chromatography	OD	Doctor of Optometry
	oral care		Officer-of-the-Day
	oral contraceptive		oligodendroglial
	osteocalcin		once daily (this is a dangerous
	osteoclast		abbreviation as it is read as right
	ovarian cancer		eye; use "once daily")
	OxyContin (oxycodone)		on duty
O & C	onset and course		optic disc
OCA	oculocutaneous albinism		oral-duodenal
	open care area		outdoor
	oral contraceptive agent		outside diameter
OCAD	occlusive carotid artery disease		ovarian dysgerminoma
OCB	obstructive chronic bronchitis		overdose
OCBZ	oxcarbazepine(Trileptal)		right eye
OCC	occasionally	Δ OD 450	deviation of optical density at 450
	occlusal	ODA	occipitodextra anterior
	old chart called		once-daily aminoglycoside
OCCC	open chest cardiac compression		osmotic driving agent
	ovarian clear cell carcinoma	ODAC	Oncologic Drugs Advisory
occl	occlusion		Committee (of the US Food and
OCCM	open chest cardiac massage		Drug Administration)
OCC PR	open chest cardiopulmonary		on-demand analgesia computer
	resuscitation	ODAT	one day at a time
OCC Th	occupational therapy	ODC	oral disease control
Occup Rx	occupational therapy		ornithine decarboxylase
OCD	obsessive-compulsive disorder		outpatient diagnostic center
	osteochondritis dissecans	ODCH	ordinary diseases of childhood
OCE	outpatient code editor	ODCs	ozone-depleting chemicals
OCG	oral cholecystogram	ODD	oculodentodigital (dysplasia)
OCI	Obsessive-Compulsive Inventory		opposition defiance disorder
OCL®	oral colonic lavage	OD'd	overdosed
OCME	Office of the Chief Medical	ODECL	open-door expansile cervical
	Examiner		laminoplasty
OCN	obsessive-compulsive neurosis	ODed	overdosed
	Oncology Certified Nurse	ODM	occlusion dose monitor
OCNS	Obsessive-Compulsive Neurosis		ophthalmodynamometry
	Scale	ODMP	on-going data management plan
O-CNV	occult choroidal neovascularization	ODN	optokinetic nystagmus
OCOR	on-call to operating room	ODP	occipitodextra posterior
OCP	ocular cicatricial pemphigoid		offspring of diabetic parents

O

OD/P	right eye patched
ODQ	on direct questioning
ODS	Office of Drug Safety (FDA)
	organized delivery system
	osmotic demyelination syndrome
ODSS	Office of Disability Support Services
ODSU	oncology day stay unit
	One-Day Surgery Unit
ODT	occipitodextra transerve
	optical Doppler tomography
	orally disintegrating tablet
ODTS	organic dust toxic syndrome
OE	on examination
	orthopedic examination
	otitis externa
O-E	standard observed minus expected
O&E	observation and examination
OEC	outer ear canal
OEI	opioid escalation index
O$_2$EI	oxygen extraction index
OEL	occupational exposure level
OENT	oral endotracheal tube
OEP	Office of Emergency Preparedness
	oil of evening primrose (evening primrose oil)
OEPA	vincristine (Oncovin), etoposide, prednisone, and doxorubicin (Adriamycin)
OER	oxygen extraction ratios
O$_2$ER	oxygen extraction ratio
OERR	order entry/results-reports (Veterans Administration's physician computer order entry system)
OET	oral esophageal tube
OETT	oral endotracheal tube
OF	occipital-frontal
	optic fundi
	osteitis fibrosa
	outlet forceps (delivery)
OFC	occipital-frontal circumference
	orbitofacial cleft
OFF	shoes off during weighing
OFI	other febrile illness
OFLOX	ofloxacin (Floxin)
OFLX	ofloxacin (Floxin)
OFM	open-face mask
	oral focal mucinosis
OFNE	oxygenated fluorocarbon nutrient emulsion
OFPF	optic fundi and peripheral fields
OFR	oxygen-free radicals
OFTT	organic failure to thrive
OG	Obstetrics-Gynecology
	orogastric (feeding)
	outcome goal (long-term goal)
OGC	oculogyric crisis
OGCT	ovarian germ cell tumor

OGD	oesophagogastro-duodenoscopy (United Kingdom and other countries)
	Office of Generic Drugs (of the Food and Drug Administration)
OGNP	Obstetric-Gynecology Nurse Practitioner
OGT	orogastric tube
OGTT	oral glucose tolerance test
OH	occupational history
	ocular history
	ocular hypertension
	on hand
	open-heart
	oral hygiene
	orthostatic hypotension
	outside hospital
17-OH	17-hydroxycorticosteroids
OHA	oral hypoglycemic agents
OHC	outer hair cell (in cochlea)
OH Cbl	hydroxycobalamine
17-OHCS	17-hydroxycorticosteroids
OHD	hydroxy vitamin D
	organic heart disease
25(OH)D$_3$	25-hydroxy vitamin D (calcifediol, Calderol)
OHF	old healed fracture
	Omsk hemorrhagic fever
	overhead frame
OHFA	hydroxy fatty acid
OHFT	overhead frame and trapeze
OHG	oral hypoglycemic
OHI	oral hygiene instructions
OHIAA	hydroxyindolacetic acid
OHL	oral hairy leukoplakia
7-OHMTX	7-hydroxymethotrexate
OHNS	Otolaryngology, Head, and Neck Surgery (Dept.)
OHP	obese hypertensive patient
	oxygen under hyperbaric pressure
17 OHP	17-hydroxyprogesterone
OHRP	open-heart rehabilitation program
OHR-QOL	oral health-related quality of life
OHRR	open-heart recovery room
OHS	obesity hypoventilation syndrome
	occupational health service
	ocular histoplasmosis syndrome
	ocular hypoperfusion syndrome
	open-heart surgery
OHSS	ovarian hyperstimulation syndrome
OHT	ocular hypertension
	overhead trapeze
OHTN	ocular hypertension
OHTx	orthotopic heart transplantation
OI	opportunistic infection
	osteogenesis imperfecta
	otitis interna
OIC	opioid-induced constipation

O

OIF	oil-immersion field		obtuse marginal
OIG	Office of the Inspector General		ocular melanoma
OIH	orthoiodohippurate		oral motor
OIHA	orthoiodohippuric acid		oral mucositis
OI&I	occupational injury and illness		organomegaly
OIM	optical immunoassay		osteomalacia
OINT	ointment		osteomyelitis
OIR	oxygen-induced retinopathy		otitis media
OIRDA	occipital intermittent rhythmical delta activity	O_2M	oxygen mask
		OM_1	first obtuse marginal (branch)
OIS	ocular ischemic syndrome	OM_2	second obtuse marginal (branch)
	optical intrinsic signal (imaging)	OMA	older maternal age
	optimum information size	OMAC	otitis media, acute, catarrhal
OIs	opportunistic infections	OMAS	Olerud-Molander Ankle Score
OIT	ovarian immature teratoma		otitis media, acute, suppurating
OIU	optical internal urethrotomy	OMB	obtuse marginal branch
OJ	orange juice (this is a dangerous abbreviation as it is read as OS, left eye)	OMB_1	first obtuse marginal branch
		OMB_2	second obtuse marginal branch
		OMC	open mitral commissuortomy
	orthoplast jacket		ostiomeatal complex
OK	all right	OMCA	otitis media, catarrhalis, acute
	approved	OMCC	otitis media, catarrhalis, chronic
	correct	OMD	organic mental disorder
OKAN	optokinetic after nystagmus	OME	Office of Medical Examiner
OKC	odontogenic keratocyst		otitis media with effusion
	open kinetic chain	7-OMEN	menogaril
OKN	optokinetic nystagmus	OMFS	oral and maxillofacial surgery
OKT	Ortho Kung T-cell, designation for a series of antigens	OMG	ocular myasthenia gravis
		OMI	old myocardial infarct
OL	left eye	OMIEI	oral medication induced esophageal injury
	open label (study)	
OLA	occiput left anterior	OMP	oculomotor (third nerve) palsy
	occipitolaevoanterior		open mediastinal biopsy
OLAP	online analytical processing	OMPA	otitis media, purulent, acute
OLB	open-liver biopsy	OMPC	otitis media, purulent, chronic
	open-lung biopsy	OMR	operative mortality rate
OLBPQ	Oswestry Low Back Pain Questionnaire	OMS	oral morphine sulfate
			organic mental syndrome
OLC	ouabain-like compound		organic mood syndrome
OLD	obstructive lung disease	OMSA	otitis media secretory (or suppurative) acute
OLE	olive leaf extract	
OLF	ouabain-like factor	OMSC	otitis media secretory (or suppurative) chronic
OLM	ocular larva migrans	
	ophthalmic laser microendoscope	OMT	oral mucosal transudate
OLNM	occult lymph node metastases		Osteopathic manipulative technique (treatment)
OLP	oral lichen planus	
OLR	optic labyrinthine righting	OMVC	open mitral valve commissurotomy
	otology, laryngology, and rhinology	OMVD	optimized microvessel density (analysis)
OLS	ordinary least squares	
	ouabain-like substance	OMVI	operating motor vehicle intoxicated
OLT	occipitolaevoposterior	ON	every night (this is a dangerous abbreviation)
	orthotopic liver transplantation	
OLTP	online transaction processing		optic nerve
OLTx	orthotopic liver transplantation		optic neuropathy
OLV	one-lung ventilation		oronasal
OLZ	olanzapine (Zyprexa)		Ortho-Novum®
OM	every morning (this is a dangerous abbreviation)		overnight
		ONC	Orthopedic Nurse, Certified

O

	over-the-needle catheter		operation
	vincristine (Oncovin)		organophosphorous
OND	Office of New Drugs (FDA)		oropharynx
	ondansetron (Zofran)		oscillatory potentials
	other neurologic disorder(s)		osteoporosis
ONH	optic nerve head		outpatient
	optic nerve hypoplasia		overpressure
ONM	ocular neuromyotonia	O&P	ova and parasites (stool examination)
ON RR	overnight recovery room	OPA	Office of the Public Advocate
ONS	Office for National Statistics (United		(guardians)
	Kingdom)		oral pharyngeal airway
ONSD	optic nerve sheath decompression		outpatient anesthesia
ONSF	optic nerve sheath fenestration	OPAC	opacity (opacification)
ONTD	open neural tube defect(s)	OPAT	outpatient parenteral antibiotic
ONTR	orders not to resuscitate		therapy
OO	ophthalmic ointment	OPB	outpatient basis
	oral order	OPC	operable pancreatic carcinoma
	other		oropharyngeal candidiasis
	out of		outpatient care
o/o	on account of		outpatient catheterization
O&O	off and on		outpatient clinic
OOB	out of bed	OPCA	olivopontocerebellar atrophy
OOBL	out of bilirubin light	OPCAB	off-pump coronary artery bypass
OOBBRP	out of bed with bathroom privileges		(grafting)
OOC	onset of contractions	op cit	in the work cited
	out of cast	OPCs	oligodendrocyte precursor cells
	out of control	OPCS-4	Classification of Surgical Operations
OO Con	out of control		and Procedures (4th revision)
OOD	outer orbital diameter	OPCx	oligodendrocyte progenitor cells
	out of doors	OPD	oropharyngeal dysphagia
OO-EMG	electromyographic recording of the		Orphan Products Development
	orbicularis oculi muscles		(office of)
OOF	out of facility		outpatient department
OOH	out of hospital	O'p'-DDD	mitotane (Lysodren)
OOH&NS	ophthalmology, otorhinolaryngology,	OPDRA	Office of Postmarketing Drug Risk
	and head and neck surgery		Assessment (FDA) (name changed
OOI	out of isolette		to Office of Drug Safety [ODS])
OOL	onset of labor	OPDUR	on-line prospective drug utilization
OOLR	ophthalmology, otology, laryngology,		review
	and rhinology	OPE	oral peripheral examination
OOM	onset of menarche		outpatient evaluation
OOP	out of pelvis	OPEN	vincristine (Oncovin), prednisone,
	out of plaster		etoposide, and mitoxantrone
	out on pass		(Novantrone)
OOPS	out of program status	OPERA	outpatient endometrial
OOR	out of room		resection/ablation
OORW	out of radiant warmer	OPG	ocular plethysmography
OOS	out of sequence		orthopantomogram (dental)
	out of specification (deviation from		osteoprotegerin
	standard)	OPIDP	organophosphate-induced delayed
	out of splint		polyneuropathy
	out of stock	OPKA	opsonophagocytic killing assay
OOT	out of town	OPL	oral premalignant lesion
OOW	out of wedlock		other party liability
	out of work	OPLC	optimum performance liquid
OP	oblique presentation		chromatography
	occiput posterior	OPLL	ossification of posterior latitudinal
	open		ligament

O

OPM	occult primary malignancy	ORIF	open reduction internal fixation
	oral and pharyngeal mucositis	ORL	oblique retinacular ligament
OPMD	oculopharyngeal muscular dystrophy		otorhinolaryngology (otology,
OPN	open partial nephrectomy		rhinology and laryngology)
	osteopontin	ORMF	open reduction metallic fixation
OPO	organ procurement organizations	ORN	operating room nurse
	overnight pulse oximetry		osteoradionecrosis
OPOC	oral pharynx, oral cavity	OROS	ostomotic release oral system
OPP	opposite	ORP	occiput right posterior
OPPG	oculopneumoplethysmography		open radical prostatectomy
OPPOS	opposition	ORR	overall response rate
OPPS	Outpatient Prospective Payment	ORS	oculorespiratory syndrome
	System		olfactory reference syndrome
OPQRST	onset, provocation, quality, radiation,		oral rehydration salts
	severity, and time (an EMT	ORSA	oxacillin-resistant *Staphylococcus*
	mnemonic used in initial patient		*aureus*
	questioning)	ORT	oestrogen (estrogen)-replacement
OPRDU	outpatient renal dialysis unit		therapy (United Kingdom and
OPRT	orotate phosphoribosyl transferase		elsewhere)
OPS	Objective Pain Scores		operating room technician
	operations		oral rehydration therapy
	Orpington prognostic scale		Registered Occupational Therapist
	orthogonal polarization spectral	OR XI	oriented to time
	(imaging)	OR X2	oriented to time and place
	outpatient surgery	OR X3	oriented to time, place, and person
	overnight polysomnography	OR X4	oriented to time, place, person, and
OPSI	overwhelming postsplenectomy		objects (watch, pen, book)
	infection	OS	left eye
OPSU	oblique partial sit-up		mouth (this is a dangerous abbre
	outpatient surgical unit		viation as it is read as left eye)
O PSY	open psychiatry		occipitosacral
OPT	optimal pharmacological therapy		oligospermic
	optimum		opening snap
	outpatient treatment		ophthalmic solution (this is a
OPT c CA	Ohio pediatric tent with compressed		dangerous abbreviation as it is
	air		read as left eye)
OPT c O₂	Ohio pediatric tent with oxygen		oral surgery
OPTN	Organ Procurement and		Osgood-Schlatter (disease)
	Transplantation Network		osmium
OPT-NSC	outpatient treatment, nonservice-		osteosarcoma
	connected		overall survival
OPT-SC	outpatient treatment, service-	OSA	obstructive sleep apnea
	connected		off-site anesthesia
OPV	oral polio vaccine		online sexual activities
	outpatient visit		osteosarcoma
OR	odds ratio	OSA/HS	obstructive sleep apnea/ hypopnea
	oil retention		syndrome
	open reduction	OSAS	obstructive sleep apnea syndrome
	operating room	OSC	oral self-care
	Orthodox	OSCAR	On-line Survey Certification and
	own recognizance		Reporting
ORA	occiput right anterior	OSCC	oral squamous cell carcinoma
ORC	outpatient rehabilitation centers	OSCE	Objective Structured Clinical
ORCH	orchiectomy		Examination
ORD	orderly	OSD	Osgood-Schlatter disease
OREF	open reduction, external fixation		overseas duty
ORF	open reading frame		overside drainage
OR&F	open reduction and fixation	OSE	ovarian surface epithelium

O

OSESC	opening-snap ejection systolic click	OTS	orotracheal suction
OSFT	outstretched fingertips	OTT	oral transit time
OSG	osteosonogram (osteosonogrammetry)		orotracheal tube
OSH	outside hospital	OTW	off-the-wall
OSHA	Occupational Safety & Health Administration	OU	each eye
		OUES	oxygen uptake efficiency slope
OSM S	osmolarity serum	OULQ	outer upper left quadrant
OSM U	osmolarity urine	OU/P	both eyes patched
OSN	off-service note	OURQ	outer upper right quadrant
OSP	outside pass	OUS	obstetric ultrasound
OS/P	left eye patched	OV	office visit
OSS	osseous		ovary
	over-shoulder strap		ovum
OSSI	orthognathic surgery simulating instrument	OVAL	ovalocytes
		OvCa	ovarian cancer
OST	occipitosubtemporal	OVD	occlusal vertical dimension
	optimal sampling theory		ophthalmic viscosurgical device
	osteogenic sarcoma	OVF	Octopus® visual field
OT	occiput transverse	OVLT	organum vasculosum of lamina terminalis
	Occupational Therapist		
	occupational therapy	OVR	Office of Vocational Rehabilitation
	old tuberculin	OVS	obstructive voiding symptoms (syndrome)
	on-treatment		
	oral transmucosal	OW	once weekly (this is a dangerous abbreviation)
	orotracheal		
	outlier threshold		open wound
	oxytocin (Pitocin)		oral warts
O/T	oral temperature		outer wall
OTA	open to air		out of wedlock
OTC	occult tumor cell		ova weight
	ornithine transcarbamoylase		overweight
	Orthopedic Technician, Certified	O/W	oil in water
	over-the-counter (sold without prescription)		otherwise
		OWL	out of wedlock
OTCD	ornithine-transcarbamylase deficiency	OWNK	out of wedlock, not keeping (baby)
		OWR	Osler-Weber-Rendu (disease)
OTD	optimal therapeutic dose	OWT	zero work tolerance
	organ tolerance dose	OX	oximeter
	out-the-door	O×1	oriented to time
OTE	(McMaster) Overall Treatment Evaluation	O×2	oriented to time and place
		O×3	oriented to time, place, and person
OTFC	oral transmucosal fentanyl citrate (Fentanyl Oralet; Actiq)	O×4	oriented to time, place, person, and objects (watch, pen, book)
OTH	other	OXA	oxacillinase
OTHS	occupational therapy home service		oxaliplatin (Eloxatin)
OTIS	Organization of Teratology Information Services	OXC	oxcarbazepine (Trileptal)
		Oxi	oximeter (oximetry)
		Ox-LDL	oxidized low-density lipoprotein
OTJ	on-the-job (injury; training)	OXPHOS	oxidative phosphorylation
OTO	one-time only	OxPt	oxaliplatin (Eloxatin)
	otolaryngology	OXM	pulse oximeter
	otology	OXT	oxytocin (Pitocin)
OTPT	oral triphasic tablets (contraceptive)	Oxy-5®	benzoyl peroxide
OTR	Occupational Therapist, Registered	OxyIR®	oxycodone immediate release capsules
OTRL	Occupational Therapist, Registered Licensed		
		OXZ	oxazepam (Serax)
OT/RT	occupational therapy/recreational therapy	OZ	optical zone
			ounce

O

P

P para
peripheral
phosphorus
pint
plan
Plasmodium
poor
protein
Protestant
pulse
pupil

$\overline{P}$ statistical probability value

$\overline{p}$ after

/P partial lower denture

P/ partial upper denture

P1 pilocarpine 1% ophthalmic solution

P_2 pulmonic second heart sound

P20 Ocusert® P20

^{32}P radioactive phosphorus

P40 Ocusert® P40

P53 tumor suppressive gene

PA panic attack
paranoid
peanut allergy
periapical (x ray)
pernicious anemia
phenol alcohol
physical activity
Physician Assistant
pineapple
platelet aggregometry
posterior-anterior (posteroanterior)
 (x-ray)
premature adrenarche
presents again
primary aldosteronism
professional association (similar to a
 corporation)
Pseudomonas aeruginosa
psychiatric aide
psychoanalysis
pulmonary artery

Pa pascal

P&A percussion and auscultation
phenol and alcohol
position and alignment

$P_2 > A_2$ pulmonic second heart sound greater
 than aortic second heart sound

PAAA para-anastomotic aneurysm of the
 aorta

PAAD persistently and acutely disabled

PAB premature atrial beat
pulmonary artery banding

PABA aminobenzoic acid (para-
 aminobenzoic acid)

PABD preoperative autologous blood
 donation

PAC cisplatin (Platinol), doxorubicin
 (Adriamycin), and
 cylcophosphamide
phenacemide
Physical Assessment Center
Physician Assistant, Certified
picture archiving communication
 (system)
Port-a-cath®
premature atrial contraction
prophylactic anticonvulsants
pulmonary artery catheter

PA-C Physician Assistant, Certified

PACATH pulmonary artery catheter

PACE population-adjusted clinical
 epidemiology
Programs of All-Inclusive Care for
 the Elderly

PACG primary angle-closure glaucoma

PACH pipers to after coming head

PACI partial anterior cerebral infarct

$PACO_2$ partial pressure (tension) of carbon
 dioxide, alveolar

$PaCO_2$ partial pressure (tension) of carbon
 dioxide, artery

PACS picture archiving and
 communications systems

PACT prism and alternate cover test
Program of Assertive Community
 Treatment

PAC-V cisplatin (Platinol), doxorubicin
 (Adriamycin), and
 cyclophosphamide

PACU postanesthesia care unit

PAD pelvic adhesive disease
peripheral artery disease
persistently and acutely disabled
pharmacologic atrial defibrillator
physician-assisted death
preliminary anatomic diagnosis
preoperative autologous donation
primary affective disorder

PADCAB perfusion-assisted direct coronary
 artery bypass

PADP pulmonary arterial diastolic pressure
pulmonary artery diastolic pressure

PADS Post Anesthesia Discharge Scoring
 System

PADT primary androgen deprivation
 therapy

PAE percutaneous angiographic
 embolization
postanoxic encephalopathy
postantibiotic effect

P

	pre-admission evaluation		pancuronium (Pavulon)
	progressive assistive exercise		panoral x-ray examination
PAEDP	pulmonary artery and end-diastole pressure		periodic alternating nystagmus
PAEE	physical activity energy expenditure		polyacrylonitrile (filter)
PAF	paroxysmal atrial fibrillation		polyarteritis nodosa
	platelet-activating factor		polyomavirus-associated nephropathy
	population attributable fraction	pANCA	perinuclear antineutrophil cytoplasmic antibody
PA&F	percussion, auscultation, and fremitus	PANDAS	pediatric autoimmune neuropsychiatric disorders
PAFE	postantifungal effect		associated with streptococcal infections
PAGA	premature appropriate for gestational age	PANENDO	panendoscopy
PAGE	polyacrylamide gel electrophoresis	PANESS	physical and neurological examination for soft signs
PAH	para-aminohippurate	PanIN-1	pancreatic intraepithelial neoplasm
	partial abdominal hysterectomy		(low grade); there is a 1A and 1B
	phenylalanine hydroxylase	PanIN-2	pancreatic intraepithelial neoplasm (moderate grade)
	polycyclic aromatic hydrocarbons	PanIN-3	pancreatic intraepithelial neoplasm (high grade)
	polynuclear aromatic hydrocarbon		
	predicted adult height		
	primary adrenal hyperplasia		
	pulmonary arterial hypertension		
PAHO	Pan American Health Organization	PANP	pelvic autonomic nerve preservation
PAI	penetrating abdominal injury	PANSS	Positive and Negative Syndrome Scale
	plasminogen activator inhibitor		
	platelet accumulation index	PANSS-EC	Positive and Negative Symptoms of
PAIDS	pediatric acquired immunodeficiency syndrome		Schizophrenia-Excited Component
		PAO	peak acid output
PAIgG	platelet-associated immunoglobulin G		peripheral arterial occlusion
		PAO₂	alveolar oxygen pressure (tension)
PAIR	Puncture, Aspiration, Injection,	PaO₂	arterial oxygen pressure (tension)
	Reaspiration (technique)	PAOD	peripheral arterial occlusive disease
PAIVMs	passive accessory intervertebral movements	PAOP	pulmonary artery occlusion pressure
		PAP	passive-aggressive personality
PAIVS	pulmonary atresia with intact ventricular septum		patient assistance program
			peroxidase-anti-peroxidase
PAK	pancreas and kidney		pokeweed antiviral protein
PAL	physical activity levels		positive airway pressure
	posterior axillary line		primary atypical pneumonia
	posteroanterior and lateral		prostatic acid phosphatase
	pyothorax-associated lymphoma		pulmonary alveolar proteinosis
PALA	N-phosphoacetate-L aspartate		pulmonary artery pressure
Pa Line	pulmonary artery line	PAPAW	pushrim-activated power-assisted wheelchair
PALN	para-aortic lymph node		
PALP	palpation	PAPS	primary antiphospholipid syndrome
PALS	pediatric advanced life support	Pap smear	Papanicolaou smear
	periarterial lymphatic sheath	PA/PS	pulmonary atresia/pulmonary stenosis
PAM	partial allosteric modulators		
	Payment Accuracy Measurement	PAPVC	partial anomalous pulmonary venous connection
	potential acuity meter		
	primary acquired melanosis	PAPVR	partial anomalous pulmonary venous return
	primary amebic meningoencephalitis		
	protein A mimetic	PAQLQ	Pediatric Asthma Quality of Life Questionnaire
2-PAM	pralidoxime (Protopam)		
PAMP	pulmonary arterial (artery) mean pressure	PAR	parafin
			parainfluenza (paramyxovirus) vaccine
PAN	pancreas		parallel
	pancreatic		

perennial allergic rhinitis
platelet aggregate ratio
population attributable risks
possible allergic reaction
postanesthetic recovery
procedures, alternatives, and risks
pulmonary arteriolar resistance

PARA number of pregnancies producing viable offspring
paraplegic
parathyroid

PARA 1 having borne one child
Paraflu Parainfluenza
PARC perennial allergic rhinoconjunctivitis
PAROM passive assistance range of motion
PARQ procedures, risks, alternatives and questions
PARR plasma aldosterone/renin activity ratio
postanesthesia recovery room
PARS postanesthesia recovery score
PARs participating physicians (Medicare)
PART para-aortic radiotherapy
PARU postanesthetic recovery unit
PAS aminosalicylic acid (para-aminosalicylic acid)
periodic acid-Schiff (reagent)
peripheral anterior synechia
physician-assisted suicide
pneumatic antiembolic stocking
postanesthesia score
premature auricular systole
Professional Activities Study
pulmonary artery stenosis
pulsatile antiembolism system (stockings)
PA-S Physician Assistant, Student
PASA aminosalicylic acid (para-aminosalicylic acid)
PASARR Preadmission Screening Assessment and Annual Resident Review
PA/S/D pulmonary artery systolic/diastolic
PASE Physical Activity Scale for the Elderly
Pas Ex passive exercise
PASG pneumatic antishock garment
PASI Psoriasis Area and Severity Index
PASK peripheral anterior stromal keratopathy
PASP pulmonary artery systolic pressure
PASS Pain Anxiety Symptoms Scale
PAT Paddington alcohol test
paroxysmal atrial tachycardia
passive alloimmune thrombocytopenia
patella
patient
percent acceleration time

peripheral arterial tone
platelet aggregation test
preadmission testing
pregnancy at term
PATH Physicians at Teaching Hospitals (Medicare Audit)
pituitary adrenotropic hormone
pathology
PATP preadmission testing program
PATS payment at time of service
PAV Pavulon (pancuronium bromide)
pre-admission visit (hospice care initial home visit)
PAVe procarbazine, melphalan (Alkeran), and vinblastine (Velban)
PAVF pulmonary arteriovenous fistula
PAVM pulmonary arteriovenous malformation
PAVNRT paroxysmal atrial ventricular nodal re-entrant tachycardia
PAWP pulmonary artery wedge pressure
PAX periapical x-ray
PB barometric pressure
British Pharmacopeia
parafin bath
phenylbutyrate
piggyback
powder board
power building
premature beat
Presbyterian
protein-bound
Prussian blue
pudendal block
pyridostigmine bromide (Mestinon)
Pb lead
phenobarbital
p/b postburn
P&B pain and burning
Papanicolaou and breast (examinations)
phenobarbital and belladonna
PBA percutaneous bladder aspiration
pseudobulbar affect
PBAC Pharmaceutical Benefits Advisory Committee
PBAL protected bronchoalveolar lavage
PbB whole blood lead
PBC point of basal convergence
prebed care
primary biliary cirrhosis
PBD percutaneous biliary drainage
postburn day
proliferative breast disease
PBDs psychotic and behavioral disturbances
PBE partial breech extraction
population bioequivalence

205

	power building exercise		*Pneumocystis carinii*
PBF	peripheral blood film		poor condition
	placental blood flow		politically correct
	pulmonary blood flow		popliteal cyst
PBFS	penile blood flow study		posterior canals (vestibular)
PBG	porphobilinogen		posterior chamber
	pressure breathing for G protection		prednicarbate
	pupillary block glaucoma		premature contractions
PBI	partial breast irradiation		present complaint
	protein-bound iodine		productive cough
PBK	pseudophakic bullous keratopathy		professional corporation
PBL	peripheral blood lymphocyte		psychiatric counselor
	primary breast lymphoma		pubococcygeus (muscle)
	primary brain lymphoma	*p.c.*	after meals
	problem-based learning	PCA	passive cutaneous anaphylaxis
PBLC	premature birth live child		patient care assistant (aide)
PBM	pharmacy benefit management		patient-controlled analgesia
	(manager)		penicillamine (Cuprimine)
PBMA	polybutylmethacrylate		porous coated anatomic (joint
PBMC	peripheral blood mononuclear cell		replacement)
PBMNC	peripheral blood mononuclear cell		postcardiac arrest
PBN	polymyxin B sulfate, bacitracin, and		postciliary artery
	neomycin		postconceptional age
PB:ND	problem: nursing diagnosis		posterior cerebral artery
PBNS	percutaneous bladder neck		posterior communicating artery
	stabilization		procainamide
PBO	placebo		procoagulation activity
PBP	penicillin-binding protein		prostate cancer
	phantom breast pain	PCa	prostate cancer
	protein-bound polysaccharide	PCAC	Physical Care Assessment Center
PBPC	peripheral blood progenitor cell	P-CAC	preparative continuous annular
PBPCT	peripheral blood progenitor cell		chromatography
	transplantation	PCAD	posterior circulation arterial
PBPI	penile-brachial pulse index		dissection
PBPs	penicillin-binding proteins	PCASSO	patient-centered access to secure
PBS	phosphate-buffered saline		systems online
	prune-belly syndrome	PCB	pancuronium bromide
PBSC	peripheral blood stem cells		para cervical block
PBT	primary brain tumor		placebo
PBT$_4$	protein-bound thyroxine		postcoital bleeding
PbtO$_2$	brain tissue partial pressure of		prepared childbirth
	oxygen		procarbazine (Matulane)
PBV	percutaneous balloon valvuloplasty		*Pseudomonas cepacia* bacteremia
PBZ	phenoxybenzamine (Dibenzyline)	PCBH	personal care boarding home
	phenylbutazone	PCBMN	palmar cutaneous branch of the
	pyribenzamine		median nerve
ΦBZ	phenylbutazone	PCBs	polychlorinated biphenyls
PC	after meals (*p.c.* preferred)	PCBUN	palmar cutaneous branch of the ulnar
	cisplatin (Platinol) and		nerve
	cyclophosphamide	PCC	patient care coordinator
	packed cells		petrous carotid canal
	paclitaxel; carboplatin		pheochromocytoma
	palliative care		pneumatosis cystoides coli
	pancreatic carcinoma		poison control center
	pathologic consultation		precipitated calcium carbonate
	photocoagulation		progressive cardiac care
	placebo-controlled (study)	PCCC	pediatric critical care center
	platelet concentrate	PCCI	penetrating craniocerebral injuries

P

PCCM	primary care case management	PCLS	precision-cut lung slices
	pulmonary and critical care medicine	PCM	pharmaceutical case management
PCCU	postcoronary care unit		primary cutaneous melanoma
PCD	pacer-cardioverter-defibrillator		protein-calorie malnutrition
	paroxysmal cerebral dysrhythmia		pubococcygeal muscle
	plasma cell dyscrasias	PC-MRI	phase-contrast magnetic resonance
	postmortem cesarean delivery		imaging
	primary ciliary dyskinesia	PCMX	chloroxylenol
	programmed cell death	PCN	penicillin
PCDAI	Pediatric Crohn Disease Activity		percutaneous nephrostomy
	Index		primary care nursing
PCE	physical capacities evaluation	PCNA	patient care nursing assistant
	potentially compensable event		proliferating cell nuclear antigen
	pseudophakic corneal edema	PCNL	percutaneous nephrostolithotomy
PCE®	erythromycin particles in tablets	PCNs	posterior cervical nodes
PCEA	patient-controlled epidural analgesia	PCNSL	primary central nervous system
PCEAO	postcarotid endarterectomy airway		lymphoma
	obstruction	PCNT	percutaneous nephrostomy tube
PCEC	purified chick embryo cell (culture)	PCO	patient complains of
PCECV	purified chick embryo cell vaccine		polycystic ovary
PCF	pharyngeal conjunctival fever		posterior capsular opacification
PCFL	primary cutaneous follicular	PCO₂	partial pressure (tension) of carbon
	lymphoma		dioxide, artery
PCFT	platelet complement fixation test	PCOD	polycystic ovarian disease
PCG	phonocardiogram	PCOE	prescriber (physician) computer
	plasma cell granuloma		order entry
	primary congenital glaucoma	P COMM	posterior communicating
	pubococcygeus (muscle)	A	artery
PCGG	percutaneous coagulation of	PCOS	polycystic ovary syndrome
	gasserian ganglion	PCP	Palliative Care Program
PCGLV	poorly contractile globular left		patient care plan
	ventricle		phencyclidine (phenylcyclohexyl
PCG/Ts	Primary Care Groups and Trusts		piperidine)
PCH	paroxysmal cold hemoglobinuria		*Pneumocystis carinii (jirovecii)*
	periocular capillary hemangioma		pneumonia
	personal care home		primary care person
PCHI	permanent childhood hearing		primary care physician
	impairment		primary care provider
PCHL	permanent childhood hearing loss		prochlorperazine (Compazine)
PC&HS	after meals and at bedtime		pulmonary capillary pressure
PCI	percutaneous coronary intervention	PCR	patient care report
	pneumatosis cystoides intestinalis		percutaneous coronary
	prophylactic cranial irradiation		revascularization
PCINA	patient-controlled intranasal		polymerase chain reaction
	analgesia		protein catabolic rate
PCIOL	posterior chamber intraocular lens	PCr	plasma creatinine
PC-IRV	pressure-controlled inverse-ratio	pCR	pathological complete response
	ventilation	PCRA	pure red-cell aplasia
PCKD	polycystic kidney disease	PCR/PSA	polymerase chain reaction analysis
PCL	pacing cycle length		of prostate-specific antigen
	plasma cell leukemia	PCS	patient care system
	posterior chamber lens		patient-controlled sedation
	posterior cruciate ligament		personal care service
	proximal collateral ligament		photon correlation spectroscopy
PCLD	polycystic liver disease		physical component summary
PCLI	plasma cell labeling index		portable cervical spine
PCLN	psychiatric consultation liaison nurse		portacaval shunt
PCLR	paid claims loss ratio		postconcussion syndrome

P

P c/s	primary cesarean section	2PD	two point discriminatory test
PC-SPES	an herbal refined powder preparation of eight medicinal plants	[103]Pd	palladium 103
		PDA	pancreatic ductal adenocarcinoma
PCT	parasite-clearance time		parenteral drug abuser
	percent		patent ductus arteriosus
	photochemical treatment		pathological demand avoidance (syndrome)
	poker chip tool (for rating pain)		
	porphyria cutanea tarda		personal digital assistant
	postcoital test		poorly differentiated adenocarcinoma
	posterior chest tube		
	Primary Care Trust (United Kingdom)		posterior descending (coronary) artery
	primary chemotherapy		property damage accident
	progesterone challenge test	PDAD	photodiode array detector
PCTA	percutaneous transluminal angioplasty	PDAF	platelet-derived angiogenesis factor
		PDAP	peritoneal dialysis-associated peritonitis
PCTS	patient-controlled transdermal system		
		PDB	preperitoneal distention balloon
PCU	palliative care unit	PDC	patient denies complaints
	primary care unit		poorly differentiated carcinoma
	progressive care unit		private diagnostic clinic
	protective care unit		property damage collision (crash)
PCV	packed cell volume		pyruvate dehydogenase complex
	polycythemia vera	PD&C	postural drainage and clapping
	pressure-controlled ventilation	PDCA	Plan-Do-Check-Act (process improvement)
	procarbazine, lomustine (CCNU [Cee Nu]), and vincristine		
		PDD	cisplatin (Platinol)
PCV 7	pneumococcal 7-valent conjugate vaccine (Prevnar)		Parkinson disease cases with dementia
			pervasive developmental disorder
PCV 23	pneumococcal vaccine polyvalent (Pneumovax 23; Pnu-Imune 23)		premenstrual dysphoric disorder
			primary degenerative dementia
PCVC	percutaneous central venous catheter	PDDNOS	pervasive developmental disorder, not otherwise specified
PCWP	pulmonary capillary wedge pressure		
PCX	paracervical	PDDs	pervasive developmental disorders
PCXR	portable chest radiograph	PDE	paroxysmal dyspnea on exertion
PCZ	procarbazine (Matulane)		pulsed Doppler echocardiography
	prochlorperazine (Compazine)	PDE4	phosphodiesterase type 4
PD	interpupillary distance	PDE 5	phosphodiesterase type 5
	Paget disease	PDEGF	platelet-derived epidermal growth factor
	pancreaticoduodenectomy		
	panic disorder	PDF	Portable Document Format
	Parkinson disease	PDFC	premature dead female child
	patient detected	PDGF	platelet-derived growth factor
	penile sclerosis	PDGXT	predischarge graded exercise test
	percutaneous drain	PDH	past dental history
	peritoneal dialysis		pyruvate dehydrogenase
	personality disorder	PDI	Pain Disability Index
	pharmacodynamics		phasic detrusor instability
	pocket depth (dental)		psychomotor developmental index
	poorly differentiated	PDIGC	patient dismissed in good condition
	post dates	PDL	periodontal ligament
	postural drainage		poorly differentiated lymphocytic
	pressure dressing		
	prism diopter		postures of daily living
	probing depth (dental)		preferred drug list
	progressive disease		progressively diffused leukoencephalopathy
	pupillary distance		
P/D	packs per day (cigarettes)		pulsed-dye laser

P

PDL-D	poorly differentiated lymphocytic-diffuse	PDWI	proton-density-weighted image(s)
PDL-N	poorly differentiated lymphocytic-nodular	PDX	pyridoxine (vitamin B$_6$)
		PDx	principal diagnosis
PDMC	premature dead male child	pDXA	peripheral dual energy x-ray absorptiometry
PDN	Paget disease of the nipple	PE	cisplatin (Platinol) and etoposide
	painful diabetic neuropathy		pedal edema
	prednisone		pelvic examination
	private duty nurse		pharyngoesophageal
	prosthetic disk nucleus		phenytoin equivalent (150 mg of
PDNE	poorly differentiated neuroendocrine (carcinoma)		fosphenytoin sodium is equivalent to 100 mg of phenytoin sodium)
PDOX	pegylated doxorubicin		physical education (gym)
PDP	pachydermoperiostosis		physical examination
	peak diastolic pressure		physical exercise
	prescription drug plan		plasma exchange
PD & P	postural drainage and percussion		pleural effusion
PDPH	postdural puncture headache		pneumatic equalization
PDPM	peripapillary detachment in pathologic myopia		polyethylene
			preeclampsia
PDPT	patient-delivered partner therapy		premature ejaculation
PDQ	pretty damn quick (at once)		pressure equalization
PDQ-39	Parkinson Disease Questionnaire		pulmonary edema
PDQ-R	Personality Diagnostic Questionnaire-Revised		pulmonary embolism
		P$_1$E$_1$®	epinephrine 1%, pilocarpine 1% ophthalmic solution
PDR	patients' dining room		
	Physicians' Desk Reference	P&E	prep and enema
	point of decreasing response	PE24	Preemie Enfamil 24
	postdelivery room	PEA	pelvic examination under anesthesia
	proliferative diabetic retinopathy		
	prospective drug review		phenylethylamine
PDRcVH	proliferative diabetic retinopathy with vitreous hemorrhage		pre-emptive analgesia
			pulseless electrical activity
PDRP	proliferative diabetic retinopathy	PEARL	physiologic endometrial ablation/resection loop
PDRUL	palmar distal radioulnar ligament		
PDS	pain dysfunction syndrome		pupils equal accommodation, reactive to light
	persistent developmental stuttering		
	polydioxanone suture		pupils equal and reactive to light
	power Doppler sonography	PEARLA	pupils equal and react to light and accommodation
	Progressive Deterioration Scale		
PDSA	Plan, Do, Study, and Act	PEB	cisplatin, etoposide, and bleomycin
PDSS	Postpartum Depression Screening Scale	PEC	pectoralis
			Physician Emergency Certificate (the 15 day hold certificate used in psychiatric hospitals)
PDT	percutaneous dilatational tracheostomy		
	photodynamic therapy		pulmonary ejection click
	postdisaster trauma	PECCE	planned extracapsular cataract extraction
PDTC	pyrrolidine dithiocarbamate		
PDU	PCR (polymerase chain reaction)-detectable units	PECHO	prostatic echogram
		PECHR	peripheral exudative choroidal hemorrhagic retinopathy
	pulsed Doppler ultrasonography		
PDUFA	Prescription Drug User Fee Act (1992)	PECO$_2$	mixed expired carbon dioxide tension
PDUR	postdialysis urea rebound	PED	paroxysmal exertion-induced dyskinesia
	prospective drug utilization review		
PDW	platelet distribution width		pediatrics
PDWHF	platelet-derived wound healing factors		pigment epithelial detachments
		PEDD	proton-electron dipole-dipole

P

PEDI	pediatric evaluation of disability inventory		percutaneous epidural nerve stimulator
PEDI-DEG	pediatric deglycerolized red blood cells	PEO	progressive external ophthalmoplegia
Peds	pediatrics	PEP	patient education program
PEE	punctate epithelial erosion		pharmacologic erection program
PEEP	positive end-expiratory pressure		positive expiratory pressure
PEF	cisplatin (Platinol), epirubicin, and fluorouracil		postexposure prophylaxis
			preejection period
	peak expiratory flow		primer extension preamplification
PEFR	peak expiratory flow rate		protein electrophoresis
PEFSR	partial expiratory flow static recoil curve	PEP/ET	pre-ejection period/ ejection time
		PEPI	preejection period index
PEG	pegylated	PEPP	payment error prevention program
	percutaneous endoscopic gastrostomy	PER	by
			pediatric emergency room
	pneumoencephalogram		pertussis (whooping cough) vaccine, antigens not otherwise unspecified
	polyethylene glycol		
PEG-ELS	polyethylene glycol and iso-osmolar electrolyte solution		protein efficiency ratio
		PER$_a$	pertussis, acellular antigen(s), vaccine
PEGG	Parent Education and Guidance Group	PERC	perceptual
			percutaneous
PEG-J	percutaneous endoscopic gastrojejunostomy	PERF	perfect
			perforation
PEG-JET	percutaneous endoscopic gastrostomy with jejunal extension tube	Peri Care	perineum care
		PERIO	periodontal disease
			periodontitis
PEG-SOD	polyethylene glycol-conjugated superoxide dismutase (pegorgotein)	peri-pads	perineal pads
		PERL	pupils equal, reactive to light
		PERLA	pupils equally reactive to light and accommodation
PEI	cisplatin (Platinol), etoposide, and ifosfamide		
		per os	by mouth (this is a dangerous abbreviation as it is read as left eye [OS])
	percutaneous ethanol injection		
	phosphate excretion index		
	physical efficiency index	PERR	pattern evoked retinal response
	polyethylenimine	PERRL	pupils equal, round, and reactive to light
PEIT	percutaneous ethanol injection therapy		
		PERRLA	pupils equal, round, reactive to light and accommodation
PEJ	percutaneous endoscopic jejunostomy		
		PERR-LADC	pupils equal, round, reactive to light and accommodation directly and consensually
PEK	punctate epithelial keratopathy		
PEL	permissible exposure limits		
	primary effusion lymphomas	PERRRLA	pupils equal, round, regular, react to light and accommodation
PELD	percutaneous endoscopic lumbar diskectomy		
		PERS	personal emergency response systems
PELOD	pediatric logistic organ dysfunction (score)		
		PERT	pancreatic enzyme replacement therapy
PELV	pelvimetry		
PEM	prescription event monitoring		program evaluation and review technique
	protein-energy malnutrition		
PEMA	phenylethylmalonamide	PERV	porcine endogenous retroviruses
PEMS	physical, emotional, mental, and safety	PER$_w$	pertussis, whole-cell antigens, vaccine
		PES	paclitaxel-eluting stent
	post-exercise muscle soreness		polyethersulfone
PEN	pancreatic endocrine neoplasm		preexcitation syndrome
	parenteral and enteral nutrition		programmed electrical stimulation
	Pharmacy Equivalent Name		pseudoexfoliation syndrome
PENS	percutaneous electrical nerve stimulation	PESA	percutaneous epididymal sperm aspiration

P

peSPL	peak equivalent sound pressure level	PFL+IFN	cisplatin (Platinol), fluorouracil, leucovorin, and interferon alfa 2b
PET	poor exercise tolerance		
	positron-emission tomography	PFM	peak flow meter
	preeclamptic toxemia		permanent first molars
	pressure equalizing tubes		porcelain fused to metal
	problem elicitation technique		primary fibromyalgia
PETN	pentaerythritol tetranitrate	PFME	pelvic floor muscle exercise
PEX	plasma exchange	PFO	patent foramen ovale
	pseudoexfoliation (glaucoma)	PFP	progression free probability
PEx	physical examination		proinsulin fusion protein
PEX# 3	plasma exchange number three	PFPC	Pall filtered packed cells
PF	patellofemoral	PFPS	patellofemoral pain syndrome
	peak flow	PFR	parotid flow rate
	peripheral fields		peak flow rate
	plantar flexion		pelvic floor relaxation
	Pontiac fever	PFRC	plasma-free red cells
	power factor	PFROM	pain-free range of motion
	preservative free	PFS	patellar femoral syndrome
	prostatic fluid		patient financial services
	pulmonary fibrosis		prefilled syringe
	push fluids		preservative-free solution (system)
Pf	*Plasmodium falciparum*		primary fibromyalgia syndrome
PF3	platelet factor 3		progression-free survival
PF4	platelet factor 4		prolonged febrile seizure
16PF	The Sixteen Personality Factors test		pulmonary function studies (study)
PFA	foscarnet (phosphonoformatic acid) (Foscavir)	PFSH	past, family, and social history (histories)
	patellofemoral arthritis	PFT	parafascicular thalamotomy
	platelet function analysis		pulmonary function test
	psychological first aid	PFTC	primary fallopian tube carcinoma
	pure free acid	PFU	plaque-forming unit
PFB	potential for breakdown	PFW	pHisoHex® face wash
	pseudofolliculitis barbae	PFWB	Pall filtered whole blood
PFC	patient-focused care		Psychological General Well-Being (index)
	perfluorochemical		
	permanent flexure contracture	PFWT	pain-free walking time
	persistent fetal circulation	PG	paged in hospital
	prefrontal cortex		paregoric
	prolonged febrile convulsions		performance goal (short-term goal)
P̄ FEEDS	after feedings		phosphatidylglycerol
PFFD	proximal femoral focal deficiency (defect)		picogram (pg) (10^{-12} gram)
PFFFP	Pall filtered fresh frozen plasma		placental grade (biophysical profile)
PFG	patellofemoral grind		polygalacturonate
	percutaneous fluoroscopic gastrostomy		practice guidelines
	proximal femur geometry		pregnant
	pulsed-field gradient		prostaglandin
PFGE	pulsed field gel electrophoresis		pyoderma gangrenosum
PfHRP-2	*Plasmodium falciparum* histidine-rich protein 2	PGA	prostaglandin A
			prothrombin time, **g**amma-glutamyl transpeptidase activity, and serum **a**polipoprotein AI concentration
PFHx	positive family history		
PFI	pill-free intervals	PGB	pregabalin (Lyrica)
	progression-free interval	PGBD	polyglucosan body disease
PFJ	patellofemoral joint	PGCG	peripheral giant cell granuloma
PFJS	patellofemoral joint syndrome	PGCH	postinfantile giant cell hepatitis
PFL	cisplatin (Platinol), fluorouracil, and leucovorin	PGCR	pharyngoglottal closure reflex
		PGCs	primordial germ cells

P

PGD	pelvic girdle dysfunction	PHACO	phacoemulsification
	preimplantation genetic diagnosis	PHACO OD	phacoemulsification of the right eye
3-PGDH	3-phosphoglyerate-dehdyrogenase		
PGE	partial generalized epilepsy	PHACO OS	phacoemulsification of the left eye
	posterior gastroenterostomy		
	proximal gastric exclusion	PHAL	peripheral hyperalimentation
PGE_1	alprostadil (prostaglandin E_1)	PHAR	pharmacist
PGE_2	dinoprostone (prostaglandin E_2)		pharmacy
PGED	Practice Guideline for Eating Disorders		pharynx
		Pharm	Pharmacy
PGF	paternal grandfather	PharmD	Doctor of Pharmacy
	placental growth factor	PHb	pyridoxylated hemoglobin
$PGF_{2\alpha}$	dinoprost (prostaglandin $F_{2\alpha}$)	PHC	permissive hypercapnia
PGGF	paternal great-grandfather		posthospital care
PGGM	paternal great-grandmother		primary health care
PGH	pituitary growth hormones		primary hepatocellular carcinoma
PGI	potassium, glucose, and insulin	PHCA	profound hypothermic cardiac arrest
PGI_2	epoprostenol (Prostacyclin)	PHD	paroxysmal hypnogenic dyskinesia
PGL	persistent generalized lymphadenopathy		Public Health Department
		PhD	Doctor of Philosophy
	primary gastric lymphoma	PHE	periodic health examination
PGM	paternal grandmother	PHEN-FEN	phentermine and fenfluramine
	phosphoglucomutase		
PGP	paternal grandparent	PHEO	pheochromocytoma
Pgp	P-glycoprotein	PHEP	progressive home exercise program
PGR	pulse-generated runoff	PHF	paired helical filament
PgR	progesterone receptor	PHG	portal hypertensive gastropathy
P-graph	penile plethysmograph	PHH	paraesophageal hiatus hernia
PGS	Persian Gulf syndrome		posthemorrhagic hydrocephalus
PGT	play-group therapy	PHHI	persistent hyperinsulinemic hypoglycemia of infancy
PGTC	primary generalized tonic-clonic (seizures)		
		PHI	patient health information
P±GTC	partial seizures with or without generalized tonic-clonic seizures		phosphohexose isomerase
			prehospital index
pGTD	persistent gestational trophoblastic disease		protected health information
		PHIS	posthead injury syndrome
PG-TXL	poly (L-glutamic acid)-paclitaxel	PHL	permanent hearing loss
PGU	postgonococcal urethritis		Philadelphia (chromosome)
PGW	person gametocyte week	PHLIS	Public Health Laboratory Information System
PGY-1	postgraduate year one (first year resident)		
		PHLS	Public Health Laboratory Service (United Kingdom)
pH	hydrogen ion concentration		
PH	past history	PHM	partial hydatidiform mole
	personal history		preventative health maintenance
	pinhole	PHMB	polyhexamethylene biguanine
	poor health	PHMD	polyhexamethylene (Baquacil, a pool cleaner)
	pubic hair		
	public health	PHN	postherpetic neuralgia
	pulmonary hypertension		Public Health Nurse
P&H	physical and history		Puritan® heated nebulizer
Ph^1	Philadelphia chromosome	PHNC	public health nurse coordinator
PHA	arterial pH	PHNI	pinhole no improvement
	passive hemagglutinating	PHO	Physician/Hospital Organization
	paternal history of alcoholism	PHOB	phobic anxiety
	peripheral hyperalimentation	PHONO	phonophoresis
	phenylalanine	PHP	pooled human plasma
	phytohemagglutinin antigen		postheparin plasma
	postoperative holding area		prepaid health plan

P

	pseudohypoparathyroidism	PIB	partial ileal bypass
	pyridoxalated hemoglobin		professional information brochure
	polyoxyethylene conjugate	PiB	Pittsburgh Compound B
PHPPO	Public Health Practice Program	PIBD	paucity of interlobular bile ducts
	Office	PIBF	progesterone-induced blocking factor
PHPT	primary hyperparathyroidism	PIC	penicillin-inhibitor combinations
PHPV	persistent hyperplastic primary		peripherally inserted catheter
	vitreous		personal injury collision (crash)
PHR	peak heart rate		polysaccharide-iron complex
	personal health record		postintercourse
PhRMA	Pharmaceutical Research and	PICA	Porch Index of Communicative
	Manufacturers of America		Ability
PHRN	Pre-Hospital Registered Nurse		posterior inferior cerebellar artery
PHS	partial hospitalization program		posterior inferior communicating
	US Public Health Service		artery
PHT	phenytoin (Dilantin)	PICC	peripherally inserted central
	portal hypertension		catheter
	posterior hyaloidal traction	PICHI	pulse-inversion contrast harmonic
	postmenopausal hormone therapy		imaging
	primary hyperthyroidism	PICT	pancreatic islet cell transplantation
	pulmonary hypertension	PICU	pediatric intensive care unit
PHTC	pulmonary hypertensive crises		psychiatric intensive care unit
PHV	peak height velocity	PICVA	percutaneous *in situ* coronary venous
	pediatric health visit		arterialization
PHVA	pinhole visual acuity	PICVC	peripherally inserted central venous
pHVA	plasma homovanillic acid		catheter
PHVD	posthemorrhagic ventricular dilatation	PID	pelvic inflammatory disease
PHx	past history		primary immunodeficiency
Phx	pharynx		prolapsed intervertebral disk
PHY	physician		proportional-integral-derivative
PhyO	physician's orders		(controller)
PI	package insert	PIE	pulmonary infiltration with
	pallidal index		eosinophilia
	pancreatic insufficiency		pulmonary interstitial emphysema
	Pearl Index	PIEE	pulsed irrigation for enhanced
	performance improvement		evacuation
	peripheral iridectomy	PIF	peak inspiratory flow
	persistent illness	PIFG	poor intrauterine fetal growth
	physically impaired	PIG	pertussis immune globulin
	plaque index (dental)	PIGD	postural instability and gait difficulty
	poison ivy		(disorder)
	postincident	PIGI	pregnancy-induced glucose
	postinjury		intolerance
	premature infant	PIGN	postinfectious glomerulonephritis
	present illness	PIH	pregnancy-induced hypertension
	principal investigator		preventricular intraventricular
	protease inhibitor		hemorrhage
	pulmonary infarction		prolactin-inhibiting hormone
	pulmonic insufficiency	PIIID	peripheral indwelling intermediate
PI-3	parainfluenza 3 virus		infusion device
P & I	probe and irrigation	PIIP	aminoterminal type three procollagen
PIA	personal injury accident		propeptide
	polysaccharide intercellular adhesine	PIIS	posterior inferior iliac spine
PIAF	cisplatin (Platinol), recombinant	PIL	patient information leaflet
	interferon alpha 2B, doxorubicin		purpose in life
	(Adriamycin), and fluorouracil	PILO	pilocarpine
PIAT	Peabody Individual Achievement	PIM	Program Integrity Manual
	Test		pulse-inversion mode (ultrasound)

P

PIMIA	potentiometric ionophore mediated immunoassay
PIMS	programmable implantable medication system
PIN	pain in the neck (no place for such a term in a written document)
	personal identification number
	posterior interosseous nerve
	prostatic intraepithelial neoplasia
	provider identification number
PIND	progressive intellectual and neurological deterioration
PINP	N-terminal propeptide of type I collagen
PINS	persons in need of supervision
PIO	pemoline (Cylert)
PIO$_2$	partial pressure of inspired oxygen
PIOK	poikilocytosis
PIOL	primary intraocular lymphoma
PIP	peak inspiratory pressure
	postictal psychosis
	postinfusion phlebitis
	proximal interphalangeal (joint)
	pulmonary immaturity of prematurity
	pulmonary insufficiency of the premature
PIPB	performance index phonetic balance
PI-PB	performance intensity-phonemically balanced
PIPIDA	N-para-isopropyl-acetanilide-iminodiacetic acid
PIPJ	proximal interphalangeal joint
PIPP	Premature Infant Pain Profile
PIP/TZ	piperacillin-tazobactam (Zosyn)
PIQ	Performance Intelligence Quotient (part of Wechsler tests)
PIR	pirarubicin
PIS	pregnancy interruption service
PISA	phase invariant signature algorithm
	proximal isovelocity surface area
PIT	pancreatic islet transplantation
	patellar inhibition test
	peak isometric torque
	Pitocin (oxytocin)
	Pitressin (vasopressin) (this is a dangerous abbreviation as it can be taken for Pitocin)
	pituitary
	pulsed-inotrope therapy
PITP	pseudo-idiopathic thrombocytopenic purpura
PITR	plasma iron turnover rate
PIV	peripheral intravenous
PIV-3	parainfluenza virus type 3
PIVD	protruded intervertebral disk
PIVH	periventricular-intraventricular hemorrhage

PIVKA	proteins induced in vitamin K absence
PIWT	partially impacted wisdom teeth
PIXI	Peripheral Instantaneous X-ray Imaging (dual-energy x-ray absorptiometry system)
PJ	procelin jacket (crown)
PJB	premature junctional beat
PJC	premature junctional contractions
PJI	prosthetic joint infection
PJIF	prosthetic joint implant failure
PJP	pneumocystis jirovecii pneumonia
PJRT	permanent form of junctional reciprocating tachycardia
PJS	peritoneojugular shunt
	Peutz-Jeghers syndrome
PJT	paroxysmal junctional tachycardia
PJVT	paroxysmal junctional-ventricular tachycardia
PK	penetrating keratoplasty
	pharmacokinetics
	plasma potassium
	pyruvate kinase
PKB	prone knee bend
PKC	protein kinase C
PKD	paroxysmal kinesigenic dyskinesia
	polycystic kidney disease
PKDL	post-kala-azar dermal leishmaniasis
PKI	public key infrastructure
PKND	paroxysmal nonkinesigenic dyskinesia
PKP	penetrating keratoplasty
PK/PD	pharmacokinetic/pharmacodynamic
PKR	phased knee rehabilitation
PK Test	Prausnitz-Küstner transfer test
PKU	phenylketonuria
pk yrs	pack-years (smoking one pack of cigarettes a day for one year is termed 1 pack-year of smoking, thus 2 packs a day for 20 years would be 40 pack-years)
PL	light perception
	palmaris longus
	peroneus longus
	pharyngolaryngectomy
	place
	placebo
	plantar
	plethoric (infant color)
	transpulmonary pressure
PLA	placebo
	Plasma-Lyte A
	polylactic acid
	posterolateral (coronary) artery
	potentially lethal arrhythmia
	Product License Application
	pulpolinguoaxial

P

PLAC	placenta
PLAD	proximal left anterior descending (artery)
Plan B®	levonorgestrel (a progestogen emergency contraceptive)
PLAP	placental alkaline phosphatase
PLAT C	platelet concentration
PLAT P	platelet pheresis
PLAX	parasternal long axis
PLB	phospholamban
	placebo
	posterolateral branch
	pursed-lip breathing
PLBO	placebo
PLC	peripheral lymphocyte count
	pityriasis lichenoides chronica
PLCH	pulmonary Langerhans cell histiocytosis
PLD	partial lower denture
	pegylated liposomal doxorubicin
	percutaneous laser diskectomy
PLDD	percutaneous laser disk decompression
PLE	polymorphic light eruption
	protein-losing enteropathy
PLED	periodic lateralizing epileptiform discharge
PLEVA	pityriasis lichenoides et varioliformis acuta
PLF	prior level of function
PLFC	premature living female child
PLG	plague (*Yersinia pestis*) (*la Peste*) vaccine
PLH	paroxysmal localized hyperhidrosis
PLIF	posterior lumbar interbody fusion
PLIG	posterior lumbar interbody graft
PLIL	partial laryngectomy with imbrication laryngoplasty
PLL	posterior longitudinal ligament
	prolymphocytic leukemia
PLLA	poly-l-lactic acid (Sculptra)
PLM	partial lateral meniscectomy
	periodic leg movement
	Plasma-Lyte M
	polarized-light microscope
	precise lesion measuring (device)
	product-line manager
PLMC	premature living male child
PLMD	periodic limb movement disorder
PLMS	periodic limb movements during sleep
PLN	pelvic lymph node
	popliteal lymph node
PLND	pelvic lymph node dissection
PLO	pluronic lecithin organogels
PLOF	previous level of functioning
PLOSA	physiologic low stress angioplasty
PLP	partial laryngopharyngectomy

	phantom limb pain
	protolipid protein
PLPH	postlumbar puncture headache
PLR	pupillary light reflex
PLRT	postlumpectomy radiotherapy
PLS	Papillon-Lefèvre syndrome
	phantom limb syndrome
	plastic surgery
	point locator stimulator
	Preschool Language Scale
	primary lateral sclerosis
PLs	premalignant lesions
PLSD	protected least significant difference (statistical test)
PLSO	posterior leafspring orthosis
PLST	progressively lowered stress threshold
PLSURG	plastic surgery
PLT	platelet
PLT EST	platelet estimate
PLTF	plaintiff
PLTS	platelets
PLUG	plug the lung until it grows
PLV	partial left ventriculectomy
	posterior left ventricular
PLX	plexus
PLYO	plyometric
PLZF	promyelocytic leukemia zinc finger
PM	afternoon
	evening
	pacemaker
	papillary muscles
	paraspinal mapping
	particulate matter
	petit mal
	physical medicine
	pneumomediastinum
	poliomyelitis
	polymyositis
	poor metabolizers
	postmenopausal
	postmortem
	presents mainly
	pretibial myxedema
	primary motivation
	prostatic massage
	pulpomesial
Pm	*Plasmodium malariae*
PM$_{10}$	particulate matter less than 10 micrometers diameter
PMA	positive mental attitude
	post-menstrual age
	premarket approval (application) (for medical devices)
	premenstrual asthma
	primary meningococcal arthritis
	Prinzmetal angina
	progress myoclonic ataxia

P

PMAA	Premarket Approval Application (medical devices)		Premarket Notification (medical devices)
PMB	polymorphonuclear basophil (leukocytes)	PMNL	polymorphonuclear leukocyte
	polymyxin B	PMNN	polymorphonuclear neutrophil
	postmenopausal bleeding	PMNS	postmalarial neurological syndrome
PMC	premature mitral closure	PMO	postmenopausal osteoporosis
	pseudomembranous colitis		probable medication overuse
PMCP	para-monochlorophenol	pmol	picomole
	perinatal mortality counseling program	PMP	pain management program
			previous menstrual period
PMCT	perinatal mortality counseling team		psychotropic medication plan
	postmortem computed tomography	PMPA	tenofovir (Viread)
PMCWR	post-mastectomy chest wall relapse	PMPM	per member, per month
PMD	perceptual motor development	PMPO	postmenopausal palpable ovary
	primary myocardial disease	PMPY	per member, per year
	primidone (Mysoline)	PMR	pacemaker rhythm
	private medical doctor		percutaneous revascularization
	progressive muscular dystrophy		polymorphic reticulosis
PMDD	premenstrual dysphoric disorder		polymyalgia rheumatica
pMDI	pressurized metered-dose inhaler		premedication regimen
PM/DM	polymyositis and dermatomyositis		prior medical record
PME	pelvic muscle exercise		progressive muscle relaxation
	phosphomonoester(s)		proportional mortality ratios
	polymorphonuclear esosinophil (leukocytes)	PM&R	physical medicine and rehabilitation
		PMRT	postmastectomy radiation
	postmenopausal estrogen	PMS	performance measurement system
	progressive myoclonus epilepsy		periodic movements of sleep
PMEALS	after meals		poor miserable soul
PMEC	pseudomembranous enterocolitis		postmarketing surveillance
PMF	peptide mass fingerprinting		postmenopausal syndrome
	progressive massive fibrosis		premenstrual syndrome
	pupils mid-position, fixed		pulse, motor, and sensory
PMH	past medical history	PMSF	phenylmethylsulfonyl fluoride
PMHNP	Psychiatric Mental Health Nurse Practitioner	PMT	pacemaker-mediated tachycardia
			percutaneous mechanical thrombectomy
PMHx	past medical history		point of maximum tenderness
PMI	Pain Management Index		premenstrual tension
	past medical illness	PMTS	premenstrual tension syndrome
	patient medication instructions	PMV	percutaneous mitral (balloon) valvuloplasty
	plea of mental incompetence		
	point of maximal impulse		prolapse of mitral valve
	posterior myocardial infarction	PMW	pacemaker wires
PMID	PubMed Unique Identifier (National Library of Medicine)	PMZ	postmenopausal zest
		PN	parenteral nutrition
PML	polymorphonuclear leukocytes		peanut (when testing for an allergy)
	posterior mitral leaflet		percussion note
	premature labor		percutaneous nephrosonogram
	progressive multifocal leukoencephalopathy		percutaneous nephrostomy
			percutaneous nucleotomy
	promyelocytic leukemia		periarteritis nodosa
PMLCL	primary mediastinal large-cell lymphoma		peripheral neuropathy
			pneumonia
PMMA	polymethyl methacrylate		polyarteritis nodosa
PMMF	pectoralis major myocutaneous flap		poorly nourished
			positional nystagmus
PMN	polymodal nociceptors		postnasal
	polymorphonuclear leukocyte		postnatal

P

	practical nurse	PNMT	phenylethanolamine-N-methyltransferase
	premie nipple		
	primary nurse	PNNP	Perinatal Nurse Practitioner
	progress note	PNP	peak negative pressure
	pyelonephritis		Pediatric Nurse Practitioner
P & N	pins and needles		progressive nuclear palsy
	psychiatry and neurology		purine nucleoside phosphorylase
PN$_2$	partial pressure of nitrogen	PNR	physician's nutritional recommendation
PNA	Pediatric Nurse Associate		
	pneumonia	PNRB	partial non-rebreather (oxygen mask)
	polynitroxyl albumin	PNS	partial nonprogressing stroke
PNa	plasma sodium		peripheral nerve stimulator
PNAB	percutaneous needle aspiration biopsy		peripheral nervous system
PNAC	parenteral nutrition associated cholestasis		practical nursing student
		PNSP	penicillin-nonsusceptible *Streptococcus pneumoniae*
PNAR	perennial nonallergic rhinitis	PNT	percutaneous nephrostomy tube
PNAS	prudent no added salt		
PNB	percutaneous needle biopsy		percutaneous neuromodulatory therapy
	popliteal nerve block		
	premature newborn		pneumatic trabeculoplasty
	premature nodal beat	pnthx	pneumothorax
	prostate needle biopsy	PNTML	pudendal-nerve terminal motor latency
PNC	penicillin		
	peripheral nerve conduction	PNU	pneumococcal (*Streptococcus pneumoniae*) vaccine, not otherwise specified
	postnecrotic cirrhosis		
	premature nodal contraction		
	prenatal care		protein nitrogen units
	prenatal course	PNUcn-7	pneumococcal (*Streptococcus pneumoniae*) conjugate vaccine, 7-valent vaccine (Prevnar)
	Psychiatric Nurse Clinician		
PNCV7	pneumococcal 7-valent conjugate vaccine (Prevnar)		
		PNUps23	pneumococcal (*Streptococcus pneumoniae*) polysaccharide, 23-valent vaccine (Pneumovax-23; Pnu-Imune-23)
PND	paroxysmal nocturnal dyspnea		
	pelvic node dissection		
	postnasal drip		
	pregnancy, not delivered	PNV	postoperative nausea and vomiting
PNDS	Perioperative Nursing Data Set		prenatal vitamins
	postnasal drip syndrome	Pnx	pneumonectomy
PNE	peripheral neuroepithelioma		pneumothorax
	primary nocturnal enuresis	PO	by mouth
PNES	psychogenic non-epileptic seizures		phone order
PNET	primitive neuroectodermal tumors		postoperative
PNET-MB	primitive neuroectodermal tumors-medulloblastoma		*Plasmodium ovale*
			prophylactic oophorectomy
PNEUMO	pneumothorax		punctal occlusion
PNF	primary nonfunction	Po	polonium
	proprioceptive neuromuscular fasciculation (reaction)	P/O	prosthetics and orthotics
		P&O	parasites and ova
PNFA	progressive nonfluent aphasia		prosthetics and orthotics
PNH	paroxysmal nocturnal hemoglobinuria	Po$_2$	partial pressure (tension) of oxygen, artery
	polynitroxyl-hemoglobin	PO$_4$	phosphate
	progressive nodular hyperplasia	POA	pancreatic oncofetal antigen
PNI	peripheral nerve injury		power of attorney
	Prognostic Nutrition Index		present on arrival
PNKD	paroxysmal nonkinesigenic dyskinesia		primary optic atrophy
PNL	percutaneous nephrolithotomy	POACH	prednisone, vincristine (Oncovin), doxorubicin (Adriamycin), cyclophosphamide, and cytarabine
	prenatal labs		
PNMG	persistent neonatal myasthenia gravis		

217

P

POAF	postoperative atrial fibrillation	POIB	place outpatient in inpatient bed
POAG	primary open-angle glaucoma	POIK	poikilocytosis
POB	phenoxybenzamine (Dibenzyline)	POL	physician's office laboratory
	place of birth		poliovirus vaccine, not otherwise specified
POBC	primary operable breast cancer		
POC	peri-operative chemotherapy		premature onset of labor
	plans of care	POLS	postoperative length of stay
	point-of-care	POLY	polychromic erythrocytes
	position of comfort		polymorphonuclear leukocyte
	postoperative care	POLY-CHR	polychromatophilia
	product of conception	POM	pain on motion
POCD	postoperative cognitive dysfunction		polyoximethylene
			prescription-only medication
POCT	point-of-care testing (test)	POMA	Performance-Oriented Mobility Assessment
	point-of-care therapy		
POD	pacing on demand	POMC	pro-opiomelanocortin
	place of death	POMP	prednisone, vincristine (Oncovin), methotrexate, and mercaptopurine (Purinthol)
	Podiatry		
	polycystic ovarian disease		
	progression of disease	POMR	problem-oriented medical record
POD 1	postoperative day one	POMS	Profile of Mood States
PODx	preoperative diagnosis	POMS-FI	Fatigue-Inertia Subscale of the Profile of Mood States
POE	patient-oriented evidence		
	point (portal, port) of entry	PON	postoperative note
	position of ease	PONI	postoperative narcotic infusion
	prone on elbows	PONV	postoperative nausea and vomiting
	provider order entry	POOH	postoperative open heart (surgery)
POEM	Patient-Oriented Evidence That Matters	POOL	premature onset of labor
		POP	pain on palpation
POEMS	plasma cell dyscrasia with polyneuropathy, organomegaly, endocrinopathy, monoclonal protein (M-protein), and skin changes		persistent occipitoposterior
			persistent organic pollutants
			plaster of paris
			popiliteal
			posterior oral pharynx
POEx	postoperative exercise	POp	postoperative
POF	physician's order form	POPC	Pediatric Overall Performance Category (scale)
	position of function		
	premature ovarian failure	poplit	popliteal
P of I	proof of illness	POPS	postoperative pain service
POG	Pediatric Oncology Group	POPs	persistent organic pollutants
	Penthrane,® oxygen, and gas (nitrous oxide)		progesterone-only pills
		POR	physician of record
	products of gestation		problem-oriented record
POGO	percentage of glottic opening	PORN	pornography
POH	perillyl alcohol		progressive outer retinal necrosis
	personal oral hygiene	PORP	partial ossicular replacement prosthesis
	presumed ocular histoplasmosis		
	progressive osseous heteroplasia	PORR	postoperative recovery room
	prone on hands	PORT	perioperative respiratory therapy
POHA	preoperative holding area		portable
POHI	physically or otherwise health impaired		postoperative radiotherapy
			postoperative respiratory therapy
POHS	by mouth, at bedtime		
	presumed ocular histoplasmosis syndrome	POS	parosteal osteosarcoma
			physician's order sheet
POI	Personal Orientation Inventory		point-of-service
	postoperative ileus		positive
	postoperative instructions	PoS	plane of surgery

P

POSHPATE	problem, onset, associated symptoms, previous history, precipitating factors, alleviating/aggravation factors, timing, an etiology (prompts for taking history and chief complaint)	P-P	probability-probability (plots)
		P&P	pins and plaster
			policy and procedure
		PIIIP	aminoterminal type three protocollegan propeptide
		PPIX	protoporphyrin nine
poss	possible	PPA	palpation, percussion, and auscultation
post	posterior		
	postmortem examination (autopsy)		phenylpropanolamine
PostC	posterior chamber		phenylpyruvic acid
PostCap	posterior capsule		postpartum amenorrhea
Post-M	urine specimen after prostate massage		Prescription Pricing Authority (United Kingdom)
post op	postoperative		primary progressive aphasia
Post Sag D	posterior sagittal diameter	PP&A	palpation, percussion, and auscultation
post tib	posterial tibial		
PostVD	posterior vitreous detachment	PPARg	peroxisome-proliferator-activated receptor gamma
POSYC	Pain Observation Scale for Young Children	PPARs	peroxisome proliferator-activated receptors
POT	peak occupancy time		
	plans of treatment	PPAS	postpolio atrophy syndrome
	potassium	PPB	parts per billion
	potential		pleuropulmonary blastoma
	primary orthostatic tremor		positive pressure breathing
POTS	postural tachycardia syndrome		prostate puncture biopsy
POU	placenta, ovaries, and uterus	PPBE	postpartum breast engorgment
POV	privately owned vehicle	PPBS	postprandial blood sugar
POVD	peripheral occlusive vascular disease	PPBTL	postpartum bilateral tubal ligation
POW	Powassan (virus)	PPC	plaster of paris cast
	prisoner of war		positive product control
POWSBP	pulse oximetry waveform systolic blood pressure		primary peritoneal carcinoma
			progressive patient care
POX	pulse oximeter (reading)	PPCD	posterior polymorphous corneal dystrophy
PP	near point of accommodation		
	pancreatic pseudocyst	PPCF	plasma prothrombin conversion factor
	paradoxical pulse		
	partial upper and lower dentures	PPD	packs per day
	pedal pulse		para-phenylenediamine (a dye)
	per protocol		permanent partial disability (rating)
	periodontal pockets		pinch-point density (histologic)
	peripheral pulses		posterior polymorphous dystrophy
	pin prick		postpartum day
	pink puffer (emphysema)		postpartum depression
	Planned Parenthood		probing pocket depth (dental)
	plasmapheresis		purified protein derivative (of tuberculin)
	plaster of paris		
	poor person		pylorus-sparing pancreaticoduodenectomy
	posterior pituitary		
	postpartum	P & PD	percussion & postural drainage
	postprandial	PPD-B	purified protein derivative, Battey
	presenting part	PPDR	preproliferative diabetic retinopathy
	private patient	PPD-S	purified protein derivative, standard
	prophylactics	PPE	palmar-plantar erythrodysesthesia (syndrome)
	protoporphyria		
	proximal phalanx		personal protective equipment
	psychogenic polydipsia		professional performance evaluation
	pulse pressure		
	push pills		pruritic papular eruption

219

P

PPES	palmar-plantar erythrodysesthesia syndrome	PPOB	postpartum obstetrics
	pedal pulses equal and strong	PPP	patient prepped and positioned
PPF	pellagra preventive factor		pearly penile papules
	plasma protein fraction		pedal pulse present
PPG	photoplethysmography		peripheral pulses palpable (present)
	portal pressure gradients		platelet-poor plasma
	postprandial glucose		postpartum psychosis
	pylorus-preserving gastrectomy		preferred practice patterns
PPGI	psychophysiologic gastrointestinal (reaction)		proportional pulse pressure (SBP minus DBP)/SBP
PPGSS	papular-purpuric "glove and socks" syndrome		protamine paracoagulation phenomenon
PPH	postpartum hemorrhage	PPPBL	peripheral pulses palpable both legs
	primary postpartum hemorrhage	PPPD	pylorus-preserving pancreatoduodenectomy
	primary pulmonary hypertension	PPPG	postprandial plasma glucose
	procedure for prolapse and hemorrhoids	PPPM	Parents' Postoperative Pain Measure
PPHN	persistent pulmonary hypertension of the newborn		per patient, per month
		PPPY	per patient, per year
PPHTN	portopulmonary hypertension	PPQ	Postoperative Pain Questionnaire
PPHx	previous psychiatric history	PPR	patient progress record
PPIX	protoporphyrin nine	PPr	periodontal prophylactics
PPI	patient package insert	PPRC	Physician Payment Review Commission
	permanent pacemaker insertion	pPROM	premature rupture of the membranes before 37 weeks gestation
	prepulse inhibition		
	Present Pain Intensity	PPS	pentosan polysulfate (Elmiron)
	proton-pump inhibitor		peripheral pulmonary stenosis
	Psychopathic Personality Inventory		per protocol set
PPIA	parental presence during induction of anesthesia		postpartum sterilization
			post-pericardiotomy syndrome
PPIVMs	passive physiological intervertebral movements		postperfusion syndrome
			postpoliomyelitis syndrome
PPJ	pure pancreatic juice		postpump syndrome
PPK	population pharmacokinetics		prospective payment system
PPL	pars plana lensectomy		pulses per second
Ppl	pleural pressure	PPSS	peripheral protein sparing solution
PPLO	pleuropneumonia-like organisms	PPT	parts-per-trillion
PPLOV	painless progressive loss of vision		person, place, and time
PPM	parts per million		Physical Performance Test
	permanent pacemaker		posterior pelvic tilt
	persistent pupillary membrane	PPTg	pedunculopontine tegmental nucleus
	physician practice management		
PPMA	postpoliomyelitis muscular atrophy	PPTL	postpartum tubal ligation
PPMS	primary progressive multiple sclerosis	PPTR	pulsed photothermal radiometry
		PPU	perforated peptic ulcer
	psychophysiologic musculoskeletal (reaction)	PPV	pars plana vitrectomy
			patent processus vaginalis
PPMs	potentially pathogenic microorganisms		percutaneous polymethyl-methacrylate vertebroplasty
PPN	peripheral parenteral nutrition		phakomatosis pigmentovascularis
PPNAD	primary pigmented nodular adrenocortical disease		pneumococcal polysaccharide vaccine
PPNG	penicillinase-producing *Neisseria gonorrhoeae*		positive predictive value
			positive-pressure ventilation
PPO	permanent punctal occlusion	PPVI	percutaneous pulmonary valve implantation
	preferred provider organization		
	pump-prime only	PPVT	Peabody Picture Vocabulary Test

P

PPVT-R	Peabody Picture Vocabulary Test-Revised	Pre-M	urine specimen before prostate massage
PPW	plantar puncture wound	PREMIE	premature infant
	premature P-wave	pre-op	before surgery
PPX	paclitaxel poliglumex	prep	prepare for surgery
PPY	packs per year (cigarettes)		preposition
PQ	pronator quadratus	PRERLA	pupils round, equal, react to light and accommodation
pQCT	peripheral quantitative computed tomography	prev	prevent
PQOCN	Psychiatric Questionnaire Obsessive-Compulsive Neurosis		previous
		PRFD	percutaneous radio-frequency denervation
PQRI	Product Quality Research Initiative	PRFNB	percutaneous radio-frequency facet nerve block
PR	far point of accommodation		
	pack removal	PrFP	pre-exposure prophylaxis
	panoramic radiography (dental)	PRG	phleborheogram
	partial remission	PRH	past relevant history
	partial response		postocclusive reactive hyperemia
	patient relations		preretinal hemorrhage
	perennial rhinitis	PRHO	preregistration house officer
	per rectum	PRI	Pain Rating Index
	pityriasis rosea		Patient Review Instrument
	premature	prim	primary
	profile	PRIMIP	primipara (1st pregnancy)
	progressive resistance	PR	part of the electrocardio-
	prolonged remission	interval	graphic cycle from onset of atrial
	prone		depolarization on onset of
	Protestant		ventricular depolarization
	Puerto Rican	PRISM	Pediatric Risk of Mortality Score
	pulmonic regurgitation	PRIT®	pretargeted radioimmunotherapy
	pulse rate	PRK	photorefractive keratectomy
P=R	pupils equal in size and reaction	PRL	prolactin
P & R	pelvic and rectal	PRLA	pupils react to light and accommodation
	pulse and respiration		
PR-2	Bennett pressure ventilator	PRM	partial rebreathing mask
PRA	panel reactive antibodies (organ transplants)		passive range of motion
			phosphoribomutase
	percent reactive antibody		photoreceptor membrane
	plasma renin activity		prematurely ruptured membrane
PRAFO	pressure relief ankle-foot orthosis		primidone (Mysoline)
PRAMS	Pregnancy Risk Assessment Monitoring System	PRMF	preretinal macular fibrosis
		PRMS	progressive relapsing multiple sclerosis
PRAT	platelet radioactive antiglobulin test		
		PRM-SDX	pyrimethamine; sulfadoxine (Fansidar)
PRBC	packed red blood cells		
PRC	packed red cells	PRN	plaque reduction neutralization
	peer review committee	p.r.n.	as occasion requires
	proximal row carpectomy	PRNS	phrenic repetitive nerve stimulation
PRCA	pure red cell aplasia	PRO	Professional Review Organization
PrCa	prostate cancer		proline
PRCC	papillary renal cell carcinoma		pronation
PRCT	prospective randomized controlled trial		protein
			prothrombin
PRD	polycystic renal disease	prob	probable
PRE	passive resistance exercises	PROCTO	procotoscopic
	progressive resistive exercise		proctology
	proton relaxation enhancement	PROG	prognathism
Pred	prednisone		prognosis
PREG	Pregestimil® (infant formula)		

P

	program
	progressive
PROM	passive range of motion
	premature rupture of membranes
ProMACE	prednisone, methotrexate, calcium leucovorin, doxorubicin (Adriamycin), cyclophosphamide, and etoposide
PROMM	passive range of motion machine
Promy	promyelocyte
PRO MYELO	promyelocytes
PRON	pronation
PROS	prostate
	prosthesis
PROT REL	protrusive relationship
prov	provisional
PROVIMI	proteins, vitamins, and minerals
PROX	proximal
PRP	panretinal photocoagulation
	patient recovery plan
	penicllinase-resistant penicillin
	penicillin-resistant pneumococci
	pityriasis rubra pilaris
	platelet rich plasma
	polyribose ribitol phosphate
	poor progression of R wave in precordial leads
	progressive rubella panencephalitis
PrP	prion protein
PRP-D	*Haemophilus influenzae,* type b diphtheria conjugate vaccine
PRPP	5-phosphoribosyl-1-pyrophosphate
PRP-T	polysaccharide tetanus conjugate vaccine
PRRE	pupils round, regular, and equal
PRRERLA	pupils round, regular, equal; react to light and accommodation
PRRs	proportional reporting ratios
PRS	photon radiosurgery system
	postradiation sarcoma
	prolonged respiratory support
PRSL	potential renal solute load
PRSP	penicillinase-resistant synthetic penicillins
	penicillin-resistant *Streptococcus pneumoniae*
PRSs	positive rolandic spikes
PRST	Blood Pressure, Heart Rate, Sweating, and Tears (scale to assess analgesic needs)
PRT	pelvic radiation therapy
	protamine response test
PRTCA	percutaneous rotational transluminal coronary angioplasty
PRTH-C	prothrombin time control
PRV	polycythemia rubra vera

PRVEP	pattern reversal visual evoked potentials
PRW	past relevant work
	polymerized ragweed
PRX	panoramic facial x-ray
PRZF	pyrazofurin
PS	paradoxic sleep
	paranoid schizophrenia
	pathologic stage
	patient's serum
	performance status
	peripheral smear
	physical status
	plastic surgery (surgeon)
	polysulfone (filter)
	posterior subcapsular (cataract type)
	posterior synechiae
	posterior synechiotomy
	pressure sore
	pressure support
	protective services
	Proteus syndrome
	pulmonary stenosis
	pyloric stenosis
	pyrimethamine; sulfadoxine (Fansidar)
	serum from pregnant women
P/S	polyunsaturated to saturated fatty acids ratio
P & S	pain and suffering
	paracentesis and suction
	permanent and stationary
PS I	healthy patient with localized pathological process
PS II	a patient with mild to moderate systemic disease
PS III	a patient with severe systemic disease limiting activity but not incapacitating
PS IV	a patient with incapacitating systemic disease
PS V	moribund patient not expected to live (These are American Society of Anesthesiologists' physical status patient classifications. Emergency operations are designated by "E" after the classification.)
PSA	polysubstance abuse
	power spectral analysis
	product selection allowed
	prostate-specific antigen
	Pseudomonas aeruginosa
PsA	psoriatic arthritis
PSAB	pretreatment prostate-specific antigen
PSAD	prostate-specific antigen density
PSADT	prostate-specific antigen doubling time

P

PSAG	*Pseudomonas aeruginosa*	PSO	Patient Safety Officer
PSAV	prostate-specific antigen velocity		pelvic stabilization orthosis
PSBO	partial small bowel obstruction		physician supplemental order
PSC	Pediatric Symptom Checklist		Polysporin ointment
	percutaneous suprapubic cystostomy		proximal subungual onychomycosis
	posterior semicircular canal	pSO$_2$	arterial oxygen saturation
	posterior subcapsular cataract	PSOC	Puget Sound Oncology Consortium
	primary sclerosing cholangitis	P/sore	pressure sore
	pronation spring control	PSP	pancreatic spasmolytic peptide
	pubosacrococcygeal (diameter)		phenolsulfonphthalein
PSCA	prostate stem cell antigen		photostimulable phosphor
PSCC	posterior subcapsular cataract		progressive supranuclear palsy
PSC Cat	posterior subcapsular cataract	PSPDV	posterior superior
PSCH	peripheral stem cell harvest		pancreaticoduodenal vein
PSCP	papillary serous carcinoma of the	PSR	posthumous sperm retrieval
	peritoneum		Psychiatric Status Rating (scale)
	posterior subcapsular precipitates	PSRA	pressure sore risk assessment
PSCT	peripheral stem cell transplant	PSRBOW	premature spontaneous rupture of
PSCU	pediatric special care unit		bag of waters
PSD	partial sleep deprivation	PSReA	poststreptococcal reactive arthritis
	pilonidal sinus disease	PSRT	photostress recovery test
	poststroke depression	PSS	painful shoulder syndrome
	power spectral density		pediatric surgical service
	psychosomatic disease		physiologic saline solution (0.9%
PSDA	Patient Self-Determination Act		sodium chloride)
PSDS	palmar surface desensitization		primary Sjögren syndrome
PSE	photosensitive epilepsy		progressive systemic sclerosis
	portal systemic encephalopathy	PSSP	penicillin-sensitive *Streptococcus*
	pseudoephedrine		*pneumoniae*
PSF	posterior spinal fusion	PST	paroxysmal supraventricular
PSG	peak systolic gradient		tachycardia
	polysomnogram		patient self-testing
	portosystemic gradient		Patient Service Technician
PSGN	poststreptococcal glomerulonephritis		penicillin skin testing
PSH	past surgical history		platelet survival time
	postspinal headache		postural stress test
PSHx	past surgical history	PSTT	placental site trophoblastic tumor
PSI	passenger space intrusion (motor	PSU	pseudomonas (*P. aeruginosa*)
	vehicle accident)		vaccine
	Physiologic Stability Index	PSUD	psychoactive substance use disorder
	pounds per square inch	PSUR	Periodic Safety Update Reporting
	prostate seed implant		(EMEA)
	punctate subepithelial infiltrate	PSV	peak systolic velocity
PSIC	pediatric surgical intensive care		persistent sciatic vein(s)
PSIG	pounds per square inch gauge		pressure supported ventilation
PSIS	posterior superior iliac spine	PSVT	paroxysmal supraventricular
PSM	patient self-management		tachycardia
	presystolic murmur	PSW	psychiatric social worker
PSMA	personal self-maintenance	PSWF	positive sharp wave fibrillations
	activities		(electromyograph)
	progressive spinal muscular atrophy	PSY	presexual youth
	prostate-specific membrane antigen	PsyD	psychological distress
PSMF	protein-sparing modified fasting	PSZ	pseudoseizures
	(Blackburn diet)	PT	cisplatin (Platinol)
PSM-R	Optimism-Pessimism Scale, revised		parathormone
PSMS	Physical Self Maintenance Scale		parathyroid
PSN	peripheral sensory neuropathy		paroxysmal tachycardia
PSNP	progressive supranuclear palsy		patch test

P

	patient		pseudotumor cerebri
	phacotrabeculectomy	PT-C	prothrombin time control
	phage type	PTCA	percutaneous transluminal coronary angioplasty
	phenytoin (Dilantin)		
	phototoxicity	PTCDLF	pregnancy, term, complicated delivered, living female
	physical therapy		
	pine tar	PTCDLM	pregnancy, term, complicated delivered, living male
	pint		
	posterior tibial	PTCL	peripheral T-cell lymphoma
	preterm	PTCR	percutaneous transluminal coronary recanalization
	pronator teres		
	prothrombin time	PTCRA	percutaneous transluminal coronary rotational atherectomy
Pt	platinum		
P/T	pain and tenderness	PTD	percutaneous transpedicular diskectomy
	piperacillin/tazobactam (Zosyn®)		
P1/2T	pressure one-half time		period to discharge
P&T	pain and tenderness		permanent and total disability
	paracentesis and tubing (of ears)		persistent trophoblastic disease
	peak and trough		pharmacy to dose
	permanent and total		pharyngotracheal duct
	Pharmacy and Therapeutics (Committee)		preterm delivery
			prior to delivery
PTA	pancreas transplant alone	PTDM	post-transplant diabetes mellitus
	patellar tendon autograft	PTDP	permanent transvenous demand pacemaker
	percutaneous transluminal angioplasty		
		PTE	pretibial edema
	Physical Therapy Assistant		proximal tibial epiphysis
	plasma thromboplastin antecedent		pulmonary thromboembolectomy
	posterior tibial artery		pulmonary thromboembolism
	post-traumatic amnesia	PTE-4®	trace metal elements injection (there is also a #5 and #6)
	pretreatment anxiety		
	prior to admission	PTED	pulmonary thromboembolic disease
	prior to arrival	PTER	percutaneous transluminal endomyocardial revascularization
	pure-tone average		
PTAB	popliteal-tibial artery bypass	PTF	patient transfer form
PTAS	percutaneous transluminal angioplasty with stent placement		Patient Treatment File
			pentoxifylline (Trental)
PTB	patellar tendon bearing		post-tetanic facilitation
	prior to birth	PTFE	polytetrafluoroethylene
	pulmonary tuberculosis	PTG	parathyroid gland
PTBA	percutaneous transluminal balloon angioplasty		photoplethysmogram
		PTGBD	percutaneous transhepatic gallbladder drainage
PTBD	percutaneous transhepatic biliary drain (drainage)		
		PTH	parathyroid hormone
PTBD-EF	percutaneous transhepatic biliary drainage—enteric feeding		post-transfusion hepatitis
			prior to hospitalization
PTBS	post-traumatic brain syndrome	PTHC	percutaneous transhepatic cholangiography
PTB-SC-SP	patellar tendon bearing-supracondylar-suprapatellar		
		PTHrP	parathyroid hormone-related protein
PTC	patient to call	PTHS	post-traumatic hyperirritability syndrome
	percutaneous transhepatic cholangiography		
		PTI	pressure-time integral
	Pharmacy and Therapeutics Committee		prior to induction
		PTJV	percutaneous transtracheal jet ventilation
	plasma thromboplastin components		
	post-tetanic count	PTK	pancreas-after-kidney (transplantation)
	premature tricuspid closure		
	prior to conception		phototherapeutic keratectomy

P

224

PTL	preterm labor	PTTD	posterior tibial tendonitis dysfunction
	pudding-thick liquid (diet consistency)	PTTG	pituitary tumor transforming gene
		PTTW	patient tolerated traction well
	Sodium Pentothal	PTU	pain treatment unit
PTLD	post-transplantation lymphoproliferative disorder (disease)		pregnancy, term, uncomplicated
			propylthiouracil
		PTUCA	percutaneous transluminal ultrasonic coronary angioplasty
PTLR	percutaneous transmyocardial laser revascularization	PTUDLF	pregnancy, term, uncomplicated delivered, living female
PTM	patient monitored	PTUDLM	pregnancy, term, uncomplicated delivered, living male
	posterior trabecular meshwork		
PTMC	percutaneous transvenous mitral commissurotomy	PTV	patient-triggered ventilation
			planning target volume (radiation therapy)
PTMDF	pupils, tension, media, disc, and fundus		
			posterior tibial vein
PTMR	percutaneous transmyocardial revascularization	PTWTKG	patient's weight in kilograms
		PTX	paclitaxel (Taxol)
PT-NANB	post-transfusion non-A, non-B (hepatitis C)		parathyroidectomy
			pelvic traction
PTNB	preterm newborn		pentoxifylline (Trental)
pTNM	postsurgical resection-pathologic staging of cancer		phototherapy
			pneumothorax
PTNS	percutaneous tibial nerve stimulation	PTZ	pentylenetetrazol
PTO	part-time occlusion (eye patch)		phenothiazine
	please turn over	PU	pelvic-ureteric
	proximal tubal obstruction		pelviureteral
PTP	phonation threshold pressure		peptic ulcer
	posterior tibial pulse		pregnancy urine
	post-transfusion purpura	P & U	Pharmacia & Upjohn Company
PTPM	post-traumatic progressive myelopathy	PUA	pelvic (examination) under anesthesia
PTPN	peripheral (vein) total parenteral nutrition	PUB	pubic
		PUBS	percutaneous umbilical blood sampling
P-to-P	point-to-point		
PTR	paratesticular rhabdomyosarcoma		purple urine bag syndrome
	patella tendon reflex	PUC	pediatric urine collector
	patient to return	PUD	partial upper denture
	prothrombin time ratio		peptic ulcer disease
PT-R	prothrombin time ratio		percutaneous ureteral dilatation
PTRA	percutaneous transluminal renal angioplasty	PUE	pyrexia of unknown etiology
		PUF	pure ultrafiltration
PTR-MS	proton transfer reaction mass spectrometry	PUFA	polyunsaturated fatty acids
		PUFFA	polyunsaturated free fatty acids
PTS	patellar tendon suspension	PUJ	pelviureteral junction
	Pediatric Trauma Score	pul.	pulmonary
	permanent threshold shift	PULP	pulpotomy
	post-thrombotic syndrome	Pulse A	pulse apical
	prior to surgery	PULSE OX	pulse oximetry
PTSD	post-traumatic stress disorder		
PTSD-T	post-traumatic stress disorder related to the transplant	Pulse R	pulse radial
		PULSES	(physical profile) physical condition, upper limb functions, lower limb functions, sensory components, excretory functions, and support factors
PTT	partial thromboplastin time		
	pharyngeal transit time		
	platelet transfusion therapy		
	posterior tibial tendon		
	protein truncation testing	PUN	plasma urea nitrogen
	pulse transit time	PUND	pregnancy, uterine, not delivered
PTT-C	partial thromboplastin time control		

P

PUNL	percutaneous ultrasonic nephrolithotripsy	PVDA	prednisone, vincristine, daunorubicin, and asparaginase
PUO	pyrexia of unknown origin	PVDF	polyvinylidene difluoride
PUP	percutaneous ultrasonic pyelolithotomy	PVE	perivenous encephalomyelitis
			portal vein embolization
	previously untreated patient		premature ventricular extrasystole
PU/PL	partial upper and lower dentures		prosthetic value endocarditis
PUPPP	pruritic urticarial papules and plaque of pregnancy	P vera	polycythemia vera
		PVF	peripheral visual field
PUS	percutaneous ureteral stent	PVFS	postviral fatigue syndrome
	preoperative ultrasound	PVGM	perifoveolar vitreoglial membrane
PUU	Puumala hantavirus	PVH	periventricular hemorrhage
PUV	posterior urethral valves		periventricular hyperintensity
PUVA	psoralen-ultraviolet-light (treatment)		pulmonary vascular hypertension
PUW	pick-up walker	PVI	pelvic venous incompetence
PV	papillomavirus		peripheral vascular insufficiency
	Parvovirus		portal-vein infusion
	pemphigus vulgaris		protracted venous infusion
	per vagina		pulmonary valve insufficiency
	plasma volume	PVK	penicillin V potassium
	polio vaccine	PVL	Panton-Valentine leukocidin
	polycythemia vera		peripheral vascular laboratory
	popliteal vein		periventricular leukomalacia
	portal vein	PVM	paraverteabral muscle
	postoperative vomiting		proteins, vitamins, and minerals
	postvoiding	PVMS	paravertebral muscle spasms
	prenatal vitamins	PVN	peripheral venous nutrition
	projectile vomiting	PVNS	pigmented villonodular synovitis
	pulmonary vein	PVO	peripheral vascular occlusion
Pv	*Plasmodium vivax*		portal vein occlusion
P & V	peak and valley (this is a dangerous abbreviation, use peak and trough)		pulmonary venous occlusion
		PVo	pulmonary valve opening
	pyloroplasty and vagotomy	Pvo$_2$	partial pressure (tension) of oxygen, vein
PVA	polyethylene vinyl acetate		
	polyvinyl alcohol		peripheral vascular occlusive disease
	Prinzmetal variant angina	PVOD	pulmonary vascular obstructive disease
PVAD	prolonged venous access devices		
PVAM	potential visual acuity meter	PVP	cisplatin (Platinol) and etoposide (VePesid)
PVAR	pulmonary vein atrial reversal		
PVB	cisplatin, (Platinol) vinblastine, and bleomycin		penicillin V potassium
			peripheral venous pressure
	paravertebral block		Photoselective Vaporization of the Prostate (procedure)
	porcelain veneer bridge		
	premature ventricular beat		polyvinylpyrrolidone
PVC	paclitaxel, vinblastine, and cisplatin		portal venous pressure
	polyethylene vacuum cup		posteroventral pallidotomy
	polyvinyl chloride	P-VP-B	cisplatin (Platinol), etoposide (VP-16), and bleomycin
	porcelain veneer crown		
	postvoiding cystogram	PVR	peripheral vascular resistance
	premature ventricular contraction		perspective volume rendering
	pulmonary venous congestion		postvoiding residual
PVCD	percutaneous vascular closure device		proliferative vitreoretinopathy
Pvco$_2$	partial pressure (tension) of carbon dioxide, vein		pulmonary valve replacement
			pulmonary vascular resistance
PVD	patient very disturbed		pulse-volume recording
	peripheral vascular disease	PVRI	pulmonary vascular resistance index
	posterior vitreous detachment	PVS	percussion, vibration and suction
	premature ventricular depolarization		peripheral vascular surgery

	peritoneovenous shunt		pulse-wave velocity
	persistent vegetative state	Px	physical exam
	Plummer-Vinson syndrome		pneumothorax
	pubovaginal sling		prognosis
	pulmonic valve stenosis		prophylaxis
PVT	paroxysmal ventricular tachycardia	PXAT	paroxysmal atrial tachycardia
	physical volume test	PXE	pseudoxanthoma elasticum
	portal vein thrombosis	PXF	pseudoexfoliation
	previous trouble	PXL	paclitaxel (Taxol)
	private	PXS	dental prophylaxis (cleaning)
	proximal vein thrombosis	PY	pack-years (see pk yrs)
PVTT	tumor thrombus in the portal vein		person-year
PVV	persistent varicose veins	PYAR	person-years at risk
PW	pacing wires	PYE	person-years of exposure
	patient waiting	PYHx	packs per year history
	plantar wart	PYLL	potential years of life lost
	posterior wall	PYP	pyrophosphate
	pulse width	PYP®	technetium Tc 99m pyrophosphate kit
	puncture wound		
P&W	pressures and waves	PZ	peripheral zone
PWA	persons with AIDS	PZA	pyrazinamide
	P-wave axis		pyrazoloacridine (a drug class of sedative/hypnotics)
PWACR	Prader-Willi/Angelman critical region	PZD	partial zona drilling
P wave	part of the electrocardio-graphic cycle representing atrial depolarization		partial zonal dissection
		PZI	protamine zinc insulin
		PZR	posterior zygomatic root
PWB	partial weight bearing		
	Positive Well being (scale)		
	psychological well-being		
PWBL	partial weight bearing, left		
PWBR	partial weight bearing, right		
PWC	personal watercraft		
	physical working capacity		
	powered wheelchair		
PWCA	personal watercraft accident		
PWD	patients with diabetes		
	person(s) with a disability		
	powder		
PWE	people with epilepsy		
PWI	pediatric walk-in clinic		
	perfusion-weighted (magnetic resonance) imaging		
	posterior wall infarct		
PWLV	posterior wall of left ventricle		
PWM	pokeweed mitogens		
PWMI	posterior wall myocardial infarction		
PWO	persistent withdrawal occlusion		
PWP	pulmonary wedge pressure		
PWS	plagiocephaly without synostosis		
	port-wine stain		
	Prader-Willi syndrome		
PWT	pad weight test(s)		
	posterior wall thickness		
	primary writing tremor		
PWTd	posterior wall thickness at end-diastole		
PWV	polistes wasp venom		

P

Q

Q	every
	quadriceps
QA	quality assurance
QAC	before every meal (this is a dangerous abbreviation)
QALE	quality-adjusted life expectancy
QALYs	quality-adjusted life years
QAM	every morning (this is a dangerous abbreviation because the Q can be read as a 9)
QAPI	quality assessment and performance improvement
QAS	quality-adjusted survival
QATTP	quality-adjusted time to progression
QB	blood flow
QC	quad cane
	quality checks
	quality control
	quick catheter
QCA	quantitative coronary angiography
Q compound	Chinese cucumber
QCSW	Qualified Clinical Social Worker
QCT	quantitative computed tomography
QD	dialysate flow
	every day (this is a dangerous abbreviation as it is read as four times daily-QID; use "once daily")
	quinupristin and dalfopristin (Synercid)
QDAM	once daily in the morning (this is a dangerous abbreviation)
QDAY	every day
QDNs	quantum dot nanocrystals
QDPM	once daily in the evening (This is a dangerous abbreviation)
QDS	United Kingdom abbreviation for four times a day
QE	quinidine effect
QED	every even day (this is a dangerous abbreviation as it will be read as four times daily-QID)
	quick and early diagnosis
QEE	quadriceps extension exercise
QEMG	quantitative electromyography
QF	quadriceps femoris (muscle)
QFB	Qu'mico Farmacéutico Bi-logo (Chemist Pharmacist Biologist; Pharmacist in Mexico)
QF-PCR	quantitative fluorescence polymerase chain reaction
QFV	Q fever (*Coxiella burnetii*) vaccine
QGS	quantitative gate SPECT (single photon emission computed tomography)
q4h	every four hours
q.h.	every hour
qhs	once daily at bedtime, each day (this is a dangerous abbreviation as it is read as every hour-QHR or four times daily-QID)
QIAD	Quantitative Inventory of Alcohol Disorders
q.i.d.	four times daily
QIDM	four times daily with meals and at bedtime
QIG	quantitative immunoglobulins
QIMT	quantitative intima media thickness
QIO	Quality Improvement Organization
QIW	four times a week (this is a dangerous abbreviation)
QJ	quadriceps jerk
QKD interval	Korotkoff sounds
QL	quality of life
QLI	Quality of Life Index
QLS	quality of life score
QM	every morning (this is a dangerous abbreviation as it will not be understood)
Qmax	maximal flow rate
QMB	qualified Medicare beneficiary
QMI	Q-wave myocardial infarction
QMRP	qualified mental retardation professional
QMT	quantitative muscle testing
q.n.	every night (this is a dangerous abbreviation as it is read as every hour)
q.n.s.	quantity not sufficient
qod	every other day (this is a dangerous abbreviation as it is read as every day or four times a day-QID)
qoh	every other hour (this is a dangerous abbreviation as it is read as every day or four times a day-QID)
qohs	every other day at bedtime (this is a dangerous abbreviation as it is read as every hour-QHR or four times daily-QID)
QOL	quality of life
QOLIE-31	quality of life in epilepsy
QOM	quality of motion
QON	every other night (this is a dangerous abbreviation)
QPCR	quantitative polymerase chain reaction
qpm	every evening (this is a dangerous abbreviation)
QPOS	Quality Point of Service

QP/QS	ratio of pulmonary blood to systemic blood flow
qqh	every four hours (United Kingdom)
qqs	every four hours (United Kingdom)
QR	quiet room
QRC	qualitative radiocardiography
QRDR	quinolone resistance-determining region(s)
QRE	quality-related event
QRNG	quinolone-resistant *N. gonorrhoeae*
QRS	part of electrocardio-graphic wave representing ventricular depolarization
QS	every shift
	quadriceps set
	quadrilateral socket
	Quality Services (Department)
	sufficient quantity
qs ad	a sufficient quantity to make
QS&L	quarters, subsistence, and laundry
Qs/Qt	intrapulmonary shunt fraction
QSP	physiological shunt fraction
QT	the time between the beginning of the QRS complex and the end of the T-wave
qt	quart
QTB	quadriceps tendon bearing
QTC	quantitative tip cultures
QTc	the QTc interval is the length of time it takes the electrical system in the heart to repolarize, adjusted for heart rate (normal 350-440 milliseconds)
QTL	quantitative trait locus
QTP	quetiapine fumarate (Seroquel)
Q-TWiST	quality-adjusted time without symptoms (of disease) and toxicity
QTY	quantity
QUAD	quadrant
	quadriceps
	quadriplegic
QU	quiet
QUART	quadrantectomy, axillary dissection, and radiotherapy
QUEST	Quality of Upper Extremity Skills Test
QUM	Quality Use of Medicines (Australia)
QuMA	quantitative microsatellite analysis
QUS	quantitative (bone) ultrasound
QW	every week (this is a dangerous abbreviation)
	Q-wave
q4w	every 4 weeks (this is a dangerous abbreviation)
QWB	Quality of Well-Being (scale)
QWE	every weekend (this is a dangerous abbreviation)
QWK	once a week (this is a dangerous abbreviation)
Q4wk	every four weeks (this is a dangerous abbreviation)
QWMI	Q-wave myocardial infarction

R

R   radial
rate
ratio
reacting
rectal
rectum
regular
regular insulin
resistant
respiration
reticulocyte
retinoscopy
rifampicin [part of tuberculosis regimen, see RHZ(E/S)/HR]
right (this a dangerous abbreviation; spell out "right" to avoid surgical errors)
Ritalin (methylphenidate) as in vitamin R
roentgen
rub

r   recombinant

®   rectal (rectally, rectum)
registered trademark
right (this is a dangerous abbreviation; spell out "right" to avoid surgical errors)

−R   Rinne test, negative

+R   Rinne test, positive

RA   radial artery
radiographic absorptiometry
rales
readmission
renal artery
repeat action
retinoic acid
rheumatoid arthritis
right arm
right atrium
right auricle
room air
rotational atherectomy

RAA   renin-angiotensin-aldosterone
right atrial abnormality
right atrial appendage

RAAA   ruptured abdominal aortic aneurysm

RAAS   renin-angiotensin-aldosterone system

RAB   rabies vaccine, not otherwise specified
rice (rice cereal), applesauce, and banana (diet)

RAB_DEV   rabies vaccine, duck embryo culture

RAB_FRhL-2   rabies vaccine, diploid fetal-rhesus-lung-2 cell line

RABG   room air blood gas

RAB_HDCV   rabies vaccine, human diploid cell culture

RABig   rabies immune globulin

RAB_PCEC   rabies vaccine, purified chick embryo cell culture

RAC   Recombinant DNA Advisory Committee
right antecubital
right atrial catheter

RACCO   right anterior caudocranial oblique

RACT   recalcified whole-blood activated clotting time

RACZ   a procedure of dissolving lumbar scar tissue (epidurolysis)

RAD   ionizing radiation unit
radical
radiology
rapid antigen detection
reactive airway disease
reactive attachment disorder
right axis deviation

RADCA   right anterior descending coronary artery

RADE   reactive airway disease exacerbation

RADISH   rheumatoid arthritis diffuse idiopathic skeletal hyperostosis

RADS   ionizing radiation units
rapid assay delivery systems
reactive airway disease syndrome

RADT   rapid antigen detection testing

RAE   right atrial enlargement

RAEB   refractory anemia, erythroblastic

RAEB-T   refractory anemia with excess blasts in transition

RAF   rapid atrial fibrillation

RAFF   rectus abdominis free flap

RAFT   Rehabilitative Addicted Family Treatment

RAG   room air gas

RAH   right atrial hypertrophy

RAHB   right anterior hemiblock

rAHF   antihemophilic factor (recombinant)

RAI   radioactive iodine
Resident Assessment Instrument

RAID   radioimmunodetection

RAIT   radioimmunotherapy

RAIU   radioactive iodine uptake

RALT   routine admission laboratory tests

RAM   radioactive material
rapid alternating movements
rectus abdominis myocutaneous

RA/MAC   regional anesthesia with monitored anesthesia care

RAN   resident's admission notes

R₂AN   second year resident's admission notes

RANKL   receptor activator of NFκB ligand

RANTES	regulated upon activation, normal T cell expressed and secreted	RBCV	red blood cell volume
RANZCOG	Fellows of the Royal Australian and New Zealand College of Obstetricians and Gynaecologists	RBD	REM (rapid eye movement sleep) behavior disorder
			right border of dullness
			right brain-damaged
RANZCP	Fellows of the Royal Australian and New Zealand College of Psychiatrists	RbDe	residue-based diagram editor
		RBE	relative biologic effectiveness
		RBF	renal blood flow
RAO	right anterior oblique	RBG	random blood glucose
rAOM	recurrent acute otitis media	RBILD	respiratory bronchiolitis-associated interstitial lung disease
RAP	renal artery pseudoaneurysm		
	request for advance payment	RBL	Roche Biomedical Laboratory
	right abdominal pain	RBON	retrobulbar optic neuritis
	right atrial pressure	RBOW	rupture bag of water
RAPA	radial artery pseudoaneurysm	RBP	recurrent bacterial pneumonia
RAQ	right anterior quadrant		retinol-binding protein
RAP	recurrent abdominal pain	RBRVS	Medicare resource-based relative-value scale
	request for anticipated payment		
	Resident Assessment Protocol (long-term care)	RBS	random blood sugar
			redback spider
RAPD	random amplified polymorphic DNA	RBT	rational behavior therapy
	relative afferent pupillary defect	RBV	right brachial vein
RAPs	Resident Assessment Protocols	RBVO	right brachial vein occlusion
RAR	right arm, reclining	RBX	ruboxistaurin
RARs	retinoic acid receptors	RC	race
RAS	recurrent aphthous stomatitis		radiocarpal (joint)
	renal artery stenosis		Red Cross
	renal artery stenting		report called
	renin-angiotensin system		retention catheter
	reticular activating system		retrograde cystogram
	right arm, sitting		retruded contact (position)
RASE	rapid-acquisition spin echo		right coronary
RAST	radioallergosorbent test		Roman Catholic
RAT	right anterior thigh		root canal
RA test	test for rheumatoid factor		rotator cuff
RATG	rabbit antithymocyte globulin	R/C	reclining chair
RATx	radiation therapy	R & C	reasonable and customary (charges)
RAU	recurrent aphthous ulcers		
RAVLT	Rey Auditory Verbal Learning Test	RCA	radiographic contrast agent
R(AW)	airway resistance		radionuclide cerebral angiogram
RB	relieved by		right carotid artery
	retinoblastoma		right coronary artery
	retrobulbar		rolling circle amplification
	right breast		root cause analysis
	right buttock	RC/AL	residential care, assisted living
R & B	right and below	RCBF	regional cerebral blood flow
RBA	right basilar artery	RCC	rape crisis center
	right brachial artery		resectable colon cancer
	risks, benefits, and alternatives (discussion with patient)		renal cell carcinoma
			Roman Catholic Church
RBB	right breast biopsy	RCCA	right common carotid artery
RBBB	right bundle branch block	RCCT	randomized controlled clinical trial
RBBX	right breast biopsy examination	RCD	relative cardiac dullness
RBC	ranitidine bismuth citrate	RCE	right carotid endartcrectomy
	red blood cell (count)	RCF	Reiter complement fixation
RBCD	right border cardiac dullness	RCF®	enteral nutrition product
RBCM	red blood cell mass	RCFA	right common femoral angioplasty
RBC s/f	red blood cells spun filtration		right common femoral artery

RCFE	residential care facility for the elderly		right deltoid
			ruptured disk
RCH	residential care home	RDA	recommended daily allowance
RCHF	right-sided congestive heart failure		Registered Dental Assistant
R-CHOP	rituximab (Rituxan), cyclophosphamide, doxorubicin (hydroxydaunorubicin), vincristine (Oncovin), and prednisone		representational difference analysis
		RDB	randomized double-blind (trial)
		RDCS	Registered Diagnostic Cardiac Sonographer
RCIN	radiographic-contrast-media-induced nephropathy	RDD	renal dose dopamine
			Rosai-Dorfman disease
RCIP	rape crisis intervention program	RDE	remote data entry
RCL	radial collateral ligament		respiratory disturbance events
	range of comfortable loudness	RDEA	right deviation of electrical axis
RCM	radiographic contrast media	RDEB	recessive dystrophic epidermolysis bullosa
	restricted cardiomyopathy		
	retinal capillary microaneurysm	RDG	right dorsogluteal
	right costal margin	RDH	Registered Dental Hygienist
RCN	radiocontrast-agent-induced nephrotoxicity	RDI	respiratory disturbance (distress) index
RCO	revoked court order	RDIH	right direct inguinal hernia
RCOG	Royal College of Obstetricians and Gynaecologists	RDLBBB	rate-dependent left bundle branch block
RCOT	revoked court-ordered treatment	RDM	right deltoid muscle
RCP	respiratory care plan	RDMS	Registered Diagnostic Medical Sonographer
	retrograde cerebral perfusion		
	Royal College of Physicians	RDMs	reactive drug metabolites
RCPM	raven-colored progressive matrices	RDOD	retinal detachment, right eye
RCPT	Registered Cardiopulmonary Technician	RDOS	retinal detachment, left eye
		RDP	random donor platelets
RCR	replication-competent retrovirus (assay)		right dorsoposterior
		RDPE	reticular degeneration of the pigment epithelium
	rotator cuff repair		
RCS	repeat cesarean section	RDS	research diagnostic criteria
	reticulum cell sarcoma		respiratory distress syndrome
	Royal College of Surgeons	RDT	rapid diagnostic test
RCT	randomized clinical trial		regular dialysis (hemodialysis) treatment
	Registered Care Technologist		
	root canal therapy	RDTD	referral, diagnosis, treatment, and discharge
	Rorschach Content Test		
	rotator cuff tear	RDU	recreational drug use
RCU	respiratory care unit	RDVT	recurrent deep vein thrombosis
RCV	red cell volume	RDW	red (cell) distribution width
	right colic vein	RE	concerning
RCVD	received		Rasmussen encephalitis
RCX	ramus circumflexus		rectal examination
RD	radial deviation		reflux esophagitis
	Raynaud disease		regarding
	reaction of degeneration		regional enteritis
	reading disability		reticuloendothelial
	reflex decay		retinol equivalents
	Registered Dietitian		right ear (this is a dangerous abbreviation as it can be read as right eye)
	renal disease		
	respiratory disease		
	respiratory distress		right eye (this a dangerous abbreviation as it can be read as right ear)
	restricted duty		
	retinal detachment		
	Reye disease		rowing ergometer
	rhabdomyosarcoma	^{186}Re	rhenium 186

R & E	rest and exercise		report
	round and equal	REP CK	rapid electrophoresis creatine kinase
R ↑ E	right upper extremity	REPL	recurrent early pregnancy loss
R ↓ E	right lower extremity	repol	repolarization
RE✓	recheck	REPS	repetitions
READM	readmission	REPT	Registered Evoked Potential
REAL	Revised European American		Technologist
	Lymphoma (classification)	RER	renal excretion rate
REALM	Rapid Estimation of Adult Literacy	RER+	replication error positive
	in Medicine	RES	recurrent erosion syndrome
REC	gingival recession		resection
	rear-end collision		resident
	recommend		reticuloendothelial system
	record	RESC	resuscitation
	recovery	RESP	respirations
	recreation		respiratory
	recur	REST	restoration
RECA	right external carotid artery		restriction of environmental
RECIST	Response Evaluation Criteria in		stimulation therapy
	Solid Tumors (guidelines)	RET	retention
	CR = complete response		reticulocyte
	PR = partial response		retina
	PD = progressive disease		retired
	SD = stable disease		return
RECT	rectum		right esotropia
REDA	Registered Eating Disorders	ret detach	retinal detachment
	Associate	retic	reticulocyte
REDs	reproductive endocrine diseases	RETRO	retrograde
RED SUBS	reducing substances	RETRX	retractions
REE	resting energy expenditure	REUE	resistive exercise, upper extremities
RE-ED	re-education	REV	reverse
R-EEG	resting electroencephalogram		review
REEGT	Registered Electroencephalogram		revolutions
	Technologist	RF	radiofrequency
REF	referred		reduction fixation
	refused		refill; refilled (prescriptions)
	renal erythropoietic factor		renal failure
ref→	refer to		respiratory failure
REG	radioencephalogram		restricted fluids
	regression analysis		rheumatic fever
Reg block	regional block anesthesia		rheumatoid factor
regurg	regurgitation		ring finger
rehab	rehabilitation		right foot
REL	relative		risk factor
	religion		radiofrequency
RELE	resistive exercise, lower extremities	R/F	retroflexed
REM	rapid eye movement	R&F	radiographic and fluoroscopic
	recent event memory	RF6	rejection-free survival at 6 months
	remarried	RFA	radiofrequency ablation
	remission		right femoral artery
	roentgen equivalent unit		right forearm
REMI	remifentanil (Ultiva)		right frontoanterior
REMS	rapid eye movement sleep	rFVIIa	recombinant activated coagulation
REO	respiratory and enteric orphan		factor VII (NovoSeven)
	(viruses)	RFB	retained foreign body
REP	rapid electrophoresis		radial flow chromatography
	repair		residual functional capacity
	repeat	RFC	reduced folate carrier

RFCA	radiofrequency catheter ablation	rest home
RFD	residue-free diet	retinal hemorrhage
RFDT	Reach in Four Directions Test	right hand
RFE	return flow enema	right hemisphere
RFFF	radial forearm free flap (reconstruction of pharyngeal defect)	right hyperphoria / room humidifier
		Rh+ Rhesus positive
RFFIT	rapid fluorescent focus inhibition test	Rh− Rhesus negative
rFVIII FS	antihemophilic factor (recombinant), formulated with sucrose (Kogenate)	RHA rheumatoid arthritis (therapeutic) vaccine / right hepatic artery
RFg	visual fields by Goldmann-type perimeter	rHA recombinant human albumin
rFGF-2	recombinant fibroblast growth factor-2	rhAPC recombinant human activated protein C
RFID	radio frequency identification	RHB raise head of bed / right heart border
RFIPC	Rating Form of IBD (inflammatory bowel disease) Patient Concerns	RH/BSO radial hysterectomy and bilateral salpingo-oophorectomy
RFL	radionuclide functional lymphoscintigraphy / right frontolateral	RHC respiration has ceased / right heart catheterization / right hemicolectomy / routine health care / rural health clinic
RFLF	retained fetal lung fluid	
RFLP	restriction fragment length polymorphism (patterns)	RHD radial head dislocation
RFM	rifampin (Rifadin)	relative hepatic dullness
RFP	Renal function panel (see page 298) / request for payment / request for proposal / right frontoposterior	rheumatic heart disease / right-hand dominant
		rh-DNase dornase alfa (Pulmozyme)
		rhEPO recombinant human erythropoietin
RFS	rapid frozen section / recurrence-free survival / refeeding syndrome / relapse-free survival	RHF rheumatic fever vaccine / right heart failure
		RHG right-hand grip
		rhGH recombinant human growth hormone
RFT	respiratory function test / right frontotransverse / routine fever therapy	r-hGH(m) mammalian-cell–derived recombinant human growth hormone (Serostim)
RFTA	radiofrequency thermal ablation	RHH right homonymous hemianopsia
RFTC	radiofrequency thermocoagulation	RHIA Registered Health Information Administrator
RFUT	radioactive fibrinogen uptake	
RFV	reason for visit / right femoral vein	RHINO rhinoplasty
		RHIOs regional health information organizations
RFVTR	radiofrequency volumetric tissue reduction	RHIT Registered Health Information Technician
RG	regurgitated (infant feeding) / right (upper outer) gluteus	RHL right hemisphere lesions / right heptic lobe
R/G	red/green	rhm roentgens per hour at one meter
RGA	right gastroepiploic artery	
RGCSE	refractory generalized convulsive status epilepticus	RHO right heel off
		Rho(D) immune globulin to an Rh-negative woman
RGM	rapidly growing Mycobacteria / recurrent glioblastoma multiforme / right gluteus medius	RhoGAM® Rh₀ (D) immune globulin
		RHP resting head pressure
RGO	reciprocating gait orthosis	rhPDGF recombinant human platelet-derived growth factor
RGP	rigid gas-permeable (contact lens)	
Rh	Rhesus factor in blood	RHR resting heart rate
RH	radical hysterectomy / reduced haloperidol / relative humidity	RHS right-hand side
		RHT regional hyperthermia / right hypertropia

rHuEPO	recombinant human erythropoietin	RINV	radiation-induced nausea and vomiting
Rhupus	coexistence of rheumatoid arthritis and systemic lupus erythematosus	RIO	right inferior oblique (muscle)
RHV	right hepatic vein	RIOJ	recurrent intrahepatic obstructive jaundice
RHW	radiant heat warmer		
RHZ(E/S)/	a tuberculosis treatment	R-IOL	remove intraocular lens
HR	regimen consisting of rifampicin, isoniazid, pyrazinamide, ethambutol, streptomycin, isoniazid, and rifampicin (also see 2EHRZ/6HE)	RIP	radioimmunoprecipitin test
			rapid infusion pump
			respiratory inductance plethysmograph
			rhythmic inhibitory pattern
RI	ramus intermedius (coronary artery)	RIPA	ristocetin-induced platelet agglutination
	refractive index		
	Registered Indian (Canada)	RIR	right inferior rectus
	regular insulin	RIS	responding to internal stimuli
	relapse incidence		risperidone (Risperdal)
	renal insufficiency	RISA	radioactive iodinated serum albumin
	respiratory illness	RISS	regular insulin sliding scale
	retroillumination	RIST	radioimmunosorbent test
	rooming in	RIT	radioimmunotherapy
RIA	radioimmunoassay		ritonavir (Norvir)
	reversible ischemic attack		Rorschach Inkblot Test
RIAC	rapid inflation, asymmetrical compression (device)	RITA	right internal thoracic artery
		RIVD	ruptured intervertebral disk
RIAT	radioimmune antiglobulin test	RIX	radiation-induced xerostomia
RIBA	recombinant immunoblot assay	RJ	radial jerk (reflex)
RIBC	residual infiltrating breast cancer		right jugular
RIC	reduced intensity conditioning	RK	radial keratotomy
	right iliac crest		right kidney
	right internal carotid (artery)	RKS	renal kidney stone
RICA	right internal carotid artery	RKT	Registered Kinesiotherapist
RICE	rest, ice, compression, and elevation	RL	right lateral
RICM	right intercostal margin		right leg
RICS	right intercostal space		right lower
RICU	respiratory intensive care unit		right lung
RID	radial immunodiffusion		Ringer lactate
	ruptured intervertebral disk		rotation left
RIDL	Release of Insects with a Dominant Lethal (mutations)	R → L	right to left
		RLA	right lower arm
RIE	radiation induced emesis	RLB	right lateral bending
	reactive ion etching		right lateral border
	rocket immunoelectrophoresis	RLBCD	right lower border of cardiac dullness
RIF	rifampin		
	right iliac fossa	RLC	residual lung capacity
	right index finger	RLD	reference listed drug
	rigid internal fixation		related living donor
RIG	rabies immune globulin		remaining life expectancy
RIGS	radioimmunoguided surgery		right lateral decubitus
RIH	right inguinal hernia		ruptured lumbar disk
RIHP	renal interstitial hydrostatic pressure	RLDP	right lateral decubital position
		RLE	right lower extremity
RIJ	right internal jugular	RLF	retrolental fibroplasia
RIMA	reversible inhibitor of monoamine oxidase-type A		right lateral femoral
		RLFP	Remaining Lifetime Fracture Probability
	right internal mammary anastamosis		
	right internal mammary artery	RLG	right lateral gaze
RIN	radiocontrast-induced nephropathy	RLGS	restriction landmark genomic scanning
RIND	reversible ischemic neurologic defect		

RLH	reactive lymphoid hyperplasia	RMI	Rivermead Mobility Index
RLL	right liver lobe	RMK #1	remark number 1
	right lower lid	RML	right mediolateral
	right lower lobe		right middle lobe
RLN	recurrent laryngeal nerve	RMLE	right mediolateral episiotomy
	regional lymph node(s)	RMMA	rhythmic masticatory muscle activity
RLND	regional lymph node dissection	RMO	responsible medical officer
RLQ	right lower quadrant	rMOG	recombinant myelin oligodendrocyte
RLQD	right lower quadrant defect		glycoprotein
RLR	right lateral rectus	RMP	right mentoposterior
RLRTD	recurrent lower respiratory tract		risk management program
	disease	RMR	resting metabolic rate
RLS	resonance light scattering		right medial rectus
	restless legs syndrome		root mean square residue
	Ringer lactate solution	RMRM	right modified radical mastectomy
	stammerer who has difficulty in	RMS	red-man syndrome
	enunciating R, L, and S		Rehabilitation Medicine Service
RLSB	right lower scapular border		repetitive motion syndrome
	right lower sternal border		rhabdomyosarcoma
RLT	right lateral thigh		Rocky Mountain spotted fever
RLTCS	repeat low transverse cesarean		vaccine
	section		root-mean-square
RLUs	relative light units	RMS®	rectal morphine sulfate (suppository)
RLWD	routine laboratory work done	RMSB	right middle sternal border
RLX	raloxifene (Evista)	RMSE	root-mean-square error
	right lower extremity	RMSF	Rocky Mountain spotted fever
RM	radical mastectomy	RMT	Registered Music Therapist
	repetitions maximum		right mentotransverse
	respiratory movement	RMV	respiratory minute volume
	risk manager (management)	RMW	respiratory muscle weakness
	risk model	RN	Registered Nurse
	room		right nostril (nare)
R&M	routine and microscopic	Rn	radon
1-RM	single repetition maximum lift	R/N	renew
RMA	reduction in metabolic activity	RNA	radionuclide angiography
	Registered Medical Assistant		Restorative Nursing Assistant
	right mentoanterior		ribonucleic acid
	Rivermead motor assessment		routine nursing assistance
RMB	right main bronchus	RN,BC	Registered Nurse, Board Certified
RMBPC	Revise Memory and Behavior		(many clinical specialties)
	Problems Checklist	RNC	Registered Nurse, Certified
RMCA	right main coronary artery	RNCD	Registered Nurse, Chemical
	right middle cerebral artery		Dependency
RMCAT	right middle cerebral artery	RNCNA	Registered Nurse Certified in
	thrombosis		Nursing Administration
RMCL	right midclavicular line	RNCNAA	Registered Nurse Certified in
RMD	recommended maintenance dose		Nursing Administration Advanced
	rippling muscle disease	RNCS	Registered Nurse Certified Specialist
RMDQ	Roland and Morris disability	RND	radical neck dissection
	questionnaire	RNEF	resting (radio-) nuclide ejection
RME	reasonable maximum exposure		fraction
	resting metabolic expenditure	RNF	regular nursing floor
	right mediolateral episiotomy	RNFA	registered nurse first assistant
RMEE	right middle ear exploration	RNFL	retinal nerve fiber layer
rMET	recombinant methioninase	RNFLT	retinal nerve fiber layer thickness
RMF	right middle finger	RNI	reactive nitrogen intermediates
RMGIC	resin-modified glass ionomer cement		rubella nonimmune
	(dental)	RNLP	Registered Nurse, license pending

RNP	Registered Nurse Practitioner	ROMWNL	range of motion within normal limits
	restorative nursing program	RON	radiation optic neuropathy
	ribonucleoprotein	RONTD	risk of neural tube defect
RNS	recurrent nephrotic syndrome	ROP	retinopathy of prematurity
	replacement normal saline (0.9%		right occiput posterior
	sodium chloride)	ROPS	roll-over protection structures
RNST	reactive nonstress test	ROR	the French acronym for measles-
RNUD	recurrent nonulcer dyspepsia		mumps-rubella vaccine
RNV	radionucleotide ventriculogram		reporting odds ratio
RO	reality orientation	R or L	right or left
	relative odds	ROS	review of systems
	report of		rod outer segments
	reverse osmosis		rule out sepsis
	routine order(s)	ROSA	rank-order stability analysis
	Russian Orthodox	ROSC	restoration of spontaneous
R/O	rule out		circulation
ROA	radiographic osteoarthritis	ROSS	review of signs and symptoms
	right occiput anterior	ROT	remedial occupational therapy
ROAC	repeated oral doses of activated		right occipital transverse
	charcoal		rotator
ROAD	reversible obstructive airway disease	ROU	recurrent oral ulcer
ROBE	routine operative breast endoscopy	ROUL	rouleaux (rouleau)
ROC	receiver operating characteristic	ROW	rest of (the) week
	record of contact	RP	radial pulse
	resident on call		radical prostatectomy
	residual organic carbon		radiopharmaceutical
ROCF	Rey-Osterrieth complex figure		Raynaud phenomenon
ROD	rapid opioid detoxification		responsible party
RODA	rapid opiate detoxification under		resting position
	anesthesia		restorative proctocolectomy
ROE	report of event		retinitis pigmentosa
	right otitis externa		retrograde pyelogram
ROF	review of outside films		retropubic prostatectomy
ROG	rogletimide		root plane
ROH	rubbing alcohol	RPA	radial photon absorptiometry
ROI	region of interest (radiology)		recursive partitioning analysis
	release of information		Registered Physician's Assistant
ROIDS	hemorrhoids		repolarization alternans
ROIH	right oblique inguinal hernia		restenosis postangioplasty
ROJM	range of joint motion		ribonuclease protection assay
ROL	right occipitolateral		right pulmonary artery
ROLC	roentgenologically occult lung	RPAC	Registered Physician's Assistant
	cancer		Certified
ROLL	radioguided occult lesion localization	RPC	root planing and curettage
ROM	range of motion	RPCDBM	randomized, placebo-controlled,
	rifampicin 600 mg, ofloxacin 400		double-blind, multinational (study)
	mg, and minocycline 100 mg	RPCF	Reiter protein complement fixation
	right otitis media	RPD	removable partial denture
	rupture of membranes	RPE	rating of perceived exertion
ROMA	representative oligonucleotide		retinal pigment epithelium
	microarray analysis	RPED	retinal pigment epithelium
Romb	Romberg		detachment
ROMCP	range of motion complete and	RPEP	rabies postexposure prophylaxis
	painfree		right pre-ejection period
ROMI	rule out myocardial infarction	RPF	regional progression-free
ROMSA	right otitis media, suppurative, acute		relaxed pelvic floor
ROMSC	right otitis media, suppurative,		renal plasma flow
	chronic		retroperitoneal fibrosis

RPFT	Registered Pulmonary Function Technologist	RRA	radioreceptor assay
RPG	retrograde percutaneous gastrostomy		Registered Record Administrator (for newer title, see RHIA)
	retrograde pyelogram		right radial artery
RPGN	rapidly progressive glomerulonephritis		right renal artery
		RRAM	rapid rhythmic alternating movements
RPH	retroperitoneal hemorrhage		
RPh	Registered Pharmacist	RRC	cohort relative risk
RPHA	reverse passive hemagglutination	RRCT,	regular rate, clear tones,
RPI	resting pressure index	no(m)	no murmurs
	reticulocyte production index	RRD	removable rigid dressing
RPICA	right posterior internal carotid artery		rhegmatogenous retinal detachment
RPICCE	round pupil intracapsular cataract extraction	RRE	round, regular, and equal (pupils)
		RRED®	Rapid Rare Event Detection
RPL	retroperitoneal lymphadenectomy	RREF	resting radionuclide ejection fraction
RPLC	reversed-phase liquid chromatography	RRI	renal resistive index
		RR-IOL	remove and replace intraocular lens
RPLND	retroperitoneal lymph node dissection	RRM	reduced renal mass
			right radial mastectomy
RPLS	reversible posterior leukoencephalopathy syndrome		risk-reducing mastectomy
		RRMS	relapsing-remitting multiple sclerosis
RPN	renal papillary necrosis	RRNA	Resident Registered Nurse Anesthetist
	resident's progress notes		
R₂PN	second year resident's progress notes	rRNA	ribosomal ribonucleic acid
RPO	right posterior oblique	RRND	right radical neck dissection
RPP	radical perineal prostatectomy	RROM	resistive range of motion
	rate-pressure product	R rot	right rotation
	retropubic prostatectomy	RRP	radical retropubic prostatectomy
RPPS	retropatellar pain syndrome		recurrent respiratory papillomatosis
RPR	rapid plasma reagin (test for syphilis)	RRR	recovery room routine
	Reiter protein reagin		regular rhythm and rate
RPS	rhabdoid predisposition syndrome		relative risk reduction
RPSGT	Registered Polysomnography Technician	RRRN	round, regular, and react normally
		RRRsM	regular rate and rhythm without murmur
RPT	Registered Physical Therapist		
RPTA	Registered Physical Therapist Assistant	RRSO	risk-reducing salpingo-oophorectomy
		RRT	Registered Respiratory Therapist
RPU	retropubic urethropexy	RRU	rapid reintegration unit
RPV	right portal vein	RRVO	repair relaxed vaginal outlet
	right pulmonary vein	RRVS	recovery room vital signs
RQ	respiratory quotient	RRV-TV	rhesus rotavirus tetravalent (vaccine)
RQLQ	Respiratory Quality of Life Questionnaire	RRW	rales, rhonchi or wheezes
		RS	Raynaud syndrome
RR	recovery room		rectal swab
	regular rate		recurrent seizures
	regular respirations		Reed-Sternberg (cell)
	relative risk		Reiter syndrome
	respiratory rate		remote sensing
	response rate		reschedule
	retinal reflex		restart
	rotation right		Rett syndrome
R/R	rales-rhonchi		Reye syndrome
R&R	rate and rhythm		rhythm strip
	recent and remote		right side
	recession and resection		Ringer solution
	resect and recess (muscle surgery)		rumination syndrome
	rest and recuperation	R/S	reschedule
	remove and replace		rest stress

	rupture spontaneous	RST	rapid simple tests
R & S	restraint and seclusion		rapid Streptococcal test
R/S I	resuscitation status one (full		right sacrum transverse
	resuscitative effort)	RSTs	Rodney Smith tubes
R/S II	resuscitation status two (no code,	RSV	respiratory syncytial virus
	therapeutic measures only)		right subclavian vein
R/S III	resuscitation status three (no code,	RSVC	right superior vena cava
	comfort measures only)	RSV_{IGIV}	respiratory syncytial virus immune
RSA	radiostereometric analysis		globulin, intravenous
	right sacrum anterior	RSV_{mab}	respiratory syncytial virus
	right subclavian artery		monoclonal antibody,
RSAPE	remitting seronegative arthritis with		intramuscular (palivizumab;
	pitting edema		Synagis)
RSB	right sternal border	RSVP	rapid serial visual presentation
RSBI	rapid shallow breathing index	RSW	right-sided weakness
RSBQ	Rett Syndrome Behavior	RT	radiation therapy
	Questionnaire		Radiologic Technologist
RSC	right subclavian (artery) (vein)		recreational therapy
RScA	right scapuloanterior		rectal temperature
RSCL	Rotterdam Symptom Check List		renal transplant
RScP	right scapuloposterior		repetition time
RSCS	respiratory system compliance score		resistance training
rscu-PA	recombinant, single-chain,		Respiratory Therapist
	urokinase-type plasminogen		reverse transcriptase
	activator		right
RSD	reflex sympathetic dystrophy		right thigh
	relative standard deviation		room temperature
RSDS	reflex-sympathetic dystrophy	R/t	related to
	syndrome	RTA	ready to administer
RSE	rattlesnake envenomation		renal tubular acidosis
	reactive subdural effusion		road traffic accident
	refractory status epilepticus	t-RA	tretinoin (*trans*-retinoic acid)
	right sternal edge	RTAE	right atrial enlargement
RSI	rapid sequence intubation	RTAH	right anterior hemiblock
	repetitive strain (stress) injury	RTAT	right anterior thigh
R-SICU	respiratory-surgical intensive care	RTB	return to baseline
	unit	RTC	Readiness to Change (questionnaire)
RSL	renal solute load		return to clinic
RSLR	reverse straight leg raise		round the clock
RSM	remote study monitoring	RTCA	ribavirin
RSNI	round spermatid nuclear injection	RTER	return to emergency room
RSO	right salpingoooophorectomy	rt.↑ext.	right upper extremity
	right superior oblique	RTF	ready-to-feed
rS_{02}	regional oxygen saturation		return to flow
RSOC	regular source of care	RTFS	return to flying status
RSOP	right superior oblique palsy	RTH	right total hip (arthroplasty)
RSP	rapid straight pacing	RTI	respiratory tract infection
	respirable suspended particles		reverse transcriptase inhibitor
	restriction site polymophism	RTIS	response to internal stimuli
	right sacroposterior	RTK	rhabdoid tumor of the kidney
RSR	regular sinus rhythm		right total knee (arthroplasty)
	relative survival rate	RTL	reactive to light
	right superior rectus		right temporal lobectomy
RSRI	renal:systemic renin index	RTLF	respiratory-tract lining fluids
RSS	reduced space symbologies	RTM	regression to the mean
	representative sample sectioned		routine medical care
	Russell-Silver syndrome	RTMCI	real-time myocardial contrast
RSSE	Russian spring-summer encephalitis		perfusion imaging

RTMD	right mid-deltoid	rupt.	ruptured
rTMS	repetitive transcranial magnetic stimulation	RUQ	right upper quadrant
		RUQD	right upper quadrant defect
RTN	renal tubular necrosis	RURTI	recurrent upper respiratory tract infection
RTNM	retreatment staging of cancer		
RTO	return to office	RUS	resonant ultrasound spectroscopy
RTOG	Radiation Therapy Oncology Group	RUSB	right upper scapular border
RTP	renal transplant patient		right upper sternal border
	return to pharmacy	RUT	rapid urease test
	return-to-play	RUTF	ready-to-use therapeutic food
rtPA	alteplase (recombinant tissue-type plasminogen activator) (Activase)	RUTI	recurring urinary tract infections
		RUV	residual urine volume
RT-PCR	reverse transcription polymerase chain reaction	RUX	right upper extremity
		RV	rectovaginal
RTR	renal transplant recipient(s)		residual volume
	return to room		respiratory volume
RT (R)	Radiologic Technologist (Registered)		retinal vasculitis
RTRR	return to recovery room		return visit
RTS	radial tunnel syndrome		rhinovirus
	raised toilet seat		right ventricle
	real-time scan		rubella vaccine
	Resolve Through Sharing	RVA	rabies vaccine, adsorbed
	return to school		right ventricular apex
	return to sender		right vertebral artery
	Revised Trauma Score	RVAD	right ventricular assist device
	Rothmund-Thomson syndrome	RVCD	right ventricular conduction deficit
	Rubinstein-Taybi syndrome	RVD	relative vertebral density
RTT	Respiratory Therapy Technician		renal vascular disease
RT$_3$U	resin triiodothyronine uptake	RVDP	right ventricular diastolic pressure
RTUS	realtime ultrasound	RVE	right ventricular enlargement
RTV	ritonavir (Norvir)	RVEDP	right ventricular end-diastolic pressure
	rotavirus vaccine, not otherwise specified		
		RVEDV	right ventricular end-diastolic volume
RTV$_{rr}$	rotavirus vaccine, rhesus reassortant		
RTW	return to ward	RVEF	right ventricular ejection fraction
	return to work	RVET	right ventricular ejection time
	Richard Turner Warwick (urethroplasty)	RVF	Rift Valley fever
			right ventricular function
RTWD	return to work determination		right visual field
RTX	resiniferatoxin	RVG	radionuclide ventriculography
RTx	radiation therapy		Radio VisioGraphy
	renal transplantation		right ventrogluteal
RU	residual urine	RVH	renovascular hypertension
	resin uptake		right ventricular hypertrophy
	retrograde ureterogram	RVHT	renovascular hypertension
	right upper	RVI	right ventricle infarction
	routine urinalysis	RVIDd	right ventricle internal dimension diastole
RU 486	mifepristone (Mifeprex)		
RUA	right upper arm	RVL	right vastus lateralis
	routine urine analysis	RVO	relaxed vaginal outlet
RUB	rubella virus vaccine		retinal vein occlusion
RUE	right upper extremity		right ventricular outflow
RUG	resource utilization group		right ventricular overactivity
	retrograde urethrogram	RVOT	right ventricular outflow tract
RUI	recurring urinary infections	RVOTH	right ventricular outflow tract hypertrophy
RUL	right upper lid		
	right upper lobe	RVOTO	right ventricular outflow tract obstruction
RUOQ	right upper outer quadrant		

RVP	right ventricular pressure
RVR	rapid ventricular response
	renal vascular resistance
	right ventricular rhythm
RVSP	right ventricular systolic pressure
rVSV	recombinant vesicular stomatitis virus
RVSW	right ventricular stroke work
RVSWI	right ventricular stroke work index
RVT	recurrent ventricular tachycardia
	renal vein thrombosis
RV/TLC	residual volume to total lung capacity ratio
RVU	relative-value units
RVV	rubella vaccine virus
RVVC	recurrent vulvovaginal candidiasis
RVVT	Russell viper venom time
RW	radiant warmer
	ragweed
	red welt
	respite worker
	rolling walker
R/W	return to work
RWIs	recreational water illnesses
RWM	regional wall motion
RWMA	regional wall motion abnormalities
RWP	ragweed pollen
RWS	ragweed sensitivity
RWT	relative wall thickness
Rx	drug
	medication
	pharmacy
	prescription
	radiotherapy
	take
	therapy
	treatment
RXN	reaction
RXRs	retinoid X receptors
RXT	radiation therapy
	right exotropia
RYGBP	Roux-en-Y gastric bypass (surgery)

S	sacral
	second (s)
	sensitive
	serum
	single
	sister
	son
	South (as in the location 2S would be second floor, South wing)
	sponge
	Staphylococcus
	streptomycin [part of tuberculosis regimen as in RHZ(E/S)/HR]
	subjective findings
	suicide
	suction
	sulfur
	supervision
	surgery
	susceptible
/S/	signature
$\bar{s}$	without (this is a dangerous abbreviation)
S'	shoulder
S_1	first heart sound
$S^{-1}...S^{-4}$	suicide risk classifications
S_2	second heart sound
S_3	third heart sound (ventricular filling gallop)
S_4	fourth heart sound (atrial gallop)
$S_1...S_5$	sacral vertebra or nerves 1 through 5
SI..SIV	symbols for the first to fourth heart sounds
SA	sacroanterior
	salicylic acid
	semen analysis
	Sexoholics Anonymous
	sinoatrial
	skeletal abnormalities
	sleep apnea
	slow acetylator
	Spanish American
	spinal anesthesia
	Staphylococcus aureus
	subarachnoid
	substance abuse
	suicide alert
	suicide attempt
	surface area
	surgical assistant
	sustained action
Sa	Saturday
S/A	same as
	sugar and acetone

S&A	sugar and acetone		self-articulating femoral
SAA	same as above		Spanish-American female
	serum amyloid A		subcutaneous abdominal fat
	Stokes-Adams attacks	SAFHS	sonic accelerated fracture healing
	synthetic amino acids		system
SAAG	serum-ascites albumin gradient	SAG	sodium antimony gluconate
SAANDs	selective apoptotic antineoplastic	SAGAM	Scientific Advisory Group on
	drugs		Antimicrobials (EMEA)
SAARDs	slow-acting antirheumatic drugs	Sag D	sagittal diameter
SAB	serum albumin	SAGE	serial analysis of gene expression
	sinoatrial block	SAH	subarachnoid hemorrhage
	Spanish-American Black		systemic arterial hypertension
	spontaneous abortion	SAHA	suberoylanilide hydroxamic acid
	Staphylococcus aureus bacteremia	SAHS	sleep apnea/hypopnea
	subarachnoid bleed		(hypersomnolence) syndrome
	subarachnoid block	SAI	self-administered injectable
SABA	short-acting beta-agonist		Sodium Amytal® interview
SABR	screening auditory brainstem	SAL	salicylate
	response		salmeterol (Serevent)
SABs	side air bags		*Salmonella*
SAC	school-age children		sensory acuity level
	segmental antigen challenge		sterility assurance level
	serial abdominal closure	SAL 12	sequential analysis of 12 chemistry
	serum aminoglycoside concentration		constituents (see page 298)
	short arm cast	SALK	surgical arthroscopy, left knee
	substance abuse counselor	SAM	methylprednisolone sodium
SACC	short arm cylinder cast		succinate (Solu-Medrol),
SACD	subacute combined degeneration		aminophylline, and metaproterenol
SACH	solid ankle, cushioned heel		(Metaprel)
SACT	sinoatrial conduction time		selective antimicrobial modulation
SAD	schizoaffective disorder		self-administered medication
	seasonal affective disorder		short arc motion
	Self-Assessment Depression (scale)		sleep apnea monitor
	social anxiety disorder		Spanish-American male
	source-axis distance		systolic anterior motion
	subacromial decompression	SAME	syndrome of arthralgias, myalgias,
	subacute dialysis		and edema
	sugar and acetone determination	SAMe	*S*-adenosylmethionine
	superior axis deviation		(ademetionine)
SADBE	squaric acid dibutyl ester	SAMHSA	Substance Abuse and Mental Health
SADD	Students Against Drunk Driving		Services Administration
SADL	simulated activities of daily living	SAMPLE	symptoms/signs, allergies,
SADR	suspected adverse drug reaction		medications, past medical history,
SADS	Schedule for Affective Disorders and		last oral intake, and events prior to
	Schizophrenia		arrival (an EMT mnemonic used
	sudden arrhythmic death syndrome		in initial patient
SADs	severe autoimmune diseases		questioning)
SADS-C	Schedule for Affective Disorders	SAMU	Service d'Aide Médicale Urgente
	And Schizophrenia – Change		(French prehospital emergency
	Version		system)
SAE	serious adverse event	SAN	side-arm nebulizer
	short above elbow (cast)		sinoatrial node
	splenic angioembolization		slept all night
SAEG	signal averaging electrocardiogram	SANC	short-arm navicular cast
SAEKG	signaled average electrocardiogram	SANE	Sexual Assault Nurse Examiner
SAESU	Substance Abuse valuating Screen	sang	sanguinous
	Unit	SANS	Schedule (Scale) for the Assessment
SAF	Self-Analysis Form		of Negative Symptoms

	sympathetic autonomic nervous system		sleep apnea syndrome
SAO	small airway obstruction		Social Adjustment Scale
	Southeast Asian ovalocytosis		Specific Activity Scale
SaO$_2$	arterial oxygen percent saturation		statistical applications software
SAP	Sample Accountability Program		subarachnoid space
	serum alkaline phosphate		subaxial subluxation
	serum amyloid P		sulfasalazine (Azulfidine)
	standard automated perimetry		synthetic absorbable sutures
	sporadic adenomatous polyps	SASA	Sex Abuse Survivors Anonymous
	statistical analysis plan	SASH	saline, agent, saline, and heparin
SAPD	self-administration of psychotropic drugs	SASP	sulfasalazine (salicylazo-sulfapyridine; Azulfidine)
SAPH	saphenous	SASS	Social Adaptation Self-Evaluation Scale
SAPHO	synovitis, acne, pustulosis, hyperostosis, and osteomyelitis (syndrome)	SASSAD	six area, six sign atopic dermatitis (severity score)
SAPS	Scale for the Assessment of Positive Symptoms	SAST	slide agglutination serotyping
	short-arm plaster splint	SAT	methylprednisolone sodium succinate (Solu-Medrol), aminophylline, and terbutaline
	Simplified Acute Physiology Score		saturated
SAPs	shock-absorbing pylons		saturation
SAPS II	Simplified Acute Physiology Score version II		Saturday
			self-administered therapy
SAPTA	stent-assisted percutaneous transluminal angioplasty		Senior Apperception Test
			speech awareness threshold
SAQ	saquinavir (Invirase)		subacute thyroiditis
	Sexual Adjustment Questionnaire		subcutaneous adipose tissue
	short-arc quadriceps	SATC	substance abuse treatment clinic
SAR	seasonal allergic rhinitis	SATL	surgical Achilles tendon lengthening
	Senior Assistant Resident	SATP	substance abuse treatment program
	sexual attitudes reassessment	SATS	refers to oxygen saturation levels
	structural activity relationships	SATU	substance abuse treatment unit
SARA	sexually acquired reactive arthritis	SAV	supra-annular valve
	SQUID (superconducting quantum interference device) array for reproductive assessment	SAVD	spontaneous assisted vaginal delivery
		SB	safety belt
			sandbag
	system for anesthetic and respiratory administration analysis		scleral buckling
			seat belt
SARAN	senior admitting resident's admission note		seen by
			Sengstaken-Blakemore (tube)
SARC	seasonal allergic rhinoconjunctivitis		sick boy
SARK	surgical arthroscopy, right knee		side bend
SARMs	selective androgen receptor modulators		side bending
			sinus bradycardia
S Arrh	sinus arrhythmia		slide board
SARS	severe acute respiratory syndrome		small bowel
SARS-CoV	severe acute respiratory syndrome-associated coronavirus		spina bifida
			sponge bath
SART	sexual assault response team		stand-by
	standard acid reflux test		Stanford-Binet (test)
SAS	saline, agent, and saline		sternal border
	scalenus anticus syndrome		stillbirth
	Sedation-Agitation Scale		stillborn
	see assessment sheet		stone basketing
	Self-rating Anxiety Scale	Sb	antimony
	short-arm splint	SB+	wearing seat belt
	Simpson-Angus Scale	SB−	not wearing seat belt

S

SBA	serum bactericidal activity		special baby Travesol
	standby angioplasty		spontaneous breathing trial
	standby assistant (assistance)	SBTB	sinus breakthrough beat
	Summary Basis of Approval	SBTT	small bowel transit time
SBAC	small bowel adenocarcinoma	SBV	single binocular vision
SBB	stereotactic breast biopsy	SBW	seat belts worn
SBBO	small-bowel bacterial overgrowth	SBX	symphysis, buttocks, and xiphoid
SBC	sensory binocular cooperation	SC	schizophrenia
	single base cane		Schwann cell
	standard bicarbonate		self-care
	strict bed confinement		serum creatinine
	superficial bladder cancer		service connected
SBD	sleep-related breathing disorder		sick call
	straight bag drainage		sickle cell
SBE	saturated base excess		small (blood pressure) cuff
	self-breast examination		Snellen chart
	short below-elbow (cast)		spinal cord
	shortness of breath on exertion		sport cord
	subacute bacterial endocarditis		sternoclavicular
SBF	splanchnic blood flow		subclavian
SBFT	small bowel follow through		subclavian catheter
SBG	stand-by guard		subcutaneous (this is a dangerous
SBGM	self blood-glucose monitoring		abbreviation as it can be read as
SBH	State Board of Health		SL [sublingual]. Use subcut or
SBI	silicone (gel-containing) breast		spell it out.)
	implants		succinylcholine
	systemic bacterial infection		sugar-coated (tablets)
SBJ	skin, bones, and joints		sulfur colloid
SBK	spinnbarkeit		supportive care
SBL	sponge blood loss		surveillance cultures
sBLA	supplemental Biologic License	s̄c	without correction (without glasses)
	Application	S&C	sclerae and conjunctivae
SB-LM	Stanford-Binet Intelligence Test-	SCA	sickle cell anemia
	Form LM		spinocerebellar ataxia
SBO	small bowel obstruction		subclavian artery
	specified bovine offals		subcutaneous abdominal (block)
SBOD	scleral buckle, right eye		sudden cardiac arrest
SBOE	surgical blood order equation		superior cerebellar artery
SBOH	State Board of Health	SCa	serum calcium
SBOM	soybean oil meal	ScA	*Scedosporium apiospermum*
SBOS	scleral buckle, left eye	SCA1	spinocerebellar ataxia type 1
SBP	school breakfast program	SCAD	short chain acyl-coenzyme A
	scleral buckling procedure		dehydrogenase
	small bowel phytobezoars		spontaneous cervical artery
	spontaneous bacterial peritonitis		dissection
	systolic blood pressure	SCAN	suspected child abuse and neglect
SBQC	small-based quad cane	SCAP	scapula; scapulae; scapular
SBR	sluggish blood return		stem cell apheresis
	strict bed rest	SCARMD	severe childhood autosomal recessive
SBRN	sensory branch of the radial nerve		muscular dystrophy
SBS	serum blood sugar	SCAT	sheep cell agglutination titer
	shaken baby syndrome		sickle cell anemia test
	short (small) bowel syndrome	SCB	strictly confined to bed
	sick-building syndrome	SCBC	small cell bronchogenic carcinoma
	side-by-side	SCBE	single-contrast barium enema
	small bowel series	SCBF	spinal cord blood flow
SBT	serum bactericidal titers	SCC	short course chemotherapy (for
	small bowel transplantation		tuberculosis)

	sickle cell crisis		specific COX-2 inhibitor
	small cell carcinoma		spinal cord injury
	spinal cord compression		subcoma insulin
	squamous cell carcinoma	SCID	severe combined immunodeficiency disorders (disease)
SCCA	semi-closed circle absorber		structured clinical interview for DSM-III-R
	squamous cell carcinoma antigen		
SCCa	squamous cell carcinoma	SCII	Strong-Campbell Interest Inventory
SCCB	small cell cancer of the bladder	SCIP	Screening and Crisis Intervention Program
SCCE	squamous cell carcinoma of the esophagus		
SCCHN	squamous cell carcinoma of the head and neck	SCIPP	sacrococcygeal to inferior pubic point
SCCI	subcutaneous continuous infusion	SCIT	single-chain immunotoxin
SCCOT	squamous cell carcinoma of the oral tongue		subcutaneous immunotherapy
		SCIU	spinal cord injury unit
SCC/T	squamous sell carcinoma of the oral tongue	SCIV	subclavian intravenous
		SCI-WORA	spinal cord injury without radiologic abnormalities
SCD	sequential compression device		
	service connected disability	SCJ	squamocolumnar junction
	sickle cell disease		sternoclavicular joint
	spinal cord disease	sCJD	sporadic Creutzfeldt-Jakob disease
	subacute combined degeneration	SCL	skin conductance level
	sudden cardiac death		symptom checklist
ScDA	scapulodextra anterior	SCL-90	Symptoms Checklist—90 items
SCDM	soybean-casein digest medium	ScLA	scapulolaeva anterior
ScDP	scapulodextra posterior	SCLAX	subcostal long axis
SCE	sister chromatid exchange	SCLC	small cell lung cancer
	soft cooked egg	SCLD	sickle cell lung disease
	specialized columnar epithelium	SCLE	subacute cutaneous lupus erythematosis
	spinal cord ependymoma		
SCEMIA	self-contained enzymatic membrane immunoassay	ScLP	scapulolaeva posterior
		SCLs	soft contact lenses
SCEP	somatosensory cortical evoked potential		synthetic combinatorial libraries
		SCM	scalene muscle
SCF	special care formula		sensation, circulation, and motion
	stem cell factor		spondylitic caudal myelopathy
	supra ciliochoroidal fluid		sternocleidomastoid
SCFA	short-chain fatty acid		supraclavicular muscle
SCFE	slipped capital femoral epiphysis	SCMD	senile choroidal macular degeneration
SCFGT	Southern California Figure Ground Test		
		SCMV	serogroup C meningococcal vaccine
SCG	seismocardiography	SCN	severe congenital neutropenia
	serum Chemogram		special care nursery
	sodium cromoglycate		suprachiasmatic nucleus (nuclei)
	substitute care giver	SCNs	subepidermal calcified nodules
SCH	schistosomiasis (Schistosoma sp.) vaccine	SCNT	somatic-cell nuclear transfer
		S/CO	signal-to-cut-off (ratios)
	subclinical hypothyroidism	SCOB	Schedule-Controlled Operant Behavior
SCh	succinylcholine chloride		
SCHIP	State Children's Health Insurance Program	SCOH	services to children in their own homes
SCHISTO	schistocytes	SCOP	scopolamine
SCHIZ	schizocytes	SCOPE	arthroscopy
	schizophrenia	SCP	secondary care provider
SCHLP	supracricord hemilaryngopharyn-gectomy		sodium cellulose phosphate
			standardized care plan
SCHNC	squamous cell head and neck cancer	SCPF	stem cell proliferation factor
SCI	silent cerebral infarct	S-CPK	serum creatine phosphokinase

SCPP	spinal cord perfusion pressure		step-down
SCQ	social communication questionnaire		sterile dressing
SCR	special care room (seclusion room)		straight drainage
	spondylitic caudal radioculopathy		streptozocin and doxorubicin
	standard care regimen		sudden death
	stem cell rescue		surgical drain
SCr	serum creatinine	S & D	seen and discussed
sCR	soluble complement receptor		stomach and duodenum
SCRIPT	prescription	S/D	sharp/dull
SC/RP	scaling and root planing		systolic-diastolic ratio
SC-RNV	subcutaneous radionuclide	SDA	sacrodextra anterior
	venography		same day admission
SCS	spinal cord stimulation		serotonin/dopamine antagonist
	splatter control shield		Seventh-Day Adventist
	stem cell support		steroid-dependent asthmatic
	suspected catheter sepsis	SDAT	senile dementia of Alzheimer type
SCSAX	subcostal short axis	SDB	Sabouraud dextrose broth
SCSIT	Southern California Sensory		self-destructive behavior
	Integration Tests		sleep disordered breathing
SCSVT	Southern California Space	SDBP	seated diastolic blood pressure
	Visualization Test		standing diastolic blood pressure
SCT	Secondary Care Trust (United		supine diastolic blood pressure
	Kingdom)	SDC	serum digoxin concentration
	Sertoli cell tumor		serum drug concentration
	sex chromatin test		Sleep Disorders Center
	sickle cell trait		sodium deoxycholate
	stem cell transplant	SD&C	suction, dilation, and curettage
	sugar-coated tablet	SDD	selective digestive (tract)
SCTX	static cervical traction		decontamination
SCU	self-care unit		sterile dry dressing
	special care unit		subantimicrobial dose doxycycline
SCUCP	small cell undifferentiated carcinoma		(dental; Periostat)
	of the prostate	SDDT	selective decontamination of the
SCUF	slow continuous ultrafiltration		digestive tract
SCUT	schizophrenia, chronic	SDE	subdural empyema
	undifferentiated type	SDES	symptomatic diffuse esophageal
SCV	subclavian vein		spasm
	subcutaneous vaginal (block)	SDF	sexual dysfunction
SCY	scytonemin		stromal-cell-derived factor
SD	scleroderma	SDH	spinal detrusor hyperreflexia
	senile dementia		subdural hematoma
	sensory deficit	SDHD	succinate dehydrogenase complex
	severe deficit		subunit D
	septal defect	SDI	Sandimmune (cyclosporine)
	severely disabled		State Disability Insurance
	shallow distance (aquatic therapy)	SDII	sudden death in infancy
	shoulder disarticulation	SDL	serum digoxin level
	single dose		serum drug level
	skin dose		speech discrimination loss
	sleep deprived	SDLE	sex-difference in life expectancy
	solvent-detergent		somatic dysfunction lower
	somatic dysfunction		extremity
	spasmodic dysphonia	SDM	soft drusen maculopathy
	speech discrimination		standard deviation of the mean
	spontaneous delivery	S/D/M	systolic, diastolic, mean
	stable disease	SDMC	safety and data monitoring
	standard deviation		committee
	standard diet	SD/N	signal-difference-to-noise ratio

SDNN	standard deviation of normal-to-normal beats	
SDO	surgical diagnostic oncology	
SDP	sacrodextra posterior	
	single donor platelets	
	solvent-detergent plasma	
	stomach, duodenum, and pancreas	
SDPTG	second derivative of photoplethysmogram	
SDR	selective dorsal rhizotomy	
	short-duration response	
SDS	same day surgery	
	Self-Rating Depression Scale	
	Shwachman-Diamond Syndrome	
	sodium dodecyl sulfate	
	somatropin deficiency syndrome	
	Speech Discrimination Score	
	standard deviation score	
	sudden death syndrome	
	Symptom Distress Scale	
SDSO	same day surgery overnight	
SDS-PAGE	sodium dodecyl sulfate – polyacrylamide gel electrophoresis	
SDT	sacrodextra transversa	
	speech detection threshold	
SDU	step-down unit	
SDUE	somatic dysfunction upper extremity	
SDV	single-dose vial	
SDX/PYR	sulfadoxine; pyrimethamine (Fansidar)	
SE	saline enema (0.9% sodium chloride)	
	self-examination	
	side effect	
	soft exudates	
	special education	
	spin echo	
	staff escort	
	standard error	
	Starr-Edwards (valve, pacemaker)	
	status epilepticus	
	surgical excision	
Se	selenium	
S/E	suicidal and eloper	
S & E	seen and examined	
SEA	sheep erythrocyte agglutination (test)	
	side-entry (venous) access	
	Southeast Asia	
	Staphylococcal enterotoxin A	
	subdural electrode array	
	synaptic electronic activation	
SEAR	Southeast Asia refugee	
SEB	Staphylococcus enterotoxin B	
	surrogate end-point biomarker	
SEC	second	
	secondary	
	secretary	
	size exclusion chromatography	
	spontaneous echo contrast	

	steric exclusion chromatography	
SECG	scalp electrocardiogram	
SECL	seclusion	
SECPR	standard external cardiopulmonary resuscitation	
SE-CPT	single-electrode current perception threshold	
SED	sedimentation	
	serious emotional disturbances	
	skin erythema dose	
	socially and emotionally disturbed	
	spondyloepiphyseal dysplasia	
SeDBP	seated diastolic blood pressure	
SEDDS	self-emulsifying drug-delivery system	
SED-NET	severely emotional disturbed - network	
sed rt	sedimentation rate	
SEEG	stereoelectroencephalographic	
SEER	Surveillance, Epidemiology, and End Results (program)	
SEF	spectral edge frequency (anesthesia-depth monitor)	
SEG	segment	
	sonoencephalogram	
SEGRA	selective glucocorticoid-receptor agonist	
segs	segmented neutrophils	
SEH	spinal epidural hematomas	
	subependymal hemorrhage	
SEI	subepithelial (corneal) infiltrate	
SELDI	surface enhanced laser desorption/ionization	
SELEX	systematic evolution of ligands by exponential enrichment	
SELFVD	sterile elective low forceps vaginal delivery	
SEM	scanning electron microscopy	
	semen	
	slow eye movement	
	standard error of mean	
	systolic ejection murmur	
sEMG	surface electromyography	
SEMI	subendocardial myocardial infarction	
SEN	spray each nostril	
SENS	sensitivity	
	sensorium	
SEOC	serous epithelial ovarian carcinoma	
SEP	multiple sclerosis (French)	
	separate	
	serum electrophoresis	
	somatosensory evoked potential	
	syringe exchange program	
	systolic ejection period	
SEPS	subfascial endoscopic perforator surgery	
SEQ	sequela	
SER	scanning equalization radiography	

S

	sertraline (Zoloft)	SFJ	saphenofemoral junction
	side effects records	SFM	scanning force microscopy
	signal enhancement ratio	SF-MPQ	Short-Form, McGill Pain
SERA-TEK	technetium-99m hexametazime		questionnaire
		SFNM	subfoveal neovascular membranes
SERF	Severity of Exacerbation and Risk Factors	SFP	simulated fluorescence process
			simultaneous foveal perception
Serial 7's	a mental status examination (starting with a 100, count backward by 7's)		spinal fluid pressure
		SFPT	standard fixation preference test
		SFRT	stereotactic fractionated radiotherapy
SER-IV	supination external rotation, type 4 fracture	SFS	split function studies
		SFT	solitary fibrous tumor
SERM	selective estrogen-receptor modulator	SFTR	sagittal, frontal, transverse, rotation
SERO-SANG	serosanguineous	SFTs	solitary fibrous tumors
		SFUP	surgical follow-up
SERP-ACWA	Skin Exposure Reduction Paste Against Chemical Warfare Agents	SFV	simian foamy viruses
			superficial femoral vein
		SFW	shell fragment wound
SERs	somatosensory evoked responses	SFWB	social/family well-being
SES	sick euthyroid syndrome	SFWD	symptom-free walking distance
	sirolimus-eluting stents	SG	salivary gland
	socioeconomic status		scrotography
	standard electrolyte solution		serum glucose
SeSBP	seated systolic blood pressure		side glide
SET	signal extraction technology		skin graft
	skin end-point titration		specific gravity
	social environmental therapy		Swan-Ganz (catheter)
	systolic ejection time	S/G	swallow/gag
SEV	sevoflurane (Ultane)	SGA	small for gestational age
SEWHO	shoulder-elbow-wrist-hand orthosis		subjective global assessment (dietary history and physical examination)
SF	salt-free		
	saturated fat		substantial gainful activity (employment)
	scarlet fever		
	seizure frequency	SGAs	second-generation antihistamines
	seminal fluid		second-generation antipsychotics
	skull fracture	SGB	Swiss gym ball
	small finger	SGC	Swan-Ganz catheter
	soft feces	SGCNB	stereotactic guided core-needle biopsy
	sound field		
	spinal fluid	SGD	salivary gland dysfunction
	starch-free		specific granule deficiency
	sugar-free		specific growth delay
	symptom-free		speech generating device
	synovial fluid		straight gravity drainage
S&F	slip and fall		sweat gland density
	soft and flat	SGE	significant glandular enlargement
SF-6	sulfahexafluoride	SGHL	superior glenohumeral ligament
SF 36	36-item short form health survey	s̄ gl	without correction (without glasses)
SFA	saturated fatty acids	SGM	serum glucose monitoring
	superficial femoral artery	SGOT	serum glutamic oxalo-acetic transaminase (same as AST)
SFB	single frequency bioimpedance		
SFC	spinal fluid count	SGP	Schering-Plough Corporation
	subarachnoid fluid collection	SGPT	serum glutamate pyruvate transaminase (same as ALT)
SFD	scaphoid fossa depression		
	small for dates	SGRQ-A	St. George's Respiratory Questionnaire translated into American English
SFE	supercritical fluid extraction		
SFEMG	single-fiber electromyography		
SFH	schizophrenia family history	SGS	second-generation sulfonylurea

	subglottic stenosis		seriously ill
sGS	surgical Gleason score		sexual intercourse
SGTCS	secondarily generalized tonic-clonic seizures		signal intensity
			small intestine
SH	serum hepatitis		strict isolation
	sexual harassment		stress incontinence
	short		stroke index
	shoulder		suicidal ideation
	shower	Si	silicon
	social history	S & I	suction and irrigation
	sulfhydryl (group)		support and interpretation
	surgical history	SIA	small intestinal atresia
	systemic hypertension	SIADH	syndrome of inappropriate antidiuretic hormone secretion
S&H	speech and hearing		
	suicidal and homicidal	SIAT	supervised intermittent ambulatory treatment
S/H	suicidal/homicidal ideation		
SH2	sarc homology region 2	SIB	self-inflating bulb
SHA	super-heated aerosol		self-injurious behavior
SHAFT	*shopping, housework, accounting (bills), food preparation, and transportation (driving); (instrumental activities of daily living)*	SIBC	serum iron-binding capacity
		sibs	siblings
		SIC	self-intermittent catherization
			squamous intraepithelial cells
			Standard Industrial Classification
SHAL	standard hyperalimentation	SICD	sudden infant crib death
SHAS	supravalvular hypertrophic aortic stenosis	SICOG	Southern Italy Cooperative Oncology Group
S Hb	sickle hemoglobin screen	SICT	selective intracoronary thrombolysis
SHBG	sex hormone-binding globulin	SICU	surgical intensive care unit
sHBO₂T	systemic hyperbaric oxygen therapy	*SID*	once daily (used in veterinary medicine)
SHC	subsequent hospital care		
SHEENT	skin, head, eyes, ears, nose, and throat	SIDA	French and Spanish abbreviation for AIDS
SHG	shigellosis (*Shigella* sp.) vaccine		
SHGT	somatic-cell human gene therapy	SIDAM	structured interview for the diagnosis of dementia of Alzheimer type
SHI	Self-Harm Inventory		
	standard heparin infusion	SIDAM-A	structured interview for the diagnosis of dementia of the Alzheimer type, multi-infarct dementia, and dementias of other etiology according to ICD-10 and DSM-III-R
Shig	*Shigella*		
SHIV	simian-human immunodeficiency virus		
SHL	sudden hearing loss		
	supraglottic horizontal laryngectomy		
SHMB	severe hypersensitivity to mosquito bites	SIDD	syndrome of isolated diastolic dysfunction
		SIDERO	siderocyte
SHO	Senior House Officer	SIDFF	superimposed dorsiflexion of foot
SHP	secondary hypertension, pulmonary	SIDS	sudden infant death syndrome
SHR	scapulohumeral rhythm	SIEP	serum immunoelectrophoresis
SHRC	shortened, held, resisted contraction	*SIG*	let it be marked (appears on prescription before directions for patient)
S-HRV	short-term heart rate variability		
SHS	second-hand smoke		
	student health service		sigmoidoscopy
SHV	short hepatic vein	Signal 99	patient in cardiac or respiratory distress
	sulfhydryl variant		
SHx	social history	SI/HI	suicidal/homicidal ideations
SI	International System of Units	SIJ	sacroiliac joint
	sacroiliac	SIJS	sacroiliac joint syndrome
	sagittal index	SIL	seriously ill list
	sector iridectomy		sister-in-law
	self-inflicted		squamous intraepithelial lesion
	sensory integration		

SILFVD	sterile indicated low forceps vaginal delivery	SJM	St. Jude Medical (heart valve prosthesis)
SILV	simultaneous independent lung ventilation	S-JRA	systemic juvenile rheumatoid arthritis
SIM	selective ion monitoring	SJS	Schwartz-Jampel syndrome
	Similac®		Stevens-Johnson syndrome
	surface-induced mineralization		Swyer-James syndrome
SIMCU	surgical intermediate care unit	S$_{jvo2}$	jugular venous oxygen saturation
Sim c Fe	Similac with iron®	SK	seborrheic keratosis
SIMV	synchronized intermittent mandatory ventilation		senile keratosis
			solar keratosis
SIN	salpingitis isthmica nodose		streptokinase
SIOD	Schimke immuno-osseous dysplasia	S & K	single and keeping (baby)
		SKAO	supracondylar knee-ankle orthosis
SIP	Sickness Impact Profile	SKAs	skills, knowledge, and abilities (ratings)
	stroke in progression	SKB	SmithKline Beecham
	subcutaneously implanted ports	SKC	single knee to chest
	sympathetically independent pain	SKINT	skinfold thickness
SIQ	sick in quarters	SK-SD	streptokinase streptodornase
SIQ-JR	Suicidal Ideation Questionnaire-Junior	SKU	stock keeping unit (related to product identification)
SIR	standardized incidence rate (ratio)	SKY	spectral karyotyping
SIRGE	A drug-waste collection and recycling system used in the European Union	SL	scapholunate
			secondary leukemia
			sensation level
SIRS	systemic inflammatory response syndrome		sentinel lymphadenectomy
			serious list
SIRT	selective internal radiation therapy		shortleg
SIS	sister		side-lying
	small intestinal submucosa		staging laparoscopy
	Surgical Infection Stratification (system)		slight
			sublingual
SISI	Short Increment Sensitivity Index	S/L	slit lamp (examination)
SISS	severe invasion streptococcal syndrome	SLA	sacrolaeva anterior
			sex and love addictions
SIT	serum inhibitory titers		slide latex agglutination
	silicon-intensified target		The Satisfaction with Life Areas
	Slossen Intelligence Test	SLAA	Sex and Love Addicts Anonymous
	specific immunotherapy (allergy)	SLAC	scapholunate advanced collapse
	sperm immobilization test	SLat	time to onset of sleep
	structured interrupted therapy	SLAM	Systemic Lupus Activity Measure
	supraspinatus, infraspinatus, teres (insertions)	SLAP	serum leucine amino-peptidase
			superior labral anteroposterior (shoulder lesion)
	surgical intensive therapy		
SITA	standard infertility treatment algorithm	SLB	short leg brace
		SLBB	single-living baby boy
SIT BAL	sitting balance	SLBG	single-living baby girl
SIT TOL	sitting tolerance	SLC	short leg cast
SIV	self-inflicted violence	SLCC	short leg cylinder cast
	simian immunodeficiency virus	SLCG	sulfolithocholylglycine
SIVB	self-inflicted violent behavior	SLCT	Sertoli-Leydig cell tumor
SIVD	subcortical ischemic vascular dementia (disease)	SLD	specific language disorder
			stealth liposomal doxorubicin
SIVP	slow intravenous push	SLE	slit-lamp examination
SIW	self-inflicted wound		St. Louis encephalitis
SJC	swollen joint count		systemic lupus erythematosus
SJCRH	St. Jude Children's Research Hospital	SLEDAI	Systemic Lupus Erythematosus Disease Activity Index

SLEX	slit-lamp examination (biomicroscopy)	SLUD	salivation, lacrimation, urination, and defecation
SLFVD	sterile low forceps vaginal delivery	SLUDGE	salivation, lacrimation, urination, diarrhea, gastrointestinal upset, and emesis (signs and symptoms of cholinergic excess)
SLGXT	symptom-limited graded exercise test		
SLI	specific language impairment		
SLIT	sublingual immunotherapy		
SLK	superior limbic keratoconjunctivitis	SLV	since last visit
SLL	second-look laparotomy	SLVD	systolic left ventricular dysfunction
	small lymphocytic lymphoma	SLWB	severely low birth weight
SLMFVD	sterile low midforceps vaginal delivery	SLWC	short leg walking cast
		SM	sadomasochism
SLMMS	slightly more marked since		service mark (such as The Pause that Refreshes)
SLMP	since last menstrual period		
SLN	sentinel lymph node(s)		skim milk
	superior laryngeal nerve		small
SLNB	sentinel lymph node biopsy		sports medicine
SLND	sentinel lymph node detection		Stairmaster®
SLNM	sentinel lymph node mapping		streptomycin
SLNTG	sublingual nitroglycerin		systolic motion
SLNWBC	short leg nonweight-bearing cast		systolic murmur
SLNWC	short leg nonwalking cast	^{153}Sm	samarium 153
SLO	scanning laser ophthalmoscope	SMA	severe malarial anemia
	second-look operation		smallpox vaccine, not otherwise specified
	shark liver oil		
	Smith-Lemli-Opitz (syndrome)		smooth muscle antibody
	streptolysin O		spinal muscular atrophy
SLOA	short leave of absence		superior mesenteric artery
SLOM	serous left otitis media	SMA-II	spinal muscular atrophy type II
SLOS	Smith-Lemli-Opitz syndrome	SMA 6	simultaneous multichannel autoanalyzer (page 298)
SLP	scanning laser polarimeter		
	single-limb progression	SMA-7	See page 298
	Speech Language Pathologist	SMA-12	See page 298
	speech language pathology	SMA 18	See page 298
	superficial lamina propria	SMA-23	See page 298
SLPI	secretory leukocyte protease inhibitor	SMAO	superior mesenteric artery occlusion
		SMAR	self-medication administration record
SLPMS	short-leg posterior-molded splint	SMAS	superficial musculoaponeurotic system (graft; flat)
SLR	straight-leg raising		
SLRS	stereotactic linac radiosurgery		superior mesenteric artery syndrome
SLRT	straight-leg raising tenderness	SMAST	Short Michigan Alcoholism Screening Test
	straight-leg raising test		
SLS	second-look sonography	SMAvac	smallpox (vaccinia virus) vaccine
	short leg splint	SMB	simulated moving bed (chromatography)
	shrinking lungs syndrome		
	single leg stance	SMBG	self-monitoring blood glucose
	single limb support	SMC	skeletal myxoid chondrosarcoma
SLT	sacrolaeva transversa		special mouth care
	scanning laser tomography	SMCA	sorbitol MacConkey agar
	single lung transplantation	SMCD	senile macular chorio-retinal degeneration
	Speech Language Therapist		
	spontaneous labor at term	SMCs	smooth muscle cells
	swing light test	SMD	senile macular degeneration
SLT-I	Shiga-like toxin I		standardized mean difference
SLTA	severe life-threatening asthma	SMDA	Safe Medical Device Act
	standard language test for aphasia	SME	significant medical event
SLTEC	Shiga-like toxin-producing *Escherichia coli*		surgical mediastinal exploration
		SMF	streptozocin, mitomycin, and fluorouracil
sl. tr.	slight trace		

SMFA	sodium monofluoroacetate		SMZL	splenic marginal-zone lymphoma
SMFP	sodium monofluorophosphate		SN	sciatic notch
SMFVD	sterile midforceps vaginal delivery			sinus node
SMG	submandibular gland			staff nurse
SMH	state mental hospital			student nurse
SMI	sensory motor integration (group)			suprasternal notch
	serious mental illness			superior nasal
	severely mentally impaired		Sn	tin
	service mix index		sN	sentinel lymph node
	small volume infusion		S/N	signal to noise ratio
	suggested minimum increment		SNA	specimen not available
	sustained maximal inspiration			Student Nursing Assistant
SMIDS	suppertime mixed insulin and daytime sulfonylureas		SNa	serum sodium
SMILE	safety, monitoring, intervention, length of stay and evaluation		SNAC	scaphoid nonunion advanced collapse
	sustained maximal inspiratory lung exercises		SNAE	*sustained pain-free and no adverse events*
SMIs	self-management interventions		SNAP	scheduled nursing activities program
SMIT	standard mycological identification techniques			Score for Neonatal Acute Physiology
				sensory nerve action potential
SMMVT	sustained monomorphic ventricular tachycardia			Swanson, Nolan, and Pelham (rating scale)
SMN	second malignant neoplasia		SNAP-25	synaptosome-associated protein 25 kilodaltons
SMO	Senior Medical Officer		SNAP-PE	Score for Neonatal Acute Physiology-Perinatal Extension
	site management organization(s)			
	slip made out		SNaRI	serotonin noradrenergic reuptake inhibitor
SMON	subacute myelo-opticoneuropathy			
SMORs	standardized mortality odds ratios		SNASA	Salford Needs Assessment Schedule for Adolescents
SMP	safety management plan			
	self-management program		SNAT	suspected nonaccidental trauma
	sympathetic maintained plan		SNB	scalene node biopsy
SmPC	Summary of Product Characteristics (European Union)			sentinel (lymph) node biopsy
			SNBx	sentinel node biopsy
SMPN	sensorimotor polyneuropathy		SNC	skilled nursing care
SMR	senior medical resident		SNc	substantia nigra compacta
	skeletal muscle relaxant		SNCV	sensory nerve conduction velocity
	sleeping metabolic rate		SND	selective neck dissection
	standardized mortality ratio			single needle device
	submucous resection			sinus node dysfunction
SMRR	submucous resection and rhinoplasty		SNDA	Supplemental New Drug Application
SMS	scalded mouth syndrome		SNE	subacute necrotizing encephalomyelopathy
	senior medical student			
	Smith-Magenis syndrome		SNEP	student nurse extern program
	somatostatin (Zecnil)		SnET2	tin ethyl etiopurpurin
	stiff-man syndrome		SNF	Simon nitinol filter
SMSA	standard metropolitan statistical area			skilled nursing facility
SMT	smooth muscle tumors		SnF$_2$	stannous fluoride
	sputum methylation testing		SNF/MR	skilled nursing facility for the mentally retarded
	standard medical therapy			
	study management team		SNGFR	single nephron glomerular filtration rate
SMV	stentless mitral valve			
	submentovertical		SNGP	supranuclear gaze palsy
	superior mesenteric vein		SNHL	sensorineural hearing loss
SMVT	sustained monomorphic ventricular tachycardia		SNIP	silver nitrate immunoperoxidase
				strict no information in paper
SMX-TMP	sulfamethoxazole and trimethoprim (SMZ-TMP)		SNIPS	single nucleotide polymorphism (SNP)

252

SNK	Student-Newman-Keuls (test)		sutures out
SNM	sentinel (lymph) node mapping		sympathetic ophthalmia
	serotoninergic neuroenteric	S/O	suggestive of
	modulators	S-O	salpingo-oophorectomy
	student nurse midwife	S&O	salpingo-oophorectomy
SnMp	tin-mesoporphyrin	SO_2	sulfur dioxide
SNOMED	Systematized Nomenclature of	SO_3	sulfite
	Medicine	SO_4	sulfate
SNOMED	Systemized	SOA	serum opsonic activity
CT	Nomenclature of Medicine, Clinical		shortness of air
	Terms		spinal opioid analgesia
SNOMED	Systemized		supraorbital artery
RT	Nomenclature of Medicine,		swelling of ankles
	Reference Terminology	SOAA	signed out against advice
SNOOP	Systematic Nursing Observation of	SOAM	sutures out in the morning
	Psychopathology	SOAMA	signed out against medical advice
SNOs	S-nitrosothiols	SOAP	subjective, objective, assessment, and
SNP	simple neonatal procedure		plans
	single nucleotide polymorphism	SOAPIE	subjective, objective, assessment,
	sodium nitroprusside (Nipride)		plan, implementation,
SNP-LP	single nucleotide polymorphisms –		(intervention), and evaluation
	linkage disequilibrium	SOAPIER	subjective, objective, assessment,
SNPs	single nucleotide polymorphisms		plan, intervention, evaluation, and
SNR	signal-to-noise ratio (radiology)		revision
SNr	substantia nigra reticularis	SOB	see order book
SNRB	selective nerve root block		shortness of breath (this abbreviation
SNRI	selective noradrenergic reuptake		has caused problems)
	inhibitor		side of bed
	serotonin norepinephrine reuptake	SOBE	short of breath on exertion
	inhibitor	SOBOE	short of breath on exertion
SNRT	sinus node recovery time	SOC	see old chart
SNS	sacral nerve stimulation		socialization
	sterile normal saline (0.9% sodium		stages of change
	chloride, sterile)		standard of care
	Strategic National Stockpile		start of care
	sympathetic nervous system		state of consciousness
SNSA	sympathetic nervous system		system organ class
	activity	S & OC	signed and on chart (e.g. permit)
SNT	sinuses, nose, and throat	SOD	sinovenous occlusive disease
	suppan nail technique		sphincter of Oddi dysfunction
SNU	skilled nursing unit		superoxide dismutase
SNUB	super neurotransmitter uptake		surgical officer of the day
	blocker	SODA	Severity of Dyspepsia Assessment
SNV	Sin Nombre virus	SODAS	spheriodal oral drug absorption
	skilled nursing visit		system
	spleen necrosis virus	SOE	source of embolism
SO	second opinion	SOFA	sepsis-related organ failure
	sex offender		assessment
	shoulder orthosis		Sequential Organ Failure Assessment
	significant other		(score)
	special observation	SOFAS	Social and Occupational Functioning
	sphincter of Oddi		Assessment Scale
	standing orders	SOG	suggestive of good
	suboccipital	SOGS	South Oaks Gambling Screen
	suggestive of	SOH	sexually oriented hallucinations
	superior oblique	SoHx	social history
	supraoptic	SOI	slipped on ice
	supraorbital		sudden overwhelming infection

S

surgical orthotopic implantation (implant)

syrup of ipecac

SOL solution

space occupying lesion

SOL I special observations level one (there are also SOL II and SOL III)

SOM secretory otitis media

serous otitis media

somatization

SOMI sterno-occipital mandibular immobilizer

SONK spontaneous osteonecrosis of the knee

Sono sonogram

SONP solid organs not palpable

SOOL spontaneous onset of labor

SOP standard operating procedure

SOPM sutures out in afternoon (or evening)

SOR sign own release

strength of recommendation

SORA stable on room air

SOS if there is need

may be repeated once if urgently required (Latin: *si opus sit*)

self-obtained smear

suicidal observation status

SOSOB sit on side of bed

SOT solid organ transplant

something other than

stream of thought

SOTP Sex-Offender Treatment Provider

SOW Scope of Work

SP sacrum to pubis

sequential pulse

serum protein

shoulder press

silent period (related to electromyographic responses)

spastic dysphonia

speech

Speech Pathologist

spinal

spouse

stand and pivot

stand pivot

status post

Streptococcus pneumoniae

sulfadoxine; pyrimethamine (Fansidar)

systolic pressure

sp species

S/P status post

suprapubic

SP 1 suicide precautions number 1

SP 2 suicide precautions number 2

SPA albumin human (formerly known as salt-poor albumin)

scintillation proximity assay

serum prothrombin activity

sheep pulmonary adenomatosis

single photon absorptiometry

Speech Pathology and Audiology

stimulation produced analgesia

student physician's assistant

subperiosteal abscess

suprapubic aspiration

SpA spondyloarthropathy

SP-A surfactant-specific protein A

SPAC satisfactory postanesthesia course

SPAG small-particle aerosol generator

SPAMM spatial modulation of magnetization

SPARC suprapubic sling operation

SPBE saw palmetto berry extract

SPBI serum protein bound iodine

SPBT suprapubic bladder tap

SPC saturated phosphatidylcholine

second primary cancer

sclerosing pancreatocholangitis

single-point cane

statistical process control

Summary of Product Characteristics

suprapubic catheter

SPCA serum prothrombin conversion accelerator (factor VII)

SPCT simultaneous prism and cover test

SPD schizotypal personality disorder

subcorneal pustular dermatosis

Supply, Processing, and Distribution (department)

suprapubic drainage

SPE saw palmetto extract

serum protein electrophoresis

solid-phase extraction

superficial punctate erosions

SPEB streptococcal pyrogenic exotoxins B

SPEC specimen

streptococcal pyrogenic exotoxins C

Spec Ed special education

SPECT single-photon emission computed tomography

SPEEP spontaneous positive end-expiratory pressure

SPEP serum protein electrophoresis

SPET single-photon emission tomography

SPF semipermeable film

S-phase fraction

split products of fibrin

sun protective factor

sp fl spinal fluid

SPG scrotopenogram

sphenopalatine ganglion

SpG specific gravity

SPH severely and profoundly handicapped

sighs per hour

spherocytes

SPHERO	spherocytes
SPI	speech processor interface
	surgical peripheral iridectomy
SPIA	solid phase immunoabsor-bent assay
SPIDER	steady-state projection imaging with dynamic echo-train readout
SPIF	spontaneous peak inspiratory force
SPIFE	serum protein and immunofixation electrophoresis (system)
S-PIN	Steinmann pin
SPINK1	serine protease inhibitor Kazal type 1
SPIO	superparamagnetic iron oxide
SPK	simultaneous pancreas-kidney (transplant)
	single parent keeping (baby)
	superficial punctate keratitis
SPL	sound pressure level
	superior parietal lobule
SPL®	Staphylococcal Phage Lysate
SPLATTT	split anterior tibial tendon transfer
SPM	scanning probe microscopy
	second primary malignancy
SPM96	statistical parametric mapping 96
SPMA	spinal progressive muscle atrophy
SPMD	scapuloperoneal muscular dystrophy
SPMDs	semipermeable membrane devices
SPME	solid-phase microextraction
SPMI	severely and persistently mentally ill
SPMS	secondary progressive multiple sclerosis
SPMSQ	Short Portable Mental Status Questionnaire
SPN	solitary pulmonary nodule
	student practical nurse
	superficial peroneal nerve
SPNK	single parent not keeping (baby)
SPNP	solid pseudopapillary neoplasm of the pancreas
SPO	status postoperative
SpO$_2$	oxygen saturation by pulse oximeter
spont	spontaneous
SponVe	spontaneous ventilation
SPOREs	Specialized Programs of Research Excellence (National Cancer Institute)
SPP	Sexuality Preference Profile
	single presentation phenotype
	super packed platelets
	suprapubic prostatectomy
spp	species
SPQ	Schizotypal Personality Questionnaire
SPR	surface plasmon resonance
SPRAS	Sheehan Patient Rated Anxiety Scale
SP-RIA	solid-phase radioimmunoassay
SPR-MS	surface plasmon resonance mass spectrometry

SPROM	spontaneous premature rupture of membrane
SPS	shoulder pain and stiffness
	simple partial seizure
	sodium polyethanol sulfonate
	sodium polystyrene sulfonate (Kayexalate; SPS®)
	status post surgery
	stiff-person syndrome
	systemic progressive sclerosis
SPSU	straight partial sit-up
SPT	second primary tumors
	skin prick test
	standing pivot transfer
	supportive periodontal therapy
	suprapubic tenderness
SP TAP	spinal tap
SPTL	spontaneous preterm labor
SPTs	second primary tumors
	single-patient trials
SP TUBE	suprapubic tube
SPTX	static pelvic traction
SPU	short procedure unit
SPVR	systemic peripheral vascular resistance
SPX	smallpox vaccine, not otherwise specified
SPx	spontaneous pneumothorax
SPX$_v$	smallpox vaccine (vaccinia virus)
SQ	status quo
	subcutaneous (this is a dangerous abbreviation, use subcut)
Sq CCa	squamous cell carcinoma
SQE	subcutaneous emphysema
SQM	square meter(s)
SQUID	superconducting quantum interference device
SQV	saquinavir (Fortovose; Invirase)
SR	screen
	sedimentation rate
	see report
	senior resident
	service record
	side rails
	sinus rhythm
	slow release
	smooth-rough
	social recreation
	standard risks
	stretch reflex
	superior rectus
	sustained release
	sustained response
	suture removal
	system review
S/R	strong/regular (pulse)
S&R	seclusion and restraint
	smooth and rough

^{89}Sr	strontium 89		speech reception threshold
SRA	serotonin release assay		speech recognition threshold
	steroid-resistant asthma		stereotactic radiotherapy
SRAN	surgical resident admission note		surfactant replacement therapy
SRBC	sheep red blood cells		sustained release theophylline
	sickle red blood cells	SRU	side rails up
SRBOW	spontaneous rupture of bag of waters	SRUS	solitary rectal ulcer syndrome
SRC	sclerodermal renal crisis	SRVC	subcutaneous reservoir and
SRCC	sarcomatoid renal cell carcinoma		ventricular catheter
SRCS	Division of Surveillance, Research,	SR ↑ X2	both siderails up
	and Communication Support	SS	half (this is a dangerous abbreviation
	(FDA)		as it is not understood or read as
SRD	service-related disability		sliding scale)
	smallest real difference		sacral sulcus
	sodium-restricted diet		sacrosciatic
SRE	sex and relationships education		saline soak (sodium chloride 0.9%)
	skeletal related event		saline solution (0.9% sodium
SREs	skeletal related events		chloride)
SRF	somatotropin releasing factor		saliva sample
	subretinal fluid		salt sensitivity (sensitive)
SRF-A	slow-releasing factor of anaphylaxis		salt substitute
SRGVHD	steroid-resistant graft-versus-host		serotonin syndrome
	disease		serum sickness
SRH	signs of recent hemorrhage		sickle cell
SRI	serotonin reuptake inhibitor		single-session (treatment)
SRICU	surgical respiratory intensive care		single-strength (as compared to
	unit		double-strength)
SRIF	somatotropin-release inhibiting factor		Sjögren syndrome
	(somatostatin; Zecnil)		sliding scale (this is a dangerous
SRK	smooth-rod Kaneda (implant)		abbreviation as it is not
SRMD	stress-related mucosal damage		understood or read as one half)
SRMS	sustained-release morphine sulfate		slip sent
SRMs	specified risk materials		Social Security
SR/NE	sinus rhythm, no ectopy		social service
SRNV	subretinal neovascularization		somatostatin (Zecnil)
SRNVM	subretinal neovascular membrane		stainless steel
SRO	sagittal ramus osteotomy		steady state
	single room occupancy		step stool
	smallest region of overlap		subaortic stenosis
	sustained-release oral		susceptible
SROA	sports-related osteoarthritis		suprasciatic (notch)
SROCPI	Self-Rating Obsessive-Compulsive		symmetrical strength
	Personality Inventory	S/S	Saturday and Sunday
SROM	self range of motion		sprain/strain
	serous right otitis media	SS#	Social Security number
	spontaneous rupture of membrane	S & S	shower and shampoo
SRP	scaling and root planing (dental)		signs and symptoms
	septorhinoplasty		sitting and supine
	stapes replacement prosthesis		sling and swathe
SRR	surgical recovery room		soft and smooth (prostate)
SRS	Silver-Russell syndrome		support and stimulation
	somatostatin receptor scintigraphy		swish and spit
s̄RS	without redness or swelling		swish and swallow
SRS-A	slow-reacting substance of	SSA	sagittal split advancement
	anaphylaxis		salicylsalicylic acid (salsalate)
SRSV	small round structured viruses		Sjögren syndrome antigen A
SRT	sedimentation rate test		Social Security Administration
	sleep-related tumescence		specific surface area

	Subjective Symptoms Assessment (profile)		selective sentinel lymphadenectomy
	sulfasalicylic acid (test)		subtotal supraglottic laryngectomy
SSADH	succinic semialdehyde dehydrogenase	SSLF	sacrospinous ligament fixation
SSAs	standard sedative agents	SSLR	seated straight leg raise
SSBP	sitting systolic blood pressure	SSM	short stay medical
SSC	sign symptom complex		skin-sparing mastectomy
	silver sulfadiazine and chlorhexidine		skin surface microscopy
	Similac® and special care		superficial spreading melanoma
	Special Services for Children	SSN	severely subnormal
	stainless steel crown		Social Security number
	standard straight cane	SSNB	suprascapular nerve block
SSc	systemic sclerosis (scleroderma)	SSO	second surgical opinion
SSCA	single shoulder contrast arthrography		sequence-specific oligonucleotide
SSCP	single-stranded conformational polymorphism		short stay observation (unit)
	substernal chest pain		Spanish speaking only
SSCr	stainless steel crown	SSOP	Second Surgical Opinion Program
SSCU	surgical special care unit		sequence-specific oligonucleotide probe
SSCVD	sterile spontaneous controlled vaginal delivery	SSP	sequence-specific primer
SSD	serosanguineous drainage		short stay procedure (unit)
	sickle cell disease		superior spermatic plexus
	silver sulfadiazine (Silvadene)		supragingival scaling and prophylaxis (dental)
	Social Security disability	SSPA	staphylococcal-slime polysaccharide antigens
	source to skin distance	SSPE	subacute sclerosing panencephalitis
SSDI	Social Security disability income	SSPG	steady-state plasma glucose
ss DNA	single-stranded desoxyribonucleic acid	SSPL	saturation sound pressure level
SSE	saline solution enema (0.9% sodium chloride)	SSPU	surgical short procedure unit
	skin self-examination	SSQ	Staring Speel Questionnaire
	soapsuds enema	SSR	Sleep Self-Reporting
	sterile speculum exam		substernal retractions
	subacute spongiform encephalopathy		sympathetic skin response
	systemic side effects	SSRFC	surrounding subretinal fluid cuff
SSEH	spontaneous spinal epidural hematoma	SSRI	selective serotonin reuptake inhibitor
SSEPs	somatosensory evoked potentials	SSRO	sagittal split ramus osteotomy (dental)
SSF	subscapular skinfold	SSRP	subgingival scaling and root planing (dental)
SSG	sodium stibogluconate	SSRs	simple sequence repeats
	sublabial salivary gland	SSS	layer upon layer
SSHL	sudden sensorineural hearing loss		scalded skin syndrome
SSI	sliding scale insulin		Scandinavian Stroke Scale
	Social Skills Inventory		Sepsis Severity Score
	sub-shock insulin		Severity Scoring System (Dart Snakebite)
	superior sector iridectomy		short stay service (unit)
	Supplemental Security Income		sick sinus syndrome
	surgical site infection		skin and skin structures
SSI-CCM	synthetic sentence identification with contralateral competing message		Spanish-speaking sometimes
			sphincter-saving surgery
SSI-ICM	synthetic sentence identification with ipsilateral competing message		spontaneous saliva swallowing
			Stanford Sleepiness Scale
SSKI	saturated solution of potassium iodide		sterile saline soak
		SSSB	sagittal split setback
SSL	second stage of labor	SSSDW	significant sharp, spike, or delta waves
		SSSE	self-sustained status epilepticus

SSSIs	skin and skin structure infections	STAT	immediately (or as defined by the institution)
SSSS	staphylococcal scalded skin syndrome		signal transducers and activators of transcription
SSSs	small short spikes (encephalography)	STATINS	HMG-CoA reductase inhibitors
SST	sagittal sinus thrombosis	STAXI	State-Trait Anger Expression Inventory
	Simple Shoulder Test		
	somatostatin (Zecnil)	STB	stillborn
SSTI	skin and skin structure infections	STBAL	standing balance
SSU	short stay unit	ST BY	stand by
SSX	sulfisoxazole acetyl	STC	serum theophylline concentration
S/SX	signs/symptoms		slow-transit constipation
ST	esotropic		soft tissue calcification
	sacrum transverse		special treatment center
	Schiotz tonometry		stimulate to cry
	Schirmer Test (dry-eye test)		stroke treatment center
	shock therapy		subtotal colectomy
	sinus tachycardia		sugar tongue cast
	skin tear	ST CLK	station clerk
	skin test	STD	sexually transmitted disease(s)
	slight trace		short-term disability
	slow-twitch		skin test dose
	smokeless tobacco		skin to tumor distance
	sore throat		sodium tetradecyl sulfate
	spasmodic torticollis	STD TF	standard tube feeding
	speech therapist	STE	ST-segment elevation
	speech therapy	STEAM	stimulated-echo acquisition mode
	sphincter tone	STEC	shiga toxin-producing *Escherichia coli*
	split thickness		
	spondee threshold	STEM	scanning transmission electron microscopic
	station (obstetrics)		
	stomach	STEMI	ST-segment elevation myocardial infarction
	straight		
	strength training	Stereo	steropsis
	stress testing	STEPS	The System for Thalidomide Educating and Prescribing Safety
	stretcher		
	subtotal	STET	single photon emission tomography
	Surgical Technologist		submaximal treadmill exercise test
	survival time	STETH	stethoscope
	synapse time	STF	special tube feeding
S & T	sulfamethoxazole and trimethoprim (SMZ-TMP or SMX-TMP)		standard tube feeding
		STG	short-term goals
STA	second trimester abortion		split-thickness graft
	spike-triggered averaging		superior temporal gyri
	staphylococcus vaccine, not otherwise specified	STH	soft tissue hemorrhage
			somatotrophic hormone
	superficial temporal artery		subtotal hysterectomy
STA_{aur}	*Staphylococcus aureus* vaccine		supplemental thyroid hormone
stab.	polymorphonuclear leukocytes (white blood cells, in nonmature form)	STHB	said to have been
		STI	sexually transmitted infection
STAI	State-Trait Anxiety Inventory		signal transduction inhibitor((s)
STAI-I	State-Trait-Anxiety Index—I		soft tissue injury
STA-MCA	superficial temporary artery-middle cerebral artery (anastomosis; bypass)		structured treatment interruption(s)
			sum total impression
			systolic time interval
STAPES	stapedectomy	STI-571	imatinib mesylate (Gleevec)
staph	*Staphylococcus aureus*	STILLB	stillborn
STA_{SPL}	staphylococcus vaccine, bacteriophage lysate	STIR	short TI (tau) inversion recovery

STIs	sexually transmitted infections		soft tissue swelling
	systolic time intervals		somatostatin (Zecnil)
STJ	scapulothoracic joint		standard threshold shift (audiology)
	subtalar joint		staurosporine
STK	streptokinase		superior temporal sulcus
STL	sent to laboratory		Surgical Technology Student
	serum theophylline level	STSG	split thickness skin graft
STLE	St. Louis encephalitis	STSS	streptococcal-induced toxic shock
STLI	subtotal lymphoid irradiation		syndrome
STLOM	swelling, tenderness, and limitation	STS-SPT	simple two-step swallowing
	of motion		provocation test
STLV	simian T-lymphotrophic viruses	STT	scaphoid, trapezium trapezoid
STM	scanning tunneling microscope		serial thrombin time
	short-term memory		skin temperature test
	soft tissue mobilization		soft tissue tumor
	sternocleidomastoideus		subtotal thyroidectomy
	streptomycin	STT#1	Schirmer tear test one
STMS	Short Test of Mental Status	STT#2	Schirmer tear test two
STMT	Seat Movement	STTb	basal Schirmer tear test
STN	subtalar neutral	STTOL	standing tolerance
	subthalamic nucleus	STU	shock trauma unit
STNI	subtotal nodal irradiation		surgical trauma unit
STNM	surgical evaluative staging of cancer	STV	short-term variability
STNR	symmetrical tonic neck reflex	STV+	short-term variability-present
S to	sensitive to	STV 0	short-term variability-absent
STO$_2$	microvascular oxygen saturation	STV inter	short-term variability-intermittent
STOP	sensitive, timely, and organized	STX	stricture
	programs (battered spouses)	STZ	streptozocin (Zanosar)
STORCH	syphilis, toxoplasmosis, other agents,	SU	sensory urgency
	rubella, cytomegalovirus, and		Somogyi units
	herpes (maternal infections)		stasis ulcer
STP	short-term plans		stroke unit
	sodium thiopental		sulfonylurea
	step training progression		supine
STPD	standard temperature and pressure—	Su	Sunday
	dry	S/U	shoulder/umbilicus
STPI	State-Trait Personality Inventory	S&U	supine and upright
STPS	Short-Term Performance Status	SUA	serum uric acid
STPT	second-trimester pregnancy		single umbilical artery
	termination	SUB	Skene urethra and Bartholin glands
STR	scotopic threshold response	Subcu	subcutaneous
	short tandem repeat	SUBCUT	subcutaneous
	sister	Subepi M	subepicardial myocardial
	small tandem repeat	Inj	injury
	stretcher	SUBL	sublingual
Strab	strabismus	SUB-	submandibular
strep	streptococcus	MAND	
	streptomycin	sub q	subcutaneous (this is a dangerous
STRICU	shock/trauma/respiratory intensive		abbreviation since the q is
	care unit		mistaken for every, when a
Str Post	strictly posterior		number follows)
MI	myocardial infarction	SUCC	succinylcholine
STS	serologic test for syphilis	SUCT	suction
	short-term survivors	SUD	substance use disorder(s)
	slide thin slab		sudden unexpected death
	sodium tetradecyl sulfate	SuDBP	supine diastolic blood pressure
	sodium thiosulfate	SUDEP	sudden unexpected (unexplained)
	soft tissue sarcoma		death in epilepsy

S

SUDS	Subjective Unit of Distress (Disturbance) (Discomfort) Scale	SVCS	superior vena cava syndrome
	sudden unexplained death syndrome	SVD	singular value decomposition (analysis)
SUF	symptomatic uterine fibroids	SVD	single-vessel disease
SUI	stress urinary incontinence		spontaneous vaginal delivery
	suicide		structural valve deterioration (dysfunction)
SUID	sudden unexplained infant death		
SUIOS	Simplified Urinary Incontinence Outcome Score	SVE	sterile vaginal examination
			Streptococcus viridans endocarditis
SULF-PRIM	sulfamethoxazole and trimethoprim		subcortical vascular encephalopathy
		SV&E	suicidal, violent, and eloper
SUN	serum urea nitrogen	SVG	saphenous vein graft
SUNCT	short-lasting unilateral neuraligform headache attacks with conjunctival injection and tearing	SVH	subjective visual horizontal (test)
		SVI	seminal vesicle invasion
			stroke volume index
SUNDS	sudden unexplained nocturnal death syndrome	S VISC	serum viscosity
		SVL	severe visual loss
SUO	syncope of unknown origin	SVN	small volume nebulizer
SUP	stress ulcer prophylaxis	SVO	small vessel occlusion
	superior	SVO$_2$	mixed venous oxygen saturation
	supination	SVOO	systemic ventricular outflow obstruction
	supinator		
	symptomatic uterine prolapse	SVP	spontaneous venous pulse
SUPAC	Scale-Up and Post Approval Change	SVPB	supraventricular premature beat
supp	suppository	SVPC	supraventricular premature contraction
SUPRV	supervision		
SUR	suramin (Metaret)	SV/PP	stroke volume/pulse pressure
	surgery	SVR	supraventricular rhythm
	surgical		sustained virological response
Surgi	Surgigator		systemic vascular resistance
SUUD	sudden unexpected, unexplained death	SVRI	systemic vascular resistance index
		SVT	superficial vein thrombosis
SUV	standard uptake variable		supraventricular tachycardia
SUVs	standard uptake values		symptom validity test(s)
SUX	succinylcholine	SVVD	spontaneous vertex vaginal delivery
	suction	SW	sandwich
SUZI	subzonal insertion		sea water
SV	scimitar vein		seriously wounded
	seminal vesical		shallow walk (aquatic therapy)
	severe		short wave
	sigmoid volvulus		Social Worker
	single ventricle		stab wound
	single vessel		sterile water
	snake venom		swallowing reflex
	stock volume	S&W	soap and water
	subclavian vein	S/W	somewhat
Sv	sievert (radiation unit)	SWA	Social Work Associate
SV40	simian virus 40	SWAN	statewide adoption network
SVA	small volume admixture	SWAP	short-wavelength automated perimetry
SVAS	supravalvular aortic stenosis		
SVB	saphenous vein bypass	SWAT	skin wound assessment and treatment
SVBG	saphenous vein bypass graft		
SVC	slow vital capacity	SWD	short wave diathermy
	subclavian vein compression	SWFI	sterile water for injection
	superior vena cava	SWG	standard wire gauge
SVCO	superior vena cava obstruction	SWI	sterile water for injection
SVC-RPA	superior vena cava and right pulmonary artery (shunt)		surgical wound infection
		S&WI	skin and wound isolation

SWL	shock wave lithotripsy
SWMA	segmental wall-motion abnormalities
SWME	Semmes-Weinstein monofilament examination
SWO	superficial white onychomycosis
SWOG	Southwest Oncology Group
SWOT	strengths, weaknesses, opportunities, threats (analysis)
SWP	small whirlpool
	southwest Pacific
SWR	surface wrinkling retinopathy
	surgical waiting room
SWS	sheltered workshop
	slow-wave sleep
	social work service
	student ward secretary
	Sturge-Weber syndrome
SWSD	shift-work sleep disorder
SWT	stab wound of the throat
	shuttle-walk test
SWU	septic work-up
SWW	static wall walk (aquatic therapy)
Sx	signs
	surgery
	symptom
SXA	single-energy x-ray absorptiometry
SXR	skull x-ray
SYN	synovial
SYN-D	synthadotin
SYN Fl	synovial fluid
SYPH	syphilis
SYR	syrup
SYS BP	systolic blood pressure
SZ	schizophrenic
	seizure
	suction
SZN	streptozocin (Zanosar)

T	inverted T wave
	tablespoon (15 mL) (this is a dangerous abbreviation)
	taenia
	teach (taught)
	temperature
	tender
	tension
	tesla (unit of magnetic flux density in radiology)
	testicles
	testosterone
	thoracic
	thymidine
	Toxoplasma
	trace
	transcribed
t	teaspoon (5 mL) (this is a dangerous abbreviation)
T+	increase intraocular tension
T−	decreased intraocular tension
2,4,5-T	2,4,5-trichlorophenoxyacetic acid
T°	temperature
$T_{1/2}$	half-life
T_1	tricuspid first sound
T_2	tricuspid second sound
T-2	dactinomycin, doxorubicin, vincristine, and cyclophosphamide
T_3	triiodothyronine (liothyronine)
T3	transurethral thermo-ablation therapy (Targis)
	Tylenol with codeine 30 mg (this is a dangerous abbreviation)
$T_{3/4}$ind	triiodothyronine to thyroxine index
T_4	levothyroxine
	thyroxine
T4	CD4 (helper-inducer cells)
T-7	free thyroxine factor
T-10	methotrexate, calcium leucovorin rescue, doxorubicin, cisplatin, bleomycin, cyclophosphamide, and dactinomycin
T-20	enfuvirtide (Fuzeon)
$T_1...T_{12}$	thoracic nerve 1 through 12
	thoracic vertebra 1 through 12
TA	Takayasu arteritis
	temperature axillary
	temporal arteritis
	temporal artery
	tendon Achilles
	therapeutic abortion
	tibialis anterior (muscle)
	tracheal aspirate
	traffic accident

	tricuspid atresia
	truncus arteriosus
Ta	tonometry applanation
T&A	tonsillectomy and adenoidectomy
	tonsils and adenoids
T(A)	axillary temperature
TA1	thymosin alpha-1
TA-55	stapling device
TAA	Therapeutic Activities Aide
	thoracic aortic aneurysm
	total ankle arthroplasty
	transverse aortic arch
	triamcinolone acetonide
	tumor-associated antigen (antibodies)
TAAA	thoracoabdominal aortic aneursym
TAB	tablet
	therapeutic abortion
	total androgen blockade
	triple antibiotic (bacitracin, neomycin, and polymyxin—this is a dangerous abbreviation)
TAC	docetaxel (Taxotere), doxorubicin (Adriamycin), and cyclophosphamide
	tetracaine, Adrenalin® and cocaine
	total arterial compliance
	tibial artery catheter
	total abdominal colectomy
	total allergen content
	triamicinolone cream
	trigeminal autonomic cephalgias
TACC	thoracic aortic cross-clamping
TACE	transarterial chemoembolization
TACI	total anterior cerebral infarct
tac-MRA	timed arterial compression magnetic resonance angiography
TACT	tuned aperture computed tomography
TAD	thoracic asphyxiant dystrophy
	transverse abdominal diameter
TADAC	therapeutic abortion, dilation, aspiration, and curettage
TADC	tumor-associated dendritic cells
TAE	transcatheter arterial embolization
TAF	tissue angiogenesis factor
TAG	triacylglycerol
	tumor-associated glycoprotein
TAGA	term, appropriate for gestational age
	term, average gestational age
TA-GVHD	transfusion-associated graft-versus-host disease
TAH	total abdominal hysterectomy
	total artificial heart
TAHBSO	total abdominal hysterectomy, bilateral salpingo-oophorectomy
TAHL	thick ascending limb of Henle loop
T Air	air puff tonometry
TAKE	Targeting Abnormal Kinetic Effects
TAL	tendon Achilles lengthening

	total arm length
T ALCON	Alcon® tonometry
T-ALL	T-cell acute lymphoblastic leukemia
TALP	total alkaline phosphatase
TAML	therapy-related acute myelogenous leukemia
t-AML	therapy-related acute myeloid leukemia
TAM	tamoxifen (Novaldex)
	teenage mother
	total active motion
	tumor-associated macrophages
TAN	treatment-as-needed
	Treatment Authorization Number
	tropical ataxic neuropathy
TANF	Temporary Assistance for Needy Families
TANI	total axial (lymph) node irradiation
TAO	thromboangitis obliterans
	troleandomycin
TAP	tone and positioning
	tonometry by applanation
	transabdominal preperitoneal (laparoscopic hernia repair)
	transesophageal atrial paced
	trypsinogen activation peptide
	tumor-activated prodrug
TAPP	transabdominal preperitoneal polypropylene (mesh-plasty)
T APPL	applanation tonometry
TAPVC	total anomalous pulmonary venous connection
TAPVD	total anomalous pulmonary venous drainage
TAPVR	total anomalous pulmonary venous return
TAR	thoracic aortic rupture
	thrombocytopenia with absent radius
	total ankle replacement
	total anorectal reconstruction
	treatment administration record
	treatment authorization request
TARA	total articular replacement arthroplasty
TART	tenderness, asymmetry, restricted motion, and tissue texture changes
	tumorectomy and radiotherapy
TAS	therapeutic activities specialist
	Thrombolytic Assessment System
	transabdominal sutures
	turning against self
	typical absence seizures
TAT	tandem autotransplants
	tell a tale
	tetanus antitoxin
	thematic apperception test
	thrombin-antithrombin III complex
	'til all taken

	total adipose tissue		total-body irradiation
	transactivator of transcription		traumatic brain injury
	transplant-associated	T bili	total bilirubin
	thrombocytopenia	TBK	total-body potassium
	turnaround time	tbl	tablespoon (15 mL)
	tyrosine aminotransferase	TBLB	transbronchial lung biopsy
TATT	tired all the time	TBLC	term birth, living child
TAU	tumescence activity units	TBLF	term birth, living female
TAUC	target area under the curve	TBLI	term birth, living infant
	time-averaged urea concentration	TBLM	term birth, living male
TAUSA	thrombolysis and angioplasty in	TBM	tracheobronchomalacia
	unstable angina		tuberculous meningitis
TAX	cefotaxime (Claforan)		tubule basement membrane
	paclitaxel (Taxol)	TBMg	total-body magnesium
TB	Tapes for the Blind	TBN	total-body nitrogen
	terrible burning	TBNA	transbronchial needle aspiration
	thought broadcasting		treated but not admitted
	toothbrush	TBNa	total-body sodium
	total base	TBO	toluidine blue O
	total bilirubin	TBOCS	Tale-Brown Obsessive-Compulsive
	total body		Scale
	tuberculosis	TBP	thyroxine-binding protein
TBA	to be absorbed		toe blood pressure
	to be added		total-body phosphorus
	to be administered		total-body protein
	to be admitted		tuberculous peritonitis
	to be announced	TBPA	thyroxine-binding prealbumin
	to be arranged	TBR	total-bed rest
	to be assessed	TBRF	tick-borne relapsing fever
	total body (surface) area	TBS	tablespoon (15ml)(this is a
TBAGA	term birth appropriate for gestational		dangerous abbreviation)
	age		tachycardia-bradycardia syndrome
T-bar	tracheotomy bar (a device used in		The Bethesda System (reporting
	respiratory therapy)		cervical and vagina cytology)
TBARS	thiobarbituric acid reactive		total-serum bilirubin
	substances	TBSA	total-body surface area
TBB	transbronchial biopsy		total-burn surface area
TBC	to be cancelled	tbsp	tablespoon (15 mL)
	total-blood cholesterol	TBT	tolbutamide test
	total-body clearance		tracheal bronchial toilet
	tuberculosis		transbronchoscopic balloon tipped
TBD	to be determined	TBUT	tear break-up time (dry-eye test)
TBE	tick-borne encephalitis	TBV	thiotepa, bleomycin, and vinblastine
	timed-barium esophagogram		total-blood volume
	to be evaluated		transluminal balloon valvuloplasty
TBE$_e$	tick-borne encephalitis, eastern	TBW	total-body water
	subtype (Far eastern encephalitis,	TBZ	thiabendazole (Mintezol)
	Russian spring-summer e., Taiga	TC	paclitaxel (Taxol) and cisplatin
	e.) vaccine		tactile cues
T-berg	Trendelenburg (position)		tai chi (exercise program)
TBEV	tick-borne encephalitis virus		team conference
TBE$_w$	tick-bone encephalitis, western		telephone call
	subtype (Central European		terminal cancer
	encephalitis) vaccine		testicular cancer
TBF	total-body fat		thioguanine and cytarabine
TBG	thyroxine-binding globulin		thoracic circumference
TBI	tick-borne illness(es)		throat culture
	toothbrushing instruction		tissue culture

	tolonium chloride
	tonic-clonic
	tonsillar coblation
	total cholesterol
	total communication
	to (the) chest
	tracheal collar
	trauma center
	true conjugate
	tubocurarine
Tc	technetium
T/C	telephone call
	ticarcillin-clavulanic acid (Timentin)
	to consider
3TC	lamivudine (Epivir)
TC7	Interceed®
T&C	turn and cough
	type and crossmatch
T&C#3	Tylenol with 30 mg codeine
TCA	thioguanine and cytarabine
	tissue concentrations of antibiotic(s)
	trichloroacetic acid
	tricuspid atresia
	tricyclic antidepressant
	tumor chemosensitivity assay
	tumor clonogenic assays
TCABG	triple coronary artery bypass graft
TCAD	transplant-related coronary-artery disease
	tricyclic antidepressant
TCAR	tiazofurin
TCB	to call back
	tumor cell burden
TCBS agar	thiosulfate-citrate-bile salt-sucrose agar
TCC	total cost of care
	transitional cell carcinoma
	2,3,5-triphenyl tetrazolium chloride
TCCB	transitional cell carcinoma of bladder
TC/CL	ticarcillin-clavulanate (Timentin)
$TcCO_2$	transcutaneous carbon dioxide
TCD	T-cell depleted
	transcerebellar diameter
	transcranial Doppler (ultrasonography)
	transverse cardiac diameter
	transcystic duct
TCDB	turn, cough, and deep breath
TCDD	tetrachlorodibenzo-p-dioxin (dioxin)
^{99m}Tc DTPA	technetium Tc 99m pentetate
TCE	tetrachloroethylene
	total-colon examination
	toxicity composite endpoint
	transcatheter embolotherapy
T cell	small lymphocyte
TCES	transcranial electrical stimulation
^{99m}TcGHA	technetium Tc 99m gluceptate

TCH	paclitaxel (Taxol), carboplatin, and trastuzumab (Herceptin)
	total cost of hospitalization
	turn, cough, hyperventilate
^{99m}Tc-HAS	technetium Tc 99m-labeled human serum albumin
TCHRs	traditional Chinese herbal remedies
TCI	target-control infusion
	to come in
TCID	tissue culture infective dose
TCIE	transient cerebral ischemic episode
TCIT	therapeutic crisis intervention training
TCL	tibial collateral ligament
	transverse carpal ligament
TCM	tissue culture media
	traditional Chinese medicine
	transcutaneous (oxygen) monitor
^{99m}Tc-MAA	technetium Tc 99m albumin microaggregated
TCMH	tumor-direct cell-mediated hypersensitivity
TCMS	transcranial cortical magnetic stimulation
TCMZ	trichlormethiazide (Naqua)
TCN	tetracycline
	triciribine phosphate (tricyclic nucleoside)
TCNS	transcutaneous nerve stimulator
TCNU	tauromustine
TcO_2	transcutaneous oxygen pressure
TcO_4^-	pertechnetate
TCOM	transcutaneous oxygen monitor
T Con	temporary conservatorship
TCP	thrombocytopenia
	transcutaneous pacing
	tranylcypromine (Parnate)
	tumor control probability
TCPC	total cavopulmonary connection
$TcPCO_2$	transcutaneous carbon dioxide
$TcPO_2$	transcutaneous oxygen
^{99m}TcPYP	technetium Tc 99m pyrophosphate
TCR	T-cell receptor
TCRE	transcervical resection of the endometrium
TCRFTA	temperature-controlled radiofrequency tissue ablation
TCS	tonic-clonic seizure
^{99m}TcSC	technetium Tc 99m sulfur colloid
TCT	thyrocalcitonin
	tincture
	transcatheter therapy
	triple combination tablet (abacavir, lamivudine, and zidovudine) (Trizivir)
TCU	transitional care unit
TCVA	thromboembolic cerebral vascular accident

TD	Takayasu disease
	tardive dyskinesia
	temporary disability
	terminal device
	test dose
	tetanus-diphtheria toxoids (pediatric use)
	tidal volume
	tolerance dose
	tone decay
	total disability
	transdermal
	transverse diameter
	travelers' diarrhea
	treatment discontinued
Td	tetanus-diphtheria toxoids (adult type)
TDAC	tumor-derived activated cell (cultures)
TDD	telephone device for the deaf
	thoracic duct drainage
	total daily dose
TDE	total daily energy (requirement)
TDF	tenofovir disoproxil fumarate (Virend)
	testis determining factor
	total-dietary fiber
	tumor dose fractionation
TDI	tissue Doppler imaging
	tolerable daily intake
	toluene diisocyanate
TDK	tardive diskinesia
TDL	thoracic duct lymph
TDLN	tumor-draining lymph nodes
TDM	therapeutic drug monitoring
T2DM	type 2 diabetes mellitus
TDMAC	tridodecylmethyl ammonium chloride
TDN	totally digestible nutrients
	transdermal nitroglycerin
TDNTG	transdermal nitroglycerin
TDNWB	touchdown nonweightbearing
TdP	torsades de pointes
TDPDS	temporomandibular disorder pain dysfunction syndrome
TDPWB	touchdown partial weight-bearing
TdR	thymidine
TDS	Teacher Drool Scale
	traveler's diarrhea syndrome
TDS	three times a day (United Kingdom)
TDT	tentative discharge tomorrow
	transmission disequilibrium test
	Trieger Dot Test
	tumor doubling time
TdT	terminal deoxynucleotidyl transferase
TDW	target dry weight
TDWB	touch down weight bearing

TDx®	fluorescence polarization immunoassay
TE	echo time
	tennis elbow
	terminal extension
	tooth extraction
	toxoplasmic encephalitis
	trace elements (chromium, copper, iodine, manganese, selenium, molybdenum andzinc)
	tracheoesophageal
	transesophageal echocardiography
	transrectal electroejaculation
*t*E	total expiratory time
T/E	testosterone to epitestosterone ratio
	testosterone/estrogen (ratio)
	trunk-to-extremity skinfold thickness (index)
T&E	testing and evaluation
	training and evaluation
	trial and error
TEA	thromboendarterectomy
	Time and Extent Application (FDA)
	total elbow arthroplasty
	transluminal extraction atherectomy
TEAE	treatment-emergent adverse event
TEAP	transesophageal atrial pacing
TEB	thoracic electrical bioimpedance
TEBG	testosterone-estradiol binding globulin
TeBG	testeosterone binding globulin
TeBIDA	technetium 99m trimethyl 1-bromo-imono diacetic acid
TEC	thromboembolic complication
	total eosinophil count
	toxic *Escherichia coli*
	transient erythroblastopenia of childhood
	transluminal extraction-endarterectomy catheter
	triethyl citrate
T&EC	trauma and emergency center
TECA	titrated extract of *Centella asiatica*
TECAB	totally endoscopic (off-pump) coronary artery bypass grafting
TED	thromboembolic disease
	thyroid eye disease
TEDS	thromboembolic disease stockings
	transesophageal echo-Doppler system
	Treatment Episode Data Set
TEE	total energy expended
	transnasal endoscopic ethmoidectomy
	transesophageal echocardiography
TEF	tracheoesophageal fistula
TEG	thromboelastogram (thromboelastography)

TEH	theophylline, ephedrine, and hydroxyzine	TETig	tetanus immune globulin
TEI	therapeutic equivalence interchange	TEU	token economy unit
	total episode of illness	TEV	talipes equinovarus (deformity)
	transesophageal imaging	TEVAP	transurethral electrovaporization of the prostate
TEL	telemetry	TF	tactile fremitus
	telephone		tail flick (reflex)
tele	telemetry		tetralogy of Fallot
TEM	temozolomide (Temodar)		tibiofemoral
	transanal endoscopic microsurgery		to follow
	transmission electron microscopy		tube feeding
TEMI	transient episodes of myocardial ischemia	TFA	topical fluoride application
			trans fatty acids
TEMP	temperature		trifluoroacetic acid
	temporal	TFB	trifascicular block
	temporary	TFBC	The Family Birthing Center
TEN	tension (intraocular pressure)	TFC	thoracic fluid content
	toxic epidermal necrolysis		time to following commands
TEN®	Total Enteral Nutrition	TFCC	triangular fibrocartilage complex
TENS	transcutaneous electrical nerve stimulation	TFF	tangential flow filtration
			trefoil factor family (peptides)
TEOAE	transient evoked otoacoustic emission (test)	TF-Fe	transferrin-bound iron
		TFI	total fluid intake
TEP	total endoprosthesis		treatment-free interval
	total extraperitoneal (laparoscopic hernia repair)	TFL	tensor fasciae latae
			transnasal fiberoptic laryngoscopy
	tracheoesophageal puncture		trimetrexate, fluorouracil, and leucovorin
	tubal ectopic pregnancy		
TEQ	toxic equivalents		trunk-forward lean
TER	terlipressin	TFM	transverse friction massage
	total elbow replacement	TFO	triplex-forming oligonucleotide
	total energy requirement	TFOs	triplex-forming oligonucleotides
	transurethral electroresection	TFPI	tissue-factor pathway inhibitor
TERB	terbutaline	TFR	total fertility rate
TERC	Test of Early Reading Comprehension	TFT	thin-film transistor
			Thought Field Therapy
TERM	full-term		thumb-finding test
	terminal		trifluridine (trifluorothymidine)
TERT	human telomerase reverse transcriptase (also hTRT)	TFTs	thyroid function tests
		TFV	tenofovir (Viread)
	tertiary	TG	total gym
	total end-range time		triglycerides
TES	therapeutic electrical stimulation	Tg	thyroglobulin
	thoracic endometriosis syndrome	6-TG	thioguanine
	thoracic endoscopic sympathectomy	TGA	Therapeutic Goods Administration (Australia)
	treatment emergent symptoms		
TESA	testicular sperm aspiration		third-generation antidepressant
TESE	testicular sperm extraction		transient global amnesia
TESI	thoracic epidural steroid injection		transposition of the great arteries
TESS	Toronto Extremity Salvage Score	TGAR	total graft area rejected
	Toxic Exposure Surveillance System	TGB	tiagabine (Gabatril)
	treatment emergent signs and symptoms	TGCE	temperature gradient capillary electrophoresis
	Treatment Emergent Symptom Scale	TGCT	testicular germ cell tumor(s)
TET	transcranial electrostimulation therapy	TGD	thyroglossal duct
			tumor growth delay
	treadmill exercise test	TGDC	thyroglossal duct cyst
TETE	too early to evaluate	TGE	transmissible gastroenteritis

TGFA	triglyceride fatty acid	THR	target heart rate
TGF	transforming growth factor		thrombin receptor
TGF-β	transforming growth factor-beta		total hip replacement
TGGE	temperature-gradient gel		training heart rate
	electrophoresis	THRL	total hip replacement, left
TGR	tenderness, guarding, and rigidity	THRR	total hip replacement, right
TGS	tincture of green soap		transient hyperemic response ratio
TGs	triglycerides	THS	Tolosa-Hunt syndrome
TGT	thromboplastin generation test	THTV	therapeutic home trial visit
TGTL	total glottic transverse laryngectomy	THV	therapeutic home visit
TGV	thoracic gas volume	TI	terminal ileus
	transposition of great vessels		thallium imaging
TGXT	thallium-graded exercise test		therapeutic index
TGZ	troglitazone (Rezulin)		thought insertion
TH	thrill		time following inversion pulse
	thyroid hormone		(radiology)
	total hysterectomy		transischial
Th	thorium		transverse diameter of inlet
	Thursday		tricuspid incompetence
T&H	type and hold		tricuspid insufficiency
TH1	T helper cell, type 1	TIA	transient ischemic attack
TH2	T helper cell, type 2	TIB	tibia
THA	tacrine (tetrahydroacridine; Cognex)	TIBC	total iron-binding capacity
	total hip arthroplasty	tib-fib	tibia and fibula
	transient hemispheric attack	TIC	paclitaxel (Taxol), ifosfamide, and
THAA	thyroid hormone autoantibodies		cisplain
	tubular hypoplasia aortic arch		trypsin-inhibitor capacity
THAL	thalassemia	TICOSMO	trauma, infection, chemical/drug
	thalidomide (Thalomid)		exposure, organ systems, stress,
THAT	Toronto Hospital Alertness Test		musculoskeletal, and other
THBI	thyroid hormone binding index		(prompts used during history
THBR	thyroid hormone-binding ratio		taking for possible etiologies of
THAM®	tromethamine		problems)
THBO₂	topical hyperbaric oxygen	TICS	diverticulosis
THC	tetrahydrocannabinol (dronabinol)	TICU	thoracic intensive care unit
	thigh circumference		transplant intensive care unit
	transhepatic cholangiogram		trauma intensive care unit
THCT	triple-phase helical computer	t.i.d.	three times a day
	tomography	TIDM	three times daily with meals
TH-CULT	throat culture	TIE	transient ischemic episode
tHcy	total homocysteine	TIF	tracheal intubation fiberscope
THE	total-head excursion	TIG	tetanus immune globulin
	transhepatic embolization	TIH	tumor-inducing hypercalcemia
Ther Ex	therapeutic exercise	TKI	tyrosine kinase inhibitor
THF	thymic humoral factor	TIL	tumor-infiltrating lymphocytes
THG	tetrahydrogestrinone	%tile	percentile
THg	total mercury	TIMI	Thrombolysis in Myocardial
THI	transient hypogamma-globinemia of		Infarction (studies)
	infancy	TIMP	tissue inhibitor of metalloproteinase
THKAFO	trunk-hip-knee-ankle-foot orthosis	TIMP-2	Tissue inhibitors of metallo-
THKAFO-	lockable joints using		proteinase 2
LU	trunk-hip-knee-ankle-foot orthosis	TIN	testicular intraepithelial neoplasia
THL	transvaginal hydrolaparoscopy		three times a night (this is a
THLAA	tubular hypoplasia left aortic arch		dangerous abbreviation)
THP	take home packs		tubulointerstitial nephritis
	total hip prosthesis	tinct	tincture
	transhepatic portography	TIND	Treatment Investigational New Drug
	trihexyphenidyl (Artane)		(application)

TINEM	there is no evidence of malignancy	thin layer chromatography
TIP	toxic interstitial pneumonitis	titanium linear cutter
	tubularized incised plate (urethroplasty)	T-lymphocyte choriocarcinoma
		total lung capacity
TIPS	transvenous intrahepatic portosystemic shunt (stent-shunt)	total lymphocyte count
		transitional living center
TIPSS	transjugular intrahepatic portosystemic shunt (stent)	triple lumen catheter
TIRFM	total-internal reflection microscopy	TLD	thermoluminescent dosimeter
TIS	tumor *in situ*	TLE	temporal lobe epilepsy
TISS	Therapeutic Intervention Scoring System	TLFB	timeline follow back (interview)
		T-LGLL	T-cell large granular lymphocyte leukemia
TIT	*Treponema* (*pallidum*) immobilization test	TLH	total laparoscopic hysterectomy
	triiodothyronine (liothyronine)	TLI	total lymphoid irradiation
			translaryngeal intubation
TIUP	term intrauterine pregnancy	TLIF	thoracolumbar intervertebral fusion
TIVA	total intravenous anethesia		translumbar interbody fusion
TIVC	thoracic inferior vena cava	TLK	thermal laser keratoplasty
+tive	positive	TLM	thalidomide (Thalomid)
TIW	three times a week (this is a dangerous abbreviation)		torn lateral meniscus
		TLNB	term living newborn
TJ	tendon jerk	TLOA	temporary leave of absence
	triceps jerk	TLP	transitional living program
TJA	total joint arthroplasty	TLR	target lesion reintervention
TJC	tender joint count		target-lesion revascularization
TJN	tongue jaw neck (dissection)		tonic labyrinthine reflex
	twin-jet nebulizer	TLRs	Toll-like receptors
TJR	total joint replacement	TLS	tumor lysis syndrome
TK	thymidine kinase	TLSO	thoracic lumbar sacral orthosis
	toxicokinetics	TLSP	trypsin-like serine protease
TKA	total knee arthroplasty	TLSSO	thoracolumbosacral spinal orthosis
	tyrosine kinase activity	TLT	tonsillectomy
TKD	tokodynamometer	TLTBI	treatment of latent tuberculosis infection
TKE	terminal knee extension	
TKIC	true knot in cord	TLUS	the time elapsed from ingestion of the first dose of medication to passage of the last unformed stool
TKNO	to keep needle open	
TKP	thermokeratoplasty	
	total knee prosthesis	TLV	threshold limit value
TKO	to keep (vein; intravenous line) open		total lung volume
TKR	total knee replacement	TM	temperature by mouth
TKRL	total knee replacement, left		tetrathiomolybdate
TKRR	total knee replacement, right		thalassemia major
TKVO	to keep vein open		Thayer-Martin (culture)
TL	team leader		thyromegaly
	thermoluminescence		Tibetan Medicine
	thoracolumbar		trabecular meshwork
	total laryngectomy		trademark (unregistered)
	transverse line		transcendental meditation
	trial leave		treadmill
	tubal ligation		tropical medicine
T/L	terminal latency		tumor
Tl	thallium		tympanic membrane
TLA	translumbar arteriogram (aortogram)	T & M	type and crossmatch
	transverse ligament of atlas	TMA	thrombotic microangiopathy
TLAC	triple lumen Arrow catheter		tissue microarray
TL BLT	tubal ligation, bilateral		trained medication aid
TLC	tender loving care		transcription mediated amplification
	therapeutic lifestyle changes		transmetatarsal amputation

T

	trimethylamine	TMST	treadmill stress test
T/MA	tracheostomy mask	TMT	tarsometatarsal
TMAS	Taylor Manifest Anxiety Scale		teratoma with malignant
TMA-uria	trimethylaminuria		transformation
T_{max}	temperature maximum		treadmill test
t_{max}	time of occurrence for maximum		tympanic membrane thermometer
	(peak) drug concentration	TMTC	too many to count
TMB	tetramethylberizidine	TMTX	trimetrexate (Neutrexin)
	therapeutic back massage	TMUGS	Tumor Marker Utility Grading Scale
	transient monocular blindness	TMX	tamoxifen (Novaldex)
	trimethoxybenzoates	TMZ	temazepam (Restoril)
TMC	transmural colitis		temozolomide (Temodar)
	Transtheorefical Model of Change	TN	normal intraocular tension
	trapeziometacarpal		team nursing
	triamcinolone		temperature normal
TMCA	trimethylcolchicinic acid		tree nut
TMCN	triamcinolone		trigeminal neuralgia
TMD	temporomandibular dysfunction		triple negative
	(disorder)	T&N	tension and nervousness
	treating physician		tingling and numbness
t-MDS	therapy-related myelodysplastic	TNA	total nutrient admixture
	syndrome	TNAB	transthoracic needle biopsy
TME	thermolysin-like	TNB	term newborn
	metalloendopeptidase		transnasal butorphanol
	total mesorectal excision		transrectal needle biopsy (of the
TMET	treadmill exercise test		prostate)
TMEV	Theiler murine encephalomyelitis		Tru-Cut® needle biopsy
	virus	TNBP	transurethral needle biopsy of
TMG	trimegestone		prostate
TMH	trainable mentally handicapped	TNCC	Trauma Nursing Course Certified
TMI	threatened myocardial infarction	TND	term, normal delivery
	transmandibular implant	TNDM	transient neonatal diabetes mellitus
	transmural infarct	TNF	tumor necrosis factor
T>MIC	time above minimum inhibitory	TNF-bp	tumor necrosis factor binding protein
	concentration	TNG	nitroglycerin
TMJ	temporomandibular joint		toxic nodular goiter
TMJD	temporomandibular joint dysfunction	TNI	total nodal irradiation
TMJS	temporomandibular joint syndrome	TnI	troponin I
TML	tongue midline	TNKase®	tenecteplase
	treadmill	TNM	primary tumor, regional lymph
TMLR	transmyocardial laser		nodes, and distant metastasis (used
	revascularization		with subscripts for the staging of
TMM	torn medial meniscus		cancer)
	total muscle mass	t-NNT	threshold number needed to treat
Tmm	McKay-Marg tension	TNP	time to neurologic progression
TMNG	toxic multinodular goiter	TNR	tonic neck reflex
TMO	transcaruncular medial orbitotomy	TNS	transcutaneous nerve stimulation
TMP	thallium myocardial perfusion		(stimulator)
	transmembrane pressure		transient neurologic symptoms
	trimethoprim		Trauma Nurse Specialist
TMP/SMZ	trimethoprim and sulfamethoxazole		Tullie-Niebörg syndrome
	(correct name is sulfamethoxazole	TNT	thiotepa, mitoxantrone (Novantrone),
	and trimethoprin; SMZ-TMP)		and paclitaxel (Taxol)
TMR	temporary medication refill		triamcinolone and nystatin
	trainable mentally retarded	TnT	troponin T
	transmyocardial revascularization	TNTC	too numerous to count
TMS	transcranial magnetic stimulation	TNU	tobacco nonuser
TMSI	Task Management Strategy Index	TNY	trichomonas and yeast

TO	old tuberculin	TORB	telephone order read back
	telephone order	TORC	Test of Reading Comprehension
	time off	TORCH	toxoplasmosis, others (other viruses
	tincture of opium (warning: this is		known to attack the fetus), rubella,
	NOT paregoric)		cytomegalovirus, and herpes
	total obstruction		simplex (maternal viral infections)
	transfer out	TORP	total ossicular replacement prosthesis
T(O)	oral temperature	TOS	intraocular pressure of the left eye
T/O	time out		thoracic outlet syndrome
T&O	tandem and ovoid (insertion)	TOT BILI	total bilirubin
	tubes and ovaries	TOTM	trioctyltrimellitate
TOA	time of arrival	TOV	telephone order verified
	tubo-ovarian abscess		trial of void
TOAA	to affected areas	TOW	time off work
TOB	tobacco	TOWL	Test of Written Language
	tobramycin	TOX	toxoplasmosis (*Toxoplasma gondii*)
TOC	table of contents		vaccine
	test-of-cure (post-therapy visit)	TOXO	toxoplasmosis
	total occlusal convergence	TP	teaching physician
	total organic carbon		temperature and pressure
TOCE	transcatheter oily chemoembolization		temporoparietal
TOCO	tocodynamometer		tender point
TOD	intraocular pressure of the right eye		therapeutic pass
	target organ damage		ThinPrep Pap (test)
	target-organ disease		thought process
	time of death		thrombophlebitis
	time of departure		thymidine phosphorylase
	tubal occlusion device		time to progression
TOE	transoesophageal echocardiography		Todd paralysis
	(United Kingdom and other		toe pressure
	countries)		toilet paper
TOF	tetralogy of Fallot		total protein
	time of flight (radiology)		"T" piece
	total of four		treating physician
	train-of-four		trigger point
TOFMS	time-of-flight mass spectrometry	T:P	trough-to-peak ratio
TOGV	transposition of the great vessels	T & P	temperature and pulse
TOH	throughout hospitalization		turn and position
TOI	Trial Outcome Index	TPA	alteplase, recombinant (tissue
TOL	tolerate		plasminogen activator)
	trial of labor		(Activase)
TOLD	Test of Language Development		temporary portacaval anastomosis
TOM	therapeutic outcomes monitoring		third-party administrator
	tomorrow		tissue polypeptide antigen
	transcutaneous oxygen monitor		total parenteral alimentation
ToM	theory-of-mind	TPAL	term infant(s), premature infant(s),
Tomo	tomography		abortion(s), living children
TON	tonight	TPB	Theory of Planned Behavior
TOP	termination of pregnancy	TPC	target plasma concentration
	Topografov (virus)		tender-point count
	topotecan (Hycamtin)		total patient care
TOP-8	Treatment Outcome PTSD (post-		total plate count
	traumatic stress disorder) (scale)		touch preparation cytology
TOPO	topotecan (Hycamtin)	TPD	tropical pancreatic diabetes
TOPO 1	topoisermerase		typhoid vaccine, not otherwise
TOPS	Take Off Pounds Sensibly		specified
TOPV	trivalent oral polio vaccine	TPD$_a$	typhoid vaccine, attenuated live (oral
TOR	toremifene (Faneston)		Ty21a strain)

TPD_{AKD}	typhoid vaccine, acetone-killed and dried (U.S. military)
TPD_{HP}	typhoid vaccine, heat and phenol inactivated, dried
TPD_{VI}	typhoid vaccine, *Vi* capsular polysaccharide
TPE	therapeutic plasma exchange
	total placental estrogens
	total protective environment
T-penia	thrombocytopenia
TPF	docetaxel (Taxotere), cisplatin (Platinol), and fluorouracil
	trained participating father
TPH	thromboembolic pulmonary hypertension
	trained participating husband
TPHA	*Treponema pallidum* hemagglutination
T PHOS	triple phosphate crystals
TPI	*Treponema pallidum* immobilization
	triose phosphate isomerase
TPIT	trigger point injection therapy
t_{pk}	time to peak
TPL	thromboplastin
T plasty	tympanoplasty
TPLSM	two-photon laser-scanning microscope
TPM	temporary pacemaker
	topiramate (Topamax)
TPMT	thiopurine methyltransferase
TPN	total parenteral nutrition
TPO	thrombopoietin
	thyroid peroxidase
	thyroperoxidase
	trial prescription order
TPP	thiamine pyrophosphate
TpP	thrombus precursor protein
TP & P	time, place, and person
TPPN	total peripheral parenteral nutrition
TPPS	Toddler-Preschooler Postoperative Pain Scale
TPPV	trans pars plana vitrectomy
TPR	temperature
	temperature, pulse, and respiration
	total peripheral resistance
TPRI	total peripheral resistance index
T PROT	total protein
TPS	tender point score
	typhus (*rickettsiae* sp.) vaccine
tPSA	total prostate-specific antigen
TPT	thermal perception threshold
	time to peak tension
	topotecan (Hycamtin)
	transpyloric tube
	treadmill performance test
*t*PTEF	time to peak tidal expiratory flow
TPU	tropical phagedenic ulcer
T-putty	Theraputty
TPV	tipranavir (Aptivus)
TPVA	tibioperoneal vessel angioplasty
TPVR	total peripheral vascular resistance
TPZ	tirapazamine
TQM	total quality management
TR	therapeutic recreation
	time to repeat
	time to repetition (radiology)
	tincture
	to return
	trace
	transfusion reaction
	transplant recipients
	trapezius
	treatment
	tremor
	tricuspid regurgitation
	tumor registry
T(R)	rectal temperature
T & R	tenderness and rebound
	treated and released
	turn and reposition
TRA	therapeutic recreation associate
	to run at
	tumor regression antigen
TRAb	thyrotropin-receptor antibody
TRAC	traction
TRACE	time-resolved amplified cryptate emission
TRACH	tracheal
	tracheostomy
TRAFO	tone-reducing ankle/foot orthosis
TRAIL	tumor-necrosis-factor-related apoptosis-inducing ligand
TRALI	transfusion-associated lung injury
TRAM	transverse rectus abdominis myocutaneous (flap)
	transverse rectus abdominum muscle
	Treatment Response Assessment Method
TRAMP	transversus and rectus abdominis musculo-peritoneal (flap)
TRANCE	tumor necrosis factor–related activation-induced cytokine
TRANS	transfers
Trans D	transverse diameter
TRANS Rx	transfusion reaction
TRAP	tartrate-resistant (leukocyte) acid phophatase
	Telomeric Repeat Amplification Protocol
	thrombospondin-related anonymous protein
	total radical-trapping antioxidant parameter
	trapezium
	trapezius muscle
TRAS	transplant renal artery stenosis

	trastuzumab (Herceptin)
TRB	return to baseline
TRBC	total red blood cells
TRC	tanned red cells
TRD	tongue-retaining device
	total-retinal detachment
	traction retinal detachment
	treatment-related death
	treatment-resistant depression
TRDN	transient respiratory distress of the newborn
TREC	T-cell receptor-rearrangement excision circles
Tren	Trendelenburg
TRF	terminal restriction fragment
TRH	protirelin (thyrotropin-releasing hormone) (Relefact TRH®; Thypinone®)
TRI	transient radicular irritation
	trimester
TriA	tricuspid atresia
T_3RIA	triiodothyronine level by radioimmunoassay
TRIAC	triiodothyroacetic acid
TRIC	trachoma inclusion conjunctivitis
TRICH	*Trichomonas*
TRICKS	time-resolved imaging contrast kinetics
TRIG	triglycerides
TRISS	Trauma Related Injury Severity Score
TR-LSC	time-resolved liquid scintillation counting
TRM	transplant-related mortality
	treatment-related mortality
TRM-SMX	trimethoprim-sulfamethoxazole (correct name is sulfamethoxazole and trimethoprin; SMZ-TMP; SMX-TMP)
tRNA	transfer ribonucleic acid
TRNBP	transrectal needle biopsy prostate
TRND	Trendelenburg (position)
TRNG	tetracycline-resistant *Neisseria gonorrhoeae*
TRO	to return to office
TROFO	trofosfamide
TROM	torque range of motion
	total range of motion
TrOOP	true out-of-pocket costs
TRP	tubular reabsorption of phosphate
TRP-1	tyrosine-related protein-1
TRPS	trichorhinophalangeal syndrome (types I, II, and III)
TrPs	trigger points
TRPT	transplant
TRS	Therapeutic Recreation Specialist
	the real symptom
	tremor rating scale
TRT	tangential radiation therapy

	testosterone replacement therapy
	thermoradiotherapy
	thoracic radiation therapy
	tinnitus retraining therapy
	treatment-related toxicity
TR/TE	time to repetition and time to echo in spin (echo sequence of magnetic resonance imaging)
T_3RU	triiodothyronine resin uptake
TRUS	transrectal ultrasonography
TRUSP	transrectal ultrasonography of the prostate
TRUST	toluidine red unheated serum test
TRZ	triazolam (Halcion)
TS	Tay-Sachs (disease)
	telomerase
	temperature sensitive
	test solution
	thoracic spine
	throat swab
	thymidylate synthase
	timed samplings
	toe signs
	Tourette syndrome
	transsexual
	Trauma Score
	tricuspid stenosis
	triple strength
	tuberous sclerosis
	Turner syndrome
T/S	trimethoprim/sulfamethoxazole (correct name is sulfamethoxazole and trimethoprin)
T&S	type and screen
Ts	Schiotz tension
	T suppressor cell
TSAb	thyroid stimulating antibodies
TSA	toluenesulfonic acid
	total shoulder arthroplasty
	trichostatin A
	tryptone soya (blood) agar
	tumor-specific antigen
	type-specific antibody
	tyramine signal amplification
TSAR®	tape surrounded Appli-rulers
TSAS	Total Severity Assessment Score
TSAT	transferrin saturation
TSB	total serum bilirubin
	trypticase soy broth
TSBB	transtracheal selective bronchial brushing
TSC	technetium sulfur colloid
	theophylline serum concentration
	total symptom complex
	tuberous sclerosis complex
T-score	number of standard deviations from the average bone mineral density (BMD) of a 25-30 year old woman

TSD	target to skin distance		treponemal test
	Tay-Sachs disease		triceps thickness
	total sleep deprivation		tuberculin tested
	T-(tumor) stage downstaging		tuberculoid leprosy
TSDP	tapered steroid dosing package		twitch tension
TSE	targeted systemic exposure		tympanic temperature
	testicular self-examination	T-T	time-to-time
	total skin examination	T/T	trace of ____/trace of ____
	transmissible spongiform	T&T	tobramycin and ticarcillin
	encephalopathy		touch and tone
TSEBT	total skin electron beam therapy		tympantomy and tube (insertion)
T set	tracheotomy set	TT4	total thyroxine
TSF	tricep skin fold (thickness)	TTA	total toe arthroplasty
TSGA	term, small gestational age		transtracheal aspiration
TSGs	tumor suppressor genes		trauma team activation
TSH	thyroid-stimulating hormone	TTAT	toe touch as tolerated
TSH-RH	thyrotropin-releasing hormone	TTC	transtracheal catheter
TSI	thyroid stimulating immunoglobulin	TTD	tarsal tunnel decompression
	tobramycin solution for inhalation		temporary total disability
	(TOBI®)		total tumor dose
TSIs	thymidylate synthase inhibitors		transverse thoracic diameter
T-skull	trauma skull		trichothiodystrophy
TSM	two-spotted spider mite	TTDE	touch-tone data entry
tsp	teaspoon (5 mL)		transthoracic color Doppler
TSP	thrombospondin		echocardiography
	total serum protein	TTDM	thallim threadmill
	tropical spastic paraparesis	TTDP	time-to-disease progression
TSPA	thiotepa	TTE	transthoracic echocardiography
T-spine	thoracic spine		trial terminated early
TSR	total shoulder replacement	t test	Student's t-test
TSS	total serum solids	TTF	time-to-treatment failure
	total symptom scores	TTGE	timed-temperature gradient
	toxic shock syndrome		electrophoresis
	transsphenoidal surgery	TTI	Teflon tube insertion
	tumor score system		total time to intubate
TSST	toxic shock syndrome toxin		transfer to intermediate
TST	titmus stereocuity test	TTII	thyrotropin-binding inhibitory
	total sleep time		immunoglobulins
	trans-scrotal testosterone	TTJV	transtracheal jet ventilation
	treadmill stress test	TTM	total tumor mass
	tuberculin skin test(s)		transtelephonic monitoring
TSTA	tumor-specific transplantation		transtheoretical model
	antigens		trichotillomania
TSTM	too small to measure	TTMV	Torque-TenoMiniVirus
TT	testicular torsion	TTN	time to normalization
	Test Tape®		transient tachypnea of the newborn
	tetanus toxoid	TTNA	transthoracic needle aspiration
	thiotepa (Thioplex)	TTNB	transient tachypnea of the newborn
	thoracostomy tube	TTND	time to nondetectable
	thrombin time	TTO	tea tree oil
	thrombolytic therapy		time trade-off
	thymol turbidity		to take out
	tilt table		transfer to open
	tilt testing		transtracheal oxygen
	tonometry	TTOD	tetanus toxoid outdated
	total thyroidectomy	TTOP	time to objective progression
	transit time	TTOT	transtracheal oxygen therapy
	transtracheal	TTP	tender to palpation

	tender to pressure	TULIPS	touch-up and loop incorporated primers (an alternative PCR technique)
	thrombotic thrombocytopenic purpura		
	time to pregnancy	TUMT	transurethral microwave thermotherapy
	time to tumor progression		
	time-to-progression	TUN	total urinary nitrogen
TTP/HUS	thrombotic thrombocytopenic purpura and hemolytic-uremic syndrome	TUNA	transurethral needle ablation
		TUNEL	terminal deoxynucleotidyl transferase-mediated dUTP-biotin nick-end labeling
TTR	time in therapeutic range		
	transthyretin	TUPR	transurethral prostatic resection
	triceps tendon reflex	TUR	transurethral resection
TTS	tarsal tunnel syndrome	T₃UR	triiodothyronine uptake ratio
	temporary threshold shift	TURB	transurethral resection of the bladder
	through the skin		turbidity
	Toddler Temperament Scale	TURBN	transurethral resection bladder neck
	transdermal therapeutic system	TURBT	transurethral resection bladder tumor
	transfusion therapy service	TURP	transurethral resection of prostate
TTs	tympanostomy tubes	TURV	transurethral resection valves
TTT	tilt-table test	TURVN	transurethral resection of vesical neck
	time to treatment termination		
	tolbutamide tolerance test	TUTL	transuterine tubal lavage
	total tourniquet time	TUU	transureteroureterostomy
	transpupillary thermotherapy	TUV	transurethral valve
	turn-to-turn transfusion	TUVP	transurethral vaporization of the prostate
TTTS	twin-twin transfusion syndrome		
TTUTD	tetanus toxoid up-to-date	TV	television
TTV	Torque-TenoVirus		temporary visit
	total tumor volume		thyroid volume
	transfusion-transmitted virus		tidal volume
TTVIs	transfusion-transmitted viral infections		tonic vergence
			transvenous
TTVP	temporary transvenous pacemaker		trial visit
TTWB	touch-toe weight bearing		*Trichomonas vaginalis*
TTx	thrombolytic therapy		tricuspid value
TU	Todd units	T/V	touch-verbal
	transrectal ultrasound	TVC	triple voiding cystogram
	transurethral		true vocal cord
	tuberculin units	TVc	tricuspid valve closure
	tumor	TVD	triple vessel disease
Tu	Tuesday	TVDALV	triple vessel disease with an abnormal left ventricle
1-TU	1 tuberculin unit		
5-TU	5 tuberculin units	TVF	tactile vocal fremitus
250-TU	250 tuberculin units		target vessel failure
TUB	tuberculosis vaccine, not BCG		true vocal fold
TUBS	traumatic, unidirectional instability and Bankart lesion	TVH	total vaginal hysterectomy
		TVI	time velocity integral
TUDS	temporary ureteral drainage system	TVN	tonic vibration response
TUE	transurethral extraction	TVP	tensor veli palatini (muscle)
TUF	total ultrafiltration		transvenous pacemaker
TUG	timed Up and GO (test)		transvesicle prostatectomy
	total urinary gonadotropin	TVR	target vessel revascularization (rate)
TUIBN	transurethral incision of bladder neck		tricuspid valve replacement
TUIP	transurethral incision of the prostate	TVRSS	total vasomotor rhinitis symptom score
TUL	tularemia (*Francisella tularensis*) vaccine		
		TVS	transvaginal sonography
TULIP®	transurethral ultrasound-guided laser-induced prostatectomy (system)		transvenous system
			trigemino-vascular system

TVSC	transvaginal sector scan	
TVT	tension-free vaginal tape	
	transvaginal taping	
	transvaginal tension-free	
TVU	total volume of urine	
	transvaginal ultrasonography	
TVUS	transvaginal ultrasonography	
TW	talked with	
	tapwater	
	test weight	
	thought withdrawal	
	Trophermyma whippleii	
	T-wave	

TVSC transvaginal sector scan
TVT tension-free vaginal tape
  transvaginal taping
  transvaginal tension-free
TVU total volume of urine
  transvaginal ultrasonography
TVUS transvaginal ultrasonography
TW talked with
  tapwater
  test weight
  thought withdrawal
  Trophermyma whippleii
  T-wave
T1WI T1 weighted image (magnetic resonance imaging term for short repetition time and short echo time)
T2WI T2 weighted image (magnetic resonance imaging term for long repetition time and long echo time)
TW2 Tanner-Whitehouse mark 2 (bone-age assessment)
5TW five times a week (this is a dangerous abbreviation)
TWA time-weighted average
  total wrist arthroplasty
  T-wave alternans
TWAR *Chlamydia pneumoniae*
T-wave part of the electrocardiographic cycle, representing a portion of ventricular repolarization
TWB total weight bearing
TWD total white and differential count
TWE tapwater enema
TWETC tapwater enema 'til clear
TWG total weight gain
TWH transitional wall hyperplasia
TWHW ok toe walking and heel walking all right
TWI tooth-wear index
  T-wave inversion
TWiST time without symptoms of progression or toxicity
TWOC trial without catheter
TWP twin pregnancy
TWR total wrist replacement
TWSTRS Toronto Western Spasmodic Torticollis Rating Scale
TWT timed walking test
TWWD tap water wet dressing
Tx therapist
  therapy
  traction
  transcription
  transfuse
  transplant
  transplantation
  treatment
  tympanostomy
T & X type and crossmatch
TXA$_2$ thromboxane A$_2$
TXB$_2$ thromboxane B$_2$
TXE Timoptic-XE®
TXL paclitaxel (Taxol) (this is a dangerous abbreviation as it can be read as TXT)
TXM type and crossmatch
TXS type and screen
TXT docetaxel (Taxotere) (this is a dangerous abbreviation as it can be read as TXL)
TY tympanic
T & Y trichomonas and yeast
TYCO #3 Tylenol with 30 mg of codeine (#1=7.5 mg, #2=15 mg and #4=60 mg of codeine present)
Tyl Tylenol (acetaminophen)
  tyloma (callus)
TYMP tympanogram
TYR tyrosine
TZ temozolomide (Temodar)
  transition zone
TZCS time-zone change syndrome
TZD thiazolidinedione
TZDs thiazolidinediones
TZM temozolomide (Temodar)

T

U

U	Ultralente Insulin®
	units (this is the most dan-gerous abbreviation—spell out "unit")
	unknown
	upper
	uranium
	urine
Ⓤ	Kosher
U/1	1 finger breadth below umbilicus
1/U	1 finger over umbilicus
U/	at umbilicus
24U	24-hour urine (collection)
U100	100 units per milliliters
UA	umbilical artery
	unauthorized absence
	uncertain about
	unstable angina
	upper airway
	upper arm
	uric acid
	urinalysis
UABD	upper airway bronchodilation
UAC	umbilical artery catheter
	under active
	upper airway congestion
UA/C	uric acid to creatinine (ratio)
UAD	upper airway disease
	use as directed
UADT	upper aerodigestive tract
UAE	urinary albumin excretion
	uterine artery embolization
UACEs	unplanned acute care encounters
UAER	urinary albumin excretion rate
UAL	umbilical artery line
	up *ad lib*
UA&M	urinalysis and microscopy
UA/ NSTEMI	unstable angina and non- ST-segment elevation myocardial infarction
UAO	upper airway obstruction
UAP	upper abdominal pain
UAPD	Union of American Physicians and Dentists
UAPF	upon arrival patient found
UAPs	unlicensed assistive personnel
U-ARM	upper arm
UARS	upper airway resistance syndrome
UAS	upstream activating sequence
UASA	upper airway sleep apnea
UASQ	Unstable Angina Symptoms Questionnaire
UAT	up as tolerated
UAVC	univentricular atrioventricular connection

UBAs	urethral bulking agents
UBC	University of British Columbia (brace)
UBD	universal blood donor
UBE	upper body ergometer
UBF	unknown black female
	uterine blood flow
UBI	ultraviolet blood irradiation
UBM	unknown black male
UBO	unidentified bright object
UBT	^{13}C-urea breath test
	uterine balloon therapy
UBW	usual body weight
UC	ulcerative colitis
	umbilical cord
	unchanged
	unconscious
	Unit clerk
	United Church of Christ
	urea clearance
	urinary catheter
	urine culture
	usual care
	uterine contraction
U&C	urethral and cervical
	usual and customary
UCABG	urgent coronary artery bypass graft (surgery)
UCAD	unstable coronary artery disease
UCB	umbilical cord blood
	unconjugated bilirubin (indirect)
	Unicorn Campbell Boy (orthotics)
UCBT	unrelated cord-blood transplant
UCCL	ulnocarpal collateral ligament
UCD	urine collection device
	usual childhood diseases
UCE	urea cycle enzymopathy
UCF	unexplained chronic fatigue
UCG	urinary chorionic gonadotropins
UCHD	usual childhood diseases
UCHI	usual childhood illnesses
UCHS	uncontrolled hemorrhagic shock
UCI	urethral catheter in
	usual childhood illnesses
UCL	ulnar collateral ligament
	uncomfortable loudness level
UCLP	unilateral cleft lip and palate
UCN	urocortin
UCN-01	7-hydroxystaurosporin
UCO	urethral catheter out
UCP	umbilical cord prolapse
	uncoupling protein
	urethral closure pressure
UCPs	urine collection pads
UCR	unconditioned reflex
	unconditioned response
	usual, customary, and reasonable (fees)

UCP-3	uncoupling protein −3		UGA	under general anesthesia
UCRE	urine creatinine			urogenital atrophy
UCRP	universal coagulation reference plasma		UGB	upper-gastrointestinal-tract bleeding
			UGCR	ultrasound-guided compression repair
UCS	unconscious		UGDP	University Group Diabetes Project
UC&S	urine culture and sensitivity		UGH	uveitis, glaucoma, and hyphema (syndrome)
UCTD	undifferentiated connective tissue disease			
			UGI	upper gastrointestinal series
UCVA	uncorrected visual acuity		UGIB	upper gastrointestinal bleeding
UCX	urine culture		UGIH	upper gastrointestinal hemorrhage
UD	as directed		UGIS	upper gastrointestinal series
	ulnar deviation		UGIT	upper gastrointestinal tract
	unit dose		UGI	upper gastrointestinal
	urethral dilatation		w/SBFT	(series) with small bowel follow through
	urethral discharge			
	urodynamics		UGK	urine, glucose, and ketones
	uterine distension		UGP	urinary gonadotropin peptide
u.d.	as directed		UGTI	ultrasound-guided thrombin injection
UDC	uninhibited detrusor (muscle) capacity		UGVA	ultrasound-guided vascular access
			UH	umbilical hernia
	usual diseases of childhood			unfavorable history
UDCA	ursodeoxycholic acid (Ursodiol)			University Hospital
UDN	updraft nebulizer		UHBI	upper hemibody irradiation
UDO	undetermined origin		UHDDS	Uniform Hospital Discharge Data Set
UDP	unassisted diastolic pressure			
UDPGT	uridinediphospho-glucuronyl transferase		UHDRS	Unified Huntington Disease Rating Scale
UDS	unconditioned stimulus		UHDs	ulcer-healing drugs
	urine drug screen		UHMWPE	ultra-high molecular weight polyethylene
UDT	undescended testicle(s)			
UE	under elbow		UHP	University Health Plan
	undetermined etiology		UI	urinary incontinence
	upper extremity		UIB	Unemployment Insurance Benefits
U & E	urea and electrolytes (see page 298)		UIBC	unbound iron binding capacity
UEBW	ultrasound estimated bladder weight			unsaturated iron binding capacity
UEC	uterine endometrial carcinoma		UID	once daily (this is a dangerous abbreviation, spell out "once daily")
UEDs	unilateral epileptiform discharges			
UES	undifferentiated embryonal sarcoma			
	upper esophageal sphincter		UIEP	urine (urinary) immunoelectrophoresis
UESEP	upper extremity somatosensory evoked potential			
			UIP	usual interstitial pneumonitis (pneumonia)
UESP	upper esophageal sphincter pressure			
UF	ultrafiltration		UIQ	upper inner quadrant
	until finished		UITN	Urinary Incontinence Treatment Network
UFC	urinary free cortisol			
UFF	unusual facial features		UJ	universal joint (syndrome)
UFFI	urea formaldehyde foam insulation		UK	United Kingdom
UFH	unfractionated heparin			unknown
UFN	until further notice			urine potassium
UFO	unflagged order			urokinase
	unidentified foreign object		UK IC	urokinase intracoronary
UFOV	useful field of view		UKE	unknown etiology
UFR	ultrafiltration rate		UKNDS	United Kingdom Neurological Disability Score
UFT	uracil and tegafur			
UFV	ultrafiltration volume		UKO	unknown origin
UG	until gone		UL	Unit Leader
	urinary glucose			upper left
	urogenital			

	upper lid
	upper limb
	upper lobe
U/L	upper and lower
U & L	upper and lower
ULBW	ultra low birth weight (between 501 and 750 g)
ULDT	ultra low-dose therapy
ULL	ulnolunate ligament
ULLE	upper lid, left eye
ULN	upper limits of normal
ULPA	ultra-low particulate air
ULQ	upper left quadrant
ULRE	upper lid, right eye
ULSB	upper left sternal border
ULTT1	upper limb tension test 1 (median nerve)
ULTT2a	upper limb tension test 2a (medial nerve)
ULTT2b	upper limb tension test 2b (radial nerve)
ULTT3	upper limb tension test 3 (ulnar nerve)
ULYTES	electrolytes, urine
UM	unmarried
	utilization management
Umb A Line	umbilical artery line
Umb V Line	umbilical venous line
umb ven	umbilical vein
UMCD	uremic medullary cystic disease
UMLS	Unified Medical Language System
UMN	upper motor neuron (disease)
UN	undernourished
	urinary nitrogen
UNA	urinary nitrogen appearance
UNa	urine sodium
unacc	unaccompanied
UNC	uncrossed
UNDEL	undelivered
UNDP	United Nations Development Program
UNE	ulnar neuropathy at the elbow
	urinary norepinephrine
UNG	ointment
UNHS	universal newborn hearing screening
UNK	unknown
UNL	upper normal levels
UNOS	United Network for Organ Sharing
UN/P	unpatched eye
UN/P OD	unpatched right eye
UN/P OS	unpatched left eye
UNS	universal neonatal screening
	unsatisfactory
UNSAT	unsatisfactory
uNTx	urinary N-telopeptide
UO	under observation

	undetermined origin
	ureteral orifice
	urinary output
UONx	unilateral optic nerve transection
UOP	urinary output
UOQ	upper outer quadrant
UORBC	uncrossmatched type-O packed red blood cells
UOS	upper oesophageal sphincter (United Kingdom and other countries)
Uosm	urinary osmolality
✓ up	check up
UP	unipolar
	ureteropelvic
U/P	urine to plasma (creatinine)
UPC	unknown primary carcinoma
UPD	uniparental disomy
UPDRS	Unified Parkinson Disease Rating Scale
UPEP	urine protein electrophoresis
UPG	uroporphyrinogen
UPIN	unique physician (provided) identification number
UPJ	ureteropelvic junction
UPJO	ureteropelvic junction obstruction
UPLIF	unilateral posterior lumbar interbody fusion
UPN	unique patient number
UPO	metastatic carcinoma of unknown primary origin
UPOR	usual place of residence
UPP	urethral pressure profile
	urethral pressure profilometry
	uvulopalatoplasty
UPPP	uvulopalatopharyngoplasty
U/P ratio	urine to plasma ratio
UPS	ubiquitin-dependent proteasomal system
	ubiquitin-proteasome system
UPSC	uterine papillary serous carcinoma
UPSIT	University of Pennsylvania Smell Identification Test
UPT	uptake
	urine pregnancy test
UR	unrelated
	upper respiratory
	upper right
	urinary retention
	utilization review
URA	unilateral renal agenesis
URAC	Utilization Review Accreditation Commission
UR AC	uric acid
URAS	unilateral renal artery stenosis
URD	undifferentiated respiratory disease
	unrelated donor
URE	Uniform Rules of Evidence
URG	urgent

URI	upper respiratory infection	USO	unilateral salpingo-oophorectomy
URIC A	uric acid	USOGH	usual state of good health
url	unrelated	USOH	usual state of health
UR&M	urinalysis, routine and microscopic	USP	unassisted systolic pressure
URO	urology		United States Pharmacopeia
UROB	urobilinogen	USPHS	United States Public Health Service
UROD	ultra-rapid opiate detoxification	USS	Upshaw-Schulman syndrome
	[under anesthesia]	USUCVD	unsterile uncontrolled vaginal
UROL	Urologist		delivery
	urology	USVMD	urine specimen volume measuring
URQ	upper right quadrant		device
URR	urea reduction ratio	UT	upper thoracic
URS	ureterorenoscopy	UTA	urinary tract anomaly
URSB	upper right sternal border	UTC	urinary tract calculi
URT	upper respiratory tract	UtCa	uterine cancer
	uterine resting tone	UTD	unable to determine
URTI	upper respiratory tract infection		up to date
US	ultrasonography	*ut dict*	as directed
	ultrasound	UTF	usual throat flora
	unit secretary	UTI	urinary tract infection
	United States of America	UTL	ulnotriquetral ligament
USA	unit services assistant		unable to locate
	United States Army		useful therapeutic life
	United States of America	UTM	urinary-tract malformations
	unstable angina	UTMDACC	University of Texas M.D. Anderson
USAF	United States Air Force		Cancer Center
USAMRIID	United States Army Medical	UTO	unable to obtain
	Research Institute of Infectious		upper tibial osteotomy
	Diseases	UTP	uridine triphosphate
USAN	United States Adopted Names	UTR	untranslated region
USAP	unstable angina pectoris	UTS	ulnar tunnel syndrome
USB	upper sternal border		ultrasound
USC	uterine serous carcinoma	U/U−	uterine fundus at umbilicus (usually
U-SCOPE	ureteroscopy		modified as number of finger
USCVD	unsterile controlled vaginal delivery		breadths below)
USDA	United States Department of	U/U+	uterine fundus at umbilicus (usually
	Agriculture		modified as number of finger
USED-	ureterosigmoidostomy,		breadths above)
CARP	small bowel fistula, extra chloride,	UUD	uncontrolled unsterile delivery
	diarrhea, carbonic anhydrase	UUI	urge urinary incontinence
	inhibitors, adrenal insufficiency,	UUN	urinary urea nitrogen
	renal tubular acidosis, and	UUTI	uncomplicated urinary tract
	pancreatic fistula (common causes		infections
	of nonanion gap metabolic	UV	ultraviolet
	acidosis)		umbilical vein
USEIR	United States Eye Injury Registry		ureterovesical
USG	ultrasmall gold (particles)		urine volume
	ultrasonography	UVA	ultraviolet A light
	urine specific gravity		ureterovesical angle
USH	United Services for Handicapped	UVB	ultraviolet B light
	usual state of health	UVBI	ultraviolet blood irradiation
USI	urinary stress incontinence	UVC	umbilical vein catheter
USM	ultrasonic mist		ultraviolet C light
USMC	United States Marine Corps	UVEB	unifocal ventricular ectopic beat
USMLE	United States Medical Licensing	UVGI	ultraviolet germicidal irradiation
	Examination	UVH	univentricular heart
USN	ultrasonic nebulizer	UVIB	ultraviolet irradiation of blood
	United States Navy	UVJ	ureterovesical junction

U

UVL	ultraviolet light
	umbilical venous line
UVR	ultraviolet radiation
UVT	unsustained ventricular tachycardia
UV-VIS	ultraviolet-visible (spectrometer)
U/WB	unit of whole blood
UW	unilateral weakness
UWF	unknown white female
UWM	unknown white male
	unwed mother
UXO	unexploded ordnance

U

V	five
	gas volume
	minute volume
	vaccinated
	vagina
	vein
	ventricular
	verb
	verbal
	vertebral
	very
	Viagra (sildenafil citrate) as in "vitamin V"
	viral
	vision
	vitamin
	vomiting
$\dot{V}$	ventilation (L/min)
+V	positive vertical divergence
V1	fifth cranial nerve, ophthalmic division
V2	fifth cranial nerve, maxillary division
V3	fifth cranial nerve, mandibular division
3V	3-vessel (cord)
V_1 to V_6	precordial chest leads
VA	vacuum aspiration
	valproic acid
	ventriculoatrial
	vertebral artery
	Veterans Administration
	visual acuity
V_A	alveolar gas volume
V&A	vagotomy and antrectomy
VAAESS	Vaccine-Associated Adverse Events Surveillance System (Canada)
VAB	variable atrial blockage
	vinblastine, dactinomycin (actinomycin D), bleomycin
VABS	Vineland Adaptive Behavior Scales
VAC	vacuum-assisted closure (dressings)
	ventriculoarterial conduction
	vincristine, dactinomycin (actinomycin D), and cyclophosphamide
	vincristine, doxorubicin (Adriamycin), and cyclophosphamide
VA cc	distance visual acuity with correction
VA ccl	near visual acuity with correction
VACE	*Vitex agnus-castus* extract (Chaste tree berry extract)
VAC EXT	vacuum extractor
VAC_{ig}	vaccinia immune globulin

VACIME	vincristine, doxorubicin (Adriamycin), cyclophosphamide, ifosfamide, mesna, and etoposide	VARig	varicella-zoster immune globulin
VACO	Veterans Administration Central Office	VAS	vasectomy vascular Visual Analogue Scale (Score)
VACTERL	vertebral, anal, cardiac, tracheal, esophageal, renal, and limb anomalies	VASC	Visual-Auditory Screen Test for Children
		VA sc	distance visual acuity without correction
VAD	vascular (venous) access device ventricular assist device vertebral artery dissection	VA scl	near visual acuity without correction
		VASPI	Visual Analogue Self Assessment Scales For Pain Intensity
	Veterans Administration Domiciliary vincristine, doxorubicin (Adriamycin), and dexamethasone	VAS RAD	vascular radiology
		VAT	ventilatory anaerobic threshold vertebral artery test video-assist thoracoscopy visceral adipose tissue
VaD	vascular dementia		
VADCS	ventricular atrial distal coronary sinus		
		VATER	vertebral, anal, tracheal, esophageal, and renal anomalies
VADRIAC	vincristine, doxorubicin (Adriamycin), and cyclophosphamide	VATH	vinblastine, doxorubicin (Adriamycin), thiotepa, and fluoxymesterone (Halotestin)
VAE	venous air embolism		
VAERS	Vaccine Adverse Events Reporting System	VATS	video assisted thoracic surgery
		VAVD	vacuum-assisted venous drainage
VAFD	vascular access flush device	VAX-D	vertebral axial decompression
VAG	vagina	VB	Van Buren (catheter) venous blood vinblastine (Velban) vinblastine and bleomycin virtual bronchoscopy
VAG HYST	vaginal hysterectomy		
VAH	Veterans Administration Hospital		
VAHBE	ventricular atrial His bundle electrocardiogram		
VAHRA	ventricular atrial height right atrium	VB_1	first voided bladder specimen
VAHS	virus-associated hemophagocytic syndrome	VB_2	second midstream bladder specimen
		VB_3	third voided urine specimen
VAI	vertebral artery injury	VBAC	vaginal birth after cesarean
VAIN	vaginal intraepithelial neoplasia	VBAI	vertebrobasilar artery insufficiency
VALE	visual acuity, left eye	VBAP	vincristine, carmustine (BiCNU), doxorubicin (Adriamycin), and prednisone
VALI	ventilator-associated lung injury		
VAMC	Veterans Affairs Medical Center		
VAMP®	venous-arterial management protection system	VBC	vinblastine, bleomycin, and cisplatin
		VBG	venous blood gas vertical banded gastroplasty
VAMS	Visual Analogue Mood Scale		
VANCO/P	vancomycin-peak	VBGP	vertical banded gastroplasty
VANCO/T	vancomycin-trough	VBI	vertebrobasilar insufficiency
VAOD	visual acuity, right eye	VBL	vinblastine (Velban)
VAOS	visual acuity, left eye	VBM	vinblastine, bleomycin, and methotrexate voxel-based morphometry
VA OS LP with P	visual acuity, left eye, left perception with projection		
VAP	venous access port ventilator-associated pneumonia vincristine, asparaginase, and prednisone	VBP	vinblastine, bleomycin, and cisplatin
		VBR	ventricular brain ratio
		VBS	vertebral-basilar system videofluoroscopic barium swallow (evaluation)
VAPCS	ventricular atrial proximal coronary sinus		
		VC	color vision etoposide (VePesid) and carboplatin pulmonary capillary blood volume vena cava verbal cues vincristine (Oncovin) virtual colonoscopy
VAPP	vaccine-associated paralytic poliomyelitis		
VAR	variant varicella (chickenpox) (*varicella zoster* virus) vaccine		
VARE	visual acuity, right eye		

	vital capacity
	vocal cords
	voluntary cough
Vc	bortezomib (Velcade)
3VC	3-vessel cord
V&C	vertical and centric (a bite)
VCA	vasoconstrictor assay
VCAM	vascular cell adhesion molecule
VCAP	vincristine, cyclophosphamide, doxorubicin (Adriamycin), and prednisone
Vcc	vision with correction
VCCA	velocity common carotid artery
VCD	vocal cord dysfunction
VCDR	vertical cup-to-disc ratio
VCE	vaginal cervical endocervical (smear)
VCF	Vaginal Contraception Film™
VCFS	velo-cardio-facial syndrome
VCG	vectorcardiography
	voiding cystogram
vCJD	variant Creutzfeldt-Jakob disease
VCO	ventilator CPAP oxyhood
Vco_2	carbon dioxide output
VCP	vocal cord palsy
VCPR	veterinarian-client-patient relationship
VCR	video cassette recorder
	vincristine sulfate (Oncovin)
VCT	venous clotting time
	voluntary counselling and testing
VCTS	vitreal corneal touch syndrome
VCU	voiding cystourethrogram
VCUG	vesicoureterogram
	voiding cystourethrogram
VCV	varicella virus
	volume-control ventilation
VD	vaginal delivery
	venereal disease
	vessel disease
	viral diarrhea
	voided
	voiding diary
	volume of distribution
V_D	deadspace volume
V_d	volume of distribution
V&D	vomiting and diarrhea
1-VD	one-vessel disease
VDA	venous digital angiogram
	visual discriminatory acuity
VDAC	vaginal delivery after cesarean
VDC	vincristine, doxorubicin, and cyclophosphamide
VDD	atrial synchronous ventricular inhibited pacing
VDDR I	vitamin D dependency rickets type I
VDDR II	vitamin D dependency rickets type II
VDE	vasodilatory edema
VDEPT	virus-directed enzyme prodrug therapy
VDG	venereal disease–gonorrhea
Vdg	voiding
VDH	valvular disease of the heart
VDJ	variable diversity joining
VDL	vasodepressor lipid
	visual detection level
VDO	varus derotational osteotomy
VD or M	venous distention or masses
VDP	vinblastine, dacarbazine, and cisplatin (Platinol)
VDPCA	variable-dose patient-controlled analgesia
VDR	vitamin D receptor (gene)
VDRF	ventilator dependent respiratory failure
VDRL	Venereal Disease Research Laboratory (test for syphilis)
VDRO	varus derotational osteotomy
VDRR	vitamin D-resistant rickets
VDRS	Verdun Depression Rating Scale
VDS	vasodepressor syncope
	venereal disease—syphilis
	vindesine (Eldisine)
VDT	vibration detection threshold
	video display terminal
	visual display terminal
VD/VT	dead space to tidal volume ratio
VE	vaginal examination
	vertex
	Vietnam era
	virtual endoscopy
	visual examination
	vitamin E
	vocational evaluation
V_E	minute volume (expired)
V/E	violence and eloper
VEA	ventricular ectopic activity
	viscoelastic agent
VEB	ventricular ectopic beat
VEC	vecuronium (Norcuron)
	velocity-encoded cine
VECG	vector electrocardiogram
VED	vacuum erection device
	vacuum extraction delivery
	ventricular ectopic depolarization
	vitamin E deficiency
VEE	Venezuelan equine encephalitis
VEE_a	Venezuelan equine encephalitis vaccine, attenuated live
VEE_I	Venezuelan equine encephalitis vaccine, inactivated
VEF	visually evoked field
VEG	vegetation (bacterial)
VEGF	vascular endothelial growth factor
VeIP	vinblastine (Velban), ifosfamide, and cisplatin (Platinol)
VEMP	vestibular evoked myogenic potentials

VENC	velocity encoding value (radiology)	VGKC	voltage-gated potassium channel
VENT	ventilation	VGM	vein graft myringoplasty
	ventilator	VGPO	volume-guaranteed pressure option
	ventral	VH	vaginal hysterectomy
	ventricular		Veterans Hospital
VEP	visual evoked potential		viral hepatitis
VER	ventricular escape rhythm		visual hallucinations
	visual evoked responses		vitreous hemorrhage
VERDICT	Veterans Evidence-based Research Dissemination Implementation Center		von Herrick (grading system)
		VH I	very narrow anterior chamber angles
		VH II	moderately narrow anterior chamber angles
VERP	ventricular effective refractory period	VH III	moderately wide open anterior chamber angles
VERT	velocity-enhanced resistance training		
VES	ventricular extrasystoles	VH IV	wide open anterior chamber angles
	video-endoscopic surgery	VHC	valved-holding chamber
	vitamin E succinate	VHD	valvular heart disease
VESS	video endoscopic swallowing study		vascular hemostatis device
VET	veteran	VHF	viral hemorrhagic fever
	Veterinarian	VHI	Voice Handicap Index
	veterinary	VHL	von Hippel-Lindau disease (complex)
VF	left leg (electrode)		
	ventricular fibrillation	VHP	vaporized hydrogen peroxide
	vertical float (aquatic therapy)	VI	six
	visual field		velocity index
	vocal fremitus		volume index
VFC	Vaccines for Children (program)	via	by way of
VFCB	vertical flow clean bench	vib	vibration
VFD	ventilator-free days	VIBS	Victim's Information Bureau Service
	visual fields	VICA	velocity internal carotid artery
VFFC	visual fields full to confrontation	VICP	Vaccine Injury Compensation Program
VFI	visual fields intact		
	Visual Functioning index	Vi CPs	typhoid Vi (capsular) polysaccharide vaccine (Typhim Vi)
V. Fib	ventricular fibrillation		
VFL	vinflunine	VID	videodensitometry
VFMI	vocal fold motion impairment	VIG	vaccinia immune globulin
VFP	vertical float progression (aquatic therapy)		vinblastine, ifosfamide, and gallium nitrate
	vitreous fluorophotometry		
	vocal fold paralysis	VIH	human immunodeficiency virus (Spanish and French abbreviation)
VFPN	Volu-feed premie nipple		
VFR	visiting friends and relatives (possible contacts for communicable diseases)	VIN	vibration-induced nystagmus
			vulvar intraepithelial neoplasm
		VIP	etopside (VePesid), ifosfamide, and cisplatin (Platinol)
VFRN	Volu-feed regular nipple		
VFSS	videofluoroscopic swallowing study		vasoactive intestinal peptide
VFT	venous filling time		vasoactive intracorporeal pharmacotherapy
	ventricular fibrillation threshold		
VG	vein graft		Vattikuti Institute prostatectomy
	ventricular gallop		very important patient
	ventrogluteal		vinblastine, ifosfamide, and cisplatin (Platinol)
	very good		
V&G	vagotomy and gastroenterotomy		voluntary interruption of pregnancy
VGAD	vein of Galen aneurysmal dilatation	VIPomas	vasoactive intestinal peptide-secreting tumors
VGAM	vein of Galen aneurysmal malformation		
		VIQ	Verbal Intelligence Quotient (part of Wechsler tests)
VGB	vigabatrin (Sabril)		
VGE	viral gastroenteritis	VIS	Vaccine Information Statement
VGH	very good health		Visual Impairment Service

VISA	vancomycin-intermediate-resistant *Staphylococcus aureus*		vertical maxillary deficiency
VISC	vitreous infusion suction cutter	VME	vertical maxillary excess
VISI	Vaccine Identification Standards Initiative	VMH	ventromedial hypothalamus
		VMI	vendor-managed inventory
	volar intercalated segmental instability		visual motor integration
		VMO	vaccinia melanoma oncolysate
VISN	Veterans Integrated Service Networks		vastus medialis oblique
		VMR	vasomotor rhinitis
VISs	Vaccine Information Statements	VMS	vanilla milkshake
VIT	venom immunotherapy	VMU	vertebral motion unit
	vital	VN	visiting nurse
	vitamin	VNA	Visiting Nurses' Association
	vitreous	VNB	vinorelbine (Navelbine)
Vitamin	see individual letters such as R, V, etc.	VNC	vesicle neck contracture
		VNS	vagal nerve stimulation
VIT CAP	vital capacity	VNTR	variable number of tandem repeats
VIU	visual internal urethrotomy	VO	verbal order
VIZ	namely		visual observation
V-J	ventriculo-jugular (shunt)	VO$_2$	oxygen consumption
VKA	vitamin K antagonists	VOC	vaso-occlusive crisis
VKC	vernal keratoconjunctivitis	VOCA	voice-output communication aid
VKDB	vitamin K deficiency bleeding	VOCAB	vocabulary
VKH	Vogt-Koyanagi-Harada disease	VOCOR	vaso-occlusive crisis
VL	left arm (electrode)		void on-call to operating room
	vial	VOCs	volatile organic compounds
	viral load	VOCTOR	void on-call to operating room
	visceral leishmaniasis (kala-azar)	VOD	veno-occlusive disease
VLA	very-late antigen		vision right eye
VLAD	variable life-adjusted display	VOE	vascular occlusive episode
VLAP	vaporization laser ablation of the prostate	VO$_2$I	oxygen consumption index
		VOL	Valuation of Life
VLBW	very low birth weight (less than 1500 g)		volume
			voluntary
VLBWPN	very low birth weight preterm neonate	VOM	vomited
VLCAD	very-long-chain acyl coenzyme A dehydrogenase	VOO	continuous ventricular asynchronous pacing
VLCD	very low calorie diet	VOOD	vesico-outlet obstructive disease
VLCFA	very-long-chain fatty acids	VOR	vestibular ocular reflex
VLDL	very-low-density lipoprotein	VORB	verbal order read back
VLE	vision left eye	VOS	vision left eye
VLH	ventrolateral nucleus of the hypothalamus	VOSS	visual observation shivering score
		VOT	Visual Organization Test
VLM	visceral larva migrans	VOU	vision both eyes
VLP	virus-like particle	VOV	verbal order verified
VLPP	Valsalva lead-point pressure	VP	etoposide (VePesid) and cisplatin (Platinol)
VLR	vastus lateralis release		
VM	venous malformation		vagal paraganglioma
	ventilated mask		variegate porphyria
	ventimask		venipuncture
	Venturi mask		venous pressure
	vestibular membrane		ventriculoperitoneal
VM 26	teniposide (Vumon)		visual perception
VMA	vanillylmandelic acid		voiding pressure
VMATs	Veterinary Medical Assistance Teams	V & P	vagotomy and pyloroplasty
VMCP	vincristine, melphalan, cyclophosphamide, and prednisone		ventilation and perfusion
		VP-16	etoposide
VMD	Doctor of Veterinary Medicine (DVM)	VPA	valproic acid
			ventricular premature activation

	vigorous physical activity
V-Pad	sanitary napkin
VPB	ventricular premature beat
VPC	ventricular premature contractions
VPD	ventricular premature depolarization
VPDC	ventricular premature depolarization contraction
VPDF	vegetable protein diet plus fiber
VPDs	ventricular premature depolarizations
VPI	velopharyngeal incompetence
	velopharyngeal insufficiency
VPL	ventro-posterolateral
VPLN	vaccine-primed lymph node (cells)
VPLS	ventilation-perfusion lung scan
VPM	venous pressure module
VPR	virtual patient record
	volume pressure response
VPS	valvular pulmonic stenosis
	ventriculoperitoneal shunt
VPT	vascularized patellar tendon
	vibration perception threshold
VQ	ventilation perfusion
VR	right arm (electrode) valve replacement
	venous resistance
	ventricular rhythm
	verbal reprimand
	vocational rehabilitation
$V_3R \cdots V_6R$	right sided precordial leads
VRA	visual reinforcement audiometry
	visual response audiometry
VRB	vinorelbine (Navelbine)
VRC	vocational rehabilitation counselor
VRE	vancomycin-resistant enterococci
	vision right eye
VREF	vancomycin-resistant *Enterococcus faecium*
VRI	viral respiratory infection
VRL	ventral root, lumbar
	vinorelbine (Navelbine)
VRP	vocational rehabilitation program
VRS	viral rhinosinusitis
VRSA	vancomycin-resistant *Staphylococcus aureus*
VRT	variance of resident time
	ventral root, thoracic
	vertical radiation topography
	Visual Retention Test
	vocational rehabilitation therapy
VRTA	Vocational Rehabilitation Therapy Assistant
VRU	ventilator rehabilitation unit
VS	vagal stimulation
	vegetative state
	versus (*vs*)
	very sensitive
	visit
	visited

	vital signs (temperature, pulse, and respiration)
VSA	variant surface antigens
VSADP	vocational skills assessment and development program
VSBE	very short below elbow (cast)
VSCC	vertical semicircular canal
VSD	ventricular septal defect
	vesicosphincter dyssynergia
VSGP	vertical supranuclear gaze palsy
VSI	visual motor integration
VSLI	vincristine sulfate liposomal injection
VSMC	vascular smooth muscle cell
VSN	visuospatial neglect
	vital signs normal
VSO	vertical subcondylar oblique
VSOK	vital signs normal
VSP	vertical stabilization program
VSQOL	Vital Signs Quality of Life
VSR	venous stasis retinopathy
	ventricular septal rupture
VSS	variable spot scanning
	visual sexual stimulation
	vital signs stable
V_{SS}	apparent volume of distribution
VSSAF	vital signs stable, afebrile
VST	visual search task
VSTM	visual short-term memory
VSULA	vaccination scar, upper left arm
VSV	vesicular stomatitis virus
VT	validation therapy
	ventricular tachycardia
V_t	tidal volume
VTA	vascular targeting agents
	ventral tegmentum area
VTBI	volume to be infused
v. tach.	ventricular tachycardia
VTE	venous thromboembolic events
	venous thromboembolism
VTEC	verotoxin-producing *Escherichia coli*
VTED	venous thromboembolic disease
VT-NS	ventricular tachycardia nonsu stained
VTOP	voluntary termination of pregnancy
VTP	voluntary termination of pregnancy
VTS	Volunteer Transport Service
VT-S	ventricular tachycardia sustained
VTSRS	Verdun Target Symptom Rating Scale
VT/VF	ventricular tachycardia/fibrillation
VTX	vertex
VU	venous ulcer
	vesicoureteral (reflux)
V/U	verbalize understanding
VUC	voided-urine cytology
VUD-BMT	volunteer unrelated-donor bone marrow transplantation

V

VUJ	vesico ureteral junction
VUR	vesicoureteric reflux
VV	vaccina virus
	varicose veins
	vulvar vestibulitis
V-V	ventriculovenous (shunt)
V&V	vulva and vagina
V/V	volume to volume ratio
VVB	venovenous bypass
VVC	vulvovaginal candidiasis
VVD	vaginal vertex delivery
VVETP	Vietnam Veterans Evaluation and Treatment Program
VVFR	vesicovaginal fistula repair
VVI	venous valvular insufficiency
V/VI	grade 5 on a 6 grade basis
VVI	ventricular demand pacing
VVI-40	ventricular backup pacing at 40/minute
VVIR	ventricular demand inhibited pacemaker (V = chamber paced-ventricle, V = chamber sensed-ventricle, I = response to sensing-inhibited, R = programmability–rate modulation)
VVL	varicose veins ligation
	verruca vulgaris of the larynx
VVOR	visual-vestibulo-ocular-reflex
VVR	ventricular response rate
VVS	vasovagal syncope
	vulvar vestibulitis syndrome
VVs	varicose veins
VVT	ventricular synchronous pacing
VW	vessel wall
VWD	ventral wall defect
vWD	von Willebrand disease
VWF	vibration-induced white finger (syndrome)
vWF	von Willebrand factor
VWM	ventricular wall motion
V_x	vaccination
	vitrectomy
V-XT	V-pattern exotropia
VY	surgical replacement flap
VZ	varicella zoster
VZIG	varicella zoster immune globulin
VZV	varicella zoster virus

W

W	wash
	watts
	wearing glasses
	Wednesday
	week
	weight
	well
	West (as in the location e.g. 2W, is second floor, West wing)
	white
	widowed
	wife
	with
	work
W-1	insignificant (allergies)
W-3	minimal (allergies)
W-5	moderate (allergies)
W-7	moderate-severe (allergies)
W-9	severe (allergies)
W-10	Interagency Transfer Form
W 22	Central Institute for the Deaf 22 Word List
WA	when awake
	while awake
	White American
	wide awake
	with assistance
W-A	Wyeth-Ayerst Laboratories
W & A	weakness and atrophy
W or A	weakness or atrophy
WAC	wholesale acquisition cost
WACH	wedge adjustable cushioned heel
WADA	World Anti-Doping Agency
WAF	weakness, atrophy, and fasciculation
	white adult female
WAGR	Wilm tumor, aniridia, genitourinary malformations, and mental retardation (syndrome)
WAIS	Wechsler Adult Intelligence Scale
WAIS-R	Wechsler Adult Intelligence Scale-Revised
WAL	Wyeth-Ayerst Laboratories
WALK	weight-activated locking knee (prosthesis)
WAM	white adult male
WAP	wandering atrial pacemaker
WAPRT	whole-abdominopelvic radiation therapy
WARI	wheezing associated respiratory infection
WAS	whiplash-associated disorders
	Wiskott-Aldrich syndrome
WASI	Wechsler Abbreviated Scale of Intelligence

V

WASO	wakefulness after sleep onset	WCHE	well-child health examination
WASP	Wiskott-Aldrich syndrome protein	WC/LC	warm compresses and lid scrubs
WASS	Wasserman test	WCM	whole cow's milk
WAT	word association test	WCS	work capacity specialist
WAZ	weight-for-age Z scores	WCST	Wisconsin Card Sorting Test
WB	waist belt	WCT	wide-complex tachycardia
	weight bearing	WD	ward
	well baby		well developed
	Western blot		well differentiated
	whole blood		wet dressing
WBACT	whole-blood activated clotting time		Wilson disease
WBAT	weight bearing as tolerated		word
WBC	weight bearing with crutches		working distance
	well baby clinic		wound
	white blood cell (count)	W/D	warm and dry
WBCT	whole-blood clotting time		withdrawal
WBD	weeks by dates (for gestational age)	W → D	wet to dry
WBE	weeks by examination (for	W4D	Worth four-dot (test for fusion)
	gestational age)	WDCC	well-developed collateral circulation
	whole-body extract	WDF	white divorced female
WBGD	whole-body glucose disposal	WDHA	watery diarrhea, hypokalemia, and
WBH	weight-based heparin (dosing)		achlorhydria
	whole-body hyperthermia	WDHH	watery diarrhea, hypokalemia, and
WBI	whole-bowel irrigation		hypochlorhydria
W Bld	whole blood	WDL	within defined limits
WBN	wellborn nursery	WDLL	well-differentiated lymphocytic
WBNAA	whole-brain N-acetylaspartate		lymphoma
WBOS	wide base of support	WDM	white divorced male
WBPTT	whole-blood partial thromboplastin	WDP	within defined parameters
	time	WDR	weighed dietary records
WBQC	wide-base quad cane	WDS	word discrimination score
WBR	whole-body radiation	WDTC	well-differentiated thyroid cancer
WBRT	whole-brain radiotherapy	WDWG	well dressed, well groomed
WBS	weeks by size (for gestational age)	WDWN-	well-developed, well-
	whole body scan	AAF	nourished African-American
	Williams-Beuren syndrome		female
WBTF	Waring Blender tube feeding	WDWN-	well-developed,
WBTT	weight bearing to tolerance	BM	well-nourished black male
WBUS	weeks by ultrasound	WDWN-	well-developed,
WBV	whole blood volume	WF	well-nourished white female
WC	waist circumference	WDXRF	wavelength-dispersive x-ray
	ward clerk		fluorescence
	ward confinement	WE	weekend
	warm compress		wide excision
	wet compresses	W/E	weekend
	wheelchair	WEBINO	wall-eyed bilateral internuclear
	when called		ophthalmoplegia
	white count	WE-D	withdrawal-emergent dyskinesia
	whooping cough	WEE	Western equine encephalitis
	will call	WEMINO	wall-eyed monocular internuclear
	workers' compensation		ophthalmoplegia
WCA	work capacity assessment	WEP	weekend pass
WCB	Workers' Compensation Board	WESR	Westergren erythrocyte
WCC	well-child care		sedimentation rate
	white cell count		Wintrobe erythrocyte sedimentation
WCE	white coat effect		rate
	work capacity evaluation	WEUP	willful exposure to unwanted
WCH	white coat hypertension		pregnancy

W

WF	well flexed	WID	widow
	wet film		widower
	white female	WIED	walk-in emergency department
W/F	weakness and fatigue	WIP	work in progess
WFB	wooden foreign body	WIQ	Walking Impairment Questionnaire
WFE	Williams flexion exercises	WIS	Ward Incapacity Scale
W FEEDS	with feedings		Wister Institute
WFH	white-faced hornet	WISC	Wechsler Intelligence Scale for Children
WFI	water for injection		
WFL	within full limits	WISC-R	Wechsler Intelligence Scale for Children-Revised
	within functional limits		
WFLC	white female living child	WIT	water-induced thermotherapy
WFNS	World Federation of Neurosurgical Societies (grade or scale)	WK	week
			work
WF-O	will follow in office	WKI	Wakefield Inventory
WFR	wheel-and-flare reaction	WKS	Wernicke-Korsakoff Syndrome
WG	Wegener granulomatosis	WL	waiting list
WGA	wheat germ agglutinin		wave length
	whole genome amplification		weight loss
WGL	wire-guide localization	WLE	wide local excision
WH	walking heel (cast)	WLI	weight-length index
	well healed	WLM	working level months
	well hydrated	WLQ	Work Limitation Questionnaire
	work hardening (physical therapy)	WLS	weight-loss surgery
WHA	warmed humidified air		wet lung syndrome
WHAS	Women's Health Assessment Scale	WLST	withdrawal of life-sustaining therapy
WHI	Women's Health Initiative	WLT	waterload test
WHIM	Worts, Hypogammaglobulinamia, Infections, and Myelokathexis (syndrome)	WM	Waldenstrom macroglobulinemia
			wall motion
			warm, moist
WHIS	War Head-Injury Score		weight maintenance
WHNP	Women's Healthcare Nurse Practitioner		wet mount
			white male
WHNR	well-healed, no residuals		white matter
WHNS	well-healed, no sequelae		whole milk
	well-healed, nonsymptomatic		working memory
WHO	World Health Organization	WMA	wall motion abnormality
	wrist-hand orthosis	WMD	warm moist dressings (sterile)
WHOART	World Health Organization Adverse Reaction Terms (Terminology)		weapons of mass destruction
			weighted mean differences
WHOQOL-100	World Health Organization Quality of Life 100-Item (instrument)	WMF	white married female
		WMFT	Wolf Motor Function Test
		WMH	white matter hyperintensities
WHP	whirlpool	WMH-CIDI	World Mental Health Composite International Diagnostic Interview
WHPB	whirlpool bath		
WHR	ratio of waist to hip circumference	WMI	wall motion index
WHV	woodchuck hepatitis virus		weighted mean index
WHVP	wedged hepatic venous pressure	WML	white matter lesions (cerebral)
WH/WD	withholding/withdrawal (of life support)	WMLC	white male living child
		WMM	white married male
WHZ	wheezes	WMP	warm moist packs (unsterile)
WI	ventricular demand pacing		weight management program
	walk-in	WMS	Wechsler Memory Scale
W/I	within		Wilson-Mikity syndrome
W+I	work and interest	WMT	Word Memory Test
WIA	wounded in action	WMTS	wireless medical telemetry service
WIC	Women, Infants, and Children (program)	WMX	whirlpool, massage, and exercise
		WN	well nourished

W

WND	wound	WRARU	Walter Reed AFRIMS (Armed Forces Research Institute of Medical Sciences) Research Unit
WNE	West Nile encephalitis		
WNF	well-nourished female		
	West Nile fever	WRAT	Wide Range Achievement Test
WNL	within normal limits	WRAT-R	The Wide Range Achievement Test, Revised
WNL x 4	upper and lower extremities within normal limits		
		WRBC	washed red blood cells
WNLS	weighted nonlinear least squares	WRC	washed red (blood) cells
WNM	well-nourished male	WRF	worsening renal function
WNND	West Nile neuroinvasive disease	WRIOT	Wide Range Interest-Opinion Test (for career planning)
WNR	within normal range		
WNt^{50}	Wagner-Nelson time 50 hours	WRL	World Reference Laboratory for Foot-and-Mouth Disease (Institute for Animal Health, Survey, United Kingdom)
WNV	West Nile virus		
WO	weeks old		
	wide open		
	written order	WRN	Werner syndrome protein
W/O	water-in-oil	WRT	weekly radiation therapy
	without		with respect (regards) to
WOB	work of breathing	WRUED	work-related upper-extremity disorder
WOCF	worst observation carried forward		
WOCN	Wound, Ostomy and Continence Nurses (Society)-formerly known as the International Association for Enterostomal Therapy (IEAT)	WS	walking speed
			ward secretary
			watt seconds
			Werner syndrome
			West syndrome
WOMAC	Western Ontario and McMaster Universities Osteoarthritis Index		Williams syndrome
			work simplification
WOP	without pain		work simulation
W or A	weakness or atrophy		work status
WORD	Wechsler objective reading dimensions	W&S	wound and skin
		WSCP	Williams Syndrome Cognitive Profile
WORLD/ DLROW	a test used in mental status examinations (patient is asked to spell WORLD backwards)		
		WSEP	Williams syndrome, early puberty
		WSepF	white separated female
		WSepM	white separated male
WP	whirlpool	WSF	white single female
WPAI	Work Productivity and Activity Impairment (Questionnaire)	WSLP	Williams syndrome, late puberty
		WSM	white single male
WPBT	whirlpool, body temperature	WSO	white superficial onychomycosis
WPCs	washed packed cells	WSOC	water-soluble organic compounds
WPFM	Wright peak flow meter	WSP	wearable speech processor
WPOA	wearing patch on arrival	WSW	women who have sex with women
WPP	Wechsler Preschool and Primary Scale of Intelligence	WST	Wheelchair Skills Test
			Wheelchair Skills Training
WPPSI	Wechsler Preschool and Primary Scale of Intelligence	WSTP	Wheelchair Skills Training Program
		WT	wait times
WPPSI-R	WPPSI revised		walking tank
WPR	written progress report		walking training
WPS	Worker Protection Standard		weight (wt)
WPV	within-person variability		wild type
	workplace violence		Wilms tumor
WPW	Wolff-Parkinson-White (syndrome)		wisdom teeth
		0WT	zero work tolerance
WR	Wassermann reaction	W-T-D	wet to dry
	wrist	WTP	willingness to pay
WRA	with-the-rule astigmatism	WTS	whole tomography slice
WRAIR	Walter Reed Army Institute of Research	W/U	work-up
		WV	whispered voice
WRAMC	Walter Reed Army Medical Center		

W

W/V	weight-to-volume ratio
WW	watchful waiting
	Weight Watchers
	wheeled walker
WWI	World War One
WWII	World War Two
W/W	weight-to-weight ratio
W Ø W	wet-to-wet
WWAC	walk with aid of cane
WW Brd	whole wheat bread
WWidF	white widowed female
WWidM	white widowed male
WWTP	wastewater treatment plant
WWW	World Wide Web
WYOU	women years of usage

W

X

X	break
	capecitabine (Xeloda) (This is a dangerous abbreviation)
	cross
	crossmatch
	exophoria for distance
	Ecstasy (methylenedioxy-methamphetamine; MDMA)
	extra
	female sex chromosome
	start of anesthesia
	ten
	times
	xylocaine
$\bar{x}$	except
	mean
X'	exophoria at 33 cm
X^2	chi-square
X+#	xyphoid plus number of fingerbreadths
X3	orientation as to time, place and person
X-ALD	X-linked adrenoleukodystrophy
XBT	xylose breath test
XC	excretory cystogram
XCF	aortic cross clamp off
XCO	aortic cross clamp on
XD	times daily
	xanthoma dissemination
X&D	examination and diagnosis
X2d	times two days
XDP	xeroderma pigmentosum
XE	capecitabine (Xeloda)
Xe	xenon
^{133}Xe	xenon, isotope of mass 133
XeCl	xenon chloride
XeCT	xenon-enhanced computed tomography
X-ed	crossed
XELIRI	capecitabine (Xeloda) and irinotecan
XEM	xonics electron mammography
XES	x-ray energy spectrometer
XFER	transfer
XFS	exfoliation syndrome
XGP	xanthogranulomatous pyelonephritis
XI	eleven
XII	twelve
XIAP	X-linked inhibitor of apoptosis
XIP	x-ray in plaster
XKO	not knocked out
XL	extended release (once a day oral solid dosage form)
	extra large
	forty

XLA	X-linked infantile agammaglobulinemia		**Y**	
X-leg	cross leg			
XLFDP	cross-linked fibrin degradation products	Y	male sex chromosome	
XLH	X-linked hypophos-phatemia		year	
XLJR	X-linked juvenile retinoschisis		yellow	
XLMR	X-linked mental retardation	YAC	yeast artificial chromosome	
XLP	X-linked proliferative (syndrome)	YACs	yeast artificial chromosomes	
XLRS	X-linked retinoschisis	YACP	young adult chronic patient	
XM	crossmatch	YAG	yttrium aluminum garnet (laser)	
X-mat.	crossmatch	YAS	youth action section (police)	
XMG	mammogram	Yb	ytterbium	
XML	extensible markup language	YBOCS	Yale-Brown Obsessive-Compulsive Scale	
XMM	xeromammography			
XMR	magnetic resonance and X-rays	Yel	yellow	
XMT	cross matched	YEPQ	Yale Eating Patterns Questionnaire	
XNA	xenoreactive natural antibodies	YF	yellow fever	
XOM	extraocular movements	YFH	yellow-faced hornet	
XOP	x-ray out of plaster	YFI	yellow fever immunization	
XP	xeroderma pigmentosum	YFV	yellow-fever virus	
XR	x-ray	YHL	years of healthy life	
XRF	x-ray fluorescence	YJV	yellow jacket venom	
XRT	radiation therapy	Y2K	year 2,000	
XS	excessive	YLC	youngest living child	
X-SCID	X-linked severe combined immunodeficiency	YLD	years of life with disability	
		YLL	years of life lost	
XS-LIM	exceeds limits of procedure	YMC	young male Caucasian	
XT	exotropia	YMRS	Young Mania Rating Scale	
	extract	Y/N	yes/no	
	extracted	YO	years old	
X(T')	intermittent exotropia at 33 cm	YOB	year of birth	
X(T)	intermittent exotropia	YOD	year of death	
XTLE	extratemporal-lobe epilepsy	YORA	younger-onset rheumatoid arthritis	
XU	excretory urogram	YPC	YAG (yttrium aluminum garnet) posterior capsulotomy	
XULN	times upper limit of normal			
XV	fifteen	YPLL	years of potential life lost before age 65	
3X/WK	three times a week			
XX	normal female sex chromosome type twenty	yr	year	
		YRI	Yoruba from Ibadan, Nigeria (populations included in HapMap - see HapMap)	
XX/XY	sex karyotypes			
XXX	thirty			
XY	normal male sex chromosome type	YSC	yolk sac carcinoma	
XYL	xylose	YTD	year to date	
XYLO	lidocaine (Xylocaine)	YTDY	yesterday	

Z

Z	impedance
	pyrazinamide [part of tuberculosis regimen, see RHZ(E/S)/HR]
ZAL	zaleplon (Sonata)
ZAP	zoster-associated pain
ZDV	zidovudine (Retrovir)
Z-E	Zollinger-Ellison (syndrome)
ZEEP	zero end-expiratory pressure
ZES	Zollinger-Ellison syndrome
Z-ESR	zeta erythrocyte sedimentation rate
ZIFT	zygote intrafallopian (tube) transfer
ZIG	zoster serum immune globulin
ZIP	zoster immune plasma
ZMC	zygomatic
	zygomatic maxillary compound (complex)
Zn	zinc
ZnO	zinc oxide
ZnOE	zinc oxide and eugenol
ZnPc	zinc phthalocyanine
ZnPP	zinc protoporphyrin
ZNS	zonisamide (Zonegran)
ZOI	zone of inhibition
ZOOM	Guarana
ZOT	zonula occludens toxin
ZPC	zero point of charge
	zopiclone
z-Plasty	surgical relaxation of contracture
ZPO	zinc peroxide
ZPP	zinc protoporphyrin
ZPS	Zubrod performance status
ZPT	zinc pyrithione
ZSB	zero stools since birth
ZSR	zeta sedimentation rate
ZSRDS	Zung Self-Rating Depression Scale

Z

Chapter 6
Symbols and Numbers

Symbols

↑	above	↑↑	extensor
	alive		extensor response (positive
	elevated		Babinsky)
	greater than		testes undescended
	high		
	improved	‖	parallel
	increase		parallel bars
	rising		
	up	√	check
	upper		flexion
↑g	increasing	√'d	checked
↓	dead	√'ing	checking
	decrease		
	depressed	#	fracture
	diminished		number
	down		pound
	falling		weight
	lower		
	lowered	∴	therefore
	normal plantar reflex	∵	because
	restricted		
↓g	decreasing	Δ scan	delta scan (computed tomography scan)
→	causes to		
	greater than	+	plus
	progressing		positive
	results in		present
	showed		
	to the right	–	absent
	transfer to		minus
			negative
←	less than		
	resulted from	/	extend
	to the left		extended
			slash mark signifying per, and, over, as a blood pressure of 160 over 100, or with (this is a dangerous symbol as it is mistaken for a one)
↔	same as		
	stable		
	to and from		
	unchanging	±	either positive or negative
			no definite cause
↓↓	flexor		plus or minus
	plantar response (Babinski)		very slight trace
	testes descended		

⌐ (right lower quadrant symbol)	right lower quadrant
⌐ (right upper quadrant symbol)	right upper quadrant
⌐ (left upper quadrant symbol)	left upper quadrant
⌐ (left lower quadrant symbol)	left lower quadrant
>	greater than (can be confused with <, use "greater than")
	left ear-bone conduction threshold
≥	greater than or equal to
<	caused by
	less than (can be confused with >, use "less than")
	right ear-bone conduction threshold
≤	less than or equal to
≮	not less than
≯	not more than
	above
∨	diastolic blood pressure
	increased
	below
	systolic blood pressure
≠	not equal to
≅	approximately equal to
=	equal
	equal to
′	feet
	minutes (as in 30′)
″	inches
	seconds
~	about
	approximately
	difference
≈	approximately equal to
≡	identical
×	left ear-air conduction threshold
	ten
]	left ear-masked bone conduction threshold
[	right ear-masked bone conduction
△	right ear-masked air conduction threshold
	change
○	threshold
	reversible
?	questionable
—	not tested

Ø	no
	none
	without
⊙	start of an operation
⊗	end of anesthesia
@	at
┬	one
┬┬	two
♂	male
♀	female
♂♂	gay
♀♀	lesbian
■	deceased male
●	deceased female
□	living male
	left ear-masked air conduction threshold
○	living female
	respiration
	right ear-air conduction threshold
◇	sex unknown
(□)	adopted living male
*	birth
†	dead
	death
♀ (standing symbol)	standing
○—<	recumbent position
♀ (sitting symbol)	sitting position
♥	heart

Numbers (Arabic and Roman)

1/2 and 1/2	half Dakin solution and half glycerin
1°	first degree
	primary
1:1	one-to-one (individual session with staff)
2°	second degree
	secondary
2×2	gauze dressing folded 2″×2″
222	aspirin, caffeine, and codeine (8 mg) tablets (Canada)
282	aspirin, caffeine, codeine, and meprobamate (Canada)
3°	tertiary
	third degree
3×	three times
4×4	gauze dressing folded 4″×4″

#

5+2	5 days of cytarabine and 2 days of daunorubicin leukemia therapy	
642	propoxyphene tablets (Canada)	
7+3	7 days of cytarabine and 3 days of daunorubicin leukemia therapy	
Serial 7's	a mental status examination (starting with 100, count backward by 7's)	
24°	twenty-four hours (24 hr is safer as the ° is seen as a zero)	
777	Ortho Novum 777® (a triphasic oral contraceptive)	
1500	Health Insurance Claim Form HCFA 1500	
1,000	one thousand (1×10^3)	
10,000	ten thousand (1×10^4)	
100,000	one hundred thousand (1×10^5)	
1,000,000	one million (1×10^6)	
10,000,000	ten million (1×10^7)	
100,000,000	one hundred million (1×10^8)	
1,000,000,000	one billion (1×10^9)	

i	one (Roman numerals are dangerous expressions and should not be used because they are not universally understood)
ii	two
iii	three
iiii	four
iv	four (this is a dangerous abbreviation as it is read as intravenous, use 4)
v	five
vi	six
vii	seven
viii	eight
ix	nine
x	ten
xi	eleven
xii	twelve
XL	forty
	extended release dosage form
L	fifty
C	hundred
M	thousand

Greek Letters

A α	alpha
β B	beta
Γ γ	gamma
Δ δ	anion gap
	change
	delta
	delta gap
	prism diopter

	temperature
	trimester
E ε	epsilon
Z ζ	zeta
H η	eta
Θ θ	negative
	theta
I ι	iota
K κ	kappa
Λ λ	lambda
M μ	micro
	mu
N ν	nu
Ξ ξ	xi
O o	omicron
Π π	pi
P ρ	rho
Σ σ	sigma
	sum of
	summary
T τ	tau
Y υ	upsilon
Φ φ	phenyl
	phi
	thyroid
X χ	chi
Ψ ψ	psi
	psychiatric
Ω ω	omega

Miscellaneous

L M
K O
S T   liver, kidneys, and spleen negative, no masses, or tenderness

\#

Additions, Corrections, and Suggestions are Welcomed

Please send them via any means shown below:

Neil M Davis
2049 Stout Drive, B-3
Warminster PA 18974-3861

FAX 1 888 333 4915 or 1 215 442 7432
Email med@neilmdavis.com
Web site www.medabbrev.com

Thank you for your help in the past.

Have You Used the Web-Version of This Book?

- It is instantaneously searchable for the meanings of abbreviations
- It is reverse searchable (search for all the abbreviations containing a particular word)
- Each month, about 80 new entries are added

See the preface (page vii) for access instructions. A two-year, single-user access is included in the purchase price of the book.

PDA Versions are Available

See pricing and ordering information in the pricing section on page 357.

Multi-User Site Licenses are Available

Medical facilities can substitute their own "Do Not Use" list of dangerous abbreviations for the one present. The ability also exists to list abbreviations that are unique to your region and/or organization which would normally not appear in any national list. These lists would be controlled by the facility. Demonstrations and pricing information are available by calling 1 888 333 1862 or 1 215 442 7430 or via an e-mail request to ev@neilmdavis.com

Chapter 7

Tables, Lists, and Conversions

Numbers and letters for teeth

Two adult numbering systems and a deciduous system are shown. The adult systems are shown as numbers, whereas deciduous teeth are lettered. The system commonly used in the U.S. is 1 to 32 (shown in bold face type).

1 (18)	upper right 3rd molar
2 (17) (A)	upper right 2nd molar
3 (16) (B)	upper right 1st molar
4 (15)	upper right 2nd bicuspid
5 (14)	upper right 1st bicuspid
6 (13) (C)	upper right canine (eyetooth)
7 (12) (D)	upper right lateral incisor
8 (11) (E)	upper right central incisor
9 (21) (F)	upper left central incisor
10 (22) (G)	upper left lateral incisor
11 (23) (H)	upper left canine
12 (24)	upper left 1st bicuspid
13 (25)	upper left 2nd bicuspid
14 (26) (I)	upper left 1st molar
15 (27) (J)	upper left 2nd molar
16 (28)	upper left 3rd molar
17 (38)	lower left 3rd molar
18 (37) (K)	lower left 2nd molar
19 (36) (L)	lower left 1st molar
20 (35)	lower left 2nd bicuspid
21 (34)	lower left 1st bicuspid
22 (33) (M)	lower left canine
23 (32) (N)	lower left lateral incisor
24 (31) (O)	lower left central incisor
25 (41) (P)	lower right central incisor
26 (42) (Q)	lower right lateral incisor
27 (43) (R)	lower right canine
28 (44)	lower right 1st bicuspid
29 (45)	lower right 2nd bicuspid
30 (46) (S)	lower right 1st molar
31 (47) (T)	lower right 2nd molar
32 (48)	lower right 3rd molar

UPPER

	1	2	3	4	5	6	7	8	9	10	11	12	13	14	15	16	UPPER
	18	17	16	15	14	13	12	11	21	22	23	24	25	26	27	28	
		A	B			C	D	E	F	G	H			I	J		
Right																	**Left**
		T	S			R	Q	P	O	N	M			L	K		
	48	47	46	45	44	43	42	41	31	32	33	34	35	36	37	38	
	32	**31**	**30**	**29**	**28**	**27**	**26**	**25**	**24**	**23**	**22**	**21**	**20**	**19**	**18**	**17**	

LOWER
LOWER

Laboratory Test Panels*

	Cl CO2 K Na	BUN Ca Creat Gluc	Alb Alk P AST(SGOT) ALT(SGPT) T Bili TP	ANA ESR RF Ur Ac	Calc LDL HDL T Chol Trig VLDL	Alb Phos	HAAb, IgM Ab HbcAb, IgM Ab HbsAG HCAb
Lytes (electrolyte panel)	X						
BMP (basic metabolic panel) or MBP, MPB	X	X					
CMP (comprehensive metabolic panel)	X	X	X				
HFP (hepatic function panel)			X plus D Bili				
AP (arthritis panel)				X			
LP (lipid Panel)					X		
RFP (renal function panel)	X	X				X	
AHP (acute hepatitis panel)							X

*These can vary from institution to institution and from year to year

Abbreviation Key

Ab-antibody
Alb-albumin
Alk P-alkaline phosphate
ALT (SGPT)-alanine aminotransferase (serum glutamate pyruvate)
ANA-antinuclear antibody
AST (SGOT)-aspartate-aminotransferase (serum glutamate oxaloacetic transaminase)
BUN-blood urea nitrogen
Ca-calcium
Calc LDL-calculated low-density lipoprotein
LDL-low density lipoprotein

Cl-chloride
CO2-carbon dioxide
Creat-creatinine
D Bili-direct bilirubin
ESR-erythrocyte sedimentation rate
Gluc-glucose
HAAb-hepatitis A antibody
HBcAb-hepatitis B core antibody
HBsAg-hepatitis B surface antigen
HCAb-hepatitis C antibody
HDL-high-density lipoprotein

IgM-immunoglobulin M
K-potassium
Na-sodium
Phos-phosphate
RF-rheumatoid factor
T Bili-total bilirubin
T Chol-total cholesterol
TP-total protein
Trig-triglycerides.
Ur Ac-uric acid
VLDl-very low-density lipoprotein

See text for meaning of the abbreviations shown

Complete Blood Count

$$10,000 \Big\rangle \begin{array}{c} 11.7 \\ 36.5 \end{array} \Big\langle \begin{array}{l} \text{50S, 25B, 35L, 5M 2N, 3E} \\ \text{83/29/30} \\ \text{290,00} \end{array}$$

$$\text{WBC} \Big\rangle \begin{array}{c} \text{HgB} \\ \text{HCT} \end{array} \Big\langle \begin{array}{l} \text{Segs/Bands/Lymphs/Monos/Basos/Eos} \\ \text{MCV-MCH-MCHC} \\ \text{platelet count} \end{array}$$

Electrolyte Panel

142	99	sodium		chloride
4.7	25	potassium		carbon dioxide

Blood Gases

7.4/80/48/98/25   pH/PO$_2$/PCO$_2$/% O$_2$ saturation/bicarbonate

Obstetrical shorthand

$$\frac{2 \text{ cm} | 80\%}{-2 \text{ Vtx}} \quad 2 \text{ cm} = \text{dilation of cervix}$$

80% = degree of cer-   Vtx = vertex; presen-
  vix effacement   tation of fetus,
                            (breech = Br)

−2 = station; distance
    above (+) or
    below (−) the
    spine of the ischium measured in cm

Reflexes

Reflexes are usually graded on a 0 to 4+ scale. The designations +, ++, +++, and ++++ should not be used.

4+ may indicate disease often associated with clonus
    very brisk, hyperactive
3+ brisker than average
    possibly but not necessarily indicative of disease
2+ average
    normal
1+ low normal
    somewhat diminished
0   may indicate neuropathy
    no response

Muscle strength[1]

0—No muscular contraction detected
1—A barely detectable flicker or trace of contraction
2—Active movement of the body part with gravity eliminated
3—Active movement against gravity
4—Active movement against gravity and some resistance
5—Active movement against full resistance without evident fatigue. This is normal muscle strength

Pulse[1]
0   completely absent
+1 markedly impaired (or 1+)
+2 modererately impaired (or 2+)
+3 slightly impaired (or 3+)
+4 normal (or 4+)

Gradation of intensity of heart murmurs[1]
1/6 or I/VI	may not be heard in all positions
	very faint, heard only after the listener has "tuned in"
2/6 or II/VI	quiet, but heard immediately upon placing the stethoscope on the chest
3/6 or III/VI	moderately loud
4/6 or IV/VI	loud
5/6 orV/VI	very loud, may be heard with a stethoscope partly off the chest (thrills are associated)
6/6 or VI/VI	may be heard with the stethoscope entirely off the chest (thrills are associated)

Tonsil Size
0   no tonsils
1   less than normal
2   normal
3   greater than normal
4   touching

Metric Prefixes and Symbols
Prefix	Symbol	
tera-	T	$1,000,000,000,000$ or (10^{12}) one trillion
giga-	G	$1,000,000,000$ or (10^{9}) one billion
mega-	M	$1,000,000$ or (10^{6}) one million
kilo-	k	$1,000$ or (10^{3}) one thousand
hecto-	h	100 or (10^{2}) one hundred
deka-	da	10 or (10^{1}) ten
deci-	d	0.1 or (10^{-1}) one-tenth
centi-	c	0.01 or (10^{-2}) one-hundredth
milli-	m	0.001 or (10^{-3}) one-thousandth
micro-	μ	$0.000,001$ or (10^{-6}) one-millionth
nano-	n	$0.000,000,001$ or (10^{-9}) one-billionth
pico-	p	$0.000,000,000,000,001$ or (10^{-12}) one-trillionth
femto-	f	$0.000,000,000,000,001$ or (10^{-15}) one-quadrillionth
atto-	a	$0.000,000,000,000,000,001$ or (10^{-18}) one-quintillionth

Kilograms/Pounds Conversions
To convert pounds to kilograms, divide by 2.2
To convert kilograms to pounds, multiply by 2.2

After carrying out a calculation, always make sure your answer is reasonable by checking with the table below.

kilograms	pounds
0.5	1.1
1	2.2
5	11
10	22
25	55
50	110
75	165
100	220

Fahrenheit/Centigrade Conversions
To convert Centigrade to Fahrenheit

$°F = 32$ plus $(9/5$ times $°C)$ or $°F = 32$ plus $(1.8$ times $°C)$

To convert Fahrenheit to Centigrade

$°C = 5/9$ times $(°F$ minus $32)$ or $°C ≈ 0.556$ times $(°F$ minus $32)$

After carrying out a calculation, always make sure your answer is reasonable by checking with the table below.

°Centigrade	°Fahrenheit
0	32
2	36
8	46
15	59
20	68
25	77
30	86
36	96.8
37	98.6
38	100.4
39	102.2
40	104
41	105.8
50	122
100	212

Apothecary symbols (Should never be used)

The symbols presented below are for informational use. The apothecary system should **not** be used. Only the metric system should be used. The methods of expressing the symbols, the meanings, and the equivalence are not the classic ones, nor are they accurate, but reflect the usual intended meanings when used by some older physicians in writing prescription directions.

℈ or ℈⠬ dram, teaspoonful, (5 mL)

℥ or ℥⠬ ounce, (30 mL)

gr grain (approximately 65 mg)

℈ⁱⁱ two drams, 2 tea-spoonfuls, (10 mL)

m̃ minim (approximately 0.06 mL)

℈ss half ounce, table-spoonful, (15 mL)

gtt drop

Reference

1. Adopted from Bates B. Bates' guide to physical examinations and history taking, 8th ed. Philadelphia: Lippincott Williams and Wilkins; 2003.

Additions, Corrections, and Suggestions are Welcomed

Please send them via any means shown below:

Neil M Davis
2049 Stout Drive, B-3
Warminster PA 18974-3861

FAX 1 888 333 4915 or 1 215 442 7432
Email med@neilmdavis.com
Web site www.medabbrev.com

Thank you for your help in the past.

Have You Used the Web-Version of This Book?

- It is instantaneously searchable for the meanings of abbreviations
- It is reverse searchable (search for all the abbreviations containing a particular word)
- Each month, about 80 new entries are added

See the preface (page vii) for access instructions. A two-year, single-user access is included in the purchase price of the book.

PDA Versions are Available

See pricing and ordering information in the pricing section on page 357.

Multi-User Site Licenses are Available

Medical facilities can substitute their own "Do Not Use" list of dangerous abbreviations for the one present. The ability also exists to list abbreviations that are unique to your region and/or organization which would normally not appear in any national list. These lists would be controlled by the facility. Demonstrations and pricing information are available by calling 1 888 333 1862 or 1 215 442 7430 or via an e-mail request to ev@neilmdavis.com

Chapter 8

Cross-Referenced List of Generic and Brand Drug Names

Listed below is a cross-referenced index of generic and brand drug names. Generic names begin with a lower case letter while brand names begin with a capital letter. This partial list consists of frequently prescribed drugs, new drugs, and recently discontinued drugs.

The meanings of abbreviated and coded drug names can be found in Chapter 5 (Lettered Abbreviations and Acronyms).

Complete indices of United States drug names can be found in current editions of Drug Facts and Comparisons[1] and the American Drug Index[2]. A complete list of world-wide names may be found in Martindales.[3] These and other references should be used to determine the equivalence of products, strengths, and dosage forms. Although several products may be listed under one generic name they may differ in strength, dosage form, or concentration available, as is the case with estradiol transdermal (Climara, Estraderm, and Vivelle).

Some products are marketed without a brand name, as in the case of thioguanine. In such cases only the generic name is listed. When a product is often prescribed and/or labeled generically, the generic name is shown in italics.

The following abbreviations are used in this listing:

EC	enteric coated	SR	sustained release tablets or capsules
HCl	hydrochloride		(and other forms of extended release)
IM	intramuscular	susp	suspension
IV	intravenous	(W)	withdrawn or discontinued from US market
inj	injection	(WA)	withdrawn or discontinued from US market
oint	ointment		but available under different name from another
ophth	ophthalmic		manufacturer
soln	solution		

A

abacavir sulfate	Ziagen
abarelix	Plenaxis
Abbokinase	urokinase
abciximab	ReoPro
Abelcet	amphotericin B lipid complex
Abilify	aripiprazole
Abraxane	paclitaxel, albumin-bound inj
acamprosate calcium	Campral
acarbose	Precose
Accolate	zafirlukast
AccuNeb	albuterol inhalation soln
Accupril	quinapril HCl
Accuretic	quinapril; hydrochlorothiazide
Accutane	isotretinoin
Accuzyme	papain; urea oint
acebutolol HCl	Sectral
Aceon	perindopril erbumine
acetaminophen	paracetamol Tylenol
acetaminophen 300 mg with Codeine Phosphate (15, 30, and 60 mg)	Phenaphen with Codeine (#2, 3, and 4) (WA) Tylenol with Codeine (#2, 3, and 4)
acetazolamide	Diamox

acetohexamide	Dymelor
acetohydroxamic acid	Lithostat
acetylcholine ophth	Miochol E
acetylcysteine	Mucomyst
Achromycin (WA)	tetracycline HCl
Aciphex	rabeprazole sodium
acitretin	Soriatane
Acora	argatroban
Acthar	corticotropin
ActHIB/Tripedia	*Haemophilus b* conjugate vaccine reconstituted with diphtheria and tetanus toxoids and acellular pertussis vaccine adsorbed
Acthrel	corticorellin ovine triflutate
Actifed	triprolidine HCl; pseudoephedrine HCl
Actigall	ursodiol
Actimmune	interferon gamma 1-b
Actiq	fentanyl oral transmucosal
Activase	alteplase, recombinant
Activella (WA)	norethindrone acetate; estradiol
Actonel	risedronate sodium
Actos	pioglitazone HCl
Acular	ketorolac tromethamine ophth
acyclovir	Zovirax
Adacel	diphtheria, tetanus, and acellular pertussis (TdaP) vaccine (adult type)
Adalat	nifedipine
Adalat CC	nifedipine SR
adalimumab	Humira
adapalene	Differin
Adapin	doxepin HCl
Adderall	amphetamine; dextroamphetamine mixed salts
adefovir dipivoxil	Hepsera Preveon
Adenocard	adenosine
adenosine	Adenocard
Adrenalin	epinephrine
Adriamycin	doxorubicin HCl
Advair Diskus	fluticasone propionate; salmeterol inhalation powder
Advicor	lovastatin; niacin
Advil	ibuprofen
AeroBid	flunisolide
Afrin nasal spray	oxymetazoline HCl
agalsidase beta	Fabrazyme
Agenerase (W)	amprenavir (W)

Aggrastat	tirofiban HCl
Aggrenox	aspirin; extended-release dipyridamole
Agrylin	anagrelide HCl
Akineton	biperiden
Alamast	pemirolast potassium ophth soln
alatrofloxacin mesylate IV (W)	Trovan inj (W)
albendazole	Albenza
Albenza	albendazole
albumin human	Albuminar Albutein Buminate Plasbumin
albumin (human), sonicated	Albunex
Albuminar	albumin human
Albunex	albumin (human), sonicated
Albutein	albumin human
albuterol	AccuNeb Proventil salbutamol Ventolin
albuterol SR	Proventil Repetabs Volmax
albuterol sulfate inhalation aerosol	Proventil HFA
Aldactazide	spironolactone; hydrochlorothiazide
Aldactone	spironolactone
Aldara	imiquimod cream
aldesleukin	Proleukin
Aldomet	methyldopa
Aldoril	methyldopa; hydrochlorothiazide
Aldurazyme	laronidase
alefacept	Amevive
alemtuzumab	Campath
alendronate sodium	Fosamax
Alesse	levonorgestrel; ethinyl estradiol
Alfenta	alfentanil HCl
alfentanil HCl	Alfenta
alfuzosin	UroXatral
alglucerase	Ceredase
alglucosidase alfa	Myozyme
Alimta	pemetrexed disodium
alitretinoin	Panretin
Allegra	fexofenadine HCl
Alinia	nitazoxanide
Alkeran	melphalan
allopurinol	Zyloprim

almotriptan malate — Axert

Alocril — nedocromil ophth soln

Alomide — lodoxamide tromethamine ophth soln

Alora — estradiol transdermal

alosetron — Lotronex

Aloxi — palonosetron HCl

Alphagan — brimonidine tartrate ophth

alpha₁-proteinase inhibitor (human) — Prolastin

alprazolam — Xanax

alprostadil — Caverject
Edex
Prostin VR

alprostadil urethral suppository — Muse

Alrex — loteprednol etabonate ophth susp

Altace — ramipril

alteplase, recombinant — Activase

alteplase (for catheter occlusions) — Cathflo Activase

altretamine — Hexalen

aluminum acetate — Domeboro

aluminum carbonate — Basaljel

aluminum hydroxide — Amphojel

aluminum hydroxide; magnesium hydroxide — Maalox

Alupent — metaproterenol sulfate

Alustra — hydroquinone topical susp

amantadine HCl — Symmetrel

Amaryl — glimepiride

Ambien — zolpidem tartrate

AmBisome — liposomal amphotericin B

amcinonide — Cyclocort

Amerge — naratriptan HCl

Amevive — alefacept

Amicar — aminocaproic acid

Amidate — etomidate

amifostine — Ethyol

amikacin sulfate — Amikin

Amikin — amikacin sulfate

amiloride HCl — Midamor

amiloride; hydro-chlorothiazide — Moduretic

amino acid inj — Aminosyn
Travasol
TrophAmine

amino acid with electrolytes in dextrose with calcium inj (various concentrations) — Clinimix E

aminocaproic acid — Amicar

aminocaproic acid gel — Caprogel

aminogluteth-imide — Cytadren

aminolevulinic acid HCl topical soln — Levulan Kerastick

aminophylline — aminophylline

aminosalicylic acid — Paser

Aminosyn — amino acid inj

amiodarone HCl — Cordarone

amitriptyline HCl — Elavil
Endep

AmLactin — ammonium lactate lotion

amlexanox oral paste — Aphthasol

amlodipine besylate — Norvasc

amlodipine besylate; atorvastatin calcium — Caduet

amlodipine besylate; benazepril HCl — Lotrel

ammonium lactate lotion — AmLactin

amobarbital sodium — Amytal

amoxapine — Asendin

amoxicillin — Amoxil
Trimox
Wymox

amoxicillin; clavulanic acid — Augmentin

amoxicillin; clavulanate potassium SR — Augmentin XR

Amoxil — amoxicillin

amphetamine resins (W) — Biphetamine (W)

amphetamine; dextroamphet-amine mixed salts — Adderall

Amphojel — aluminum hydroxide

Amphotec — amphotericin B cholesteryl sulfate

amphotericin B	Fungizone
amphotericin B cholesteryl sulfate	Amphotec
amphotericin B lipid complex	Abelcet
ampicillin	Principen
ampicillin sodium; sulbactam sodium	Unasyn
amprenavir (W)	Agenerase (W)
amrinone (former name)	inamrinone (new name)
amsacrine	Amsidyl
Amsidyl	amsacrine
Amvisc	sodium hyaluronate
Amytal	amobarbital sodium
Anadrol-50	oxymetholone
Anafranil	clomipramine HCl
anagrelide HCl	Agrylin
anakinra	Kineret
Anaprox	naproxen sodium
anastrozole	Arimidex
Anbesol	benzocaine
Ancef	cefazolin sodium
Ancobon	flucytosine
Androderm	testosterone transdermal system
AndroGel	testosterone gel
Androgel-DHT	dihydrotestosterone transdermal
Anectine	succinylcholine chloride
Anexsia	hydrocodone bitartrate; acetaminophen
Angiomax	bivalirudin
anidulafungin IV	Eraxis
Ansaid	flurbiprofen
Antabuse	disulfiram
Antagon	ganirelix acetate
antihemophilic factor (recombinant)	Kogenate ReFacto
Antilirium	physostigmine salicylate
antipyrine otic	Auralgan
antithrombin III (human)	Thrombate III
antithymocyte globulin, (rabbit)	Thymoglobulin
Antivert	meclizine
Antizol	fomepizole
Anturane	sulfinpyrazone
Anzemet	dolasetron mesylate
Aphthasol	amlexanox oral paste
Apidra	insulin glulisine [rDNA origin]

A.P.L.	chorionic gonadotropin
apligraf	Graftskin
Aplisol	tuberculin skin test
Apokyn	apomorphine HCl inj
apomorphine HCl	Uprima
apomorphine HCl inj	Apokyn
Aposyn	exisulind
aprepitant	Emend
Apresazide	hydralazine HCl; hydrochloro-thiazide
Apresoline	hydralazine HCl
aprotinin	Trasylol
Aptivus	tipranavir
AquaMEPHY-TON	phytonadione
Aralen	chloroquine phosphate
Aramine	metaraminol bitartrate
Aranesp	darbepoetin alfa
Arava	leflunomide
arbutamine HCl	GenEsa
arcitumomab	CEA-Scan
ardeparin sodium (W)	Normiflo (W)
Arduan (W)	pipecuronium bromide (W)
Aredia	pamidronate disodium
Arestin	minocycline HCl dental microspheres
Arfonad (W)	trimethaphan camsylate (W)
argatroban	argatroban
arginine HCl	R-Gene
Aricept	donepezil HCl
Arimidex	anastrozole
aripiprazole	Abilify
Aristocort	triamcinolone acetonide
Arixtra	fondaparinux sodium
Aromasin	exemestane
arsenic trioxide	Trisenox
Artane (W)	trihexyphenidyl HCl (W)
Arthrotec	diclofenac; misoprostol
Asacol	mesalamine
Asendin	amoxapine
Aslera	prasterone
asparaginase	Elspar
aspirin 325 mg with codeine phosphate (30 and 60 mg)	Empirin with codeine #3 and #4
aspirin buffered	Bufferin
aspirin EC	Ecotrin
Astelin	azelastine HCl nasal spray
astemizole (W)	Hismanal (W)
Atacand	candesartan cilexetil
Atarax (WA)	hydroxyzine HCl
atazanavir sulfate	Reyataz
atenolol	Tenormin

atenolol; chlorthalidone	Tenoretic
Atgam	lymphocyte imimmune globulin
articaine; epinephrine	Septocaine
aspirin; extended-release dipyridamole	Aggrenox
Atacand HCT	candesartan cilexetil; hydrochlorothiazide
atazanavir	Revetaz
Ativan	lorazepam
Atomoxetine HCl	Strattera
atorvastatin calcium	Lipitor
atovaquone	Mepron
atovaquone; proguanil HCl	Malarone
atracurium besylate	Tracrium
Atridox	doxycycline hyclate gel
Atripla	efavirenz, emtricitabine, and tenofovir
Atromid-S (W)	clofibrate (W)
atropine sulfate tablets	Sal-Tropine
Atrovent	ipratropium bromide
Augmentin	amoxicillin; clavulanic acid
Augmentin XR	amoxicillin; clavulanate potassium SR
Auralgan	antipyrine otic
auranofin	Ridaura
Aurolate	gold sodium thiomalate
aurothioglucose	Solganal
Avalide	irbesartan; hydro-chlorothiazide
Avandamet	rosiglitazone maleate; metformin HCl
Avandia	Rosiglitazone maleate
Avanir	docosanol cream
Avapro	irbesartan
Avastin	bevacizumab
Avelox	moxifloxacin HCl
Aventyl	nortriptyline HCl
Avinza	morphine sulfate tab SR
Avita	tretinoin cream 0.025%
Avitene	collagen hemostat
Avodart	dutasteride
Avonex	interferon beta-la
Axert	almotriptan malate
Axid	nizatidine
azacitidine	Vidaza
Azactam	aztreonam
azatadine maleate	Optimine
azathioprine	Imuran
azelaic acid cream	Azelex Finevin

azelastine HCl nasal spray	Astelin
azelastine HCl ophth soln	Optivar
Azelex	azelaic acid cream
azithromycin	Zithromax
Azmacort	triamcinolone acetonide aerosol
Azopt	brinzolamide ophth susp
aztreonam	Azactam
Azulfidine	sulfasalazine

B

Baciguent	bacitracin ointment
bacitracin ointment	Baciguent
baclofen	Lioresal
Bactrim	sulfamethoxazole; trimeth-oprim
Bactroban	mupirocin nasal ointment
BAL in Oil	dimercaprol
Baraclude	entecavir
Basaljel	aluminum carbonate
balsalazide disodium	Colazal
basiliximab	Simulect
Baycol (W)	cerivastatin sodium (W)
BCG intravesical	Pacis TheraCys TICE BCG
becaplermin gel	Regranex
beclomethasone dipropionate	Beclovent Beconase AQ Nasal Qvar Vancenase Vancenase AQ Nasal Vanceril
Beclovent	beclomethasone dipropionate
Beconase AQ Nasal	beclomethasone dipropionate
belladonna alkaloids; phenobarbital	Donnatal (W)
Bellergal-S	phenobarbital; ergotamine; belladonna
Benadryl	diphenhydramine HCl
benazepril HCl	Lotensin
BeneFix	factor IX, (recombinant)
Benemid	probenecid
Benicar	olmesartan medoxomil
Benicar HCT	olmesartan medoxomil; hydrochlorothiazide
bentoquatam	IvyBlock
Bentyl	dicyclomine HCl

Right margin: B R̪

Benzamycin	erythromycin; benzoyl peroxide topical gel	Bicillin L-A	penicillin G benzathine (for IM use only)
benzocaine	Anbesol	Bicitra	sodium citrate; citric acid
	Hurricaine	BiCNU	carmustine
	Orabase	BiDil	isosorbide dinitrate;
	Orajel		hydralazine
benzocaine; tetracaine HCl	Cetacaine	Bilopaque	tyropanoate sodium
benztropine mesylate	Cogentin	bimatoprost ophth soln	Lumigan
bepridil (W)	Vascor (W)	biperiden	Akineton
beractant	Survanta	Biphetamine (W)	amphetamine resins (W)
Berroca	vitamin B complex; folic acid; vitamin C	bisacodyl	Dulcolax
Betadine	povidone iodine	bismuth subsalicylate; metronidazole; tetracycline HCl	Helidac
17β-estradiol; norgestimate	Ortho-Prefest		
Betagan	levobunolol HCl		
betaine anhydrous	Cystadane	bisoprolol fumarate; hydrochlorothi-azide	Ziac
betamethasone	Celestone		
betamethasone dipropionate	Diprosone		
betamethasone; clotrimazole cream	Lotrisone	bitolterol mesylate	Tornalate
		bivalirudin	Angiomax
betamethasone valerate (foam)	Luxiq	Blenoxane	bleomycin sulfate
		bleomycin sulfate	Blenoxane
Betapace	sotalol	Blocadren	timolol maleate
Betaseron	interferon beta-1b	Boniva	ibandronate
betaxolol	Kerlone	bortezomib	Velcade
betaxolol HCl ophth soln	Betoptic	bosentan	Tracleer
		B & O Supprettes	opium; belladonna suppositories
betaxolol HCl ophth susp	Betoptic S	Botox	botulinum toxin type A
betaxolol HCl; pilocarpine HCl ophth soln	Betoptic Pilo	botulinum toxin type A	Botox
		botulinum toxin type B	Myobloc
bethanechol chloride	Urecholine	Bravelle	urofollitropin
Betoptic	betaxolol HCl ophth soln	Brethaire	terbutaline sulfate aerosol
Betoptic Pilo	betaxolol HCl; pilocarpine HCl, ophth soln	Brethine	terbutaline sulfate tablets and inj
		bretylium tosylate	Bretylol
Betoptic S	betaxolol HCl ophth suspension	Bretylol	bretylium tosylate
bevacizumab	Avastin	Brevibloc	esmolol HCl
bexarotene gel	Targretin	Brevital Sodium	methohexital sodium
Bextra (W)	valdecoxib (W)	Bricanyl	terbutaline sulfate tablets and inj
Bexxar	tositumomab and I-131 tositumomab	brimonidine tartrate ophth	Alphagan
Biaxin	clarithromycin	brinzolamide ophth suspension	Azopt
Biaxin XL	clarithromycin SR		
bicalutamide	Casodex		
Bicillin C-R	penicillin G benzathine; penicillin G procaine (for IM use only)	bromfenac ophth soln	Xibrom

bromocriptine mesylate — Parlodel

brompheniramine maleate — Dimetane

brompheniramine maleate; phenylpropanolamime — Dimetapp Extentabs

Bronkometer — isoetharine HCl aerosol

Bronkosol — isoetharine HCl soln

Bucladin-S — buclizine HCl

buclizine HCl — Bucladin-S

budesonide capsule SR — Entocort EC

budesonide inhalation powder — Pulmicort Turbuhaler

budesonide nasal inhaler — Rhinocort

Bufferin — aspirin buffered

bumetanide — Bumex

Bumex — bumetanide

Buminate — albumin human

Buphenyl — phenylbutyrate sodium

bupivacaine HCl — Marcaine HCl

buprenorphine HCl — Subutex

buprenorphine HCl; naloxone HCl — Suboxone

bupropion HCl — Wellbutrin

bupropion HCl SR — Wellbutrin SR Zyban

BuSpar — buspirone HCl

buspirone HCl — BuSpar

busulfan — Myleran

busulfan inj — Busulfex

Busulfex — busulfan inj

butabarbital sodium — Butisol

butalbital; acetaminophen; caffeine — Fioricet

butalbital; aspirin; caffeine — Fiorinal

butenafine HCl — Mentax

Butisol — butabarbital sodium

butoconazole nitrate vaginal cream — Gynazole

butorphanol tartrate inj — Stadol

butorphanol tartrate nasal spray — Stadol NS

Byetta — exenatide inj

C

cabergoline — Dostinex

Ca-DTPA — calcium trisodium (trisodium calcium diethylenetriaminepentaacetate)

Caduet — amlodipine besylate; atorvastatin calcium

Cafcit — caffeine citrate inj

Cafergot — ergotaminetartrate; caffeine

caffeine citrate inj — Cafcit

Calan SR — verapamil HCl SR

Calciferol — ergocalciferol

Calcimar — calcitonin

calcipotriene cream — Dovonex

calcitonin — Calcimar

calcitonin-salmon — Miacalcin

calcitriol — Rocaltrol

calcium carbonate — Os-Cal 500 Tums

calcium carbonate; vitamin D and K chewable — Viactiv

calcium trisodium (trisodium calcium diethylenetriaminepentaacetate) — Ca-DTPA

calfactant intratracheal susp — Infasurf

Campath — alemtuzumab

camphorated tincture of opium — paregoric

Campral — acamprosate calcium

Camptosar — irinotecan HCl

candesartan cilexetil — Atacand

candesartan cilexetil; hydrochlorothiazide — Atacand HCT

Cancidas — caspofungin acetate

Capastat Sulfate — capreomycin sulfate

capecitabine — Xeloda

Capital w/ Codeine Suspension — codeine phosphate; acetaminophen suspension

Capitrol	chloroxine	cefepime HCl	Maxipime
Capoten	captopril	cefixime (W)	Suprax (W)
capreomycin sulfate	Capastat Sulfate	Cefizox	ceftizoxime sodium
Caprogel	aminocaproic acid gel	Cefobid	cefoperazone sodium
capromab pendetide	ProstaScint	cefonicid sodium (W)	Monocid (W)
captopril	Capoten	cefoperazone sodium	Cefobid
Carafate	sucralfate	Cefotan	cefotetan
carbachol	Isopto Carbachol	cefotaxime sodium	Claforan
carbamazepine	Tegretol	cefotetan	Cefotan
carbamazepine SR	Carbatrol Tegretol-XR	cefoxitin sodium	Mefoxin
carbamide peroxide otic	Debrox	cefpodoxime proxetil	Vantin
Carbatrol	carbamazepine SR	cefprozil	Cefzil
carbenicillin	Geocillin	ceftazidime	Ceptaz
Carbex	selegiline		Fortaz
Carbocaine	mepivacaine HCl		Tazicef
carboplatin	Paraplatin		Tazidime
Cardene	nicardipine HCl	ceftibuten	Cedax
Cardiolite	technetium Tc99m sestamibi	Ceftin	cefuroxime axetil
Cardiotec	technetium Tc-99m teboroxime kit	ceftizoxime sodium	Cefizox
Cardizem	diltiazem HCl	ceftriaxone sodium	Rocephin
Cardizem CD	diltiazem HCl SR	cefuroxime axetil	Ceftin
Cardura	doxazosin mesylate		
carisoprodol	Soma		
carmustine	BiCNU	cefuroxime sodium	Kefurox Zinacef
carmustine implantable wafer	Gliadel	Cefzil	cefprozil
		Celebrex	celecoxib
Carnitor	levocarnitine	celecoxib	Celebrex
Cartia XR	diltiazem HCl SR	Celestone	betamethasone
carvedilol	Coreg	Celexa	citalopram hydrobromide
Casodex	bicalutamide	CellCept	mycophenolate mofetil
caspofungin acetate	Cancidas	Cenestin	synthetic conjugated estrogens, A
Cataflam	diclofenac potassium	Centrum	vitamins; minerals
Catapres	clonidine HCl	cephalexin	Keflex
Cathflo Activase	alteplase (for catheter occlusions)	cephalexin HCl	Keftab
Caverject	alprostadil	cephalothin sodium (W)	Keflin (W)
CEA-SCAN	arcitumomab	cephapirin sodium (W)	Cefadyl (W)
Ceclor	cefaclor		
Cedax	ceftibuten	cephradine (W)	Velosef (W)
CeeNu	lomustine	Cephulac	lactulose
cefaclor	Ceclor	Ceptaz	ceftazidime
cefadroxil	Duricef	Cerebyx	fosphenytoin sodium
Cefadyl (W)	cephapirin sodium	Ceredase	alglucerase
cefamandole nafate (W)	Mandol (W)	Cerezyme	imiglucerase
cefazolin sodium	Ancef Kefzol (WA)	cerivastatin sodium (W)	Baycol (W)
cefdinir	Omnicef	Cernevit-12	multivitamins for infusion
cefditoren pivoxil	Spectracef	Cerubidine	daunorubicin HCl
		Cervidil	dinoprostone vaginal insert

Cesamet	nabilone
Cetacaine	benzocaine; tetracaine HCl
cetirizine HCl	Zyrtec
cetirizine HCL; pseudoephedrine HCl SR	Zyrtec-D
cetrorelix	Cetrotide
Cetrotide	cetrorelix
cetuximab	Erbitux
cevimeline HCl	Evoxac
Chantix	varenicline
Chirocaine	levobupivacaine
chloral hydrate	chloral hydrate
chlorambucil	Leukeran
chloramphenicol	Chloromycetin
chloramphenicol ophth (W)	Chloroptic ophth (W)
chlordiazepoxide HCl	Librium
chlordiazepoxide HCl; amitriptyline HCl	Limbitrol
chlorhexidine gluconate	Hibiclens PerioChip
chlorhexidine gluconate mouth rinse	Peridex
Chloromycetin	chloramphenicol
chloroprocaine HCl	Nesacaine
Chloroptic ophth (W)	chloramphenicol ophth (W)
chloroquine phosphate	Aralen
chlorothiazide	Diuril
chloroxine	Capitrol
chlorpheniramine maleate	Chlor-Trimeton
chlorpheniramine maleate SR	Teldrin
chlorpromazine	Thorazine
chlorpropamide	Diabinese
chlorthalidone	Hygroton
chlorthalidone; reserpine	Regroton
Chlor-Trimeton	chlorpheniramine maleate
chlorzoxazone 250 mg	Paraflex
chlorzoxazone 500 mg	Parafon Forte DSC
Cholebrine	iocetamic acid
Choledyl	oxtriphylline
cholestyramine	Questran
choline chloride inj	Intrachol
choline magnesium trisalicylate	Trilisate
Choloxin (W)	dextrothyroxine sodium (W)
chorionic gonadotropin	A.P.L.
choriogona- dotropin alfa	Ovidrel
Chronulac	lactulose
Chymodiactin	chymopapain
chymopapain	Chymodiactin
Cialis	tadalafil
Cibalith-S	lithium citrate
ciclopirox cream and lotion	Loprox
ciclopirox soln	Penlac Nail Lacquer
cidofovir	Vistide
cilostazol	Pletal
Ciloxan	ciprofloxacin ophth soln
cimetidine HCl	Tagamet
cinacalcet HCl	Sensipar
Cipro	ciprofloxacin HCl
ciprofloxacin HCl	Cipro
ciprofloxacin; hydrocortisone otic	Cipro HC Otic
ciprofloxacin ophth soln	Ciloxan
Cipro HC Otic	ciprofloxacin; hydrocortisone otic
cisapride (W)	Propulsid (W)
cisatracurium besylate	Nimbex
cisplatin	*cisplatin*
citalopram hydrobromide	Celexa
cladribine	Leustatin
Claforan	cefotaxime sodium
Clarinex	desloratadine
clarithromycin	Biaxin
clarithromycin SR	Biaxin XL
Claritin	loratadine
Claritin D	loratadine; pseudoephed- rine sulfate
clemastine fumarate	Tavist
Cleocin	clindamycin HCl
clidinium (W) bromide	Quarzan (W)
clidinium; chlordiaze- poxide	Librax
Climara	estradiol transdermal
clindamycin; benzoyl peroxide gel	BenzaClin
clindamycin HCl	Cleocin
clindamycin phosphate pledgets	Clindets

Clindets	clindamycin phosphate pledgets	colistimethate sodium	Coly-Mycin M
Clinimix E	amino acid with electrolytes in dextrose with calcium inj (various concentrations)	colistin sulfate; hydrocortisone, and neomycin otic soln	Coly-Mycin S
Clinoril	sulindac	collagen	Avitene
clioquinol	Vioform	hemostat	
clobetasol foam	Olux	collagenase	Santyl
clobetasol propionate gel	Clobevate	Collyrium	tetrahydrozoline HCl ophth
		Colomed	short chain fatty acids enema
Clobevate	clobetasol propionate gel	Coly-Mycin M	colistimethate sodium
		Coly-Mycin S	colistin sulfate; hydrocortisone, and neomycin otic soln
clofarabine	Clolar		
clofibrate (W)	Atromid-S (W)		
Clolar	clofarabine	CoLyte	polyethylene glycol-electrolyte soln
Clomid	clomiphene citrate		
clomiphene citrate	Clomid	CombiPatch	norethindrone acetate; estradiol transdermal
clomipramine HCl	Anafranil	Combivent	ipratropium bromide; albuterol sulfate
clonazepam	Klonopin	Combivir	lamivudine; zidovudine
clonidine HCl	Catapres	Combunox	oxycodone HCl, ibuprofen
clonidine HCl inj	Duraclon	Compazine	prochlorperazine
clopidogrel bisulfate	Plavix	Comtan	entacapone
		Comvax	Haemophilus b conjugate; Hepatitis B vaccine
clorazepate dipotassium	Tranxene		
		Concerta	methylphenidate HCl SR
Clorpactin WCS-90	oxychlorosene sodium	Condylox	podofilox gel
		conivaptan	Vaprisol
clotrimazole	Gyne-Lotrimin Lotrimin Mycelex	Copaxone	glatiramer acetate
		Cordarone	amiodarone HCl
		Coreg	carvedilol
clozapine	Clozaril	Corgard	nadolol
Clozaril	clozapine	Corlopam	fenoldopam mesylate
coagulation factor IX (recombinant)	BeneFix	Cortef	hydrocortisone
		corticorellin ovine triflutate	Acthrel
coagulation factor VII a (recombinant)	NovoSeven	corticotropin	Acthar
		cortisone acetate	Cortone Acetate
coal tar product	Zetar	Cortone Acetate	cortisone acetate
codeine phosphate; acetaminophen suspension	Capital w/ Codeine Suspension	Cortrosyn	cosyntropin
		Corvert	ibutilide fumarate
		Cosmegen	dactinomycin
		Cosopt	dorzolamide HCl; timolol maleate ophth soln
coenzyme Q10	UbiQGel		
Cogentin	benztropine mesylate	cosyntropin	Cortrosyn
Cognex	tacrine HCl	Cotazym	pancrelipase
Colace	docusate sodium	Cotazym-S	pancrelipase EC
Colazol	balsalazide disodium	Cotrim	sulfamethoxazole; trimethoprim
ColBENEMID (W)	probenecid; colchicine (W)	co-trimoxazole	Bactrim Cotrim Septra sulfamethoxazole; trimethoprim
colchicine	colchicine		
colesevelam HCl	Welchol		
Colestid	colestipol HCl		
colestipol HCl	Colestid	Coumadin	warfarin sodium

C
R℟

Covera HS	verapamil HCl SR bedtime formulation	Cytosar-U	cytarabine
		Cytotec	misoprostol
Cozaar	losartan potassium	Cytovene	ganciclovir
Crestor	rosuvastatin calcium	Cytoxan	cyclophosphamide
Crinone	progesterone gel		
Crixivan	indinavir		
CroFab	crotalidae polyvalent immune fab (ovine)	**D**	
cromolyn sodium	Gastrocrom		
	Nasalcrom	dacarbazine	DTIC-Dome
	Opticrom	daclizumab	Zenapax
crotalidae polyvalent immune fab (ovine)	CroFab	Dacogen	decitabine inj
		dactinomycin	Cosmegen
		Dalmane	flurazepam HCl
		dalteparin sodium	Fragmin
crotamiton	Eurax		
Cubicin	daptomycin	danaparoid sodium	Orgaran
Cuprimine	penicillamine		
Curosurf	poractant alpha intratracheal susp	danazol (W)	Danocrine (W)
		Danocrine (W)	danazol (W)
Cutivate	fluticasone propionate cream & ointment	Dantrium	dantrolene sodium
		dantrolene sodium	Dantrium
cyanocobalamin nasal gel	Nascobal		
		dapsone	dapsone
cyclobenzaprine HCl	Flexeril	daptomycin	Cubicin
		Daranide (W)	dichlorphenamide (W)
Cyclocort	amcinonide	Daraprim	pyrimethamine
Cyclogyl	cyclopentolate HCl	darbepoetin alfa	Aranesp
cyclopentolate HCl	Cyclogyl	darifenacin	Enablex
		Darvocet-N 100	propoxyphene napsylate; acetaminophen
cyclophospha-mide	Cytoxan		
	Neosar	Darvon	propoxyphene HCl
cycloserine	Seromycin	Darvon Compound 65	propoxyphene HCl; aspirin; caffeine
cyclosporine	Sandimmune		
cyclosporine capsules (modified) and oral soln	Neoral	dasatinib	Sprycel
		daunorubicin citrate liposomal	DaunoXome
		daunorubicin HCl	Cerubidine
cyclosporine capsules, (modified)	Gengraf		
		DaunoXome	daunorubicin citrate liposomal
cyclosporine ophth emulsion	Restasis	Daypro	oxaprozin
		DDAVP	desmopressin acetate
Cycrin	medroxyprogesterone acetate	Debrox	carbamide peroxide otic
		Decadron	dexamethasone
Cylert (WA)	pemoline	Deca-Durabolin	nandrolone decanoate
Cymbalta	duloxetine HCl	decitabine inj	Dacogen
Cypher stent	sirolimus-eluting stent	Declomycin	demeclocycline HCl
cyproheptadine HCl	Periactin	deferoxamine mesylate	Desferal
Cystadane	betaine anhydrous	delavirdine mesylate	Rescriptor
Cystospaz-M	hyoscyamine sulfate SR		
Cytadren	aminoglutethimide	Delestrogen	estradiol valerate
cytarabine	Cytosar-U	Deltasone	prednisone
cytarabine, liposomal inj	DepoCyt	Demadex	torsemide
		demecarium bromide (W)	Humorsol (W)
Cytomel	liothyronine sodium		

demeclocycline HCl	Declomycin
Demerol	meperidine HCl
Demser	metyrosine
Demulen	ethynodiol diacetate; ethinyl estradiol
Denavir	penciclovir cream
denileukin diftitox	Ontak
Depacon	valproate sodium inj
Depakene	valproic acid
Depakote	divalproex sodium
Depakote ER	divalproex sodium SR
DepoCyt	cytarabine, liposomal inj
DepoDur	morphine sulfate extended-release liposome inj
Depo-Medrol	methylprednisolone acetate SR
Depo-Provera	medroxyprogesterone acetate SR
Depo-Testosterone	testosterone cypionate SR
Desferal	deferoxamine mesylate
desflurane	Suprane
desipramine HCl	Norpramin
Desirudin	iprivask
desloratadine	Clarinex
desmopressin acetate	DDAVP
Desogen	desogestrel; ethinyl estradiol
desogestrel; ethinyl estradiol	Desogen Ortho-Cept
desogestrel and ethinyl estradiol; ethinyl estradiol	Mircette
desonide	Tridesilon
desoximetasone	Topicort
Desoxyn	methamphetamine HCl
Desyrel	trazodone HCl
Detrol	tolterodine tartrate
Detrol LA	tolterodine tartrate (SR)
dexamethasone	Decadron Hexadrol
dexamethasone-eluting stent	Dexamet stent
Dexamet stent	dexamethasone-eluting stent
dexchlorphenir-amine maleate SR	Polaramine Repetabs
Dexedrine	dextroamphetamine sulfate
dexfenfluramine HCl (W)	Redux (W)
Dexferrum	iron dextran inj

dexmedetomidine HCl inj	Precedex
dexmethyl-phenidate HCl	Focalin
dexrazoxane	Zinecard
dextro-amphetamine sulfate	Dexedrine
dextrothyroxine sodium (W)	Choloxin (W)
D.H.E. 45	dihydroergotamine mesylate inj
DiaBeta	glyburide
Diabinese	chlorpropamide
Diamox	acetazolamide
Diapid (W)	lypressin (W)
Diastat	diazepam rectal gel
diazepam	Valium
diazepam emulsified inj	Dizac
diazepam rectal gel	Diastat
diazoxide	Hyperstat
Dibenzyline	phenoxybenzamine HCl
dibucaine	Nupercainal
dichlorphena-mide (W)	Daranide (W)
diclofenac gel	Solaraze
diclofenac potassium	Cataflam
diclofenac sodium	Voltaren
diclofenac sodium; misoprostol	Arthrotec
diclofenac sodium SR	Voltaren-XR
dicloxacillin sodium	Dynapen
dicyclomine HCl	Bentyl
didanosine	Videx
didanosine SR	Videx EC
Didronel	etidronate disodium
diethylcarbama-zine citrate	Hetrazan
diethylpropion HCl	Tenuate
Differin	adapalene
diflorasone diacetate	Florone
Diflucan	fluconazole
diflunisal	Dolobid
Digibind	digoxin immune fab
digoxin	Lanoxin
digoxin capsules	Lanoxicaps
digoxin immune fab	Digibind

D
R̸

dihydroergota-mine mesylate inj	D.H.E. 45	Dizac	diazepam emulsified inj
		dobutamine HCl	Dobutrex
		Dobutrex	dobutamine HCl
dihydroergota-mine mesylate nasal spray	Migranol	docetaxel	Taxotere
		docosanol cream	Avanir
		docusate sodium	Colace
dihydrotestoster-one transdermal	Androge12DHT	docusate sodium; casanthranol	Peri-Colace
		dofetilide	Tikosyn
Dilacor XR	diltiazem HCl SR	dolasetron mesylate	Anzemet
Dilantin	phenytoin		
Dilaudid	hydromorphone HCl	Dolobid	diflunisal
diltiazem HCl	Cardizem	Dolophine	methadone HCl
diltiazem HCl SR	Cardizem CD	Domeboro	aluminum acetate
	Cartia XR	donepezil HCl	Aricept
	Dilacor XR	Donnatal (W)	belladonna alkaloids; phenobarbital
	Tiazac		
diltiazem maleate SR	Tiamate	dopamine HCl	Intropin (WA)
		Dopar	levodopa
dimenhydrinate	Dramamine	Dopram	doxapram HCl
dimercaprol	BAL in Oil	dornase alpha	Pulmozyme
Dimetane	brompheniramine maleate	dorzolamide HCI	Trusopt
dinoprostone gel	Prepidil		
dinoprostone vaginal insert	Cervidil	dorzolamide HCl; timolol maleate ophth soln	Cosopt
dinoprostone vaginal suppositories	Prostin E2		
Diovan	valsartan	Dostinex	cabergoline
Diovan HCT	valsartan; hydrochloro-thiazide	Dovonex	calcipotriene cream
		doxacurium chloride	Nuromax
Dipentum	olsalazine sodium		
diphenhydramine HCl	Benadryl	doxapram HCl	Dopram
		doxazosin mesylate	Cardura
diphenoxylate HCl; atropine sulfate	Lomotil	doxepin HCl	Adapin Sinequan
		doxepin HCl cream	Prudoxin
diphtheria, tetanus, and acellular pertussis (TdaP) vaccine (adult type)	Adacel	doxercalciferol	Hectorol
		Doxil	doxorubicin, liposomal
		doxorubicin HCl	Adriamycin Rubex
dipivefrin	Propine		
Diprivan	propofol	doxorubicin, liposomal	Doxil
Diprosone	betamethasone dipropionate		
dipyridamole	Persantine	*doxycycline hyclate*	Vibramycin
dirithromycin	Dynabac		
Disalcid	salsalate	doxycycline hyclate 20 mg tab & cap	Periostat
disopyramide phosphate	Norpace		
disulfiram	Antabuse	doxycycline hyclate gel	Atridox
Ditropan	oxybutynin chloride		
Diulo (WA)	metolazone	Dramamine	dimenhydrinate
Diuril	chlorothiazide	Drisdol	ergocalciferol
divalproex sodium	Depakote	Dristan Long Lasting	oxymetazoline HCl
divalproex sodium SR	Depakote ER	Drixoral Syrup	pseudoephedrine HCl; bromphiramine maleate

dronabinol | Marinol
droperidol | Inapsine
drospirenone; ethinyl estradiol | Yasmin
drotrecogin alfa | Xigris
Droxia | hydroxyurea
DTIC-Dome | dacarbazine
Dulcolax | bisacodyl
duloxetine HCl | Cymbalta
Durabolin (W) | nandrolone phenpropionate (W)
Duraclon | clonidine HCl inj
Duragesic | fentanyl transdermal
Duramorph | morphine sulfate inj
Duranest | etidocaine HCl
Duricef | cefadroxil
dutasteride | Avodart
Dyazide | triamterene 37.5 mg; hydrochlorothiazide 25 mg
Dymelor | acetohexamide
Dynabac | dirithromycin
DynaCirc | isradipine
Dynapen | dicloxacillin sodium
dyphylline | Lufyllin
Dyrenium | triamterene

E

EchoGen | perflenapent emulsion
echothiophate iodide (W) | Phospholine Iodide (W)
Ecotrin | aspirin EC
Edecrin | ethacrynic acid
edetate disodium | Endrate
Edex | alprostadil inj
edrophonium chloride | Tensilon
E.E.S. 400 | erythromycin ethylsuccinate
efalizumab | Raptiva
efaproxiral | Efaproxyn
Efaproxyn | efaproxiral
efavirenz | Sustiva
efavirenz, emtricitabine, and tenofovir | Atripla
Effexor | venlafaxine HCl
Effexor XR | venlafaxine HCl SR
eflornithine HCl cream | Vaniqa
Efudex | fluorouracil cream; soln
Elavil | amitriptyline HCl
Eldepryl | selegiline HCl
Eldisine | vindesine sulfate
Elestat | epinastine

eletriptan hydrobromide | Relpax
Elidel | pimecrolimus cream
Eligard | leuprolide acetate
Elitek | rasburicase
Elixophyllin | theophylline
Ellence | epirubicin HCl
Elmiron | pentosan polysulfate sodium
Elocon | mometasone furoate topical
Eloxatin | oxaliplatin
Elspar | asparaginase
Emadine | emedastine difumarate opthth soln
Emcyt | estramustine phosphate sodium
emedastine difumarate opthth soln | Emadine
Emend | aprepitant
EMLA Cream | lidocaine; prilocaine cream
Empirin with codeine #3 and #4 | aspirin 325 mg with codeine phosphate (30 and 60 mg)
emtricitabine | Emtriva
emtricitabine, efavirenz, and tenofovir | Atripla
emtricitabine; tenofovir disoproxil | Truvada
Emtriva | emtricitabine
E-Mycin | erythromycin
Enablex | darifenacin
enalapril maleate | Vasotec
enalapril maleate; diltiazem malate | Teczem
enalapril maleate; felodipine SR | Lexxel
enalapril maleate; hydrochlorothiazide | Vaseretic
Enbrel | etanercept
encainide HCl | Enkaid
Endep | amitriptyline HCl
Endocet | oxycodone HCl; acetaminophen
Endrate | edetate disodium
Enduron | methyclothiazide
enflurane | Ethrane
enfuvirtide | Fuzeon
Engerix-B | hepatitis B vaccine
Enkaid | encainide HCl

enoxaparin sodium	Lovenox
entacapone	Comtan
entecavir	Baraclude
Entex LA	phenylpropanolamine HCl; guaifenesin SR
Entocort EC	budesonide capsule SR
epinastine	Elestat
epinephrine	Adrenalin
epinephrine racemic	Vaponefrin
epirubicin HCl	Ellence
Epivir	lamivudine
Epivir HBV	lamivudine
eplerenone	Inspra
epoetin alfa	Epogen Procrit
Epogen	epoetin alfa
epoprostenol sodium	Flolan
eprosartan mesylate	Teveten
eprosartan mesylate; hydrochloro-thiazide	Teveten HCT
eptifibatide	Integrilin
Epzicom	lamivudine; abacavir sulfate
Equanil (WA)	meprobamate
Eraxis	anidulafungin IV
Erbitux	cetuximab
Ergamisol (W)	levamisole HCl (W)
ergocalciferol	Calciferol Drisdol
ergoloid mesylates	Hydergine
ergotamine tartrate; caffeine	Cafergot
ergotamine tartrate	Ergostat
Ergotrate	ergonovine maleate
erlotinib	Tarceva
Ertaczo	sertaconazole
ertapenem sodium	Invanz
Ery-Tab	erythromycin EC
Erythrocin Stearate	erythromycin stearate
erythromycin	E-Mycin
erythromycin base coated particles	PCE Dispertab
erythromycin; benzoyl peroxide topical gel	Benzamycin

erythromycin EC	Ery-Tab
erythromycin estolate	Ilosone
erythromycin ethylsuccinate	E.E.S. 400
erythromycin ethylsuccinate; sulfisoxazole	Pediazole
erythromycin stearate	Erythrocin Stearate
escitalopram oxalate	Lexapro
Esclim	estradiol transdermal
Eserine Sulfate	physostigmine ophth ointment
Esidrix (WA)	hydrochlorothiazide
Esimil	guanethidine monosulfate; hydrochlorothiazide
Eskalith	lithium carbonate
esmolol HCl	Brevibloc
esomeprazole magnesium	Nexium
estazolam	ProSom
Estinyl	ethinyl estradiol
Estrace	estradiol
Estraderm	estradiol transdermal
estradiol	Estrace
estradiol hemihydrate vaginal tab	Vagifem
estradiol transdermal	Alora Climara Esclim Estraderm FemPatch Menostar Vivelle
estradiol vaginal ring	Estring
estradiol valerate	Delestrogen
estramustine phosphate sodium	Emcyt
Estratest	estrogens, esterified; methyltestosterone
Estratest H.S.	estrogens, esterified; methyltestosterone, half strength
Estring	estradiol vaginal ring
estrogens, conjugated	Premarin
estrogens conjugate, A synthetic	Cenestin
estrogens, conjugated; medroxyproges-terone acetate	Premphase Prempro

estrogens, esterified; methyltestosterone — Estratest

estrogens, esterified methyltestosterone, half strength — Estratest H.S.

estropipate — Ogen

Estrostep — norethindrone acetate; ethinyl estradiol

eszopiclone — Lunesta

etanercept — Enbrel

ethacrynic acid — Edecrin

ethambutol HCl — Myambutol

ethchlorvynol (W) — Placidyl (W)

Ethezyme — papain; urea oint

ethinyl estradiol — Estinyl

ethinyl estradiol; levonorgestrel (91 day cycle) — Seasonale

ethionamide — Trecator-SC

Ethmozine — moricizine

ethopropazine HCl — Parsidol

ethosuximide — Zarontin

Ethrane — enflurane

ethyl chloride — ethyl chloride

ethynodiol diacetate; ethinyl estradiol — Demulen

Ethyol — amifostine

etidocaine HCl — Duranest

etidronate disodium — Didronel

etodolac — Lodine

etodolac SR — Lodine XL

etomidate — Amidate

etonogestrel; ethinyl estradiol vagina ring — NuvaRing

etonogestrel implant — Implanon

Etopophos — etoposide phosphate diethanolate

etoposide — VePesid

etoposide phosphate diethanolate — Etopophos

Etrafon — perphenazine; amitriptyline HCl

Eulexin (W) — flutamide (W)

Eurax — crotamiton

Euthroid (WA) — liotrix

Eutonyl — pargyline HCl

Evista — raloxifene HCl

Evoxac — cevimeline HCl

Exelon — rivastigmine tartrate

exemestane — Aromasin

exenatide inj — Byetta

exisulind — Aposyn

Ex-Lax — sennosides

Extraneal — icodextrin 7.5% with electrolyte peritoneal dialysis soln

ezetimibe — Zetia

ezetimibe; simvastatin — Vytorin

F

Fabrazyme — agalsidase beta

Factive — gemifloxacin mesylate

factor IX, concentrate — BeneFix

Factrel — gonadorelin HCl

famciclovir — Famvir

famotidine — Pepcid

famotidine, oral disintegrating tablet — Pepcid RPD

Famvir — famciclovir

Fansidar — sulfadoxine; pyrimethamine

Fareston — toremifene citrate

Faslodex — fulvestrant

Fastin — phentermine HCl

fat emulsion — Intralipid
Liposyn II and III

felbamate — Felbatol

Felbatol — felbamate

Feldene — piroxicam

felodipine — Plendil

Femara — letrozole

Femhrt — norethindrone acetate; ethinyl estradiol

FemPatch — estradiol transdermal

fenfluramine HCl (W) — Pondimin (W)

fenofibrate — Tricor

fenoldopam mesylate — Corlopam

fenoprofen calcium — Nalfon

fentanyl citrate — Sublimaze

fentanyl citrate; droperidol — Innovar

Fentanyl Oralet — fentanyl transmucosal

fentanyl transdermal — Duragesic

fentanyl transmucosal — Actiq
Fentanyl Oralet

Feosol	ferrous sulfate	fluorescein	Fluor-I-Strip
Fer-In-Sol	ferrous sulfate	sodium strips	
Fergon	ferrous gluconate	Fluorescite	fluorescein sodium soln
Feridex	ferumoxide HCl	fluorometholone	FML
Ferrlecit	sodium ferric gluconate	Fluoroplex	fluorouracil cream; soln
	complex in sucrose inj	*fluorouracil inj*	*fluorouracil inj*
ferrous gluconate	Fergon	fluorouracil	Efudex
ferrous sulfate	Feosol	cream; soln	Fluoroplex
	Fer-In-Sol	Fluothane	halothane
ferrous sulfate	SlowFe	fluoxetine HCl	Prozac
SR			Sarafem
Fertinex	urofollitropin for inj	fluoxymesterone	Halotestin
ferumoxetil oral	Gastromark	fluphenazine HCl	Permitil
suspension			Prolixin
ferumoxide HCl	Feridex	flurazepam HCl	Dalmane
fexofenadine	Allegra	flurbiprofen	Ansaid
HCl		flutamide (W)	Eulexin (W)
filgrastim	Neupogen	fluticasone	Flonase
finasteride	Propecia 1 mg tablet	propionate	Flovent (WA)
	Proscar 5 mg tablet	spray	
Finevin	azelaic cream	fluticasone	Cutivate
Fioricet	butalbital; acetaminophen;	propionate	
	caffeine	cream &	
Fiorinal	butalbital; aspirin; caffeine	ointment	
Flagyl	metronidazole	fluticasone	Advair Diskus
Flagyl ER	metronidazole SR	propionate;	
flavocoxid	Limbrel	salmeterol	
flavoxate HCl	Urispas	inhalation	
Flaxedil	gallamine triethiodide	powder	
flecainide acetate	Tambocor	fluvastatin	Lescol
Flexeril	cyclobenzaprine HCl	sodium	
Flolan	epoprostenol sodium	fluvoxamine	Luvox
Flomax	tamsulosin HCl	maleate	
Flonase	fluticasone propionate spray	FML	fluorometholone
Florinef	fludrocortisone acetate	Focalin	dexmethylphenidate HCl
Florone	diflorasone diacetate	Folex PFS	methotrexate inj
Floropryl	isoflurophate	*folic acid*	Folvite
Florotag	synopinine	Follistim	follitropin beta
Flovent (WA)	fluticasone propionate spray	follitropin alfa	Gonal-F
Floxin	ofloxacin	follitropin beta	Follistim
Floxin Otic	ofloxacin otic soln	Folvite	folic acid
floxuridine	FUDR	fomepizole	Antizol
fluconazole	Diflucan	fomivirsen	Vitravene
flucytosine	Ancobon	sodium inj	
Fludara	fludarabine phosphate	fondaparinux	Arixtra
fludarabine	Fludara	sodium	
phosphate		Foradil	formoterol fumarate
fludrocortisone	Florinef	Forane	isoflurane
acetate		formoterol	Foradil
Flumadine	rimantadine	fumarate	
flumazenil	Romazicon	Fortaz	ceftazidime
flunisolide	Aero Bid	Forteo	teriparatide
fluocinolone	Synalar	Fortovase	saquinavir soft gel capsule
acetonide		Fosamax	alendronate sodium
fluocinonide	Lidex	fosamprenavir	Lexiva
Fluor-I-Strip	fluorescein sodium strips	calcium	
fluorescein	Fluorescite	foscarnet	Foscavir
sodium soln		Foscavir	foscarnet

F
Rx

fosfomycin tromethamine — Monurol
fosinopril sodium — Monopril
fosphenytoin sodium — Cerebyx
Fosrenol — lanthanum carbonate
Fragmin — dalteparin sodium
Frova — frovatriptan succinate
frovatriptan succinate — Frova
FUDR — floxuridine
fulvestrant — Faslodex
Fulvicin P/G — griseofulvin
Fungizone — amphotericin B
Furacin — nitrofurazone
furosemide — Lasix
Fuzeon — enfuvirtide

G

gabapentin — Neurontin
Gabitril — tiagabine HCl
gadoteridol — ProHance
gadoversetamide — OptiMark
galantamine HBr — Razadyne (formerly called Reminyl)
gallamine triethiodide — Flaxedil
gallium nitrate — Ganite
galsulfase — Naglazyme
Galzin — zinc acetate
Gamimune N — immune globulin intravenous
Gammagard S/D — immune globulin intravenous
ganciclovir — Cytovene
ganciclovir ophthalmic implant — Vitrasert
ganirelix acetate — Antagon
Ganite — gallium nitrate
Gantanol (W) — sulfamethoxazole (W)
Garamycin — *gentamicin sulfate*
Gastrocrom — cromolyn sodium
Gastromark — ferumoxetil oral suspension
gatifloxacin — Tequin
gatifloxacin ophth soln — Zymar
gefitinib — Iressa
gemcitabine HCl — Gemzar
gemfibrozil — Lopid
gemifloxacin mesylate — Factive

gemtuzumab ozogamicin — Mylotarg
Gemzar — gemcitabine HCl
GenEsa — arbutamine HCl
Gengraf — cyclosporine capsules, (modified)
Genotropin — somatropin for inj
gentamicin sulfate — Garamycin
Geocillin — carbenicillin
Geodon — ziprasidone HCl
Geref — sermorelin acetate
glatiramer acetate — Copaxone
Gleevec — imatinib mesylate
Gliadel — carmustine implantable wafer
glimepiride — Amaryl
glipizide — Glucotrol
glipizide SR — Glucotrol XL
glipizide; metformin — Metaglip
GlucaGen — glucagon (rDNA origin)
glucagon — glucagon
glucagon (rDNA origin) — GlucaGen
Glucophage — metformin HCl
Glucophage XR — metformin HCl SR
Glucotrol — glipizide
Glucotrol XL — glipizide SR
Glucovance — glyburide; metformin HCl
glyburide — DiaBeta
Micronase
glyburide; metformin HCl — Glucovance
glyburide micronized — Glynase
glycerin ophth soln — Ophthalgan
glycopyrrolate — Robinul
Glynase — glyburide micronized
Glyset — miglitol
gold sodium thiomalate — Aurolate
GoLYTELY — polyethylene glycol-electrolyte soln
gonadorelin HCl — Factrel
Gonal-F — follitropin alfa
goserelin acetate implant — Zoladex
graftskin — Apligraf
granisetron HCl — Kytril
grepafloxacin HCl (W) — Raxar (W)
Grifulvin V (W) — griseofulvin (W)
griseofulvin (W) — Fulvicin P/G (W)
Grifulvin V

guaifenesin	Organidin NR
	Robitussin
guaifenesin;	Robitussin A-C
codeine	Tussi-Organidin
phosphate	NR
guaifenesin;	Robitussin-DM
dextromethor-	
phan	
guanabenz	Wytensin
acetate	
guanadrel sulfate	Hylorel
guanethidine	Ismelin (W)
monosulfate (W)	
guanethidine	Esimil
monosulfate;	
hydrochlorothi-	
azide	
guanfacine HCl	Tenex
Gynazole	butoconazole nitrate vaginal
	cream
Gyne-Lotrimin	clotrimazole

H

Habitrol	nicotine transdermal system
Haemophilus b	ActHIB/Tripedia
conjugate	
vaccine	
reconstituted	
with	
diphtheria and	
tetanus toxoids	
and acellular	
pertussis	
vaccine	
adsorbed	
Haemophilus b	Comvax
conjugate;	
Hepatitis B	
vaccine	
haemophilus b	Hib-Immune (W)
vaccine	HibTITER
	PedvaxHIB
	ProHIBiT
halcinonide	Halog
Halcion	triazolam
Haldol	haloperidol
Halfan	halofantrine HCl
halofantrine HCl	Halfan
Halog	halcinonide
haloperidol	Haldol
haloprogin	Halotex
Halotestin	fluoxymesterone
Halotex	haloprogin
halothane	Fluothane

Havrix	hepatitis A vaccine,
	inactivated
Healon	sodium hyaluronate
Hectorol	doxercalciferol
Helidac	bismuth subsalicylate;
	metronidazole;
	tetracycline HCl
heparin sodium	*heparin sodium*
hepatitis A	Twinrix
inactivated;	
hepatitis B	
(recombinant)	
vaccine	
hepatitis A	Havrix
vaccine,	Vaqta
inactivated	
hepatitis B	NABI-HB
immune	
globulin	
(human)	
hepatitis B	Engerix-B
vaccine	Recombivax HB
Hepsera	adefovir dipivoxil
Herceptin	trastuzumab
Herplex (W)	idoxuridine (W)
Hespan	hetastarch
hetastarch	Hespan
hetastarch in	Hextend
lactated	
electrolyte inj	
Hetrazan	diethylcarbamazine citrate
Hexadrol	dexamethasone
Hexalen	altretamine
Hextend	hetastarch in lactated
	electrolyte inj
Hib-Immune (WA)	haemophilus b vaccine
Hibiclens	chlorhexidine gluconate
HibTITER	haemophilus b vaccine
Hiprex	methenamine hippurate
Hismanal (W)	astemizole (W)
Hivid	zalcitabine
homatropine	Isopto
hydrobromide	Homatropine
ophth	
Humalog	insulin, lispro (human)
Humalog	insulin lispro
Mix75/25	protamine susp 75%;
	insulin lispro inj 25%
	[rDNA origin]
Humatin	paromomycin sulfate
Humatrope	somatropin
Humira	adalimumab
Humorsol (W)	demecarium bromide (W)
Humulin 70/30	isophane insulin suspension
	70%, insulin
	inj 30% (human)
Humulin L	insulin zinc suspension
	(Lente) (human)

H
R⃓

Humulin N	isophane insulin suspension (NPH) (human)	hydromorphone HCl SR (W)	Palladone XL (W)
Humulin R	insulin inj (human)	Hydromox (W)	quinethazone (W)
Humulin U Ultralente	insulin zinc suspension, extended, (human)	hydroquinone topical susp	Alustra
Hurricane	benzocaine	hydroquinone; tretinoin; fluocinolone cream	Tri-Luma
Hyalgan	sodium hyaluronate		
hyaluronidase	Wydase		
Hycamtin	topotecan HCl	hydroxychloro- quine sulfate	Plaquenil
Hydergine	ergoloid mesylates		
hydralazine HCl	Apresoline	hydroxyurea	Droxia Hydrea
hydralazine HCl; hydrochlorothi- azide	Apresazide	hydroxyzine HCl	Atarax (WA)
hydralazine; hydrochlorothi- azide; reserpine	Ser-Ap-Es	hydroxyzine pamoate	Vistaril
		Hygroton	chlorthalidone
		hylan G-F 20	Synvisc
Hydrea	hydroxyurea	Hylorel	guanadrel sulfate
hydrochlorothi- azide	Esidrix (WA) HydroDIURIL Microzide Oretic (WA)	hyoscyamine sulfate orally disintegrating tab	NuLev
hydrocodone bitartrate; acetaminophen	Anexsia 5/500 Anexsia 7.5/650 Lorcet 10/650 Lorcet-HD (5/500) Lorcet plus (7.5/650) Lortab 2.5/500; 5/500; 7.5/500; 10/500 Norco Vicodin Vicodin ES Zydone 5/400, 7.5/400, 10/400	hyoscyamine sulfate SR	Cystospaz-M Levbid
		Hyperab (W)	rabies immune globulin, human
		Hyperstat	diazoxide
		Hyper-Tet (W)	tetanus immune globulin (human) (W)
		Hytrin	terazosin HCl
		Hyzaar	losartan potassium; hydrochlorothiazide
hydrocodone bitartrate 7.5 mg; ibuprofen 200 mg	Vicoprofen		

I-J

hydrocodone polistirex; chlorphenira- mine	Tussionex	ibandronate	Boniva
		ibritumomab tiuxetan	Zevalin
hydrocortisone	Cortef Hydrocortone	*ibuprofen*	Advil Motrin Nuprin
hydrocortisone buteprate cream	Pandel	ibutilide fumarate	Corvert
hydrocortisone sodium succinate	Solu-Cortef	icodextrin 7.5% with electro- lyte peritoneal dialysis soln	Extraneal
Hydrocortone	hydrocortisone	Idamycin	idarubicin
HydroDIURIL	hydrochlorothiazide	idarubicin	Idamycin
hydroflumethia- zide	Saluron	idoxuridine (W)	Herplex (W)
		IFEX	ifosfamide
hydromorphone HCl	Dilaudid	ifosfamide	IFEX
		iloprost	Ventavis

Ilosone	erythromycin estolate
Imagent GI	perflubron
imatinib mesylate	Gleevec
imciromab pentetate	Myoscint
Imdur	isosorbide mononitrate SR
imiglucerase	Cerezyme .
imipenem-cilastatin sodium	Primaxin
imipramine HCl	Tofranil
imiquimod cream	Aldara
Imitrex	sumatriptan
immune globulin intravenous	Gamimune N Gammagard S/D Sandoglobulin
Imodium	loperamide HCl
Imogam	rabies immune globulin, human
Implanon	etonogestrel implant
Imuran	azathioprine
inamrinone	Inocor
Inapsine	droperidol
indapamide	Lozol
Inderal	propranolol HCl
Inderide	propranolol HCl; hydrochlorothiazide
indinavir	Crixivan
indium In-111 pentetreotide	OctreoScan
Indocin	indomethacin
indomethacin	Indocin
Infasurf	calfactant intratracheal susp
INFeD	iron dextran inj
Infergen	interferon alfacon-1
infliximab	Remicade
Innohep	tinzaparin sodium
Innovar	fentanyl citrate; droperidol
Inocor	inamrinone
INOmax	nitric oxide for inhalation
Inspra	eplerenone
insulin aspart (rDNA origin)	NovoLog
insulin detemir [rDNA origin]	Levemir
insulin glargine (rDNA origin)	Lantus
insulin glulisine [rDNA origin]	Apidra
insulin inj (human)	Humulin R Novolin R Velosulin Human
insulin lispro (human)	Humalog

insulin lispro protamine susp 75%; insulin lispro inj 25% [rDNA origin]	Humalog Mix75/25
insulin zinc suspension (Lente) (human)	Humulin L Novolin L (WA)
insulin zinc suspension, extended (beef)	Ultralente U
insulin zinc suspension, extended, (human)	Humulin U Ultralente
Integrilin	eptifibatide
interferon alfa-2a	Roferon-A
interferon alfa-2b	Intron A
interferon alfa-n[1] lymphoblastoid	Wellferon
interferon alfa-n3 (human leukocyte derived)	Alferon
interferon alfacon-1	Infergen
interferon beta-la	Avonex Rebif
interferon beta-1b	Betaseron
interferon gamma 1-b	Actimmune
Intrachol	choline chloride inj
Intralipid	fat emulsion
Intron A	interferon alfa-2b
Intropin (WA)	dopamine HCl
Invanz	ertapenem sodium
Inversine	mecamylamine HCl
Invirase	saquinavir mesylate
iocetamic acid	Cholebrine
iodamide meglumine	Renovue 65
iodixanol	Visipaque
iohexol	Omnipaque
Ionamin	phentermine resin
iopamidol	Isovue
iopanoic acid	Telepaque
iopromide	Ultravist
iotrolan	Osmovist
ioversol	Optiray
ioxilan	Oxilan
Ipol	poliovirus vaccine inactivated
ipratropium bromide	Atrovent

I R

ipratropium bromide; albuterol sulfate	Combivent
iprivask	Desirudin
irbesartan	Avapro
irbesartan; hydrochlorothi- azide	Avalide
Iressa	gefitinib
irinotecan HCl	Camptosar
iron dextran inj	INFeD Dexferrum
iron sucrose inj	Venofer
Ismelin	guanethidine monosulfate
ISMO	isosorbide mononitrate
isocarboxazid	Marplan
isoetharine HCl aerosol	Bronkometer
isoetharine HCl soln	Bronkosol
isoflurane	Forane
isoflurophate	Floropry l
isoniazid	Nydrazid
isoniazid; rifampin	Rifamate
isophane insulin suspension (NPH) (human)	Humulin N Novolin N
isophane insulin suspension (NPH) 70%, insulin inj 30% (human)	Humulin 70/30 Novolin 70/30
isoproterenol HCl	Isuprel
Isoptin	verapamil HCl
Isopto Carbachol	carbachol ophth
Isopto Carpine	pilocarpine HCl ophth
Isopto Homatropine	homatropine hydrobromide ophth
Isopto Hyoscine	scopolamine hydrobromide ophth
Isordil	isosorbide dinitrate
isosorbide dinitrate	Isordil
isosorbide dinitrate; hydralazine	BiDil
isosorbide mononitrate	ISMO
isosorbide mononitrate SR	Imdur
isotretinoin	Accutane
Isovue	iopamidol
isoxsuprine HCl	Vasodilan
isradipine	DynaCirc
Isuprel	isoproterenol HCl

itraconazole	Sporanox
ivermectin	Stromectol
IvyBlock	bentoquatam

K

Kadian	morphine sulfate SR
Kaletra	lopinavir; ritonavir
kanamycin sulfate	Kantrex
Kantrex	kanamycin sulfate
Kaon	potassium gluconate
Kaon-Cl	potassium chloride SR
Kayexalate	polystyrene sulfonate sodium
K-Dur	potassium chloride SR
Keflex	cephalexin
Keflin (W)	cephalothin sodium (W)
Keftab	cephalexin HCl
Kefurox	cefuroxime sodium
Kefzol (WA)	cefazolin sodium
Kemadrin	procyclidine HCl
Kenalog	triamcinolone acetonide
Kepivance	palifermin
Keppra	levetiracetam
Kerlone	betaxolol
Ketalar	ketamine HCl
ketamine HCL	Ketalar
Ketek	telithromycin
ketoconazole	Nizoral
ketoprofen (W)	Orudis (W)
ketoprofen SR	Oruvail
ketorolac tromethamine	Toradol
ketorolac tromethamine ophth	Acular
ketotifen fumarate ophth soln	Zaditor
Kineret	anakinra
Klaron	sodium sulfacetamide lotion
Klonopin	clonazepam
Klor-Con 10	potassium chloride SR
K-Lyte	potassium bicarbonate; potassium citrate effervescent
K-Lyte/Cl	potassium chloride potassium bicarbonate effervescent
Kogenate	antihemophilic factor (recombinant)
Kolyum	potassium chloride; potassium gluconate
Konsyl-D	psyllium
Kwell (WA)	lindane
Kytril	granisetron HCl

L

labetalol HCl — Normodyne
Trandate

Lac-Hydrin — lactic acid; ammonium lactate lotion

lactic acid; ammonium lactate lotion — Lac-Hydrin

lactulose — Cephulac
Chronulac

Lamictal — lamotrigine

Lamisil — terbinafine HCl

lamivudine — Epivir
Epivir HBV

lamivudine; abacavir sulfate — Epzicom

lamivudine; zidovudine — Combivir

lamivudine; zidovudine; abacavir sulfate — Trizivir

lamotrigine — Lamictal

Lanoxicaps — digoxin capsules

Lanoxin — digoxin

lansoprazole — Prevacid

lansoprazole; amoxicillin; clarithromycin — Prevpac

lanthanum carbonate — Fosrenol

Lantus — insulin glargine (rDNA origin)

Lariam — mefloquine HCl

Larodopa — levodopa

laronidase — Aldurazyme

Lasix — furosemide

latanoprost — Xalatan

leflunomide — Arava

lepirudin — Refludan

Lescol — fluvastatin sodium

letrozole — Femara

leucovorin calcium — Wellcovorin (WA)

Leukeran — chlorambucil

Leukine — sargramostim

leuprolide acetate — Eligard
Lupron

leuprolide acetate implant — Viadur

Leustatin — cladribine

levalbuterol HCl inhalation soln — Xopenex

levamisole HCl (W) — Ergamisol (W)

Levaquin — levofloxacin

Levbid — hyoscyamine sulfate SR

Levemir — insulin detemir [rDNA origin]

levetiracetam — Keppra

Levitra — vardenafil HCl

Levlite — levonorgestrel; ethinyl estradiol

levobupivacaine — Chirocaine

levocabastine HCl ophth susp (W) — Livostin (W)

Levo-Dromoran — levorphanol tartrate

levobunolol HCl — Betagan

levocarnitine — Carnitor

levodopa — Dopar
Larodopa

levodopa; carbidopa — Parcopa
Sinemet

levodopa; carbidopa SR — Sinemet CR

levodopa, carbidopa, and entacapone — Stalevo

levofloxacin — Levaquin

levofloxacin ophth soln — Quixin

levomethadyl acetate HCl (W) — Orlaam (W)

levonorgestrel — Plan B

levonorgestrel; ethinyl estradiol — Alesse
Levlite
Nordette
Preven Emergency Contraceptive Kit
Tri-Levlen
Triphasil

levonorgestrel implant (W) — Norplant (W)

levonorgestrel-releasing intrauterine system — Mirena

Levophed — norepinephrine bitartrate

levorphanol tartrate — Levo-Dromoran

levothyroxine sodium — Levoxyl
Synthroid

Levoxyl — levothyroxine sodium

Levulan Kerastick — aminolevulinic acid HCl topical soln

Lexapro — escitalopram oxalate

Lexiva — fosamprenavir calcium

Lexxel	enalapril maleate; felodipine SR	lopinavir; ritonavir	Kaletra
Librax	clidinium; chlordiaz-epoxide	Lopressor	metoprolol tartrate
		Loprox	ciclopirox cream and lotion
Librium	chlordiazepoxide HCl	Lorabid	loracarbef
Lidex	fluocinonide	loracarbef	Lorabid
lidocaine HCl	Xylocaine HCl	loratadine	Claritin
lidocaine patch	Lidoderm	loratadine; pseudoephe-drine sulfate	Claritin D
lidocaine; prilocaine cream	EMLA Cream		
Lidoderm	lidocaine patch	lorazepam	Ativan
Limbitrol	chlordiazepoxide HCl; amitriptyline HCl	Lorcet (various combinations)	hydrocodone bitartrate; acetaminophen
Limbrel	flavocoxid	Lortab (various combinations)	hydrocodone bitartrate; acetaminophen
Lincocin	lincomycin HCl		
lincomycin HCl	Lincocin	losartan potassium	Cozaar
lindane	Kwell (WA) lindane	losartan potassium; hydrochlorothi-azide	Hyzaar
linezolid	Zyvox		
Lioresal	baclofen		
liothyronine sodium	Cytomel	Lotemax	loteprednol etabonate ophth susp
liothyronine sodium inj	Triostat	Lotensin	benazepril HCl
liotrix	Thyrolar	loteprednol etabonate ophth susp	Alrex Lotemax
Lipitor	atorvastatin calcium		
liposomal am-photericin B	AmBisome	Lotrel	amlodipine besylate; benazepril HCl
Liposyn II and III	fat emulsion	Lotrimin	clotrimazole
lisinopril	Prinivil Zestril	Lotrisone	betamethasone; clotrimazole cream
lisinopril; hydrochloro-thiazide	Zestoretic	Lotronex (W)	alosetron (W)
		lovastatin	Mevacor
lithium carbonate	Eskalith Lithobid	lovastatin; niacin	Advicor
lithium citrate	Cibalith-S	Lovenox	enoxaparin sodium
Lithobid	lithium carbonate	loxapine succinate	Loxitane
Lithostat	acetohydroxamic acid	Loxitane	loxapine succinate
Livostin (W)	levocabastine HCl ophth susp (W)	Lozol	indapamide
		Lucentis	ranibizumab inj
Lodine	etodolac	Ludiomil (W)	maprotiline HCl (W)
Lodine XL	etodolac SR	Lufyllin	dyphylline
lodoxamide tromethamine ophth soln	Alomide	LumenHance	manganese chloride
		Lunelle	medroxyprogesterone acetate; estradiol cypionate inj
Loestrin	norethindrone acetate; ethinyl estradiol	Lunesta	eszopiclone
lomefloxacin	Maxaquin	Lupron	leuprolide acetate
Lomotil	diphenoxylate HCl; atropine sulfate	Luride	sodium fluoride
		lutropin alfa	Luveris
lomustine	CeeNu	Luveris	lutropin alfa
Loniten (W)	minoxidil tablets (W)	Luvox	fluvoxamine maleate
Lo/Ovral	norgestrel; ethinyl estradiol	Luxiq	betamethasone valerate (foam)
loperamide HCl	Imodium		
Lopid	gemfibrozil	Lyrica	pregabalin

Lyme disease vaccine (W)	LYMErix (W)
LYMErix (W)	Lyme disease vaccine (W)
lymphocyte immune globulin	Atgam
lypressin (W)	Diapid (W)
Lysodren	mitotane

M

Maalox	aluminum hydroxide; magnesium hydroxide
Macrobid	nitrofurantoin macrocrystals and monohydrate
Macrodantin	nitrofurantoin macrocrystals
Macugen	pegaptanib
magaldrate	Riopan
manganese chloride	LumenHance
magnesium chloride SR	Slow-Mag
magnesium oxide	MAG-OX 400
magnesium sulfate	magnesium sulfate
MAG-OX 400	magnesium oxide
Malarone	atovaquone; proguanil HCl
Mandol	cefamandole nafate
mangofodipir trisodium	Teslascan
maprotiline HCl (W)	Ludiomil (W)
Marcaine HCl	bupivacaine HCl
Marinol	dronabinol
Marplan	isocarboxazid
Matulane	procarbazine HCl
Mavik	trandolapril
Maxalt	rizatriptan benzoate
Maxalt-MLT	rizatriptan oral disintegrating tablet
Maxaquin	lomefloxacin
Maxipime	cefepime HCl
Maxzide	triamterene 75 mg; hydrochlorothiazide 50 mg
Maxzide-25MG	triamterene 37.5 mg; hydrochlorothiazide 25 mg
mazindol	Sanorex
measles, mumps, rubella vaccines, combined	M-M-R II
Mebaral	mephobarbital
mebendazole	Vermox
mecamylamine HCl	Inversine

mechlorethamine HCl	Mustargen
Meclan	meclocycline sulfosalicylate
meclizine	Antivert
meclocycline sulfosalicylate	Meclan
meclofenamate sodium	Meclomen
Meclomen	meclofenamate sodium
Medrol	methylprednisolone
medroxyprogesterone acetate	Cycrin Provera
medroxyprogesterone acetate; estradiol cypionate inj (W)	Lunelle (W)
medroxyprogesterone acetate SR	Depo-Provera
mefenamic acid	Ponstel
mefloquine HCl	Lariam
Mefoxin	cefoxitin sodium
Megace	megestrol acetate
megestrol acetate	Megace
Mellaril (WA)	thioridazine HCl
meloxicam	Mobic
melphalan	Alkeran
memantine HCl	Namenda
Menactra	meningococcal vaccine
menadiol sodium diphosphate	Synkayvite
meningococcal vaccine	Menactra Menomune
Menomune	meningococcal vaccine
Menostar	estradiol transdermal system
menotropins	Pergonal (WA) Repronex
Mentax	butenafine HCl
meperidine HCl	Demerol
mephentermine sulfate	Wyamine
mephenytoin	Mesantoin
mephobarbital	Mebaral
mepivacaine HCl	Carbocaine
meprobamate	Equanil (WA) Miltown
Mepron	atovaquone
mequinol; tretinoin	Solage
mercaptopurine	Purinethol
Meridia	sibutramine HCl monohydrate
meropenem	Merrem
Merrem	meropenem
Meruvax II	rubella virus vaccine live attenuated

mesalamine	Asacol
	Rowasa
Mesantoin	mephenytoin
mesna	Mesnex
Mesnex	mesna
mesoridazine	Serentil
Mestinon	pyridostigmine bromide
Metadate ER	methylphenidate HCl SR
Metaglip	glipizide;
	metformin
Metamucil	psyllium
Metaprel	metaproterenol sulfate
metaproterenol	Alupent
sulfate	Metaprel
metaraminol	Aramine
bitartrate	
Metaret	suramin
Metastron	strontium-89 chloride inj
metformin HCl	Glucophage
metformin	Glucophage XR
HCl SR	
methadone HCl	Dolophine
methampheta-	Desoxyn
mine HCl	
methazolamide	Neptazane
methenamine	Urised
combination	
methenamine	Hiprex
hippurate	
Methergine	methylergon-ovine maleate
methicillin	Staphcillin (W)
sodium (W)	
methimazole	Tapazole
methocarbamol	Robaxin
methohexital	Brevital Sodium
sodium	
methotrexate	Mexate
	Rheumatrex
	Trexall
methotrexate,	Folex PFS
preservative-	
free inj	
methoxamine	Vasoxyl (W)
HCl (W)	
methoxsalen	Oxsoralen
methoxsalen	Uvadex
extracorporeal	
administration	
methscopolamine	Pamine
bromide	
methyclothiazide	Enduron
methyldopa	Aldomet
methyldopa;	Aldoril
hydrochlorothi-	
azide	
methylergonovine	Methergine (W)
maleate (W)	
Methylin	methylphenidate HCl

Methylin ER	methylphenidate HCl SR
methylphenidate	Methylin
HCl	Ritalin
methylphenidate	Concerta
SR	Metadate ER
	Methylin ER
	Ritalin SR
methylpredniso-	Medrol
lone	
methylpredniso-	Depo-Medrol
lone acetate	
SR inj	
methylpredniso-	Solu-Medrol
lone sodium	
succinate inj	
methyltestoster-	*methyltestosterone*
one	
methysergide	Sansert (W)
maleate (W)	
Meticorten	prednisone
metoclopramide	Reglan
HCl	
metolazone	Mykrox
	Zaroxolyn
Metopirone	metyrapone
metoprolol	Toprol XL
succinate SR	
metoprolol	Lopressor
tartrate	
MetroGel-	metronidazole
Vaginal	vaginal gel
metronidazole	Flagyl
metronidazole SR	Flagyl ER
metronidazole	MetroGel-
vaginal gel	Vaginal
metyrapone	Metopirone
metyrosine	Demser
Mevacor	lovastatin
Mexate	methotrexate
mexiletine HCl	Mexitil
Mexitil	mexiletine HCl
Mezlin (W)	mezlocillin (W)
mezlocillin (W)	Mezlin (W)
Miacalcin	calcitonin-salmon
mibefradil	Posicor (W)
dihydrochloride	
(W)	
micafungin	Mycamine
sodium	
Micardis	telmisartan
Micro K	potassium chloride SR
miconazole	Monistat
nitrate	
Micronase	glyburide
Micronor	norethindrone
Microzide	hydrochlorothiazide
Midamor	amiloride HCl
midazolam HCl	Versed

midodrine HCl	ProAmatine	Monocid (W)	cefonicid sodium (W)
Mifeprex	mifepristone	Monopril	fosinopril sodium
mifepristone	Mifeprex	montelukast	Singulair
miglitol	Glyset	sodium	
miglustat	Zavesca	Monurol	fosfomycin tromethamine
Migranol	dihydroergotamine mesylate	moricizine	Ethmozine
	nasal spray	morphine sulfate	Roxanol
milrinone lactate	Primacor	morphine sulfate	DepoDur
Miltown	meprobamate	extended-	
Minipress	prazosin HCl	release	
Minocin	minocycline HCl	liposome inj	
minocycline HCl	Minocin	morphine sulfate,	Roxanol-T
minocycline HCl	Arestin	immediate	
dental		release	
microspheres		concentrated	
minoxidil tablets	Loniten (W)	oral soln	
(W)		*morphine sulfate*	Duramorph
minoxidil topical	Rogaine	*inj*	
Mintezol	thiabendazole	*morphine sulfate*	Avinza
Miochol E	acetylcholine ophth	*SR*	Kadian
MiraLax	polyethylene glycol 3350		MS Contin
	powder		Oramorph SR
Mirapex	pramipexole		Roxanol SR
	dihydrochloride	Motrin	ibuprofen
Mircette	desogestrel; ethinyl	moxifloxacin	Avelox
	estradiol and ethinyl	HCl	
	estradiol	MS Contin	morphine sulfate SR
Mirena	levonorgestrel-releasing	Mucomyst	acetylcysteine
	intrauterine system	multivitamins	Cernevit-12
mirtazapine	Remeron	for infusion	Multi-12 (vial 1 and vial 2)
misoprostol	Cytotec	mupirocin nasal	Bactroban
Mithracin (W)	plicamycin (W)	ointment	
mitomycin	Mutamycin	muromonab-CD3	Orthoclone OKT3
mitotane	Lysodren	Muse	alprostadil urethral
mitoxantrone	Novantrone		suppository
HCl		Mustargen	mechlorethamine HCl
Mivacron	mivacurium chloride	Mutamycin	mitomycin
mivacurium	Mivacron	M.V.I.-12	vitamin, multiple inj
chloride		Myambutol	ethambutol HCl
M-M-R II	measles, mumps, rubella	Mycamine	micafungin sodium
	vaccines, combined	Mycelex	clotrimazole
Moban	molindone HCl	Mycifradin	neomycin sulfate
Mobic	meloxicam	Sulfate	oral soln
modafinil	Provigil	Myciguent	neomycin sulfate ointment
Moduretic	amiloride HCl;		and cream
	hydrochlorothiazide	Mycolog Cream	nystatin; triamcinolone
moexipril HCl	Univasc		cream
moexipril HCl;	Uniretic	mycophenolate	CellCept
hydrochloro-		mofetil	
thiazide		mycophenolic	Myfortic
molindone HCl	Moban	acid	
mometasone	Elocon	Mycostatin	nystatin
furoate topical		Mydriacyl	tropicamide
Mometasone	Nasonex	Myfortic	mycophenolic acid
furoate		Mykrox	metolazone
monohydrate		Myleran	busulfan
nasal spray		Mylicon	simethicone
Monistat	miconazole nitrate	Mylotarg	gemtuzumab ozogamicin

M
℞

Myobloc — botulinum toxin type B
Myochrysine (WA) — gold sodium thiomalate
Myoscint — imciromab pentetate
Myozyme — alglucosidase alfa
Mysoline — primidone

N

NABI-HB — hepatitis B immune globulin (human)
nabilone — Cesamet
nabumetone — Relafen
nadolol — Corgard
Nafcil (W) — nafcillin sodium
nafcillin sodium (W) — Nafcil (W) Unipen (W)
Naglazyme — galsulfase
nalbuphine HCl — Nubain
Nalfon — fenoprofen calcium
nalidixic acid — NegGram
nalmefene HCl — Revex
naloxone HCl — Narcan (WA)
naltrexone — ReVia
Namenda — memantine HCl
nandrolone phenpropionate (W) — Durabolin (W)
nandrolone decanoate — Deca-Durabolin
naphazoline ophth soln — Vasocon
Naprelan — naproxen sodium SR
Naprosyn — naproxen
naproxen — Naprosyn
naproxen sodium — Anaprox
naproxen sodium SR — Naprelan
naratriptan HCl — Amerge
Narcan (WA) — naloxone HCl
Nardil — phenelzine sulfate
Naropin — ropivacaine HCl
Nasacort — triamcinolone acetonide nasal inhaler
Nasalcrom — cromolyn sodium
Nascobal — cyanocobalamin nasal gel
Nasonex — Mometasone furoate monohydrate nasal spray
natalizumab — Tysabri
nateglinide — Starlix
Natrecor — nesiritide
Navane — thiothixene
Navelbine — vinorelbine tartrate
Nebcin — tobramycin sulfate
NebuPent — pentamidine isethionate aerosol

nedocromil inhalation — Tilade
nedocromil ophth soln — Alocril
nefazodone HCl (W) — Serzone (W)
NegGram — nalidixic acid
nelfinavir mesylate — Viracept
Nembutal — pentobarbital sodium
Neo-Synephrine — phenylephrine HCl
neomycin sulfate ointment and cream — Myciguent
neomycin sulfate oral soln — Mycifradin Sulfate
Neoral — cyclosporine capsules (modified) and oral soln
Neosar — cyclophosphamide
Neosporin Cream — polymyxin; neomycin
Neosporin Ointment — polymyxin; neomycin; bacitracin
Neosporin ophth Ointment — polymyxin; neomycin; bacitracin
Neosporin ophth soln — polymyxin; neomycin
neostigmine methylsulfate — Prostigmin
nepafenac — Nevanac
Neptazane — methazolamide
Nesacaine — chloroprocaine HCl
nesiritide — Natrecor
netilmicin sulfate — Netromycin
Netromycin — netilmicin sulfate
Neulasta — pegfilgrastim
Neumega — oprelvekin
Neupogen — filgrastim
Neurolite — technetium Tc-99m bicisate kit
Neurontin — gabapentin
Neutrexin — trimetrexate glucuronate
Nevance — nepafenac
nevirapine — Viramune
Nexavar — sorafenib tosylate
Nexium — esomeprazole magnesium
niacin SR — Niaspan Nicobid
Niaspan — niacin SR
nicardipine HCl — Cardene
Niclocide — niclosamide
niclosamide — Niclocide
Nicobid — niacin SR
Nicorette — nicotine polacrilex
nicotine nasal spray — Nicotrol NS
nicotine polacrilex — Nicorette

nicotine transdermal	Habitrol
	Nicotrol
	Prostep
Nicotrol	nicotine transdermal
Nicotrol NS	nicotine nasal spray
nifedipine	Adalat
	Procardia
nifedipine SR	Adalat CC
	Procardia XL
Nilandron	nilutamide
nilutamide	Nilandron
Nimbex	cisatracurium besylate
nimodipine	Nimotop
Nimotop	nimodipine
Nipent	pentostatin inj
Nipride	nitroprusside sodium
nisoldipine SR	Sular
nitazoxanide	Alinia
nitisinone	Orfadin
Nitrek	nitroglycerin transdermal
nitric oxide for inhalation	INOmax
Nitro-Bid	nitroglycerin oint
Nitro-Dur	nitroglycerin transdermal
nitrofurantoin macrocrystals	Macrodantin
nitrofurantoin macrocrystals and monohydrate	Macrobid
nitrofurazone	Furacin
nitroglycerin transdermal	Transderm-Nitro
nitroglycerin inj	Tridil
	Nitro-Bid IV
nitroglycerin ointment	Nitrol
	Nitro-Bid
nitroglycerin sublingual tablets	Nitrostat
nitroglycerin transdermal	Nitrek
	Nitro-Dur
Nitro-BID	nitroglycerin ointment
nitroprusside sodium	Nipride
Nitrostat	nitroglycerin sublingual tablets
Nix	permethrin
nizatidine	Axid
Nizoral	ketoconazole
nofetumomab	Verluna
nolatrexed dihydrochloride	Thymitaq
Nolvadex	tamoxifen citrate
Norco	hydrocodone bitartrate; acetaminophen

Norcuron	vecuronium bromide
Nordette	levonorgestrel; ethinyl estradiol
Norditropin	somatropin inj
norelgestromin; ethinyl estradiol transdermal system	Ortho Evra
norepinephrine bitartrate	Levophed
norethindrone	Micronor
norethindrone acetate; ethinyl estradiol	Estrostep
	Loestrin
norethindrone; ethinyl estradiol (or mestranol)	Femhrt
	Ortho-Novum (products)
norethindrone acetate; estradiol transdermal	CombiPatch
Norflex	orphenadrine citrate
norfloxacin	Noroxin
Norgesic	orphenadrine citrate; aspirin; caffeine
norgestimate; ethinyl estradiol	Ortho Tri-Cyclen
norgestrel; ethinyl estradiol	Lo/Ovral
	Ovral
Normiflo (W)	ardeparin sodium (W)
Normodyne	labetalol HCl
Noroxin	norfloxacin
Norpace	disopyramide phosphate
Norplant (W)	levonorgestrel implant (W)
Norpramin	desipramine HCl
nortriptyline HCl	Aventyl
	Pamelor
Norvasc	amlodipine besylate
Norvir	ritonavir
Novantrone	mitoxantrone HCl
Novocain HCl	procaine HCl
Novolin 70/30	isophane insulin suspension (NPH) 70%, insulin inj 30% (human)
Novolin N	isophane insulin suspension (NPH) (human)
Novolin R	insulin inj (human)
NovoLog	insulin aspart (rDNA origin)
NovoSeven	coagulation factor VII a (recombinant)
Nubain	nalbuphine HCl
NuLev	hyoscyamine sulfate orally disintegrating tab

Numorphan	oxymorphone HCl	Ontak	denileukin diftitox
Nupercainal	dibucaine	Onxol	paclitaxel inj
Nuromax	doxacurium chloride	Opana	oxymorphone HCl
Nuprin	ibuprofen	Opana ER	oxymorphone HCl extended
Nutropin	somatropin for inj		release tablets
Nutropin AQ	somatropin inj	Ophthaine (WA)	proparacaine
NuvaRing	etonogestrel; ethinyl	Ophthalgan	glycerin ophth soln
	estradiol vagina ring	Ophthetic	proparacaine HCl
Nydrazid	isoniazid	opium;	B & O
nystatin	Mycostatin	belladonna	Supprettes
nystatin topical	Nystop	suppositories	
powder		oprelvekin	Neumega
nystatin;	Mycolog Cream	Opticrom	cromolyn sodium
triamcinolone		OptiMark	gadoversetamide
cream		Optimine	azatadine maleate
Nystop	nystatin topical powder	Optiray	ioversol
		Optivar	azelastine HCl ophth soln
		Orabase	benzocaine
		Orajel	benzocaine
	O	Oramorph SR	morphine sulfate SR
		Orap	pimozide
		Oretic	hydrochlorothiazide
OctreoScan	indium In-111 pentetreotide	Orfadin	nitisinone
octreotide acetate	Sandostatin	Organidin NR	guaifenesin
octreotide acetate	Sandostatin LAR	Orgaran	danaparoid sodium
susp for inj	Depot	Orinase	tolbutamide
ofloxacin	Floxin	Orlaam	levomethadyl acetate HCl
ofloxacin otic	Floxin Otic	orlistat	Xenical
soln		Ornade	phenylpropanol-
Ogen	estropipate	Spansules	amine HCl; chlorphenir-
olanzapine	Zyprexa		amine maleate SR
olanzapine;	Symbyax	orphenadrine	Norflex
fluoxetine		citrate	
olmesartan	Benicar	orphenadrine	Norgesic
medoxomil		citrate; aspirin;	
olmesartan	Benicar HCT	caffeine	
medoxomil;		Ortho-Cept	desogestrel; ethinyl
hydrochloro-			estradiol
thiazide		Orthoclone	muromonab-CD3
olopatadine HCl	Patanol	OKT3	
ophth soln		Ortho Evra	norelgestromin; ethinyl
olsalazine	Dipentum		estradiol transdermal
sodium			system
Olux	clobetasol foam	Ortho-Novum	norethindrone;
Omacor	omega-3-acid ethyl esters	(products)	ethinyl estradiol (or
omalizumab	Xolair		mestranol)
omega-3-acid	Omacor	Ortho-Prefest	17β-estradiol; norgestimate
ethyl ester		Ortho Tri-Cyclen	norgestimate; ethinyl
omeprazole	Prilosec		estradiol (combinations)
Omnicef	cefdinir	Orudis (W)	ketoprofen (W)
Omnipaque	iohexol	Oruvail	ketoprofen SR
Oncaspar	pegaspargase	Os-Cal 500	calcium carbonate
OncoScint	satumomab pendetide	oseltamivir	Tamiflu
Oncovin	vincristine sulfate	phosphate	
ondansetron	Zofran	Osmovist	iotrolan
ondansetron	Zofran ODT	Otrivin	xylometazoline
orally		Ovidrel	choriogonadotropin alfa
disintegrating		ovine	Vitrase
tab		hyaluronidase	

Ovral   norgestrel; ethinyl estradiol
oxaliplatin   Eloxatin
Oxandrin   oxandrolone
oxandrolone   Oxandrin
oxaprozin   Daypro
oxazepam   Serax
oxcarbazepine   Trileptal
oxiconazole   Oxistat
   nitrate cream
Oxilan   ioxilan
Oxistat   oxiconazole nitrate cream
Oxsoralen   methoxsalen
oxtriphylline   Choledyl
oxybate sodium   Xyrem
oxybutynin   Ditropan
   chloride
oxychlorosene   Clorpactin
   sodium   WCS-90
oxycodone HCl   Percolone (WA)
     Roxicodone
oxycodone HCl   OxyContin
   SR
oxycodone HCl;   Percocet 5/325;
   acetaminophen   7.5/500; 10/650
     Endocet
     Roxicet
oxycodone HCl;   Percodan
   aspirin
oxycodone HCl;   Combunox
   ibuprofen
OxyContin   oxycodone HCl SR
oxymetazoline   Afrin nasal spray
   HCl   Dristan Long Lasting
oxymetholone   Anadrol-50
oxymorphone   Numorphan
   HCl   Opana tablets
oxymorphone HCl   Opana ER
   extended release
   tablets
oxytocin   Pitocin

P

Pacis   BCG intravesical
paclitaxel   Onxol
     Taxol
paclitaxel,   Abraxane
   albumin-bound
   inj
paclitaxel-eluting   Taxus Express2 stent
   stent   V-Flex plus PTX stent
palifermin   Kepivance
palivizumab   Synagis
Palladone XL   hydromorphone HCl SR
palonosetron   Aloxi
   HCl

Pamelor   nortriptyline HCl
pamidronate   Aredia
   disodium
Pamine   methscopolamine bromide
Pancrease   pancrelipase EC
pancrelipase   Cotazym
pancrelipase EC   Cotazym-S
     Pancrease
pancuronium   Pavulon
   bromide
Pandel   hydrocortisone buteprate
     cream
Panretin   alitretinoin
pantoprazole   Protonix
papain; urea oint   Accuzyme
     Ethezyme
papaverine HCl   Pavabid (W)
   SR (W)
paracetamol   acetaminophen
Paradione   paramethadione
Paraflex   chlorzoxazone 250 mg
Parafon Forte   chlorzoxazone
   DSC   500 mg
paramethadione   Paradione
Paraplatin   carboplatin
Parathar   teriparatide acetate
Parcopa   levodopa; carbidopa
paregoric   camphorated tincture of
     opium
pargyline HCl   Eutonyl
paricalcitol   Zemplar
Parlodel   bromocriptine mesylate
Parnate   tranylcypromine sulfate
paromomycin   Humatin
   sulfate
paroxetine HCl   Paxil
Parsidol   ethopropazine HCl
Paser   aminosalicylic acid
Patanol   olopatadine HCl ophth soln
Pavabid (W)   papaverine HCl SR (W)
Pavulon   pancuronium bromide
Paxil   paroxetine HCl
PBZ   tripelennamine HCl
PCE Dispertab   erythromycin base coated
     particles
Pediazole   erythromycin
     ethylsuccinate;
     sulfisoxazole
PedvaxHIB   haemophilus b vaccine
pegaptanib   Macugen
pegaspargase   Oncaspar
Pegasys   peginterferon
     alfa-2a
pegfilgrastim   Neulasta
peginterferon   Pegasys
   alfa-2a
peginterferon   PEG-Intron
   alfa-2b
   (recombinant)

P
R

PEG-Intron	peginterferon alfa-2b (recombinant)	Percocet 5/325; 7.5/500; 10/650	oxycodone HCl; acetaminophen
pegvisomant	Somavert	Percodan	oxycodone HCl; aspirin
pemetrexed disodium	Alimta	Percolone (WA)	oxycodone HCl
pemirolast potassium ophth soln	Alamast	perflenapent emulsion	EchoGen
		perflubron	Imagent GI
pemoline	Cylert (WA)	Pergonal (WA)	menotropins
penicillamine	Cuprimine	Periactin	cyproheptadine HCl
penciclovir cream	Denavir	Peri-Colace (W)	docusate sodium; casanthranol (W)
penicillin G benzathine	Bicillin L-A (for IM use only) Permapen (for IM use only)	Peridex	chlorhexidine gluconate mouth rinse
		perindopril erbumine	Aceon
penicillin G benzathine; penicillin G procaine	Bicillin C-R (for IM use only)	PerioChip	chlorhexidine gluconate
		Periostat	doxycycline hyclate 20 mg tab & cap
		Peritrate	pentaerythritol tetranitrate
penicillin G procaine	Wycillin (for IM use only)	Permapen	penicillin G benzathine (for IM use only)
penicillin V potassium	Pen Vee K	permethrin	Nix
Penlac Nail Lacquer	ciclopirox soln	Permitil	fluphenazine HCl
		perphenazine	Trilafon (WA)
pentaerythritol tetranitrate	Peritrate	perphenazine; amitriptyline HCl	Etrafon Triavil (WA)
pentagastrin	Peptavlon	Persantine	dipyridamole
Pentam 300	pentamidine isethionate inj	petrolatum, white	Vaseline
pentamidine isethionate aerosol	NebuPent	Phenaphen with Codeine (#2, 3, and 4) (WA)	acetaminophen 300 mg with Codeine Phosphate (15, 30, and 60 mg)
pentamidine isethionate inj	Pentam 300		
Pentaspan	pentastarch	phenazopyridine HCl	Pyridium
pentastarch	Pentaspan		
pentazocine HCl	Talwin	phendimetrazine tartrate	Plegine
pentazocine HCl; naloxone HCl	Talwin Nx	phenelzine sulfate	Nardil
pentetate zinc trisodium (tri-sodium zinc diethylenetri-aminepentaacetate)	Zn-DTPA	Phenergan	promethazine HCl
		phenobarbital	phenobarbital
		phenobarbital, ergotamine; belladonna	Bellergal-S
pentobarbital sodium	Nembutal		
pentosan polysulfate sodium	Elmiron	phenoxybenza-mine HCl	Dibenzyline
		phentermine HCl	Fastin
pentostatin inj	Nipent		
Pentothal	thiopental sodium	phentermine resin	Ionamin
pentoxifylline	Trental		
Pen Vee K	penicillin V potassium	phentolamine mesylate (W)	Regitine (W)
Pepcid	famotidine		
Pepcid RPD	famotidine, oral disintegrating tablet	phenylbutyrate sodium	Buphenyl
Peptavlon	pentagastrin		

phenylephrine HCl   Neo-Synephrine

phenylpropanol-amine HCl; chlorphenir-amine maleate SR   Ornade

phenylpropanol-amine HCl; guaifenesin SR   Entex LA

Phenytek   phenytoin sodium extended

phenytoin   Dilantin

phenytoin sodium extended   Phenytek

Pholpholine Iodide (W)   echothiophate iodide (W)

Photofrin   porfimer sodium

physostigmine ophth ointment   Eserine Sulfate

physostigmine salicylate   Antilirium

phytonadione   AquaMEPHYTON

pilocarpine HCl ophth   Isopto Carpine

pilocarpine HCl tablet   Salagen

pimecrolimus cream   Elidel

pimozide   Orap

pindolol   Visken

pioglitazone HCl   Actos

pipecuronium bromide (W)   Arduan (W)

piperacillin sodium (W)   Pipracil (W)

piperacillin sodium; tazobactam sodium   Zosyn

Pipracil (W)   piperacillin sodium (W)

piroxicam   Feldene

Pitocin   oxytocin

Pitressin   vasopressin

Placidyl (W)   ethchlorvynol (W)

Plan B   levonorgestrel

Plaquenil   hydroxychloroquine sulfate

Plasbumin   albumin human

plasma protein fraction   Plasma-Plex
   Plasmanate
   Plasmatein
   Protenate

Plasma-Plex   plasma protein fraction

Plasmanate   plasma protein fraction

Plasmatein   plasma protein fraction

Platinol AQ (WA)   cisplatin

Plavix   clopidogrel bisulfate

Plegine   phendimetrazine tartrate

Plenaxis   abarelix

Plendil   felodipine

Pletal   cilostazol

Plexion   sulfacetamide sodium and sulfur lotion

plicamycin (W)   Mithracin (W)

pneumococcal vaccine   Pneumovax

pneumococcal 7-valent conjugate vaccine   Prevnar

Pneumovax   pneumococcal vaccine

podofilox gel   Condylox

Polaramine Repetabs   dexchlorpheniramine-maleate SR

poliovirus vaccine inactivated   Ipol

polyethylene glycolelectro-lyte soln   CoLyte
   GoLYTELY

polyethylene glycol 3350 powder   MiraLax

poly-l-lactic acid   Sculptra

polymyxin B sulfate; trimethoprim ophth soln   Polytrim

polymyxin; neomycin   Neosporin Cream
   Neosporin ophth soln

polymyxin; neomycin; bacitracin   Neosporin Ointment
   Neosporin ophth Ointment

polystyrene sulfonate sodium   Kayexalate

polythiazide (W)   Renese (W)

Polytrim   polymyxin B sulfate; trimethoprim ophth soln

Pondimin (W)   fenfluramine HCl (W)

Ponstel   mefenamic acid

Pontocaine   tetracaine HCl

poractant alpha intratracheal susp   Curosurf

porfimer sodium   Photofrin

Posicor (W)   mibefradil dihydrochloride (W)

P
Rx

potassium bicarbonate; potassium citrate effervescent	K-Lyte
potassium chloride; potassium bicarbonate effervescent	K-Lyte/Cl
potassium chloride SR	Kaon-Cl K-Dur Klor-Con 10 Slow-K Micro K
potassium chloride; potassium gluconate	Kolyum
potassium citrate tab	Urocit-K
potassium gluconate	Kaon
povidone iodine	Betadine
pralidoxime chloride	Protopam
pramipexole dihydrochloride	Mirapex
pramlintide acetate	Symlin
pramoxine HCl	Tronothane HCl
Prandin	repaglinide
prasterone	Aslera
Pravachol	pravastatin sodium
pravastatin sodium	Pravachol
prazosin HCl	Minipress
Precedex	dexmedetomidine HCl inj
Precose	acarbose
prednisolone syrup	Prelone
prednisone	Deltasone Meticorten
pregabalin	Lyrica
Prelone	prednisolone syrup
Premarin	estrogens, conjugated
Premphase	estrogens, conjugated; medroxyprogesterone acetate
Prempro	
Prepidil	dinoprostone gel
Preven Emergency Contraceptive Kit	levonorgestrel; ethinyl estradiol
Prevacid	lansoprazole
Prevnar	pneumococcal 7-valent conjugate vaccine

Preveon	adefovir dipivoxil
Prevpac	lansoprazole; amoxicillin; clarithromycin
Prialt	ziconotide
Priftin	rifapentine
Prilosec	omeprazole
Primacor	milrinone lactate
Primaxin	imipenemcilastatin sodium
primidone	Mysoline
Primsol (W)	trimethoprim (W)
Principen	ampicillin
Prinivil	lisinopril
Priscoline (W)	tolazoline (W)
ProAmatine	midodrine HCl
Pro-Banthine	propantheline bromide
probenecid	Benemid
probenecid; colchicine	ColBENEMID (W)
procainamide	Pronestyl
procainamide HCl SR	Procan SR Procanbid
procaine HCl	Novocain HCl
Procan SR	procainamide HCl SR
Procanbid	procainamide HCl SR
procarbazine HCl	Matulane
Procardia	nifedipine
Procardia XL	nifedipine SR
Prochieve	progesterone gel
prochlorperazine	Compazine
Procrit	epoetin alfa
procyclidine HCl	Kemadrin
progesterone gel	Crinone Prochieve
progesterone micronized	Prometrium
Prograf	tacrolimus
ProHance	gadoteridol
ProHIBiT	haemophilus b vaccine
Prokine (WA)	sargramostim
Prolastin	alpha$_1$-proteinase inhibitor (human)
Proleukin	aldesleukin
Prolixin	fluphenazine HCl
Proloid (W)	thyroglobulin (W)
promethazine HCl	Phenergan
Prometrium	progesterone micronized
Pronestyl	procainamide
Propacet-100	propoxyphene napsylate; acetaminophen
propafenone HCl	Rythmol
propantheline bromide	Pro-Banthine
proparacaine HCl	Ophthaine (WA) Ophthetic
Propecia	finasteride tablets 1 mg

Propine	dipivefrin
propofol	Diprivan
propoxyphene HCl	Darvon
propoxyphene HCl; acetaminophen	Wygesic
propoxyphene HCl; aspirin; caffeine	Darvon Compound 65
propoxyphene napsylate; acetaminophen	Darvocet-N 100 Propacet-100
propranolol HCl	Inderal
propranolol HCl; hydrochlorothiazide	Inderide
Propulsid (W)	cisapride (W)
Proscar	finasteride tablets 5 mg
ProSom	estazolam
ProstaScint	capromab pendetide
Prostep	nicotine transdermal system
Prostigmin	neostigmine methylsulfate
Prostin E$_2$	dinoprostone vaginal suppositories
Prostin VR	alprostadil
protamine sulfate	protamine sulfate
Protenate	plasma protein fraction
Protonix	pantoprazole
Protopam	pralidoxime chloride
Protopic	tacrolimus oint
protriptyline HCl	Vivactil
Protropin	somatrem
Protropin II	somatropin for inj
Proventil	albuterol
Proventil HFA	albuterol sulfate inhalation aerosol
Proventil Repetabs	albuterol SR
Provera	medroxyprogesterone acetate
Provigil	modafinil
Prozac	fluoxetine HCl
Prudoxin	doxepin HCl cream
Prussian blue	Radiogardase
pseudoephedrine HCl	Sudafed
pseudoephedrine HCl; bromphiramine maleate	Drixoral Syrup
psyllium	Konsyl-D Metamucil
Pulmicort Turbuhaler	budesonide inhalation powder
Pulmozyme	dornase alfa
Purinethol	mercaptopurine
Pyridium	phenazopyridine HCl

pyridostigmine bromide	Mestinon
pyrimethamine	Daraprim
pyrimethamine; sulfadoxine	Fansidar

Q

Quadramet	samarium SM 153 lexidronam
Quarzan (W)	clidinium bromide (W)
Questran	cholestyramine
quetiapine fumerate	Seroquel
Quinaglute	quinidine gluconate SR
quinapril HCl	Accupril
quinapril; hydrochlorothiazide	Accuretic
quinethazone (W)	Hydromox (W)
Quinidex Extentabs	quinidine sulfate SR
quinidine gluconate SR	Quinaglute
quinidine sulfate	quinidine sulfate
quinidine sulfate SR	Quinidex Extentabs
quinupristin; dalfopristin	Synercid
Quixin	levofloxacin ophth soln
Qvar	beclomethasone diproprionate inhalation aerosol

R

RabAvert	rabies vaccine for human use
rabeprazole sodium	Aciphex
rabies immune globulin, human	Hyperab (W) Imogam
rabies vaccine, adsorbed	rabies vaccine, adsorbed
rabies vaccine for human use	RabAvert
Radiogardase	Prussian blue
raloxifene HCl	Evista
ramelteon	Rozerem
ramipril	Altace
ranibizumab inj	Lucentis
ranitidine bismuth citrate	Tritec
ranitidine HCl	Zantac

rapacuronium bromide (W)	Raplon (W)
Rapamune	sirolimus
Raplon (W)	rapacuronium bromide (W)
Raptiva	efalizumab
rasburicase	Elitek
rattlesnake anti-venom	CroFab
Raxar (W)	grepafloxacin HCl (W)
Razadyne	galanthamine HBr
Rebetol	ribavirin
Rebetron	ribavirin; interferon alfa-2b
Rebif	interferon beta-1a
reboxetine mesylate	Vestra
Recombivax HB	hepatitis B vaccine
Redux (W)	dexfenfluramine HCl (W)
Refacto	antihemophilic factor (recombinant)
Refludan	lepirudin
Regitine (W)	phentolamine mesylate (W)
Reglan	metoclopramide HCl
Regranex	becaplermin gel
Regroton	chlorthalidone; reserpine
Relafen	nabumetone
Relenza	zanamivir for inhalation
Relpax	eletriptan hydrobromide
Remeron	mirtazapine
Remicade	infliximab
remifentanil HCl	Ultiva
Reminyl	name changed to Razadyne
Remodulin	treprostinil sodium
Renagel (W)	sevelamer HCl (W)
Renese (W)	polythiazide (W)
Renova	tretinion topical
Renovue 65	iodamide meglumine
ReoPro	abciximab
repaglinide	Prandin
Repronex	menotropins
Requip	ropinirole HCl
Rescriptor	delavirdine mesylate
Rescula (W)	unoprostone isopropyl ophth soln (W)
reserpine	Serpasil (WA)
RespiGam	respiratory syncytial virus immune globulin intravenous (human)
respiratory syncytial virus immune globulin intravenous (human)	RespiGam
Restasis	cyclosporine ophth emulsion
Restoril	temazepam

Retavase	reteplase
reteplase	Retavase
Retin-A	tretinoin topical
Retin-A Micro	tretinoin gel
Retrovir	zidovudine
Revex	nalmefene HCl
ReVia	naltrexone
Reyataz	atazanavir sulfate
Rezulin (W)	troglitazone (W)
R-Gene	arginine HCl
Rheumatrex	methotrexate tablets
Rhinocort	budesonide nasal inhaler
RH$_O$ (D) immune globulin	RhoGAM
RH$_O$ (D) immune globulin IV (human)	WinRho SD
RhoGAM	RH$_O$ (D) immune globulin
ribavirin	Rebetol
	Virazole
ribavirin; interferon alfa-2b	Rebetron
Ridaura	auranofin
Rifadin	rifampin
Rifamate	isoniazid; rifampin
rifampin	Rifadin
	Rimactane
rifapentine	Priftin
rifaximin	Xifaxan
Rilutek	riluzole
riluzole	Rilutek
Rimactane	rifampin
rimantadine	Flumadine
rimexolone	Vexol
Riopan	magaldrate
risedronate sodium	Actonel
Risperdal	risperidone
risperidone	Risperdal
Ritalin	methylphenidate HCl
Ritalin SR	methylphenidate SR
ritodrine HCl (W)	Yutopar (W)
ritonavir	Norvir
Rituxan	rituximab
rituximab	Rituxan
rivastigmine tartrate	Exelon
rizatriptan benzoate	Maxalt
rizatriptan oral disintegrating tablet	Maxalt-MLT
Robaxin	methocarbamol
Robinul	glycopyrrolate
Robitussin	guaifenesin
Robitussin A-C	guaifenesin; codeine phosphate
Robitussin-DM	guaifenesin; dextromethorphan

R
Rx

Rocaltrol	calcitriol
Rocephin	ceftriaxone sodium
rofecoxib (W)	Vioxx (W)
Roferon-A	interferon alfa-2a
Rogaine	minoxidil topical
Romazicon	flumazenil
ropinirole HCl	Requip
ropivacaine HCl	Naropin
Rosiglitazone maleate	Avandia
rosiglitazone maleate; metformin HCl	Avandamet
rosuvastatin calcium	Crestor
Rotashield (W)	rotavirus (W) vaccine, live, oral, tetravalent
rotavirus vaccine, live, oral, (W) tetravalent	Rotashield (W)
Rowasa	mesalamine
Roxanol	morphine sulfate
Roxanol SR	morphine sulfate SR
Roxanol-T	morphine sulfate, immediate release concentrated oral soln
Roxicet	oxycodone HCl; acetaminophen
Roxicodone	oxycodone HCl
Rozerem	ramelteon
rubella virus vaccine live attenuated	Meruvax II
Rubex	doxorubicin HCl
Rythmol	propafenone HCl

S

sacrosidase	Sucraid
Saizen	somatropin
Salagen	pilocarpine HCl tablet
salbutamol sulfate	albuterol sulfate
salmeterol xinafoate	Serevent
salmeterol xinafoate inhalation powder	Serevent Diskus
salsalate	Disalcid
Sal-Tropine	atropine sulfate tablets
Saluron	hydroflumethiazide
samarium SM 153 lexidronam	Quadramet

Sanctura	trospium chloride
Sandimmune	cyclosporine
Sandoglobulin	immune globulin intravenous
Sandostatin	octreotide acetate
Sandostatin LAR Depot	octreotide acetate susp for inj
Sanorex	mazindol
Sansert (W)	methysergide maleate (W)
Santyl	collagenase
saquinavir mesylate	Invirase
saquinavir soft gel capsule	Fortovase
Sarafem	fluoxetine
sargramostim	Leukine Prokine (WA)
satumomab pendetide	OncoScint
Sclerosol	talc, sterile aerosol
Scopace	scopolamine hydrobromide, soluble tab
scopolamine hydrobromide ophth	Isopto Hyoscine
scopolamine hydrobromide, soluble tab	Scopace
scopolamine transdermal	Transderm Scop
Sculptra	poly-l-lactic acid
Seasonale	ethinyl estradiol; levonorgestrel (91 day cycle)
Sectral	acebutolol HCl
Seldane (W)	terfenadine (W)
Seldane D (W)	terfenadine; pseudoephedrine HCl (W)
selegiline HCl	Carbex Eldepryl
selenium sulfide	Selsun Blue
Selsun Blue	selenium sulfide
Sensipar	cinacalcet
sennosides	Ex Lax
sennosides	Senokot
sennosides; docusate sodium	Senokot-S
Senokot	senna concentrates
Senokot-S	sennosides; docusate sodium
Sensipar	cinacalcet HCl
Septocaine	articaine; epinephrine
Septra	sulfamethoxazoletrimethoprim
Ser-Ap-Es	hydralazine; hydrochlorothiazide; reserpine

S
R

Serax	oxazepam	sodium	Klaron
Serentil (W)	mesoridazine (W)	sulfacetamide	
Serevent	salmeterol xinafoate	lotion	
Serevent Diskus	salmeterol xinafoate inhalation powder	sodium tetradecyl	Sotradecol
Serlect	sertindole	sulfate	
sermorelin acetate	Geref	Solage	mequinol; tretinoin
Seromycin	cycloserine	Solaraze	diclofenac gel
Seroquel	quetiapine fumerate	Solganal	aurothioglucose
Serostim	somatropin (rDNA origin) for inj	solifenacin succinate	Vesicare
Serpasil (WA)	*reserpine*	Solu-Cortef	hydrocortisone sodium succinate
sertaconazole	Ertaczo		
sertindole	Serlect	Solu-Medrol	methylprednisolone sodium succinate
sertraline HCl	Zoloft		
Serzone (W)	nefazodone HCl (W)	Soma	carisoprodol
sevelamer HCl	Renagel	somatostatin	Zecnil
sevoflurane	Ultane	somatrem	Protropin
short chain fatty acids enema	Colomed	somatropin for inj	Genotropin Humatrope
sibutramine HCl monohydrate	Meridia		Norditropin Nutropin
sildenafil citrate	Viagra		Protropin II
Silvadene	silver sulfadiazine		Saizen
silver sulfadiazine	Silvadene	somatropin inj	Nutropin AQ
		somatropin (rDNA origin) for inj	Serostim
simethicone	Mylicon		
Simulect	basiliximab		
simvastatin	Zocor	Somavert	pegvisomant
Sinemet	levodopa; carbidopa	Sonata	zaleplon
Sinemet CR	levodopa; carbidopa SR	sorafenib tosylate	Nexavar
Sinequan	doxepin HCl	Soriatane	acitretin
Singulair	montelukast sodium	sotalol	Betapace
sirolimus	Rapamune	Sotradecol	sodium tetradecyl sulfate
sirolimus-eluting stent	Cypher stent	sparfloxacin	Zagam
		stavudine	Zerit
Skelid	tiludronate disodium	spectinomycin HCl	Trobicin
Slo-bid	theophylline SR		
Slo-Phyllin	theophylline	Spectracef	cefditoren pivoxil
Slow Fe	ferrous sulfate SR	Spiriva HandiHaler	tiotropium bromide inhalation powder
Slow-K	potassium chloride SR		
Slow-Mag	magnesium chloride SR		
sodium citrate; citric acid	Bicitra	spironolactone	Aldactone
		spironolactone; hydrochloroth- iazide	Aldactazide
sodium ferric gluconate complex in sucrose inj	Ferrlecit		
		Sporanox	itraconazole
		Sprycel	dasatinib
sodium fluoride	Luride	Stadol	butorphanol tartrate inj
sodium hyaluronate	Amvisc Healon	Stadol NS (W)	butorphanol tartrate nasal spray (W)
	Hyalgan	Stalevo	levodopa; carbidopa; entacapone
sodium oxybate	Xyrem		
sodium phenylbutyrate	Buphenyl	stanozolol	Winstrol
		Staphcillin	methicillin sodium
sodium phosphate tab	Visicol	Starlix	nateglinide
		Stelazine	trifluoperazine HCl

Strattera	Atomoxetine HCl
Streptase	streptokinase
streptokinase	Streptase
streptomycin sulfate	streptomycin sulfate
streptozocin	Zanosar
Striant	testosterone buccal
Stromectol	ivermectin
strontium-89 chloride inj	Metastron
Sublimaze	fentanyl citrate
Suboxone	buprenorphine HCl; naloxone HCl
Subutex	buprenorphine HCl
succinylcholine chloride	Anectine
Sucraid	sacrosidase
sucralfate	Carafate
Sudafed	pseudoephedrine HCl
Sufenta	sufentanil citrate
sufentanil citrate	Sufenta
Sulamyd sodium	sulfacetamide sodium ophth
Sular	Nisoldipine SR
sulfacetamide sodium and sulfur lotion	Plexion
sulfacetamide sodium ophth	Sulamyd sodium
sulfadoxine; pyrimethamine	Fansidar
sulfamethoxazole (W)	Gantanol (W)
sulfamethoxazole-trimethoprim	Bactrim
	Cotrim
	co-trimoxazole
	Septra
sulfasalazine	Azulfidine
sulfinpyrazone	Anturane
sulindac	Clinoril
Sultrin	triple sulfa vaginal cream
sumatriptan	Imitrex
Sumycin	tetracycline HCl
Suprane	desflurane
Suprax (W)	cefixime (W)
suramin	Metaret
Surmontil	trimipramine maleate
Survanta	beractant
Sustiva	Efavirenz
Symbyax	olanzapine; fluoxetine
Symlin	pramlintide acetate
Symmetrel	amantadine HCl
Synagis	palivizumab
Synalar	fluocinolone acetonide
Synercid	quinupristin; dalfopristin
Synkayvite	menadiol sodium diphosphate
synopinine	Florotag

synthetic conjugated estrogens, A	Cenestin
Synthroid	levothyroxine sodium
Synvisc	hylan G-F 20

T

tacrine HCl	Cognex
tacrolimus	Prograf
tacrolimus oint	Protopic
tadalafil	Cialis
Tagamet	cimetidine HCl
talc, sterile aerosol	Sclerosol
Talwin	pentazocine HCl
Talwin Nx	pentazocine HCl; naloxone HCl
Tambocor	flecainide acetate
Tamiflu	oseltamivir phosphate
tamoxifen citrate	Nolvadex
tamsulosin HCl	Flomax
Tapazole	methimazole
Tarceva	erlotinib
Targretin	bexarotene gel
Tarka	trandolapril; verapamil SR
tarzarotene gel	Tazorac
Tasmar	tolcapone
tasosartan	Verdia
Tavist	clemastine fumarate
Taxol	paclitaxel
Taxotere	docetaxel
Taxus Express2 stent	paclitaxel-eluting stent
Tazicef	ceftazidime
Tazidime	ceftazidime
Tazorac	tarzarotene gel
technetium Tc-99m bicisate kit	Neurolite
technetium Tc-99m red blood cell kit	Ultratag
technetium Tc-99m	Cardiotec
technetium Tc99m sestamibi	Cardiolite
technetium Tc99m teboroxime kit	
Teczem	enalapril maleate; diltiazem malate
tegaserod maleate	Zelnorm
Tegretol	carbamazepine

Teldrin	chlorpheniramine maleate SR
Telepaque	iopanoic acid
telithromycin	Ketek
telmisartan	Micardis
temazepam	Restoril
Temodar	temozolomide
temozolomide	Temodar
tenecteplase	TNKase
Tenex	guanfacine HCl
teniposide	Vumon
tenofovir disoproxil fumarate	Viread
tenofovir, efavirenz, and emtricitabine	Atripla
Tenoretic	atenolol; chlorthalidone
Tenormin	atenolol
Tensilon	edrophonium chloride
Tenuate	diethylpropion HCl
Tequin	gatifloxacin
Terazol	terconazole
terazosin HCl	Hytrin
terbinafine HCl	Lamisil
terbutaline sulfate aerosol	Brethaire
terbutaline sulfate tablets and inj	Brethine Bricanyl
terconazole	Terazol
terfenadine (W)	Seldane (W)
terfenadine; pseudoephedrine HCl (W)	Seldane D (W)
teriparatide	Forteo
teriparatide acetate	Parathar
Teslac	testolactone
Teslascan	mangofodipir trisodium
Testim	testosterone gel
Testoderm (W)	testosterone transdermal (W)
Testoderm TTS (W)	testosterone transdermal (W)
testolactone	Teslac
testosterone buccal	Striant
testosterone cypionate SR	DEPO-Testosterone
testosterone gel	AndroGel Testim
testosterone transdermal	Androderm Testoderm Testoderm TTS
tetracaine HCl	Pontocaine
tetracycline HCl	Achromycin (WA) Sumycin
tetrahydrozoline HCl ophth	Collyrium Visine Extra
Teveten	eprosartan mesylate
Teveten HCT	eprosartan mesylate; hydrochlorothiazide
thalidomide	Thalomid
Thalomid	thalidomide
Tham	tromethamine
Theo-Dur (WA)	theophylline SR
theophylline	Elixophyllin Slo-Phyllin
theophylline SR	Slo-bid Theo-Dur (WA) Uniphyl
TheraCys	BCG intravesical
Theragran-M	vitamins; minerals
thiabendazole	Mintezol
thiethylperazine maleate	Torecan
thioguanine	thioguanine
thiopental sodium	Pentothal
Thioplex	thiotepa
thioridazine HCl	Mellaril (WA)
thiotepa	Thioplex
thiothixene	Navane
Thorazine	chlorpromazine
Thrombate III	antithrombin III (human)
thymalfasin	Zadaxin
Thymitaq	nolatrexed dihydrochloride
Thymoglobulin	anti-thymocyte globulin, (rabbit)
thyroglobulin (W)	Proloid (W)
thyroid	thyroid
Thyrogen	thyrotropin alpha
Thyrolar	liotrix
thyrotropin (W)	Thytropar (W)
thyrotropin alpha	Thyrogen
Thytropar (W)	thyrotropin (W)
tiagabine HCl	Gabitril
Tiamate	diltiazem maleate SR
Tiazac	diltiazem HCl SR
Ticar	ticarcillin disodium
ticarcillin disodium	Ticar
ticarcillin; clavulanic acid	Timentin
TICE BCG	BCG intravesical
Ticlid	ticlopidine
ticlopidine	Ticlid
Tigan	trimethobenzamide HCl
tigecycline inj	Tygacil
Tikosyn	dofetilide
Tilade	nedocromil inhalation
tiludronate disodium	Skelid

Timentin	ticarcillin; clavulanic acid	Tonocard	tocainide HCl
timolol maleate ophth soln	Timoptic	Topamax	topiramate
		Topicort	desoximetasone
timolol maleate ophth soln, gel forming	Timoptic-XE	topiramate	Topamax
		topotecan HCl	Hycamtin
		Toprol XL	metoprolol succinate SR
timolol maleate	Blocadren	Toradol	ketorolac tromethamine
timolol maleate; dorzolamide HCl	Cosopt	Torecan	thiethylperazine maleate
		toremifene citrate	Fareston
Timoptic-XE	timolol maleate ophth soln, gel forming	Tornalate	bitolterol mesylate
		torsemide	Demadex
Timoptic	timolol maleate ophth soln	tositumomab and I-131 tositumomab	Bexxar
Tinactin	tolnaftate		
Tindamax	tinidazole		
Tine Test Tuberculin Old	tuberculin, old	Totacillin-N	ampicillin sodium
		Tracleer	bosentan
		Tracrium	atracurium besylate
Tine Test PPD	tuberculin, purified protein derivative	tramadol; acetaminophen	Ultracet
tinidazole	Tindamax	tramadol HCl	Ultram
tinzaparin sodium	Innohep	Trandate	labetalol HCl
TNKase	tenecteplase	trandolapril	Mavik
tioconazole	Vagistat-1	trandolapril; verapamil SR	Tarka
tiotropium bromide inhalation powder	Spiriva HandiHaler		
		Transderm Scop	scopolamine transdermal
		Transderm-Nitro	nitroglycerin transdermal
		Tranxene	clorazepate dipotassium
tipranavir	Aptivus	tranylcypromine sulfate	Parnate
tirofiban HCl	Aggrastat		
tizanidine HCl	Zanaflex	trastuzumab	Herceptin
TOBI	tobramycin soln for inhalation	Trasylol	aprotinin
		Travasol	amino acid inj
TobraDex	tobramycin; dexamethasone oint and susp	Travatan	travoprost ophth soln
		travoprost ophth soln	Travatan
tobramycin sulfate	Nebcin	trazodone HCl	Desyrel
		Trecator-SC	ethionamide
tobramycin sulfate ophth	Tobrex	Trelstar Depot	triptorelin pamoate
tobramycin; dexamethasone oint and susp	TobraDex	Trelstar LA	triptorelin pamoate (3 month inj)
		Trental	pentoxifylline
tobramycin soln for inhalation	TOBI	treprostinil sodium	Remodulin
Tobrex	tobramycin sulfate ophth	tretinoin cream 0.025%	Avita
tocainide HCl	Tonocard		
Tofranil	imipramine HCl	tretinoin gel	Retin-A Micro
tolazamide	Tolinase	tretinion topical	Renova Retin-A
tolazoline (W)	Priscoline (W)		
tolbutamide	Orinase	tretinoin capsules	Vesanoid
tolcapone	Tasmar	Trexall	methotrexate tablets
Tolectin	tolmetin sodium	triamcinolone acetonide	Aristocort Kenalog
Tolinase (W)	tolazamide (W)		
tolmetin sodium	Tolectin	triamcinolone acetonide aerosol	Azmacort
tolnaftate	Tinactin		
tolterodine tartrate	Detrol		
		triamcinolone acetonide nasal inhaler	Nasacort
tolterodine tartrate (SR)	Detrol LA		

T
R

triamcinolone acetonide nasal spray	Tri-Nasal	triptorelin pamoate (3 month inj)	Trelstar LA
triamterene	Dyrenium	Trisenox	arsenic trioxide
triamterene 37.5 mg; hydro-chlorothiazide 25 mg	Maxzide -25MG Dyazide	Tritec Tri-Vi-Flor	ranitidine bismuth citrate vitamins A, D, & C; fluoride
triamterene 75 mg; hydro-chlorothiazide 50 mg	Maxzide	Trizivir Trobicin troglitazone (W)	lamivudine; zidovudine; abacavir sulfate spectinomycin HCl Rezulin (W)
Triavil (WA)	perphenazine; amitriptyline HCl	tromethamine Tronothane HCl	Tham pramoxine HCl
triazolam	Halcion	TrophAmine	amino acid inj
Tricor	fenofibrate	Tropicacyl	tropicamide
Tri-Cyclen	norgestimate; ethinyl estradiol	tropicamide	Mydriacyl Tropicacyl
Tridesilon	desonide	trospium chloride	Sanctura
Tridil	nitroglycerin inj	trovafloxacin (W)	Trovan tablets (W)
Tridione	trimethadione	Trovan tablet (W)	trovafloxacin mesylate (W)
trifluoperazine HCl	Stelazine	Trovan inj (W)	alatrofloxacin mesylate IV (W)
trifluridine	Viroptic	Trusopt	dorzolamide HCl
trihexyphenidyl HCl (W)	Artane (W)	Truvada	emtricitabine; tenofovir disoproxil
Trileptal	oxcarbazepine	trypan blue ophth soln	VisionBlue
Trilafon (WA)	perphenazine	tuberculin, old	Tine Test, Tuberculin Old
Tri-Levlen	levonorgestrel; ethinyl estradiol	tuberculin, purified protein derivative	Tine Test PPD
Trilisate	choline magnesium trisalicylate		
Tri-Luma	hydroquinone; tretinoin; fluocinolone cream	tuberculin skin test	Aplisol
trimethadione	Tridione	tubocurarine	tubocurarine
trimethaphan camsylate (W)	Arfonad (W)	Tucks Tums	witch hazel pads calcium
trimethobenza-mide HCl	Tigan	Tussi-Organidin	carbonate guaifenesin;
trimethoprim (W)	Primsol (W)	NR	codeine phosphate
trimetrexate glucuronate	Neutrexin	Tussionex	hydrocodone polistirex; chlorpheniramine
trimipramine maleate	Surmontil	Twinrix	hepatitis A
Trimox	amoxicillin		inactivated; hepatitis B (recombinant) vaccine
Tri-Nasal	triamcinolone acetonide nasal spray	Tylenol Tylenol with	acetaminophen acetaminophen
Triostat	liothyronine sodium inj	Codeine (#2,	300 mg with
tripelennamine HCl	PBZ	3, and 4)	Codeine Phosphate (15, 30, and 60 mg)
Triphasil	levonorgestrel; ethinyl estradiol	Typhim Vi	typhoid Vi polysaccharide vaccine
triple sulfa vaginal cream	Sultrin	typhoid Vi polysaccharide	Typhim Vi
triprolidine HCl; pseudoephe-drine HCl	Actifed	vaccine	
triptorelin pamoate	Trelstar Depot	tyropanoate sodium	Bilopaque

Tygacil	tigecycline inj
Tysabri	natalizumab

U

UbiQGel	coenzyme Q10
Ultane	sevoflurane
Ultiva	remifentanil HCl
Ultracet	tramadol HCl; acetaminophen
Ultralente U	insulin zinc suspension, extended (beef)
Ultram	tramadol HCl
Ultratag	technetium Tc-99m red blood cell kit
Ultravist	iopromide
Unasyn	ampicillin sodium; sulbactam sodium
Unipen (W)	nafcillin sodium (W)
Uniphyl	theophylline SR
Uniretic	moexipril HCl; hydrochlorothiazide
Univasc	moexipril HCl
Urecholine	bethanechol chloride
Urised	methenamine combination
Urispas	flavoxate HCl
urofollitropin	Bravelle
urofollitropin for inj	Fertinex
urokinase	Abbokinase
unoprostone isopropyl ophth soln (W)	Rescula (W)
UroXatral	alfuzosin
Uprima	apomorphine HCl
Urocit-K	potassium citrate tab
URSO	ursodiol
ursodiol	Actigall URSO
Uvadex	methoxsalen extracorporeal administration

V

Vagifem	estradiol hemihydrate vaginal tab
Vagistat-1	tioconazole
valacyclovir	Valtrex
Valcyte	valganciclovir
valdecoxib (W)	Bextra (W)
valganciclovir	Valcyte
Valium	diazepam
valproate sodium inj	Depacon

valproic acid	Depakene
valrubicin, (for intravesical use)	Valstar
valsartan	Diovan
valsartan; hydrochlorothiazide	Diovan HCT
Valstar	valrubicin, (for intravesical use)
Valtrex	valacyclovir
Vancenase	beclomethasone dipropionate
Vancenase AQ Nasal	beclomethasone dipropionate
Vanceril	beclomethasone dipropionate
Vancocin	vancomycin HCl
vancomycin HCl	Vancocin
Vaniqa	eflornithine HCl cream
Vantin	cefpodoxime proxetil
Vaponefrin	epinephrine racemic
Vaprisol	conivaptan
Vaqta	hepatitis A vaccine, inactivated
vardenafil HCl	Levitra
varicella virus vaccine	Varivax
varenicline	Chantix
Varivax	varicella virus vaccine
Vascor (W)	bepridil (W)
Vaseline	petrolatum, white
Vaseretic	enalapril maleate; hydrochlorothiazide
Vasocon	naphazoline ophth soln
Vasodilan	isoxsuprine HCl
vasopressin	Pitressin
Vasotec	enalapril maleate
Vasoxyl (W)	methoxamine HCl (W)
vecuronium bromide	Norcuron
Velban	vinblastine sulfate
Velcade	bortezomib
Velosef (W)	cephradine (W)
Velosulin Human	insulin inj (human)
venlafaxine HCl	Effexor
venlafaxine HCl SR	Effexor XR
Venofer	iron sucrose inj
Ventavis	iloprost
Ventolin	albuterol
VePesid	etoposide
verapamil HCl	Isoptin
verapamil HCl SR	Calan SR Verelan
verapamil HCl SR bedtime formulation	Covera HS Verelan PM
Verdia	tasosartan

V
R

Verelan	verapamil HCl SR
Verelan PM	verapamil HCl SR bedtime formulation
Verluna	nofetumomab
Vermox	mebendazole
Versed	midazolam HCl
verteporfin inj	Visudyne
Vesanoid	tretinoin capsules
Vesicare	solifenacin succinate
Vestra	reboxetine mesylate
Vexol	rimexolone
Vfend	voriconazole
V-Flex plus PTX stent	paclitaxel-eluting stent
Viactiv	calcium carbonate; vitamin D and K chewable
Viadur	leuprolide acetate implant
Viagra	sildenafil citrate
Vibramycin	doxycycline hyclate
Vicodin	hydrocodone bitartrate; acetaminophen
Vicoprofen	hydrocodone bitartrate 7.5 mg; ibuprofen 200 mg
vidarabine monohydrate (W)	Vira-A (W)
Vidaza	azacitidine
Videx	didanosine
Videx EC	didanosine SR
vinblastine sulfate	Velban
vincristine sulfate	Oncovin
vindesine sulfate	Eldisine
vinorelbine tartrate	Navelbine
Vioform	clioquinol
Vioxx (W)	rofecoxib (W)
Vira-A (W)	vidarabine monohydrate (W)
Viracept	nelfinavir mesylate
Viramune	nevirapine
Virazole	ribavirin
Viread	tenofovir disoproxil fumarate
Viroptic	trifluridine
Visicol	sodium phosphate tab
Visine Extra	tetrahydrozoline HCl ophth
VisionBlue	trypan blue ophth soln
Visipaque	iodixanol
Visken	pindolol
Vistaril	hydroxyzine pamoate
Vistide	cidofovir
Visudyne	verteporfin inj
Vitrase	ovine hyaluronidase
Vitravene	fomivirsen sodium inj
Vivelle	estradiol transdermal system
Volmax	albuterol SR

Voltaren	diclofenac sodium
Voltaren-XR	diclofenac sodium SR
voriconazole	Vfend
Vumon	teniposide
Vytorin	ezetimibe; simvastatin

W

warfarin sodium	Coumadin
Welchol	colesevelam HCl
Wellbutrin	bupropion HCl
Wellbutrin SR	bupropion HCl SR
Wellcovorin (WA)	*leucovorin calcium*
Wellferon	interferon ALFA-n[1] lymphoblastoid
WinRho SD	RH$_O$·(D) immune globulin IV (human)
Winstrol	stanozolol
witch hazel pads	Tucks
Wyamine	mephentermine sulfate
Wycillin (for IM use only)	penicillin G procaine (for IM use only)
Wydase	hyaluronidase
Wygesic	propoxyphene HCl; acetaminophen
Wymox	amoxicillin
Wytensin	guanabenz acetate

XYZ

Xalatan	latanoprost
Xanax	alprazolam
Xeloda	capecitabine
Xenical	orlistat
Xibrom	bromfenac ophth soln
Xifaxan	rifaximin
Xigris	drotrecogin alfa
Xolair	omalizumab
Xopenex	levalbuterol HCl inhalation soln
Xylocaine HCl	lidocaine HCl
xylometazoline	Otrivin
Xyrem	oxybate sodium
Yasmin	drospirenone; ethinyl estradiol
Yutopar (W)	ritodrine HCl (W)
Zadaxin	thymalfasin
Zaditor	ketotifen fumarate ophth soln
zafirlukast	Accolate
Zagam	sparfloxacin

V
R

References

1. Facts and Comparisons. St. Louis: Facts and Comparisons, Inc. (published monthly and online)

2. Billup NF, Billup SM. American drug index. St. Louis: Facts and Comparisons. Inc.yw (published yearly)

3. Sweetman SC. Ed. Martindale: 34th edition. The Pharmaceutical Press. London, 2005.

Additions, Corrections, and Suggestions are Welcomed

Please send them via any means shown below:

Neil M Davis
2049 Stout Drive, B-3
Warminster PA 18974-3861

FAX 1 888 333 4915 or 1 215 442 7432
Email med@neilmdavis.com
Web site www.medabbrev.com

Thank you for your help in the past.

Have You Used the Web-Version of This Book?

- It is instantaneously searchable for the meanings of abbreviations
- It is reverse searchable (search for all the abbreviations containing a particular word)
- Each month, about 80 new entries are added

See the preface (page vii) for access instructions. A two-year, single-user access is included in the purchase price of the book.

PDA Versions are Available

See pricing and ordering information in the pricing section on page 357.

Multi-User Site Licenses are Available

Medical facilities can substitute their own "Do Not Use" list of dangerous abbreviations for the one present. The ability also exists to list abbreviations that are unique to your region and/or organization which would normally not appear in any national list. These lists would be controlled by the facility. Demonstrations and pricing information are available by calling 1 888 333 1862 or 1 215 442 7430 or via an e-mail request to ev@neilmdavis.com

Chapter 9

Normal Adult Laboratory Values*

In the following tables, normal reference values for commonly requested laboratory tests are listed in traditional units and in SI units. The tables are a guideline only. Values are method dependent and "normal values" may vary between laboratories.

Blood, Plasma or Serum		
	Reference Value	
Determination	Conventional Units	SI Units
Ammonia (NH₃) − diffusion	20–120 mcg/dl	12–70 mcmol/L
Ammonia Nitrogen	15–45 mcg/dl	11–32 μmol/L
Amylase	35–118 IU/L	0.58–1.97 mckat/L
Anion Gap (Na⁺ − [Cl⁻ + HCO₃⁻]) (P)	7–16 mEq/L	7–16 mmol/L
Antinuclear antibodies	negative at 1:10 dilution of serum	negative at 1:10 dilution of serum
Antithrombin III (AT III)	80–120 units/dl	800–1200 units/L
Bicarbonate: Arterial Venous	21–28 mEq/L 22–29 mEq/L	21–28 mmol/L 22–29 mmol/L
Bilirubin: Conjugated (direct) Total	≤0.2 mg/dl 0.1–1 mg/dl	≤4 mcmol/L 2–18 mcmol/L
Calcitonin <100 pg/mL	<100 ng/L	
Calcium: Total Ionized	8.6–10.3 mg/dl 4.4–5.1 mg/dl	2.2–2.74 mmol/L 1–1.3 mmol/L
Carbon dioxide content (plasma)	21–32 mmol/L	21–32 mmol/L
Carcinoembryonic antigen	<3 ng/mL	<3 mcg/L
Chloride 95–110 mEq/L	95–110 mmol/L	
Coagulation screen: Bleeding time Prothrombin time Partial thromboplastin time (activated) Protein C Protein S	3–9.5 min 10–13 sec 22–37 sec 0.7–1.4 μ/mL 0.7–1.4 μ/mL	180–570 sec 10–13 sec 22–37 sec 700–1400 units/mL 700–1400 units/mL
Copper, total 70–160 mcg/dl	11–25 mcmol/L	
Corticotropin (ACTH adrenocorticotropic hormone) − 0800 hr	<60 pg/mL	<13.2 pmol/L
Cortisol: 0800 hr 1800 hr 2000 hr	5–30 mcg/dl 2–15 mcg/dl ≤50% of 0800 hr	138–810 nmol/L 50–410 nmol/L ≤50% of 0800 hr
Creatine kinase: Female Male	20–170 IU/L 30–220 IU/L	0.33–2.83 mckat/L 0.5–3.67 mckat/L
Creatine kinase isoenzymes, MB fraction	0–12 IU/L	0–0.2 mckat/L
Creatinine	0.5–1.7 mg/dl	44–150 mcmol/L
Fibrinogen (coagulation factor I)	150–360 mg/dl	1.5–3.6 g/L

Normal Adult Laboratory Values (Cont.) Blood*

Blood, Plasma or Serum (Cont.)		
	Reference Value	
Determination	Conventional Units	SI Units
Follicle-stimulating hormone (FSH):		
Female	2–13 mIU/mL	2–13 IU/L
Midcycle	5–22 mIU/mL	5–22 IU/L
Male	1–8 mIU/mL	1–8 IU/L
Glucose, fasting	65–115 mg/dl	3.6–6.3 mmol/L
Glucose Tolerance Test (Oral)	mg/dL	mmol/L
	Normal	Normal
Fasting	70–105	3.9–5.8
60 min	120–170	6.7–9.4
90 min	100–140	5.6–7.8
120 min	70–120	3.9–6.7
	Diabetic	Diabetic
Fasting	>140	>7.8
60 min	≥200	≥11.1
90 min	≥200	≥11.1
120 min	≥140	≥7.8
(γ) − Glutamyltransferase (GGT):		
Male	9–50 units/L	9–50 units/L
Female	8–40 units/L	8–40 units/L
Haptoglobin	44–303 mg/dl	0.44–3.03 g/L
Hematologic tests:		
Fibrinogen	200–400 mg/dl	2–4 g/L
Hematocrit (Hct), female	36%–44.6%	0.36–0.446 fraction of 1
male	40.7%–50.3%	0.4–0.503 fraction of 1
Hemoglobin A_{1C}	5.3%–7.5% of total Hgb	0.053–0.075
Hemoglobin (Hb), female	12.1–15.3 g/dl	121–153 g/L
male	13.8–17.5 g/dl	138–175 g/L
Leukocyte count (WBC)	3800–9800/mcl	$3.8–9.8 \times 10^9$/L
Erythrocyte count (RBC), female	$3.5–5 \times 10^6$/mcl	$3.5–5 \times 10^{12}$/L
male	$4.3–5.9 \times 10^6$/mcl	$4.3–5.9 \times 10^{12}$/L
Mean corpuscular volume (MCV)	80–97.6 mcm³	80–97.6 fl
Mean corpuscular hemoglobin (MCH)	27–33 pg/cell	1.66–2.09 fmol/cell
Mean corpuscular hemoglobin concentrate (MCHC)	33–36 g/dl	20.3–22 mmol/L
Erythrocyte sedimentation rate (sedrate, ESR)	≤30 mm/hr	≤30 mm/hr
Erythrocyte enzymes: Glucose-6-phosphate dehydrogenase (G-6-PD)	250–5000 units/10^6 cells	250–5000 mcunits/cell
Ferritin	10–383 ng/mL	23–862 pmol/L
Folic acid: normal	>3.1–12.4 ng/mL	7–28.1 nmol/L
Platelet count	$150–450 \times 10^3$/mcl	$150–450 \times 10^9$/L
Reticulocytes	0.5%–1.5% of erythrocytes	0.005–0.015
Vitamin B_{12}	223–1132 pg/mL	165–835 pmol/L
Iron: Female	30–160 mcg/dl	5.4–31.3 mcmol/L
Male	45–160 mcg/dl	8.1–31.3 mcmol/L
Iron binding capacity	220-420 mcg/dl	39.4–75.2 mcmol/L
Isocitrate Dehydrogenase	1.2–7 units/L	1.2–7 units/L
Isoenzymes		
Fraction 1	14%–26% of total	0.14–0.26 fraction of total
Fraction 2	29%–39% of total	0.29–0.39 fraction of total
Fraction 3	20%–26% of total	0.20–0.26 fraction of total
Fraction 4	8%–16% of total	0.08–0.16 fraction of total
Fraction 5	6%–16% of total	0.06–0.16 fraction of total
Lactate dehydrogenase	100–250 IU/L	1.67–4.17 mckat/L

Blood, Plasma or Serum (Cont.)		
	Reference Value	
Determination	**Conventional Units**	**SI Units**
Lactic acid (lactate)	6–19 mg/dl	0.7–2.1 mmol/L
Lead	≤50 mcg/dl	≤2.41 mcmol/L
Lipase	10–150 units/L	10–150 units/L
Lipids:		
Total Cholesterol		
Desirable	<200 mg/dl	<5.2 mmol/L
Borderline-high	200–239 mg/dl	<5.2–6.2 mmol/L
High	>239 mg/dl	>6.2 mmol/L
LDL		
Desirable	<130 mg/dl	<3.36 mmol/L
Borderline-high	130–159 mg/dl	3.36–4.11 mmol/L
High	>159 mg/dl	>4.11 mmol/L
HDL (low)	<35 mg/dl	<0.91 mmol/L
Triglycerides		
Desirable	<200 mg/dl	<2.26 mmol/L
Borderline-high	200–400 mg/dl	2.26–4.52 mmol/L
High	400–1000 mg/dl	4.52–11.3 mmol/L
Very high	>1000 mg/dl	>11.3 mmol/L
Magnesium	1.3–2.2 mEq/L	0.65–1.1 mmol/L
Osmolality	280–300 mOsm/kg	280–300 mmol/kg
Oxygen saturation (arterial)	94%–100%	0.94–1 fraction of 1
PCO$_2$, arterial	35–45 mm Hg	4.7–6 kPa
pH, arterial	7.35–7.45	7.35–7.45
PO$_2$, arterial: Breathing room air[1]	80–105 mm Hg	10.6–14 kPa
On 100% O$_2$	<500 mm Hg	
Phosphatase (acid), total at 37°C	0.13–0.63 IU/L	2.2–10.5 IU/L or 2.2–10.5 mckat/L
Phosphatase alkaline[2]	20–130 IU/L	20–130 IU/L or 0.33–2.17 mckat/L
Phosphorus, inorganic,[3] (phosphate)	2.5–5 mg/dl	0.8–1.6 mmol/L
Potassium	3.5–5 mEq/L	3.5–5 mmol/L
Progesterone		
Female	0.1–1.5 ng/mL	0.32–4.8 nmol/L
Follicular phase	0.1–1.5 ng/mL	0.32–4.8 nmol/L
Luteal phase	2.5–28 ng/mL	8–89 nmol/L
Male	<0.5 ng/mL	<1.6 nmol/L
Prolactin	1.4–24.2 ng/mL	1.4–24.2 mcg/L
Prostate specific antigen	0–4 ng/mL	0–4 ng/mL
Protein: Total	6–8 g/dl	60–80 g/L
Albumin	3.6–5 g/dl	36–50 g/L
Globulin	2.3–3.5 g/dl	23–35 g/L
Rheumatoid factor	<60 IU/mL	<60 kIU/L
Sodium	135–147 mEq/L	135–147 mmol/L
Testosterone: Female	6–86 ng/dl	0.21–3 mmol/L
Male	270–1070 ng/dl	9.3–37 nmol/L

[1] Age dependent
[2] Infants and adolescents up to 104 IU/L
[3] Infants in the first year up to 6 mg/dl

Normal Adult Laboratory Values (Cont.) Blood*

Blood, Plasma or Serum (Cont.)		
	Reference Value	
Determination	Conventional Units	SI Units
Thyroid Hormone Function Tests:		
Thyroid-stimulating hormone (TSH)	0.35–6.2 mcU/mL	0.35–6.2 mU/L
Thyroxine-binding globulin capacity	10–26 mcg/dl	100–260 mcg/L
Total triiodothyronine (T_3)	75–220 ng/dl	1.2–3.4 nmol/L
Total thyroxine by RIA (T_4)	4–11 mcg/dl	51–142 nmol/L
T_3 resin uptake	25%–38%	0.25–0.38 fraction of 1
Transaminase, AST (aspartate aminotransferase, SGOT)	11–47 IU/L	0.18–0.78 mckat/L
Transaminase, ALT (alanine aminotransferase, SGPT)	7–53 IU/L	0.12–0.88 mckat/L
Transferrin	220–400 mg/dL	2.20–4.00 g/L
Urea nitrogen (BUN)	8–25 mg/dl	2.9–8.9 mmol/L
Uric acid	3–8 mg/dl	179–476 mcmol/L
Vitamin A (retinol)	15–60 mcg/dl	0.52–2.09 mcmol/L
Zinc	50–150 mcg/dl	7.7–23 mcmol/L

Normal Laboratory Values—Urine

Urine		
	Reference Value	
Determination	Conventional Units	SI Units
Calcium[1]	50–250 mcg/day	1.25–6.25 mmol/day
Catecholamines: Epinephrine	<20 mcg/day	<109 nmol/day
Norepinephrine	<100 mcg/day	<590 nmol/day
Catecholamines, 24-hr	<110 mcg	<650 nmol
Copper[1]	15–60 mcg/day	0.24–0.95 mcmol/day
Creatinine: Child	8–22 mg/kg	71–195 μmol/kg
Adolescent	8–30 mg/kg	71–265 μmol/kg
Female	0.6–1.5 g/day	5.3–13.3 mmol/day
Male	0.8–1.8 g/day	7.1–15.9 mmol/day
pH	4.5–8	4.5–8
Phosphate[1]	0.9–1.3 g/day	29–42 mmol/day
Potassium[1]	25–100 mEq/day	25–100 mmol/day
Protein Total	1–14 mg/dL	10–140 mg/L
At rest	50–80 mg/day	50–80 mg/day
Protein, quantitative	<150 mg/day	<0.15 g/day
Sodium[1]	100–250 mEq/day	100–250 mmol/day
Specific Gravity, random	1.002–1.030	1.002–1.030
Uric Acid, 24-hr	250–750 mg	1.48–4.43 mmol

[1] Diet dependent

Normal Adult Laboratory Values—Drug Levels*

		Drug Levels†	
		Reference Value	
	Drug Determination	**Conventional Units**	**SI Units**
Aminoglycosides	Amikacin		
	(trough)	1–8 mcg/mL	1.7–13.7 mcmol/L
	(peak)	20–30 mcg/mL	34–51 mcmol/L
	Gentamicin		
	(trough)	0.5–2 mcg/mL	1–4.2 mcmol/L
	(peak)	6–10 mcg/mL	12.5–20.9 mcmol/L
	Kanamycin		
	(trough)	5–10 mcg/mL	nd
	(peak)	20–25 mcg/mL	nd
	Netilmicin		
	(trough)	0.5–2 mcg/mL	nd
	(peak)	6–10 mcg/mL	nd
	Streptomycin		
	(trough)	<5 mcg/mL	nd
	(peak)	5–20 mcg/mL	nd
	Tobramycin		
	(trough)	0.5–2 mcg/mL	1.1–4.3 mcmol/L
	(peak)	5–20 mcg/mL	12.8–21.8 mcmol/L
Antiarrhythmics	Amiodarone	0.5–2.5 mcg/mL	1.5–4 mcmol/L
	Bretylium	0.5–1.5 mcg/mL	nd
	Digitoxin	9–25 mcg/L	11.8–32.8 nmol/L
	Digoxin	0.8–2 ng/mL	0.9–2.5 nmol/L
	Disopyramide	2–8 mcg/mL	6–18 mcmol/L
	Flecainide	0.2–1 mcg/mL	nd
	Lidocaine	1.5–6 mcg/mL	4.5–21.5 mcmol/L
	Mexiletine	0.5–2 mcg/mL	nd
	Procainamide	4–8 mcg/mL	17–34 mcmol/mL
	Propranolol	50–200 ng/ml	190–770 nmol/L
	Quinidine	2–6 mcg/mL	4.6–9.2 mcmol/L
	Tocainide	4–10 mcg/mL	nd
	Verapamil	0.08–0.3 mcg/mL	nd
Anti-convulsants	Carbamazepine	4–12 mcg/mL	17–51 mcmol/L
	Phenobarbital	10–40 mcg/mL	43–172 mcmol/L
	Phenytoin	10–20 mcg/mL	40–80 mcmol/L
	Primidone	4–12 mcg/mL	18–55 mcmol/L
	Valproic acid	40–100 mcg/mL	280–700 mcmol/L
Antidepressants	Amitriptyline	110–250 ng/mL[3]	500–900 nmol/L
	Amoxapine	200–500 ng/mL	nd
	Bupropion	25–100 ng/mL	nd
	Clomipramine	80–100 ng/mL	nd
	Desipramine	115–300 ng/mL	nd
	Doxepin	110–250 ng/mL[3]	nd
	Imipramine	225–350 ng/mL[3]	nd
	Maprotiline	200–300 ng/mL	nd
	Nortriptyline	50–150 ng/mL	nd
	Protriptyline	70–250 ng/mL	nd
	Trazodone	800–1600 ng/mL	nd
Antipsychotics	Chlorpromazine	50–300 ng/mL	150–950 nmol/L
	Fluphenazine	0.13–2.8 ng/mL	nd
	Haloperidol	5–20 ng/mL	nd
	Perphenazine	0.8–1.2 ng/mL	nd
	Thiothixene	2–57 ng/mL	nd

†The values given are generally accepted as desirable for treatment without toxicity for most patients. However, exceptions are not uncommon.
[3]Parent drug plus N-desmethy7l metabolite
nd — No data available

Normal Adult Laboratory Values (Cont.) Drug Levels*

	Drug Levels†		
		Reference Value	
Drug Determination		**Conventional Units**	**SI Units**
Miscellaneous	Amantadine	300 ng/mL	nd
	Amrinone	3.7 mcg/mL	nd
	Chloramphenicol	10–20 mcg/mL	31–62 mcmol/L
	Cyclosporine[1]	250–800 ng/mL (whole blood, RIA)	nd
		50–300 ng/mL (plasma, RIA)	nd
	Ethanol[2]	0 mg/dl	0 mmol/L
	Hydralazine	100 ng/mL	nd
	Lithium	0.6–1.2 mEq/L	0.6–1.2 mmol/L
	Salicylate	100–300 mg/L	724–2172 mcmol/L
	Sulfonamide	5–15 mg/dl	nd
	Terbutaline	0.5–4.1 ng/mL	nd
	Theophylline	10–20 mcg/mL	55–110 mcmol/L
	Vancomycin		
	(trough)	5–15 ng/mL	nd
	(peak)	20–40 mcg/mL	nd

†The values given are generally accepted as desirable for treatment without toxicity for most patients. However, exceptions are not uncommon.
[1]24 hour trough values
[2]Toxic: 50–100 mg/dl (10.9–21.7 mmol/L)
nd — No data available

Reorder and Prices for the 13th Edition

Medical Abbreviations: 28,000 Conveniences at the
Expense of Communication and Safety
by Neil M Davis
(ISBN 0-931431-13-1)

1–19 copies	$26.95 each plus S&H
20 or more copies	$18.90 each plus S&H

Plus U.S. Shipping and Handling Charges

Number of Books Ordered	U.S. S&H charges to be added to each **order**
1	$5.00 + price shown above
2	$7.00 + price shown above
3–6	$9.00 + price shown above
7–11	$12.00 + price shown above
12–20	$16.00 + price shown above
21–40	$28.00 + price shown above
41 or more	$42.00 + price shown above

Orders shipped to Pennsylvania must add 6% sales tax.
No sales tax for other states (subject to change).
Purchase orders are accepted.

Payable by–

Visa   MasterCard   Discover
American Exp.   Check   Money Order

Order from and make check payable to–

Neil M. Davis Associates
2049 Stout Drive, B-3
Warminster PA 18974-3861

Orders may be mailed to above address or

Phone 215 442 7430 or 888 333 1862
Fax 215 442 7432 or 888 333 4915
Secure Web site www.medabbrev.com
E-mail med@neilmdavis.com

Where applicable, please have ready credit card number and expiration date, phone
number, and mailing address. A PO box address is <u>not</u> acceptable for orders as they
are shipped via UPS.

Reorder and Price Information—continued

Outside of the United States

- Pay by credit card (VISA, MasterCard, Discover, American Express), or in U.S. dollars through a corresponding U.S. bank, or an International Money Order in U.S. currency.
- Prices as shown on the previous page plus shipping costs.
- To obtain shipping cost, fax query to 1 215 442 7432 or E-mail to ev@neilmdavis.com

Information Needed on Order Form

PLEASE PRINT OR TYPE

Name _____

Address (PO Box addresses not acceptable) _____

_____

City _____ State _____ Zip Code _____

Phone (___) _____

Attention (If Applicable) _____

Number of copies ordered _____ PO # (If Applicable) _____

Method of payment:

_____ Check or money order enclosed

_____ Visa _____ MasterCard

_____ Discover _____ American Express

Card Number _____

Exp. Date _____

Cardholder's Name _____

Signature _____

Internet Access

Each book purchased includes, at no extra cost, a single-user access license for the website version of this 13th edition, which is updated monthly (see preface page vii). This license is valid for 24 months from the date of the initial log-in. Multi-User Site Licenses are available. To obtain a copy of the Multi-User Site License, call 1 888 333 1862, FAX 1 888 333 4915 or E-mail to ev@neilmdavis.com

To Order the PDA Versions

Palm OS or Pocket PC PDA versions of "Medical Abbreviations: 28,000 Conveniences at the Expense of Communication and Safety," the 13th edition, 2007, by Neil M Davis, are available from Lexi-Comp Inc., at either:

Their website	www.lexi.com
Phone	1 800 837 5394
Fax	1 330 656 4307

The PDA versions are updated with 80 new entries per month. The Palm version is approximately 1.7MB. The Pocket PC version is approximately 2.2MB.

Pricing: If you list on the Lexi-Comp website order form or mention on the telephone or FAX order, the Promotion Code **"KT8BK"** you will be given a 10% discount, lowering the price to $31.50 for one year. The normal price is $35.00.

Lexi-Comp is currently developing a smart cell-phone version. Call Lexi-Comp for details.

Additions

Please forward additional meanings for these abbreviations, additional abbreviations and their meanings, or corrections to the author so that the web-version, PDA versions, and book can be updated. Thank you. Dr. Neil M Davis, 2049 Stout Drive, B-3, Warminster, PA 18974. FAX 215 442 7432 or 888 333 4915. E-mail med@neilmdavis.com

Additions

(See the preface (page vii) for instructions on how to access to the web-version of this book which is updated each month with about 80 new entries. Your suggestions are appreciated.)

Additions, Corrections, and Suggestions are Welcomed

Please send them via any means shown below:

Neil M Davis
2049 Stout Drive, B-3
Warminster PA 18974-3861

FAX 1 888 333 4915 or 1 215 442 7432
Email med@neilmdavis.com
Web site www.medabbrev.com

Thank you for your help in the past.

Have You Used the Web-Version of This Book?

- It is instantaneously searchable for the meanings of abbreviations
- It is reverse searchable (search for all the abbreviations containing a particular word)
- Each month, about 80 new entries are added

See the preface (page vii) for access instructions. A two-year, single-user access is included in the purchase price of the book.

PDA Versions are Available

See pricing and ordering information in the pricing section on page 357.

Multi-User Site Licenses are Available

Medical facilities can substitute their own "Do Not Use" list of dangerous abbreviations for the one present. The ability also exists to list abbreviations that are unique to your region and/or organization which would normally not appear in any national list. These lists would be controlled by the facility. Demonstrations and pricing information are available by calling 1 888 333 1862 or 1 215 442 7430 or via an e-mail request to ev@neilmdavis.com